Herbs, Spices and Medicinal Plants: Processing, Health Benefits and Safety

About the IFST Advances in Food Science Book Series

The Institute of Food Science and Technology (IFST) is the leading qualifying body for food professionals in Europe and the only professional organization in the UK concerned with all aspects of food science and technology. Its qualifications are internationally recognized as a sign of proficiency and integrity in the industry. Competence, integrity, and serving the public benefit lie at the heart of the IFST philosophy. IFST values the many elements that contribute to the efficient and responsible supply, manufacture and distribution of safe, wholesome, nutritious and affordable foods, with due regard for the environment, animal welfare and the rights of consumers. *IFST Advances in Food Science* is a series of books dedicated to the most important and popular topics in food science and technology, highlighting major developments across all sectors of the global food industry. Each volume is a detailed and in-depth edited work, featuring contributions by recognized international experts, and which focuses on new developments in the field. Taken together, the series forms a comprehensive library of the latest food science research and practice, and provides valuable insights into the food processing techniques that are essential to the understanding and development of this rapidly evolving industry. The IFST Advances series is edited by Dr. Brijesh Tiwari, who is Senior Research Officer at Teagasc Food Research Centre in Ireland.

Forthcoming Titles in the IFST Series

Innovative Processing Technologies for Healthy Grains edited by Milica Pojic and Uma Tiwari

Food Formulation: Novel Ingredients and Processing Techniques edited by Shivani Pathania and Brijesh Tiwari

Recent Advances in Micro and Macroalgal Processing: Food and Health Perspectives edited by Gaurav Rajauria and Yvonne V. Yuan.

Oil and Oilseed Processing: Opportunities and Challenges edited by Ingrid Aguiló, Tomás Lafarga and Gloria Bobo.

Herbs, Spices and Medicinal Plants: Processing, Health Benefits and Safety

Edited by

Mohammad B. Hossain
Teagasc Food Research Centre
Ashtown, Ireland

Nigel P. Brunton
School of Agriculture and Food Science
University College Dublin
Dublin, Ireland

Dilip K. Rai
Teagasc Food Research Centre
Ashtown, Ireland

WILEY Blackwell

This edition first published 2020

Registered Offices
John Wiley & Sons, Inc., 111 River Street, Hoboken, NJ 07030, USA
John Wiley & Sons Ltd, The Atrium, Southern Gate, Chichester, West Sussex, PO19 8SQ, UK

Editorial Office
The Atrium, Southern Gate, Chichester, West Sussex, PO19 8SQ, UK

For details of our global editorial offices, customer services, and more information about Wiley products visit us at www.wiley.com.

Wiley also publishes its books in a variety of electronic formats and by print-on-demand. Some content that appears in standard print versions of this book may not be available in other formats.

Library of Congress Cataloging-in-Publication Data

Names: Hossain, Mohammad B., 1978- editor. | Brunton, Nigel P., editor. | Rai, Dilip K., 1972- editor.
Title: Herbs, spices and medicinal plants : processing, health benefits and safety / edited by Mohammad B. Hossain, Nigel P. Brunton, and Dilip K. Rai
Description: Hoboken, NJ : Wiley-Blackwell, 2020. | Series: IFST advances in food science book series | Includes bibliographical references and index.
Identifiers: LCCN 2019058270 (print) | LCCN 2019058271 (ebook) | ISBN 9781119036616 (hardback) | ISBN 9781119036647 (adobe pdf) | ISBN 9781119036630 (epub)
Subjects: LCSH: Pharmacognosy. | Medicinal plants–Preservation. | Spices–Therapeutic use. | Herbs–Therapeutic use. | Plant extracts.
Classification: LCC RS164 .H386 2020 (print) | LCC RS164 (ebook) | DDC 615.3/21–dc23
LC record available at https://lccn.loc.gov/2019058270
LC ebook record available at https://lccn.loc.gov/2019058271

Cover Design: Wiley
Cover Images: Yellow flowers © LFRabanedo/Shutterstock,
Spices and herbs © fcafotodigital/Getty Images,
Plums © Helmut Meyer zur Capellen/Getty Images

Set in 9.5/11.5pt TimesTenLTstd-Roman by SPi-Global, Chennai, India

10 9 8 7 6 5 4 3 2 1

Contents

List of Contributors

Ramón Aznar, Department of Food BioSciences, Teagasc Food Research Centre Ashtown, Dublin, Ireland

Nigel P. Brunton, School of Agriculture and Food Science, University College Dublin, Dublin, Ireland

Alka Choudhary, Department of Food BioSciences, Teagasc Food Research Centre Ashtown, Dublin, Ireland

Shweta Deotale, Indian Institute of Food Processing Technology, Thanjavur, India

Ambrose Furey, Department Physical Sciences, Cork Institute of Technology, Cork, Ireland

Deirdre Gilroy, Department of Biological Sciences, Cork Institute of Technology, Bishopstown, Cork, Co. Cork, Ireland

Maria Glibetic, Center of Research Excellence in Nutrition and Metabolism, Institute for Medical Research, University of Belgrade, Serbia

M. Herrero, Laboratory of Foodomics, Institute of Food Science Research (CIAL-CSIC), Madrid, Spain

E. Ibáñez, Laboratory of Foodomics, Institute of Food Science Research (CIAL-CSIC), Madrid, Spain

Wei Jin, State Key Laboratory of Food Science and Technology, Jiangnan University, Wuxi, Jiangsu, China

Anna-Maria Keaveney, Department Physical Sciences, Cork Institute of Technology, Cork, Ireland

Ciara-Ruth Kenny, Department of Biological Sciences, Cork Institute of Technology, Cork, Ireland

Rosari Kingston, West Cork Herb Farm, Knockeens, Churchcross, Co. Cork, Ireland

Anjali H. Kurup, Indian Institute of Food Processing Technology, Thanjavur, India

Mary Lehane, Mass Spectrometry Research Centre (MSRC), Department of Physical Science, Cork Institute of Technology, Cork, Ireland

Brigid Lucey, Department of Biological Sciences, Cork Institute of Technology, Cork, Ireland

Jose A. Mendiola, Laboratory of Foodomics, Institute of Food Science Research (CIAL-CSIC), Madrid, Spain

Lidia Montero, Laboratory of Foodomics, Institute of Food Science Research (CIAL-CSIC), Madrid, Spain

Arun S. Mujumdar, Department of Chemical and Biochemical Engineering, Western University, London, Ontario, Canada

Ankit Patras, Department of Agricultural and Environmental Sciences, College of Agriculture, Tennessee State University, Nashville, USA

Camila A. Perussello, Technological University Dublin, Environmental Sustainability and Health Institute, Grangegorman Campus, Dublin, Ireland

Dilip K. Rai, Department of Food BioSciences, Teagasc Food Research Centre Ashtown, Dublin, Ireland

Ashish Rawson, Indian Institute of Food Processing Technology, Thanjavur, India

Celia Rodríguez-Pérez, Department of Nutrition and Food Science, University of Granada, Campus of Cartuja, Granada, Spain

Andrea P. Sánchez-Camargo, Laboratory of Foodomics, Institute of Food Science Research (CIAL-CSIC), Madrid, Spain

Weifeng Shi, Nestlé R&D Centre Shanghai Ltd., Shanghai, China

Md Abu Bakar Siddique, School of Agriculture and Food Science, University College Dublin, Dublin, Ireland

Mary C. Tassell, Mass Spectrometry Research Centre (MSRC), Department of Physical Science, Cork Institute of Technology, Cork, Ireland

Katerina Tzima, Department of Food BioSciences, Teagasc Food Research Centre Ashtown, Dublin, Ireland

Manja Zec, Center of Research Excellence in Nutrition and Metabolism, Institute for Medical Research, University of Belgrade, Belgrade, Serbia

Min Zhang, State Key Laboratory of Food Science and Technology, Jiangnan University, Wuxi, Jiangsu, China

1
Thermal Processing of Herbs and Spices

Anjali H. Kurup[1], Shweta Deotale[1], Ashish Rawson[1], and Ankit Patras[2]
[1]*Indian Institute of Food Processing Technology, Thanjavur, TN 613005, India*
[2]*Department of Agricultural and Environmental Sciences, College of Agriculture, Tennessee State University, Nashville, TN 37209, USA*

1.1 Introduction

Herbs and spices are fresh or dried aromatic products obtained from a plant used to impart flavor to foods of plant and animal origin (Shelef 1984; Sung et al. 2012). More than 100 varieties of spices exist across the globe, which are significantly affected by the climatic conditions of the region (Gottardi et al. 2016). Asia is the leading producer of spices, particularly cinnamon, pepper, nutmeg, cloves, and ginger, while in Europe mainly basil, bay leaves, celery leaves, chives, coriander (cilantro), dill tips, thyme, and watercress are produced. America produces spices which include pepper, nutmeg, ginger, allspice, and sesame seed (Prasad et al. 2012; Gottardi et al. 2016). From ancient times, spices and herbs have been used not only for flavoring and preserving foods, but also for medicinal and cosmetic purposes (Simmonds 1982; Subbulakshmi and Naik 2002; Srinivasan 2005). As spices possess antimicrobial, antiviral, and strong flavoring properties, they are used to mask spoilage or off-flavor in many food products (Risch 1997). India is the largest producer and exporter of spices, which include pepper, followed by Capsicum fruits, turmeric, ginger, cardamom seed spices, curry powders, spice oils, and oleoresins (Risch 1997; Subbulakshmi and Naik 2002; Srinivasan 2005).

The term "herb" is referred to as a subset of spice or leafy spice and belongs to plant sources with aromatic leaves valued for its medicinal and aromatic properties (Zheng and Wang 2001). Spices and herbs are considered rich sources of powerful antioxidants with high bioactivity (Sackewitz 1956; Embuscado 2015). Spices and herbs have also been used for preservation of foods and beverages primarily due to the presence of bioactive phytochemicals (Peter 2006; Singhal et al. 2017). Spices and herbs have been used as antioxidants in the form of whole or ground spice/herb, extracts, encapsulated or as emulsions (Embuscado 2015). Spices and herbs are classified and selected on the basis of their characteristics, such as flavor and color, that they impart to foods, i.e. hot

Herbs, Spices and Medicinal Plants: Processing, Health Benefits and Safety, First Edition.
Edited by Mohammad B. Hossain, Nigel P. Brunton, and Dilip K. Rai.

(pepper), pungent (garlic), aromatic (cinnamon, clove), herbaceous (sage, rosemary), and coloring (turmeric) (Clark 1970). By flavor characteristics, spice concentrations in foods are determined, normally ranging from 0.5% to 1% in finished food products (Fischetti 1980). Some of the common spices along with their functional component, parts used, and common names are tabulated in Table 1.1.

1.2 Thermal Processing of Spices

1.2.1 Cooking and Roasting of Spices

Spices are important ingredients in the preparation of food formulations for improved flavors and acceptability. Hence, spices can be added to food in different forms comprising different unit operations – such as slicing, roasting, grinding, frying, boiling, or cooking – to release their characteristic aromatic components. During cooking, spices contribute taste, aroma, texture, and color to the food or beverage. Additionally, some herbs and spices act as an antimicrobial agent which increases the shelf life of packed food (Billing and Sherman 1998) and some spices act as an antioxidant agent which prevents the oxidation of oils and fat (Tiwari et al. 2006). Many herbs and spices have health benefits when consumed with food. (Table 1.2). It is observed that depending upon the time and temperature, the method of cooking helps to stabilize and enhance the quality of stored foods, retaining the special aroma, flavor of the spice, texture, and nutritional content of the food (James and James 2005).

The essential component or flavoring component from herbs and spices leaches out during cooking. As the material is soaked in the water during cooking, it swells due to permeation of water from outside to inside the cell membrane of the herb/spice, which is followed by rupturing on the surface of the cell; finally, due to the concentration gradient, the essential component comes out as cell breakage happens and imparts delicious flavor to the food during cooking. The schematic mechanism is shown in Figure 1.1. A similar mechanism occurs during the extraction and distillation process to obtain the essential component from herbs and spices (Douglas et al. 2005).

During cooking there is a loss of the active component of some spices. In one study, tur dal (split red gram) was prepared by adding a known quantity of curry powder, turmeric powder, red pepper, and black pepper powder. By using the thin-layer chromatographic (TLC) method, the effect of cooking on the active principle component was studied. It was observed that the cooking time and pH had a significant effect on the active components of spices (Srinivasan et al. 1992) Table 1.3.

The objectives should be clear when spices are used in cooking. The basic function of the spices used in cooking can be divided into four categories: flavoring, pungency, coloring, and deodorizing/masking. Out of these, the first three are direct functions of spices and deodorizing/masking overlaps with them showing complex functions (Hirasa and Takemasa 1998). Sometimes food possesses an undesirable odor, for example freshwater fish, and in such circumstances spices play an important role in masking the smell during cooking. The volatile compound present in ginger and the sulfur-containing compound in garlic possess a strong ability to reduce the off odor (Li, J. et al. 2016). Many studies have reported that the combination of caraway, cassia, clove, ginger, laurel, mace, nutmeg, onion, pepper, sage, and thyme helps to mask the off odor/flavor of raw material during cooking (Kikuchi et al. 1968; Yoshida et al. 1984; Kasahara and Osawa 1998).

Table 1.1 Nomenclature of spices and herb its part which is used as spice and its active component

Common name	Botanical name/Scientific name	Part used	Active/principle component	Uses
Ajowan	*Trachyspermum ammi*	Whole seed	Thymol (35–60%) α-pinene, ρ-cymene	Spice blend, chat masala
Allspice (clove pepper)	*Pimento dioica*	Whole or ground seed	Eugenol (80–90%)	Baked goods, chewing gums, candy, ice cream, fruit soups, tea.
Anise/Aniseed (sweet cumin)	*Pimpinella anisum*	Spice: whole or ground Herb: leaf, fresh or dried.	Trans-anethol (80–90%)	Sweet rolls, cakes, marinated meat and fish, beef stew, salad dressing, sausages
Annatto	*Bixa orellana*	Seed	Bixin	Butter, margarine, ice cream, sausages, cheese
Asafoetida (hing)	*Ferula asa-foetida L*	Resin, dried granules, chunks or powder	2-butyl-1-propenyl disulfide, Sulfur compounds, ferulic ester	Spice blend, chat masala
Basil (tulsi)	Sweet basil: *Ocimum basilicum* Holi basil: *Ocimum sanctum*	Herb: fresh dried leaves Spice: paste	Linalool (40%), methyl chavicol (25%)	Spice blend
Bay/ Laurel leaf (tejpatta)	*Laurus nobilis*	leaf	1–8-cineole (35%), methyl eugenol (4%), α-pinene (12%)	Spice blend, curry blends
Caraway (shai jeera)	*Carum carvi*	Herb: leaf Spice: dried, ripe fruit, root, seed	d-carvone (50–85%) and limonene (20–30%)	Soups and salads, pickle blend, spice blend
Cardamom (false or greater)	*Amomum subulatum* Linn.	Fruit and seed	1–8-cineole (70%)	Garam masala, curry powder

(continued)

Table 1.1 *(continued)*

Common name	Botanical name/Scientific name	Part used	Active/principle component	Uses
Cardamom (true or lesser)	*Elettaria cardamomum*	Fruit and seed	1-8-cineole (25–45%), α-terpineol acetate (28–34%)	Cakes, cookies, breads
Celery	*Apium graveolens*	Herb: leaf (fresh and dried) Spice: seed, stalks or stem, root.	Limonene (68%) B-selinene (8%)	Foods and beverage, tomato juice blend, curry blend, pickling blend
Chervil	*Anthriscus cerefolium*	Herb: leaf (fresh and dried)	Iso-anethole	Fine herbs, sauce blend
Chile peppers (chili)	*Capsicum annum*	Ground, crushed, chili powder	Capsaicin (50–70%) Dihydrocapasaicin (20–25%)	Chili powder, periperi sauce
Chives	*Allium schoenoprasum*	Herb: stem and leaves (fresh, frozen and dried)	Dipropyl disulfide, methyl pentyl disulfide and Pentanethiol	Cottage cheese, egg dishes, cocktail sauces, dried soups
Cinnamon (dalchini)	*Cinnamomum zeylanicum*	Bark, leaves, buds, roots, flower	Cinnamic aldehyde (65–75%), Eugenol (5–10%), linalool (2–3%)	Sweets, soup, pastries, wines, tea, garam masala
Clove	*Syzyium aromaticum*	Dried unopened flower buds	Eugenol (81%)	Garam masala, curry blends, ketchup blend
Coriander	*Coriandrum sativum*	Herb: fresh and dried leaf Spice: dried seeds, stem, roots	d-linalool (60–70%)	Curries, pickle, snacks, curry powder, garam masala
Cumin and black cumin	*Cuminium cyminum, Cuminium ni-grum*	Dried and ripe fruits or seed	Cumin: cuminic aldehyde (33%) Black cumin: carvone (45–60%)	Yogurts, chutneys, curries, biryanies, garam masala, snacks

Dill and Dillweed	*Anethum graveolens*	Dill: seeds Dillweed: leaves (fresh or dried)	Dillapiole (52%) Carvone (21%)	Sauerkraut blend, pickling blend, salad dressing
Fennel seed	*Foeniculum vulgare*	Spice: Seeds Herb: leaf, stalk	Limonene	Cakes, baked goods, curry blends
Fenugreek	*Trigonella foenum-graceum*	Spice: seed Herb: leaf (fresh or dried)	*n*-alkanes, sesquiterpenes and alkanoles	Fish, meat, chicken curries
Greater galangal (mild ginger)	*Alpinia galanga*	Spice: fresh, frozen and canned Rhizome Herb: fresh leaves, flower	1,8-cineol, α-pinene, eugenol, methyl cinnamate	Thai red curry paste blend, meat marinades
Garlic	*Allilum sativum*	Bulb	Diallyl disulfide (60%), Allicin	Soups, curries, stews
Ginger	*Zingiber officinale*	Rhizome	Zingiberene (70%), curcumene	Curry blends, snacks, tea, desserts
Juniper berry	*Juniperus communis*	Dried berry	α-and β-pinene (80%)	Cheese, goose, pot roasts, pickled meat, seafoods
Kari leaf	*Murraya koenigi*	Herb: leaf (fresh or dried)	Cabinene (34%), α-pinene (27%) and dipentene (16%)	Curry blends, chutney blends, fish curry blends
Lemongrass	*Cymbopogon flexuosus*	Herb: dried, fresh and frozen leaves	Citral (80–85%)	Soups, stews, curries, sauces, tea
Mace	*Myristica fragrans*	Aril or mace blades	Monoterpenes (87.5%)	Garam masala, curry blends, cakes, cookies, doughnuts
Marjoram	*Origanum hortensis*	Herb: fresh and dried leaves	*Cis*-sabinene hydrate (8–40%), terpinen 4-ol (18–48%)	Sauces, salad, vinegar, mushroom, tomato based sauces

(continued)

Table 1.1 (*continued*)

Common name	Botanical name/Scientific name	Part used	Active/principle component	Uses
Mint	Peppermint: *Menthe piperita* Spearmint: *Menthe spicata*	Herb: fresh and dried leaves	Menthol (26–46%), menthone (16–36%)	Salad, fish and poultry curries, seasoned rice, sauces, soups
Mustard	*Brassica nigra*	Whole seeds	Allyl isothiocynate (95–99%)	Cold meat, sausages, salad dressing, hot sauces, chutneys, curries
Nigella (kalonji)	*Nigella sativa*	seed	Thymoquinone (54%)	Salad, cottage cheese, lamb, pickles, poultry
Nutmeg	*Myristica fragrans*	Nut and seed	Sainene (15–50%)	Rice dishes, pastas, soups, biscuits
Onion	*Allium cepa*	Bulb, stems (dried or powder)	d-n-prpyl disulfide	Soups, curries, pickles
Oregano	*Origanum vulgare*	Herb: fresh and dried leaves	Phenols (60–70%), thymol, carvacrol	Salads, sauces, soup, pizza sauce blend, roasts
Paprika	*Capsicum annum*	Dried Fruits	Capsanthin (35–60%)	Sausages, condiments, salad dressings
Parsley (Chinese coriander)	*Petroselinum satiuum*	Herb: fresh and dried leaves	Myristicin (20.6%), apiole (18.3%)	Salad, soups
Pepper	*Pepper nigrum*	Dried berry	Monoterpenes (80%)	Soup, salads, cheese
Poppy seeds	*Papaver somniferum*	seeds	Linoleic acid (30%), oleic acid (30%), and linolenic acid (30%)	Salad dressings, soups, cooked vegetables
Rosemary	*Rosmarinus offinialis*	Herb: Fresh and dried leaves	1,8-cineol (30%), borneol (16–20%), camphor (15–25%)	Salad, fruit fillings, meat, pizza sauce blend

Saffron	*Crocus sativus*	Dried stigma of flower	Monoterpene aldehydes (safranal)	Cakes, ice-creams, milkshakes
Sage	*Salvia officinalis*	Herb: leaves (fresh or dried)	Thujone (28%), 1,8-cineol (12%), borneol (4%).	Herb salad, tea, processed meat, pizza
Savory	*Satureja hortensis*	Herb: leaves (fresh or dried)	Carvacrol (3.4–50.4%), thymol (22.5%), γ-terpinene (2–60.3%)	Liqueurs, gravy, soup mixes, confections
Sesame	*Sesamum indicum*	seeds	Oleic acid (40%), linoleic acid (45%), and saturated acid (10%).	Breads, cakes, sweet, sauces, rice, meat, steamed vegetables
Sweet flag	*Acorus calamus*	Rhizome	β-asarone	Soups, sauces
Star anise	*Illicium verum*	Dried fruit	Anethole (85–90%)	Curries, soups, sauces
Tamarind	*Tamarindus indica*	Dried ripe fruits	Tartaric acid (12%)	Curry blend, chutney blend
Tarragon	*Artemisia dracunculus*	Herb: leaves (fresh or dried)	Estragol (60–75%), anethole (10%)	Vinegar, tartar sauce, eggs, chicken, seafoods
Thyme	*Thymus vulgaris*	Herb: leaves (fresh or dried)	Thymol (12–61%), carvacrol (0.4–20.6%)	Tomato sauce, stuffings, roast, fish, vegetable soup
Turmeric	*Curcuma longa*	Rhizome	Turmerone (30%), dihydro-turmerone and zingiberene (25%), sabinene (58–60%)	Pickles, soup, lentils, vegetables, fried fish, pullaos, desserts
Zedoary (white turmeric)	*Curcuma zedoarea*	Fresh, dried, sliced or ground rhizome	Sesquiterpenes (79%)	Pickle blend, fish marinade, chicken curry blend

Source: NIIR Board of Consultants and Engineers (2006), Gottardi et al. (2016), Sorensen (2015).

Table 1.2 Properties of the selected herbs and spices

Property	Herbs and spices
Taste	Basils, black pepper, cardamom, jalapeno, asafoetida, lemongrass, star anise, vanilla, kokum
Aroma	Clove, kari leaf, mint, ginger, rosemary, nutmeg, tarragon, cardamom
Texture	Garlic, onion, mustard, sesame seed
Color	Annatto, paprika, parsley, turmeric, saffron, basil
Antimicrobial	Ginger, fenugreek, cinnamon, clove, cumin, oregano, sage, rosemary, thyme, chili pepper
Antioxidant	Ginger, turmeric, sage, clove, mace, oregano, rosemary
Health benefit	Ginger, turmeric, garlic, caraway, clove, cinnamon, chili pepper, fenugreek.
Deodorizing/masking	Garlic, savory, bay leaves, clove, leek, thyme, rosemary, caraway, sage, oregano, onion, coriander
Pungency	Garlic, savory, bay leaves, clove, leek, thyme, rosemary, caraway, sage, oregano, onion, coriander, red pepper, mustard, ginger

Source: NIIR Board of Consultants and Engineers (2006), Tiwari et al. (2006), Ravindran et al. (2002).

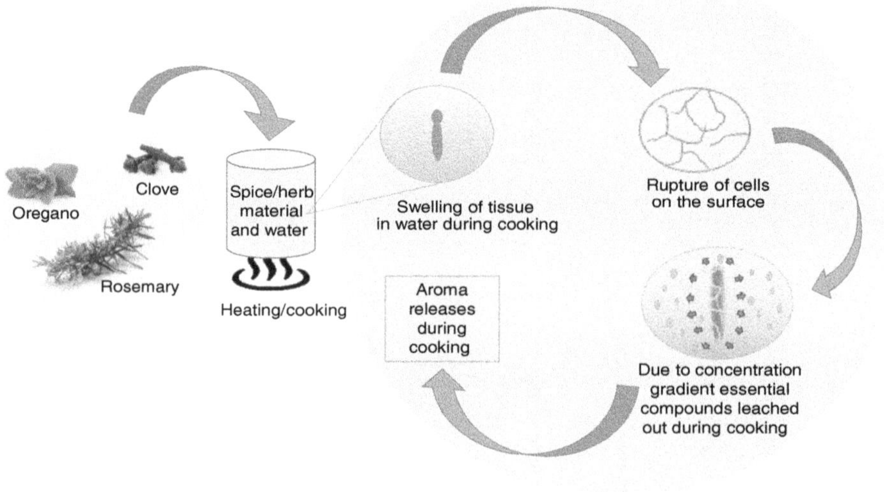

Figure 1.1 Schematic representation of leaching of essential component from the herb/spices during cooking.

Many spices have a harsh and bitter taste when fresh due to the presence of alkaloids, glycosides, and organic and inorganic salt. Cooking techniques such as frying in oil or boiling in water help to reduce the harshness/bitterness of the compound-containing spices and makes the product tastier. Coloring pigments are present in spices in the form of carotenoids, flavonoids, and chlorophyll. As carotenoid is an oil-soluble pigment it can be used during cooking; but in the case of

Table 1.3 Effect of cooking on active principle component at different pH condition

	15 min cooking	30 min cooking
Curry powder I	86% curcumin loss at pH 6.1 88.2% curcumin loss at pH 5.1	87.2% curcumin loss at pH 6.1 90.7% curcumin loss at pH 5.1
Turmeric powder	86.6% curcumin loss at pH 6.1 89.4% curcumin loss at pH 5.1	87.2% curcumin loss at pH 6.1 89.7% curcumin loss at pH 5.1
Curry powder II	No capsaicin loss at pH 6.1 19.2% capsaicin loss at pH 5.1	33.2% capsaicin loss at pH 6.1 28.8% capsaicin loss at pH 5.1
Red pepper powder	3.5% capsaicin loss at pH 6.1 19.2% capsaicin loss at pH 5.1	19.2% capsaicin loss at pH 6.1 31.3% capsaicin loss at pH 5.1
Curry powder II	56.9% piperine loss at pH 6.1 53.4% piperine loss at pH 5.1	60.3% piperine loss at pH 6.1 62.1% piperine loss at pH 5.1
Black pepper powder	13.2% piperine loss at pH 6.1 49.6% piperine loss at pH 5.1	17.1% piperine loss at pH 6.1 54% piperine loss at pH 5.1

chlorophyll it will react during cooking and give a brown pigmentation on heating. So in the case of chlorophyll-containing green leaves, the cooking time should be shortened to retain the green color of herbs, which should be added at the end of cooking process (Hirasa and Takemasa 1998). The active components of spices come from the volatile and nonvolatile oils present. Most of the flavor component is generated during the heating and cooking of spices. With an increase in temperature, the flavor components of spices become more volatile, and by controlling cooking conditions, including temperature and time, the flavor sensation of each spice can be changed (Hirasa and Takemasa 1998).

1.2.2 Blanching

Blanching, an essential operation in spice processing, is a minimal temperature heat treatment (80–90 °C) generally applied to spices primarily to inactivate the natural enzymes before processing or storage (Akintunde et al. 2011). Prior to processing techniques like freezing and drying, blanching is generally carried out as a pretreatment process (Rawson et al. 2011).

Innovative blanching technologies include the application of thermal, hot water, microwave, steam, ohmic and infrared blanching. Blanching is important for spices that are to be frozen (like freeze-dried spice products) because freezing just slows enzyme action, it does not destroy or completely stop it. If spices are not blanched before freezing, they will slowly develop off-flavors, off-colors, and other kinds of enzymatic damage to the product (Thane and Reddy 1997; Vaclavik and Christian 2014). Blanching gelatinizes the surface starch and forms a compact appearance with fewer pores and air cells. Hence it can be used as a pretreatment so that the oil uptake during the process can be reduced.

Spices are blanched for the following purposes: inactivation of enzymes, enhancement of drying rate and product quality, removal of certain pesticide residues, expelling air from the tissues, decreasing microbial load, minimizing non-enzymatic browning reactions, easy removal of outer layer/covering, and increasing the extraction efficiency of bioactive compounds (Xiao et al. 2017).

1.2.2.1 Applications Garlic, a spice in the onion genus, *Allium,* is blanched in steam or hot water for five to seven minutes to prevent the enzymatic activity of peroxidase, polyphenol oxidase, and inulinase, which are responsible for flavor alterations that lead to the deterioration of the product during transportation, storage, and processing (Fante and Noreña 2012). To retain the natural characteristics of nutmeg and mace, mild blanching for one minute is carried out. It helps in the retention of color without affecting the flavor principles accompanied by sulfitation. Blanching increases glossiness and decreases mold growth. Green pepper, which is superior among all products in flavor, aroma, texture, and color – but expensive – is blanched to avoid browning during processing and storage. The carotenoid content is increased in blanched red chili compared to unblanched.

The effectiveness of blanching is mostly assessed based on the degree of inactivation of the peroxidase (POD) and polyphenol oxidase (PPO) enzyme, color, and texture. The severity of heat treatment can be measured by evaluating color (Ling et al. 2015). Texture indicates the physiochemical characteristic of change in the cell wall, which corresponds to quality degradation. Ascorbic acid is used as an indicator for the evaluation of nutrients lost during blanching (Gupta et al. 2008). Since the water soluble ascorbic acid is prone to leaching from cells and is also thermally liable, light sensitive, and can be easily degraded by ascorbic acid oxidase, it is selected as the most frequently measured nutrient to evaluate nutrient loss during blanching. Vitamin C retention was found to be significantly higher in microwave-blanched bell pepper than hot-water blanched ones (Ramesh et al. 2001). The reason was low leaching losses of vitamin C in the microwave blanching. For the production of high-quality paprika and chili powders, complete inactivation of deteriorative enzymes such as POD, LOX (lipoxygenase), and PPO is a necessary prerequisite (Xiao et al. 2017). These enzymes can negatively affect taste, pungency, color intensity, and stability during long storage periods. The residual activity of these enzymes after steam and hot water blanching were studied by (Schweiggert et al. 2006), who determined that PPO showed the lowest heat stability and was completely inactivated, while POD activities decreased by around 98% in chili and paprika powder at 80 °C for 10 minutes. Thermal blanching is mostly used for the blanching of garlic. It inactivates the POD and PPO enzymes responsible for undesirable changes in quality, mainly rapid browning in peeled garlic slices. From the investigation of Fante and Noreña 2012, the best result was given by steam blanching for four minutes, which reduced the enzymatic activities of these enzymes with no changes in texture.

1.2.3 High-Pressure Steam Treatment

It is this natural "organic" sterilization process that is the most effective method for reducing or eliminating bacteria, pathogens, and other food-borne pathogens by the application of steam. Effective steam treatment will remove *Listeria monocytogenes, Salmonella enterica, Escherichia coli*, and a variety of plant pathogens (Studer et al. 2013). In addition, steam treatment is effective in the deactivation of enzymes, e.g. amylase and lipase, which have been shown to cause a breakdown of fat and starch components in sauces, salads, and many ready-made meals. This cannot be done with irradiation or ethylene oxide treatment. Since the heart of the nut is left natural and alive, it will still germinate. This supports the "organic" food label to be applied.

The process works by feeding and discharging the product through a self-cleaning pressure rotary valve that isolates an autoclave from the ambient room. Inside this autoclave, a shaking table transports the product through a steam-pressurized chamber at a specific speed and creates a thin layer of product. Condensation builds on the product surface and this imparts high energy into the surface of the product. This kills unwanted bacteria and pathogens (Grasso et al. 2014).

With this system, a continuous "inflow" of high-pressure steam results in the elimination of undesired microorganisms while causing minimum harm to the organoleptic characteristics (flavor, color, texture, or taste) of spices, herbs, and nuts. It can be used to process chili powders, whole and ground pepper, paprika, garlic, cloves, and a variety of herbs, seeds, and other spices (Lilie et al. 2007). Leafy spices can also be sterilized by this method without any damage to the leaf due to the gentle shaking action applied.

Decontamination is a crucial step in spice processing. Application of a suitable sterilization technology and the selection of appropriate conditions are of great importance. The third world origin of many spices can pose a potential microbial risk. Total counts of food-borne pathogens like Salmonella are found to be in excess in food products, which are likely to be present in nearly 10% of batches imported (Peter 2006). In recent years, the use of ethylene oxide for fumigation in spices has led to anxiety over the residues left by this treatment, and thus bans on its use (Vajdi and Pereira 1973). This has led to the use of an alternative heat treatment for decontamination and sterilization of spices, generally using high-pressure steam in highly specialized equipment.

High-pressure steam treatment is a sterilization technique used for microbial decontamination as well as the sterilization of spices. Sterilization of spices is performed by chemical or physical treatments. High-pressure steam treatment is a physical sterilization technique. Usually, a high-temperature treatment is applied to the whole spice before grinding. The moisture that condenses on the surface of the particles needs to be removed for the prevention of unwanted mold growth in the steam-treated spices. If the optimal pressure and temperature condition of the steam is not maintained, the treatment may affect the volatile profile, color, functionality, and physical state (caking may occur) (Ramos 2003; Grasso et al. 2014). This advance in spice processing proved its application in various spice products such as straight spice powders, culinary powders, masala blends, seasonings, and tastemakers. Effective decontamination of spices can be achieved by this continuous steam sterilization system process which results in the simultaneous reduction of the microbial load and inactivation of enzymes (Rico et al. 2010). The raw materials are heavily contaminated with molds, yeasts, spore formers, and Enterobacteriaceae from the soil that can easily lead to spoilage (Rawat 2015). Steam treatment does not use chemicals and hence chemical residual effects are not found in the treated products. Also, steam is an ideal gas as it is nontoxic, cheap, and there is an unlimited supply. Since high-pressure steam is used, it is the fastest possible way of the product heating to an exact preset condition. Steam condenses on the product and provides the water activity required for effective sterilization, while the steam that condensed on the product surface will protect the product against burning. Hence the system concept complies with the condition that the product is subjected to the minimum heat load for adequate decontamination with a minimum adverse effect on flavor, color, and loss of volatile oil (Kiss and Farkas 1988). The continuous inflow application of saturated high-pressure steam provides the ideal environment for the inactivation of enzymes and elimination of certain microorganisms, while causing minimum harm to the organoleptic characteristics of spices (Grasso et al. 2014).

1.2.4 Electromagnetic Energy (Microwave) Treatment

It is well known that spices can be heavily contaminated with microorganisms because of the processing conditions and environment under which they are produced. The microbial load has to be lowered before they are incorporated safely into food products. Since high-temperature treatment can cause loss of volatile oils from spices, it can also lead to significant loss of flavor and aroma. Steam also results in the loss of volatile components and color changes at same time as increasing moisture levels. So, steam treatment can be substituted by a better alternative method: electromagnetic energy treatment (Chew 2011). A successful application of electromagnetic heating (like microwave, radiofrequency, and ohmic heating) offers great volumetric heating under continuous flow situations. This could motivate many industries to replace certain heat exchangers that transfer heat quite slowly and are susceptible to fouling. Electromagnetic heating methods directly transfer energy from its source without heating up the heat-transferring surface of the processing equipment into the food (Awuah et al. 2007). Microwave energy is the most used application of electromagnetic energy in the field of spice processing.

Microwaves are electromagnetic waves with wavelengths ranging from 1 mm to 1 m that have corresponding frequencies ranging from 300 MHz to 300 GHz (Thostenson and Chou 1999; Das et al. 2009). The applications of microwaves in modern society include communication, radar, radio astronomy, navigation, and food processing. Since the Federal Communications Commission (FCC) of the USA wants to prevent certain devices from interfering with communication signals, only 915 MHz and 2450 MHz microwaves are allowed for industrial, scientific, and medical (ISM) heating applications (Kumbhar 2017). Microwave (MW) treatment has been successfully used in drying, pasteurization, blanching, thawing, tempering, and baking and serves as a good preservation technique that solves deterioration problems to a great extent. This aids in increasing the activity of the bioactive compounds present, release of flavonoids, and also improves the chemical extraction of these compounds. Spices are treated with a microwave prior to extraction processes (expression, steam/hydro distillation, soxhlet extraction, distillation), for the production of various spice products (essential oil, resinoid, oleoresins, resins, and balms) with increased value in the market to meet the expectations of consumers (Ramanadhan 2005).

In microwave heating, the principle of dielectric heating caused by molecular dipole rotation and agitation of charged ions within a high-frequency alternating electric field is applied, in which the heated materials absorb microwave energy and convert it into heat by dielectric heating effect (Chandrasekaran et al. 2013). When the oscillating electric field interacts with high water content materials, the dipolar water molecules will align in the direction of the electromagnetic field alternates at 915 or 2450 MHz (Thostenson and Chou 1999). The internal resistance, due to rotating molecules that collide with other adjacent molecules or atoms, produces volumetric heating (Zhang et al. 2006) and agitation of charged ions in the alternating electrical field also provides microwave heating. It takes place both on the surface of wet biological materials and within them. Compared to conventional heating methods applied in the food industry, in which energy transfer mainly depends on the temperature gradient and the thermal conductivity of the product, microwave heating has several advantages such as volumetric heating, high heating rates, and short processing times. Here, the direct interaction between the electromagnetic field and food materials for heating generation significantly reduces the amount of nutrients lost through leaching (Kidmose and Martens 1999; Ramesh et al. 2002; Brewer and Begum 2003).

Since natural drying leads to quality deterioration by way of contamination, artificial methods, such as drying with the help of hot air or a microwave oven, have been widely adopted. Microwave treatment is a technique that produces spices with a good flavor and acceptable level of contamination (Ramanadhan 2005). Bendini et al. (1998) identified that the essential oil which can also act as a preservative extracted from the microwaved fruits of anise seed exhibits good antioxidant properties. Singh et al. (1996) observed microwave blanching of marjoram gave the maximum retention of ascorbic acid. Raghavan et al. (1997) found that microwave drying had a great impact on the preservation of the flavor quality of marjoram. *Cis*-sabinene hydrate, one of the major components responsible for the flavor characteristics of marjoram, was retained in microwave (175 W) dried samples to a great extent (Novak et al. 2000). Microwave treatment plays a vital role in the production of essential oils from spices, which is one of the most demanded and valuable spice products (Krishnakumar and Potty 2012). Its application is widespread, not only in the flavor industry (food and beverages, tobacco industry), but also in personal care (cosmetics, dental, and household), pharmaceutical (medicinal and veterinary), and other industries (pesticide industry, motor industry, paper and print, rubber and plastics, textile industry, paints, and adhesives).

Cumin seeds are roasted in a conventional dryer and simultaneously subjected to microwave heating to extract the essential oil. Essential oil is extracted from both conventionally roasted and microwave heated samples; then the results are compared. The optimum condition in the conventional dryer method was found to be 125 °C for 10 minutes, while in case of microwave heating method, the best condition was found to be 730 W for 10 minutes. Under these conditions, similar yields of volatile oils were obtained in both cases. Gas chromatography (GC) and gas chromatography–mass spectrometry (GC–MS) analysis of both optimized condition samples showed that microwave heated samples gave better retention of the characteristic flavor compounds of cumin (i.e. total aldehydes) than conventionally-roasted samples. From this case study it is observed that there is loss of the volatile component during roasting of cumin seed (Behera et al. 2004).

1.3 Thermal Processing of Herbs

The leafy parts of the plant that are more habitually utilized for medicinal or therapeutic purposes are termed herbs (Farkas 2000). Fennel, oregano, mint, coriander (cilantro), ginger, rosemary, asparagus, garlic chives, lemon balm, thyme, marjoram, and parsley are some of the common herbs generally used in the day-to-day life. Herbs are marketed in an array of forms, including fresh herbs, dried herbs, herbs in a paste format that have been heat treated, and other ingredients packaged with fresh herbs in a tube format. The centers of origin and the leading global suppliers for most of these traditionally used herbs are developing countries like China, India, and South East Asian countries (Kosalec et al. 2009).

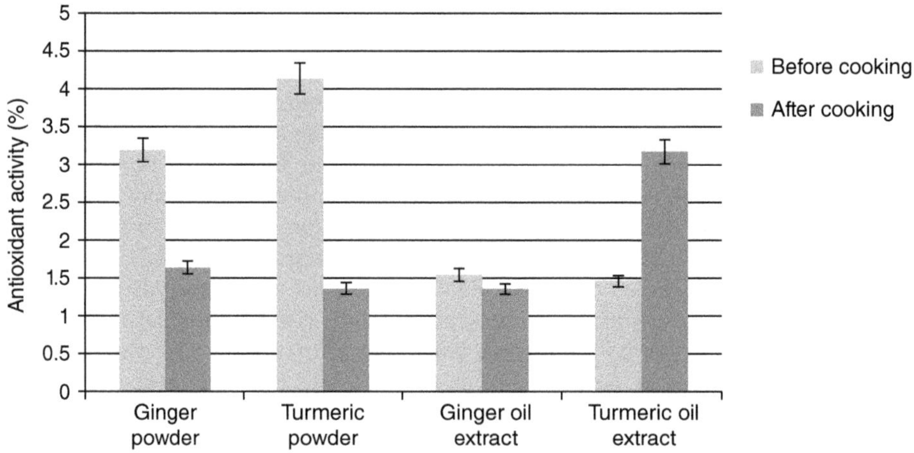

Figure 1.2 Effect of cooking on antioxidant activity of ginger and turmeric.

Herbs that are a source of natural colors and flavors are also used for their volatile aromatic oils and biological principles. Hence, improving the safety of herbs by detecting and controlling the chance of contamination, and controlling pesticide and other residues during harvesting and sun drying – specifically the production of mycotoxins by mold contamination – are of great concern. In order to prevent fungal infection, the moisture levels for most herbs and spices should be reduced to below 11% (Peter 2006). Herbs and spices are a rich source of antioxidants which uphold their pharmaceutical value (Dragland et al. 2003). Thermal processing has a significant effect on the antioxidant activity of these herbs (Figure 1.2). In Indian cooking, ginger and turmeric are commonly used herbs in food preparations. During cooking, temperatures may rise higher than 100 °C, which may lead to the apparent change in antioxidant activity of the dry powder of ginger and turmeric and their oil extracts. In the case of dry powder, antioxidant activity reduced after cooking in both cases. While in turmeric oil extract it increased and for ginger oil extracts it reduced after cooking (Tiwari et al. 2006).

Msaada et al. (2017) suggested coriander fruit as a new potential source of natural antioxidant and also as a food additive. Quality is one of the most superior factors in the world food market. Traders place growing magnitude on "clean" herbs and spices rather than "cleaned" herbs and will never trade in goods that are contaminated even after cleaning.

Thermal treatments like microwave processing, steam sterilization, and blanching are some of the common solutions that aid in the preservation of herbs. Moreover, handling of these herbs by food manufactures comprises washing, cooking, canning, freezing, and drying, which will also decrease the residue levels. Steam sterilization is ideal for both whole and ground herbs and spices because no chemical residue is left on account of this treatment. Sterilization leads to changes in the bioactive compounds of the food stuffs (Rawson et al. 2011). For an effective treatment, steam must be applied under pressure with high precision. Maintenance of the pressure at the specific level should be achieved or else due to the temperature rise the essential oil will be lost. As soon as the treatment is over, the moisture in the system should be completely removed in order to prevent clogging and mold growth (Anon 1991). Since this system is expensive, only a few processing industries use it.

Some common herbs used in day-to-day life

Young plant leaves which are used in cooking are considered culinary herbs; while dried parts of plants comprising essential volatile oils or aromatic flavors, such as buds (cloves), bark (cinnamon), roots (ginger), berries (peppercorns), aromatic seeds (cumin), and the stigma of a flower (saffron), are referred to as spices (Tantipopipat et al. 2010; Banchob 2000a,b). Sometimes, depending upon the parts of the plant, a single plant gives a herb as well as a spice; for example, fennel leaf is a herb, while its dried seed is a spice. In northeast Thai diets, people prefer herb extracts due to the presence of high content polyphenols which have a number of health benefits (Tantipopipat et al. 2010).

1.3.1.1 Coriander (*Coriandrum sativum*) Coriander, which is also known as cilantro, is an annual herb which belongs to the Apiacae family. These are broadly used in cooking throughout the world. Aflatoxin B1 (AFB1) (Majerus et al. 1985) and Ochratoxin A (OTA) (Thirumala-Devi et al. 2001) are the two types of mycotoxins that contaminate coriander. The research done by Selim et al. (1996) found that aflatoxin in the coriander sample was below detectable levels following thermal treatment. Thermal degradation kinetics of chlorophyll in coriander leaf puree was investigated by Rudra et al. (2008) at varying pH levels ranging from 4.5 to 8.5 and processing temperatures from 80–145 °C. The result indicated that chlorophylls were more stable at alkaline pH during thermal processing.

The final quality of the thermally processed herb is usually determined by the degree of greenness, which is naturally gained from chlorophyll (Ahmed et al. 2004). The major findings of this study were that both pigment and visual color degradation during thermal processing follow first-order kinetics which indicate the severity of the process.

Since microwave treatment does not leave harmful residues and does not destroy the heat liable aroma and bioactive constituents of spices and herbs, this justifies the microwave's application in spice processing (Rahath Kubra et al. 2016).

1.3.1.2 Fennel (*Foeniculum vulgare*) Rawson et al. (2013) studied the effect of roasting and boiling on the polyacetylene and polyphenol content of fennel bulb. The study shows that boiling decreases these phytochemicals due to the leaching of essential components in water, whereas roasting also shows a significant decrease in polyacetylenes when compare to the raw bulb. This study indicates that thermal processing affects the antioxidant activity of fennel due to the loss of polyphenol.

In Jordanian diet, raw plants as well as some wild plants are used because of their therapeutic uses and nutrition value. They use large numbers of wild edible plants in their local meals by means of cooking/boiling with water, frying, baking or roasting, and sometimes eaten raw in the form of salads. Fennel is used raw without preparation in green salad, as a bread ingredient (fresh leaves), in seasoning, and is considered a vitamin and mineral rich plant. Along with fennel, coriander, mint, celery, and thyme are also used for seasonings. For preservation purposes, these plants are sun dried and used in cooking throughout the year (Tukan et al. 1998).

Gardeli et al. (2010) conducted a comparative study on the effect of oven drying and freeze drying on fennel plant. It was observed that air and oven drying changes the physiochemical properties as well as aroma of the leaves when compared to freeze drying. Furthermore, this study focused on the essential oil obtained from dried fennel and the effect of drying retention on its flavoring components, such as trans-anethole and isoanethole. They observed that a freeze drying time from 7 to 24 hours resulted in increased amounts of trans-anethole in the freeze-dried herb, while isoanethole decreased. The freeze-dried herb was reported to show a nearly similar aroma profile when compared to fresh herb and better than air or oven drying (Gardeli et al. 2010).

1.3.1.3 Ginger (*Zingiber officinale*) Koch et al. (2016) studied the influence of thermal processing on the antioxidant potential of ginger and ginger-containing products and observed a significant effect on its antioxidant capacity. Autoclaving and microwave energy increased the antioxidant capacity, whereas drying and boiling decreased its bioavailability. Li, J. et al. (2016) observed that weakening in antioxidant potential in thermally processed samples might be due to the oxidation or dehydration of the phenolics present in ginger (like gingerols) and an increased concentration of shogaols, which possess lower antiradical activity. In spite of this, some studies have suggested the creation of new metabolites and other new derivatives of volatile components in thermal processing (Jolad et al. 2005; Höferl et al. 2015). Dahmke et al. (2014) explained an uplifted anticancer potential of turmeric tubers that were initially thermally processed.

1.3.1.4 Oregano (*Origanum vulgare*) Oregano is a perennial herb flowering plant which belongs to the mint family, Lamiaceae. This aromatic herb is often used as fresh seasoning to garnish food, as dry seasoning, or for extracted essential oils, which consist of Carvacrol and Thymol (Marcinčák et al. 2008). Kulišić et al. (2006) developed an aqueous tea infusion prepared from oregano, thyme, and wild thyme. A comparative study conducted revealed that among these teas, based on antioxidant activity, total phenolic, flavonoid, catechin, and anthocyanin content, oregano aqueous tea infusion had the highest number of total phenols (12 500 mg/l GAE) and flavonoids (9000 mg/l GAE). Oregano aqueous tea showed the highest amount of antioxidant and also the dominant presence of rosmarinic acid. Marcinčák *et al.* (2008) showed that compared to the controlled diet at all time points, the essential oil extracted from oregano was more effective in delaying lipid oxidation. This property of oregano can be enhanced by some pretreatments with the microwave or ohmic treatments.

1.4 Conclusion

The key role of herbs and spices is indisputable, due to the presence of aromatic/flavor components. However, initial processing of herbs and spices is required to inactivate microorganisms as well as to improve the extraction yield of their flavor components, color, etc. in food. Herbs and spices are rich in bioactive phytochemicals which may promote health if consumed regularly. These herbs and spices in turn are also responsible for extending the shelf life of food products. Moreover, recent research also suggests that herbs and spices used alone or in combination can lead to a reduction of salt and sugar in foods.

References

Ahmed, J., Shivhare, U.S., and Singh, P. (2004). Colour kinetics and rheology of coriander leaf puree and storage characteristics of the paste. *Food Chemistry* **84** (4): 605–611.

Akintunde, T.T., Akintunde, B.O., and Fagbeja, A. (2011). Effect of blanching methods on drying kinetics of bell pepper. *African Journal of Food, Agriculture, Nutrition and Development* **11** (7): 5457–5474.

Anon (1991). *Hand Book on Spices*. Delhi: National Institute of Industrial Research, Asia Pacific Business Press Inc.

Awuah, G.B., Ramaswamy, H.S., and Economides, A. (2007). Thermal processing and quality: principles and overview. *Chemical Engineering and Processing: Process Intensification* **46** (6): 584–602.

Banchob, M. (2000a). *Indigenous Northeast Thailand Herbs Book* No.1-2. Institute of Herbal Research, National Institute of Health, Thanacharoensin Printing (Thai).

Banchob, M. (2000b). *Indigenous Northeast Thailand Herbs Book* Bo. 3. Institute of Herbal Research, National Institute of Health of Thailand, AR Printing Mass Product Ltd (Thai).

Behera, S., Nagarajan, S., and Rao, L.J.M. (2004). Microwave heating and conventional roasting of cumin seeds (*Cuminum cyminum* L.) and effect on chemical composition of volatiles. *Food Chemistry* **87** (1): 25–29.

Bendini, A., Toschi, T.G., and Lercker, G. (1998). Influence of γ-irradiation and microwaves on the linear unsaturated hydrocarbon fraction in spices. *Zeitschrift für Lebensmitteluntersuchung und-Forschung A* **207** (3): 214–218.

Billing, J. and Sherman, P.W. (1998). Antimicrobial functions of spices: why some like it hot. *The Quarterly Review of Biology* **73** (1): 3–49.

Brewer, M.S. and Begum, S. (2003). Effect of microwave power level and time on ascorbic acid content, peroxidase activity and color of selected vegetables. *Journal of Food Processing and Preservation* **27** (6): 411–426.

Chandrasekaran, S., Ramanathan, S., and Basak, T. (2013). Microwave food processing—a review. *Food Research International* **52** (1): 243–261.

Chew, H.H. and Mass Technology (HK) Ltd. (2011). Method and device for water treatment using an electromagnetic field. US Patent 7 887 708.

Clark, W.R.E. (1970). Modern trends in the application of spice. *Food Manufacture* **45** (1): 53–66.

Dahmke, I.N., Boettcher, S.P., Groh, M., and Mahlknecht, U. (2014). Cooking enhances curcumin anti-cancerogenic activity through pyrolytic formation of "deketene curcumin". *Food Chemistry* **151**: 514–519.

Das, S., Mukhopadhyay, A.K., Datta, S., and Basu, D. (2009). Prospects of microwave processing: an overview. *Bulletin of Materials Science* **32** (1): 1–13.

Douglas, M., Heyes, J., and Smallfield, B. (2005). *Herbs, Spices and Essential Oils: Post-Harvest Operations in Developing Countries*, 61. UNIDO and FAO.

Dragland, S., Senoo, H., Wake, K. et al. (2003). Several culinary and medicinal herbs are important sources of dietary antioxidants. *The Journal of Nutrition* **133** (5): 1286–1290.

Embuscado, M.E. (2015). Spices and herbs: natural sources of antioxidants–a mini review. *Journal of Functional Foods* **18**: 811–819.

Fante, L. and Noreña, C.P.Z. (2012). Enzyme inactivation kinetics and colour changes in garlic (*Allium sativum* L.) blanched under different conditions. *Journal of Food Engineering* **108** (3): 436–443.

Farkas, J. (2000). The microbiological safety and quality of food. In: *Spices and Herbs*, vol. **I**, 897–913. Gaithersburg, Maryland: Apsen Publishers.

Fischetti, F. Jr. (1980). Natural and artificial flavors. In: *CRC Handbook of Food Additives*, vol. **2**, 229–326. CRC press: Boca Raton, Florida.

Gardeli, C., Evageliou, V., Poulos, C. et al. (2010). Drying of fennel plants: oven, freeze drying, effect of freeze-drying time, and use of biopolymers. *Drying Technology* **28** (4): 542–549.

Gottardi, D., Bukvicki, D., Prasad, S., and Tyagi, A.K. (2016). Beneficial effects of spices in food preservation and safety. *Frontiers in Microbiology* **7**: 1394.

Grasso, E.M., Stam, C.N., Anderson, N.M., and Krishnamurthy, K. (2014). Heat and steam treatments. In: *The Microbiological Safety of Low Water Activity Foods and Spices*, 403–424. New York: Springer.

Gupta, S., Lakshmi, A., and Prakash, J. (2008). Effect of different blanching treatments on ascorbic acid retention in green leafy vegetables. *Natural Product Radiance* **7** (2): 111–116.

Hirasa, K. and Takemasa, M. (1998). *Spice Science and Technology*. CRC Press.

Höferl, M., Stoilova, I., Wanner, J. et al. (2015). Composition and comprehensive antioxidant activity of ginger (*Zingiber officinale*) essential oil from Ecuador. *Natural Product Communications* **10** (6): 1085–1090.

James, S.J. and James, C. (2005). Minimal processing of ready meals. In: *Emerging Technologies for Food Processing*, 717–732. London: Elsevier Academic.

Jolad, S.D., Lantz, R.C., Chen, G.J. et al. (2005). Commercially processed dry ginger (*Zingiber officinale*): composition and effects on LPS-stimulated PGE2 production. *Phytochemistry* **66** (13): 1614–1635.

Kasahara, K. and Osawa, C. (1998). Combination effects of spices on masking of odor in boiled sardine. *Fisheries Science* **64** (3): 415–418.

Kidmose, U. and Martens, H.J. (1999). Changes in texture, microstructure and nutritional quality of carrot slices during blanching and freezing. *Journal of the Science of Food and Agriculture* **79** (12): 1747–1753.

Kikuchi, T., Hirai, K., and Sudarso, A.S. (1968). Suppressing effect of spice for fishy odor: a model experiment with the mixture of trimethylamine and spice. *Eiyo to Shokuryo* **21**: 253–256.

Kiss, I. and Farkas, J. (1988). Irradiation as a method for decontamination of spices. *Food Reviews International* **4** (1): 77–92.

Koch, W., Kukula-Koch, W., Dziedzic, M. et al. (2016). Influence of thermal processing and in vitro digestion on the antioxidant potential of ginger and ginger containing products. *Natural Product Communications* **11** (8): 1153–1156.

Kosalec, I., Cvek, J., and Tomić, S. (2009). Contaminants of medicinal herbs and herbal products. *Arhivzahigijenuradaitoksikologiju* **60** (4): 485–500.

Krishnakumar, V. and Potty, S.N. (2012). Marjoram. In: *Handbook of Herbs and Spices*, 2e, vol. **1**, 336–365. Woodhead Publishing.

Kulišić, T., Dragović-Uzelac, V. and Miloš, M. (2006). Antioxidant activity of aqueous tea infusions prepared from oregano, thyme and wild thyme.

Kumbhar, A. (2017). Overview of ISM bands and software-defined radio experimentation. *Wireless Personal Communications* **97** (3): 3743–3756.

Li, J., Tu, Z., Zhang, L. et al. (2016). The effect of ginger and garlic addition during cooking on the volatile profile of grass carp (*Ctenopharyngodon idella*) soup. *Journal of Food Science and Technology* **53** (8): 3253–3270.

Li, Y., Hong, Y., Han, Y. et al. (2016). Chemical characterization and antioxidant activities comparison in fresh, dried, stir-frying and carbonized ginger. *Journal of Chromatography B* **1011**: 223–232.

Lilie, M., Hein, S., Wilhelm, P., and Mueller, U. (2007). Decontamination of spices by combining mechanical and thermal effects–an alternative approach for quality retention. *International Journal of Food Science & Technology* **42** (2): 190–193.

Ling, B., Tang, J., Kong, F. et al. (2015). Kinetics of food quality changes during thermal processing: a review. *Food and Bioprocess Technology* **8** (2): 343–358.

Majerus, P., Woller, R., Leevivat, P., and Klintrimas, T. (1985). Gewürze-schimmelpilzbefall und gehalt an aflatoxinen, ochratoxinA und stergmatocysin. *Fleischwirtschaft* **65** (9): 1155–1158.

Marcinčák, S., Cabadaj, R., Popelka, P., and Šoltýsová, L. (2008). Antioxidative effect of oregano supplemented to broilers on oxidative stability of poultry meat. *Slovenian Veterinary Research* **45** (2): 61–66.

Msaada, K., Jemia, M.B., Salem, N. et al. (2017). Antioxidant activity of methanolic extracts from three coriander (*Coriandrum sativum* L.) fruit varieties. *Arabian Journal of Chemistry* **10**: S3176–S3183.

NIIR board of consultants and engineers (2006). *The Complete Book on Spices & Condiments (with Cultivation, Processing & Uses)*. Delhi: Asia Pacific Business Press.

Novak, J., Bitsch, C., Langbehn, J. et al. (2000). Ratios of cis-and trans-sabinene hydrate in *Origanum majorana* L. and *Origanum microphyllum* (Bentham) Vogel. *Biochemical Systematics and Ecology* **28** (7): 697–704.

Peter, K.V. (ed.) (2006). *Handbook of Herbs and Spices*, vol. **3**. Cambridge, England: Woodhead Publishing.

Prasad, S., Gupta, S.C., and Aggarwal, B.B. (2012). Micronutrients and cancer: add spice to your life. In: *Nutrition, Diet and Cancer*, 23–48. Dordrecht: Springer.

Raghavan, B., Rao, L.J., Singh, M., and Abraham, K.O. (1997). Effect of drying methods on the flavour quality of marjoram (*Oreganum majorana* L.). *Molecular Nutrition & Food Research* **41** (3): 159–161.

Rahath Kubra, I., Kumar, D., and Jagan Mohan Rao, L. (2016). Emerging trends in microwave processing of spices and herbs. *Critical Reviews in Food Science and Nutrition* **56** (13): 2160–2173.

Ramanadhan, B. (2005). Microwave extraction of essential oils (from black pepper and coriander) at 2.46 Ghz. Doctoral dissertation. University of Saskatoon, Saskatchewan.

Ramesh, M.N., Wolf, W., Tevini, D., and Jung, G. (2001). Influence of processing parameters on the drying of spice paprika. *Journal of Food Engineering* **49** (1): 63–72.

Ramesh, M.N., Wolf, W., Tevini, D., and Bognar, A. (2002). Microwave blanching of vegetables. *Journal of Food Science* **67** (1): 390–398.

Ramos, L.P. (2003). The chemistry involved in the steam treatment of lignocellulosic materials. *Química Nova* **26** (6): 863–871.

Ravindran, P.N., Johny, A.K., and Nirmal, B.K. (2002). Spices in our daily life. *Satabdi Smaranika* Souvenir **2**: 227–242.

Rawat, S. (2015). Food spoilage: microorganisms and their prevention. *Asian Journal of Plant Science and Research* **5** (4): 47–56.

Rawson, A., Patras, A., Tiwari, B.K. et al. (2011). Effect of thermal and non thermal processing technologies on the bioactive content of exotic fruits and their products: review of recent advances. *Food Research International* **44** (7): 1875–1887.

Rawson, A., Hossain, M.B., Patras, A. et al. (2013). Effect of boiling and roasting on the polyacetylene and polyphenol content of fennel (*Foeniculum vulgare*) bulb. *Food Research International* **50** (2): 513–518.

Rico, C.W., Kim, G.R., Ahn, J.J. et al. (2010). The comparative effect of steaming and irradiation on the physicochemical and microbiological properties of dried red pepper (*Capsicum annum* L.). *Food Chemistry* **119** (3): 1012–1016.

Risch, S.J. (1997). Spices: sources, processing, and chemistry. In: *Spices Flavour Chemistry and Anitoxidant Properties*, vol. **660** (eds. S.J. Risch and C.T. Ho), 2–6. Washington DC: American Chemical Society.

Rudra, S.G., Sarkar, B.C., and Shivhare, U.S. (2008). Thermal degradation kinetics of chlorophyll in pureed coriander leaves. *Food and Bioprocess Technology* **1** (1): 91–99.

Sackewitz, P. (1956). The Story of Spices von JW Parry, Chemical Publishing Co., New York, (1953). 1. Aufl., VIII, 208 S., geb. *Angewandte Chemie* **68** (22): 720–720.

Schweiggert, U., Schieber, A., and Carle, R. (2006). Effects of blanching and storage on capsaicinoid stability and peroxidase activity of hot chili peppers (*Capsicum frutescens* L.). *Innovative Food Science & Emerging Technologies* **7** (3): 217–224.

Selim, M.I., Popendorf, W., and Ibrahim, M.S. (1996). Aflatoxin B1 in common Egyptian foods. *Journal of AOAC International* **79** (5): 1124–1129.

Shelef, L.A. (1984). Antimicrobial effects of spices. *Journal of Food Safety* **6** (1): 29–44.

Simmonds, N.W. (1982). Spices. By J. W. Purseglove, E. G. Brown, C. L. Green and S. R. J. Robbins. London and New York: Longman (1981), Vol. 1, pp. 1–439, Vol. 2, pp. 447–813. *Experimental Agriculture*. Cambridge University Press **18** (3): 330–330.

Singh, M., Raghavan, B., and Abraham, K.O. (1996). Processing of marjoram (*Majorana hortensis Moench.*) and rosemary (*Rosmarinus Officinalis* L.). Effect of blanching methods on quality. *Molecular Nutrition & Food Research* **40** (5): 264–266.

Singhal, P., Singla, N., Sakhare, D., and K Sharma, A. (2017). A comparative evaluation of in-vitro antioxidant activity of some commonly used spices of northern India. *The Natural Products Journal* **7** (2): 131–136.

Sorensen N.J. (2015). Herb and spice chart. http://www.foodandnutrition.com/Appendix/spice_chart.htm (accessed 17 December 2019).

Srinivasan, K. (2005). Role of spices beyond food flavoring: nutraceuticals with multiple health effects. *Food Reviews International* **21**: 167–188.

Srinivasan, K., Sambaiah, K., and Chandrasekhara, N. (1992). Loss of active principles of common spices during domestic cooking. *Food Chemistry* **43** (4): 271–274.

Studer, P., Heller, W.E., Hummerjohann, J., and Drissner, D. (2013). Evaluation of aerated steam treatment of alfalfa and mung bean seeds to eliminate high levels of *Escherichia coli* O157: H7 and O178: H12, *Salmonella enterica*, and *Listeria monocytogenes*. *Applied and Environmental Microbiology* **79** (15): 4613–4619.

Subbulakshmi, G. and Naik, M. (2002). Nutritive value and technology of spices: current status and future perspectives. *Journal of Food Science & Technology* **39**: 319–344.

Sung, B., Prasad, S., Yadav, V.R., and Aggarwal, B.B. (2012). Cancer cell signaling pathways targeted by spice-derived nutraceuticals. *Nutrition and Cancer* **64** (2): 173–197.

Tantipopipat, S., Boonpraderm, A., Charoenkiatkul, S. et al. (2010). Dietary intake of spices and herbs in habitual northeast thai diets. *Malaysian Journal of Nutrition* **16** (1): 137–148.

Thane, C. and Reddy, S. (1997). Processing of fruit and vegetables: effect on carotenoids. *Nutrition & Food Science* **97** (2): 58–65.

Thirumala-Devi, K., Mayo, M.A., Reddy, G. et al. (2001). Occurrence of ochratoxin A in black pepper, coriander, ginger and turmeric in India. *Food Additives & Contaminants* **18** (9): 830–835.

Thostenson, E.T. and Chou, T.W. (1999). Microwave processing: fundamentals and applications. *Composites Part A: Applied Science and Manufacturing* **30** (9): 1055–1071.

Tiwari, V., Shanker, R., Srivastava, J., and Vankar, P.S. (2006). Change in antioxidant activity of spices-turmeric and ginger on heat treatment. Electron. *Journal of Environmental, Agricultural and Food Chemistry* **5** (2): 1313–1317.

Tukan, S.K., Takruri, H.R., and Al-Eisawi, D.M. (1998). The use of wild edible plants in the Jordanian diet. *International Journal of Food Sciences and Nutrition* **49** (3): 225–235.

Vaclavik, V.A. and Christian, E.W. (2014). Food preservation. In: *Essentials of Food Science*, 323–342. New York, NY: Springer.

Vajdi, M. and Pereira, R.R. (1973). Comparative effects of ethylene oxide, gamma irradiation and microwave treatments on selected spices. *Journal of Food Science* **38** (5): 893–895.

Xiao, H.W., Pan, Z., Deng, L.Z. et al. (2017). Recent developments and trends in thermal blanching–a comprehensive review. *Information Processing in Agriculture* **4** (2): 101–127.

Yoshida, A., Sasaki, K., and Ohshiba, K. (1984). Suppressing experiments for fishy odor. II. Seikatsu Esei. *Journal of Urban Living and Health Association* **28** (4): 211–218.

Zhang, M., Tang, J., Mujumdar, A.S., and Wang, S. (2006). Trends in microwave-related drying of fruits and vegetables. *Trends in Food Science & Technology* **17** (10): 524–534.

Zheng, W. and Wang, S.Y. (2001). Antioxidant activity and phenolic compounds in selected herbs. *Journal of Agricultural and Food Chemistry* **49** (11): 5165–5170.

2
Non-Thermal Processing of Herbs and Spices

Camila A. Perussello
Technological University Dublin, Environmental Sustainability and Health Institute, Grangegorman Campus, Dublin, D07 H6K8, Ireland

2.1 Introduction

Herbs, spices, and their essential oils have been used in foods, beverages, cosmetics, and medicines since ancient times. Differently from regular vegetables, culinary herbs (e.g., thyme, oregano, mint, fennel, rosemary, parsley, sage, basil, coriander) are fresh and dried leaves used in small amounts to provide flavor rather than substance to food. Egypt is the main producer of aromatic herbs, especially basil, marjoram, parsley, dill, coriander (cilantro), spearmint, and peppermint, followed by Morocco (thyme and rosemary), Turkey (oregano, sage, and laurel), and Albania (sage). The global market for herbs has grown 23% from 2012 to 2016, corresponding to USD 299 million in the 52-week period ending in May 2016, with oregano alone accounting for USD 44 million (FAO 2018). Some plants are used either as herbs or spices, such as coriander leaves and seeds. Spices are usually the flowers, fruits, seeds, bark, and roots of tropical plants that are used as seasonings or to add color, aroma or both to a wide range of foods and beverages. Examples are black pepper, white pepper, cardamom, powdered mustard, paprika, cardamom seeds, celery seeds, coriander seeds, cloves, vanilla, and cinnamon. With a market worth USD 927 million in 2016, 19% higher compared to 2012, the largest producers of spices are India (1 407 500 tonnes in 2015–2016), Turkey (241 053 tonnes), and Bangladesh (163 497 tonnes) (FAO 2018).

Herbs and spices are rich in phytochemicals (e.g., flavonoids, carotenoids, plant sterols, phthalides, and glucosinolates), dietary fibers, proteins, minerals, vitamins, and unsaturated fatty acids (Embuscado 2015). Scientific studies have confirmed their effects against several diseases (e.g., cardiovascular ailments, cancer, cataract, macular degeneration, diabetes, obesity, hypertension, dyslipidaemia, stroke, inflammation, arthritis, Alzheimer's, and cognition impairment) either in animals or humans (Bi et al. 2017; Ribeiro-Santos et al. 2017a; Sánchez-Camargo and Herrero 2017; Srinivasan 2017; Kaefer and Milner 2008; Srivastav et al. 2017). Herbs and spices have also been used as natural antioxidants and antimicrobials either in food formulations

Herbs, Spices and Medicinal Plants: Processing, Health Benefits and Safety, First Edition.
Edited by Mohammad B. Hossain, Nigel P. Brunton, and Dilip K. Rai.

or in food biodegradable packaging (i.e., edible films and coatings) to delay lipid oxidation and microbial growth (Ribeiro-Santos et al. 2017b).

The increasing demand for spices and herbs is a result of population growth, rising income, globalization, change in food preferences and lifestyle (i.e. home cooking), and greater awareness of the relationship between diet and health. A more frequent consumption of spices can reduce the amounts of sodium, sweeteners, and fats people use to flavor their recipes. The largest overseas markets are European countries (particularly Germany, the Netherlands, and the UK) followed by the United States (US). The boost in the imports of spices and herbs has led to safety and toxicity concerns. Approximately 7% of the imports of spices in 2007–2009 were contaminated by salmonella (Van Doren et al. 2013), the most common bacterial pathogen associated with product recalls and outbreaks in spices (ASTA 2011). As most spices are cooked before being consumed, salmonella contamination may not pose a health problem, but some spices are often eaten raw, such as pepper. Shipments from Mexico and India are the most frequently contaminated (Harris 2013).

National food laws and regulations specify maximum permissible limits of contaminants in herbs and spices, which include extraneous matter, microbial infection, insect infestation, bird and animal excrements, mycotoxins, pesticide residues, and heavy metals. Herbs and spices are exposed to a variety of microbial contaminants before, during, and after processing, especially when sun-dried on the floor (McKee 1995). Herbs and spices can carry a significant amount of microbial contaminants, especially xerophilic storage molds, mesophilic bacteria, and enterobacteria, but also pathogens, such as *Salmonella* spp., *Staphylococcus aureus, Yersinia intermedia, Shigella* spp., *Enterobacter* spp., and others (Sospedra et al. 2010). The most frequent molds in these products are *Aspergillus* spp. and *Penicillium* spp., some of their species being potential producers of mycotoxins that exhibit toxic and carcinogenic effects in humans and animals, i.e. aflatoxins, ochratoxins, and sterigmatocystine (Fogele et al. 2018; Kabak and Dobson 2017). The initial level of bacterial contamination depends basically on the hygienic handling conditions of the raw materials and final products, and the processing conditions.

While European Union (EU) legislation has no definite microbiological standards for spices and herbs, *Salmonella* spp. should be completely absent in 25 g of sample (European Commission (EC) 2004). Additionally, the sample cannot exceed the following levels according to EC (2004): *Escherichia coli* $\leq 10^2$ CFU/g, *Bacillus cereus* $\leq 10^4$ CFU/g, *Clostridium perfringens* $\leq 10^3$ CFU/g, and total molds $\leq 10^6$ CFU/g. Different mandatory microbiological standards are established by national authorities of different countries. Depending on public and private requirements, these products must comply with limits for mycotoxins, molds, yeasts, food pathogens (i.e. *Salmonella enterica, B. cereus,* and *S. aureus*), indicators of hygiene practices (i.e. *Enterococcus faecalis* and *E. coli*), additives and illegal colorants, pesticides, and polycyclic aromatic hydrocarbons (Schaarschmidt 2016).

The most widely used methods for decontamination of spices are steaming, irradiation, and ethylene oxide fumigation. Steaming involves the application of dry steam at 100–200 °C to the product for 6–120 seconds (Molnár et al. 2018; Almela et al. 2002). While it is a natural, renewable process that provides decontamination of bacteria and pathogens typically at two to five log-reduction levels, unfavorable color changes of chlorophyll- and carotenoid-containing materials occur following steaming, as well as lowering of the contents of bioactive compounds and volatile oil (Molnár et al. 2018; Duncan et al. 2017). Additionally, this procedure is not recommended for powdered

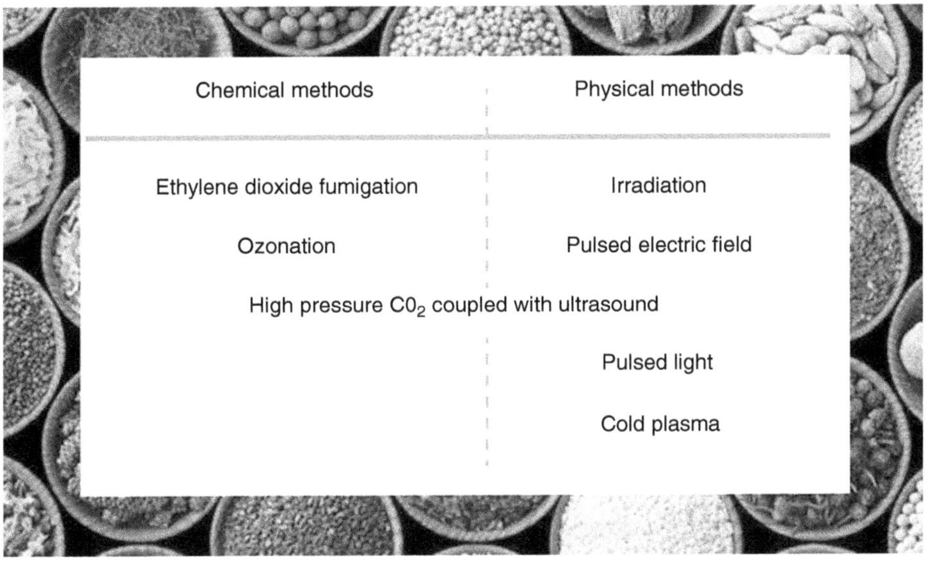

Figure 2.1 Non-thermal decontamination methods for herbs and spices.

materials, as they become clumped. While fumigation with ethylene oxide gas is prohibited in the EU due to its carcinogenic potential to humans, it is commonly used in the US because it is effective against bacteria, viruses, and fungi. Furthermore, the local legislation does not require labeling. Gamma irradiation is authorized in the EU provided the maximum absorbed dose does not exceed 10 kGy (Farkas 2006). Despite the high efficiency against microorganisms, irradiation may impair the sensory and antioxidant properties of the final product (Schweiggert et al. 2007). In addition, irradiated products are usually not socially accepted.

There is no technology alone able to decontaminate all types of herbs and spices with minimal loss of nutrients and sensory properties. The decontamination technology must rather be chosen based on legislation standards, purchaser requirements, production budget, product specificities (i.e., powder, leaves, seeds), and desirable product sensory quality. There is a trend toward non-thermal processing in the food industry, aiming at reduced energy demand and better preservation of heat-labile components. This chapter discusses chemical and physical non-thermal technologies currently used to decontaminate herbs and spices (Figure 2.1), namely ozonation, radiation, pulsed electric field (PEF), pulsed light, fumigation with ethylene dioxide (ETO), high pressure CO_2 coupled with ultrasound, and cold plasma.

2.2 Ozone

Gaseous ozone (O_3), a triatomic form of oxygen, is regarded as a green treatment against microbial contamination of food, water, and food processing surfaces. O_3 is a potent oxidant, with an oxidizing potential of 2.07 V compared to 1.36 V of chlorine, a strong disinfectant. Ozone has high reactivity and penetrability, and liberates innocuous ordinary oxygen as the major end product, hence does not leave residual

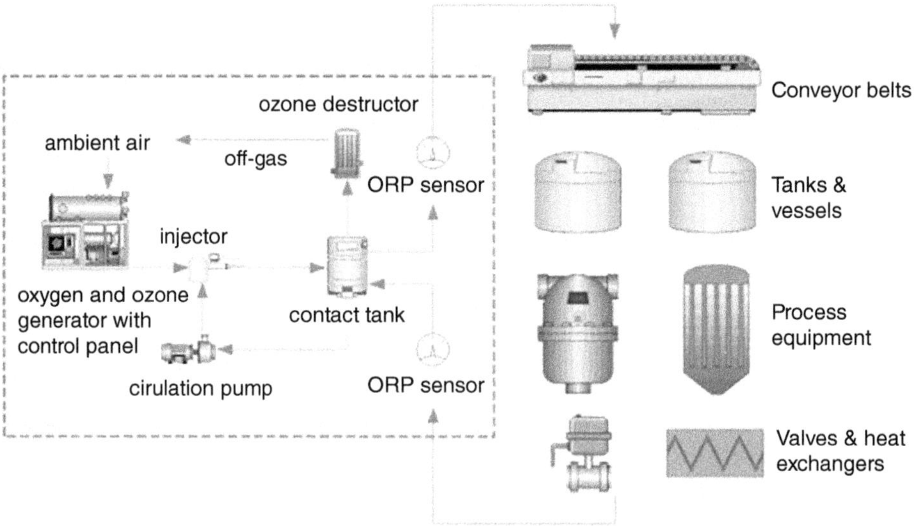

Figure 2.2 Ozone sterilization equipment for food and beverages. *Source:* Ozonotech 2018.

components on products (Kim et al. 1999; Guzel-Seydim et al. 2004; Novak et al. 2008; Torlak et al. 2013). Meshophilic and pathogenic bacteria (i.e. *Listeria monocytogenes, S. aureus, E. coli, S. typhimurium*), viruses, yeasts, and bacterial spores (i.e. *B. cereus*) are destroyed by ozone by oxidation in the following order of vulnerability: gram-positive bacteria > gram-negative bacteria > fungi > spores (Brodowska and Śmigielski 2014).

Ozone gas is generally created onsite from ambient air or from pure oxygen bottles in laboratory scale, either by a generator via corona discharge, ultraviolet light, or electrochemical methods (Figure 2.2). In the contact tank (solid and liquid foods), fixed or dynamic bed (solid foods), or bubble column (liquid foods), the gas is pumped directly onto the food or alternatively into water, which is used as a rinse, spray or bath. Ozone sensors are installed to allow the monitoring of ozone concentrations. An ozone destructor is placed at the end of the line to ensure elimination of innocuous gas back to the atmosphere. In an industrial setup, the ozone treatment zone is connected to the production line. Ozonation parameters are usually ozone concentration, exposure time, temperature, and relative humidity (Brodowska et al. 2015; Torlak et al. 2013; Cullen et al. 2009).

Ozone is approved by the US Food and Drug Administration (FDA 2001) as GRAS (generally recognized as safe) and has been used for decades as an antimicrobial agent for direct application on food products such as fruit juices, drinking water, fruits, and vegetables (de Souza et al. 2018; Cullen et al. 2009). Some studies have recommended ozonation for decontamination of herbs and spices, since reductions higher than 2 log were obtained, as proposed by food safety regulatory bodies in relation to antimicrobial agents (Tiwari and Rice 2012). Although different countries have established different microbial population limits for spices and herbs, in summary, the microbiological contamination should be low enough to ensure safety for consumers.

Torlak et al. (2013) applied a continuous ozone stream to dried oregano under different concentrations (2.8 and 5.3 mg/L) and times up to 120 minutes. Considerable reductions of microbial counts – including aerobic bacteria, yeasts, molds, and salmonella – were obtained without hindering taste, flavor, and appearance when an ozone concentration of 2.8 mg/L was used. Reductions reached 2.7 log in aerobic plate counts and 1.8 log in yeast and mold counts at 2.8 mg/L for 120 minutes, and 3.2 log in aerobic plate counts at 5.3 mg/L for 90 minutes. The population of three *Salmonella* serotypes (*S. typhimurium, S. newport,* and *S. montevideo*) treated for 120 minutes was reduced by 2.8 log at 5.3 mg/L and by 3.7 log at 2.8 mg/L. Only the higher concentration at maximum time (120 minutes) interfered negatively on overall appearance, which is closely related to color.

Inan et al. (2007) decontaminated red peppers with ozone and obtained 80–93% aflatoxin B1 reduction levels. Different ozone concentrations (16, 33, 66 mg/L) and exposure times (7.5, 15, 30, 60 minutes) at 25 °C and 60% relative humidity were tested in flaked and chopped dried samples naturally contaminated with 20 and 32 μg/kg of aflatoxin B1, respectively. Longer treatments and higher ozone concentrations resulted in greater destruction levels. The final aflatoxin population (4 and 2 mg/kg at 66 mg/L after 30 and 60 minutes, respectively) complied with national legislation standards, and the color remained similar to that of the untreated product.

Akbas and Ozdemir (2008) treated flaked red peppers inoculated with *E. coli, B. cereus,* and *B. cereus* spores with gaseous ozone at 20 °C and 70% relative humidity at different ozone concentrations (0.1–9.0 ppm) for 360 minutes. *B. cereus* and *E. coli* populations were reduced by 1.5 log and 2.0 log at 1.0 ppm, respectively, whereas ozone concentrations ≥5.0 ppm were required to reduce *B. cereus* spores. *E. coli* was more sensitive to ozone than *B. cereus* in all treatments, which is in accordance with the higher resistance to ozone of gram-positive bacteria compared to gram-negative bacteria (Brodowska and Śmigielski 2014). As expected, spores of *B. cereus* were more resistant than vegetative cells, with the highest reduction of 1.5 log at 7.0 ppm for 360 minutes. Differently from *E. coli* and *B. cereus*, higher ozone concentrations did not increase the destruction rate of *B. cereus* spores significantly. The greater the exposure time, the higher the inactivation level for either viable cells or spores. Slight but significant sensory changes related to flavor, appearance, and overall palatability were detected at 5–9 ppm.

Brodowska et al. (2015) published a comprehensive study on the ozone treatment of juniper fruits (*Juniperus communis* L.), which are used as a spice in Northern Europe. The treatment was repeated nine times using different ozone concentrations (100, 130, and 160 g O_3/m^3) and exposure times (30, 60, and 90 minutes). The microbiological profile, phenolic profile, total phenolic content (TPC), beta-carotene bleaching power, and antioxidant activity of the essential oil were determined after each replicate. The initial contamination of the samples comprising total mesophilic bacteria and total fungi was extremely high (>10^5 CFU/g). A 30 minute-treatment yielded a 1 log reduction in the levels of total meshophilic bacteria and total fungi. The lethality was in general not proportional to exposure time and ozone concentration: the 60-minute treatment led to activation of bacteria and fungi, which suggests resistance of these microorganisms to ozone. In addition, longer treatments (90 minutes) were not statistically more effective than shorter ones (30 minutes). *Bacillus cereus* was found in 20% of the control samples at populations of 1.7×10^5 CFU/g, which were reduced to10^5–10^3 CFU/g after ozonation – lower than the infective dose of 10^5–10^6 CFU/g related to food outbreaks according to EFSA (2016). Nevertheless, populations in the range 10^3–10^5 CFU/g can still cause emesis and diarrhea in adults (EFSA 2016). Enterobacteria were not found before or after ozonation. The essential oil from juniper berries exhibited greater losses at the highest ozone concentrations (130 and 160 g O_3/m^3) and the longest treatments (90 minutes) since ozone is a strong oxidant. In these cases, there was approximately 50% loss of α-pinene (the predominant component in the essential oil) compared to the untreated sample. Longer ozone exposure caused degradation of phenolics due to cleavage of glycosidic linkages with sugars or oxidation of polyphenols to carbonyl groups; however, TPC increased after 30-minute treatments (for instance, 15.47 mg catechin equivalent/g of extract for treatment 100/30 versus 9.81 mg CE/g of extract in control samples). The 2,2-diphenyl-1-picryl-hydrazyl-hydrate (DPPH) antioxidant capacity was statistically similar before and after ozonation (IC_{50} varied from 7.63 to 6.86–13.68 μg/L), but the Ferric Reducing Antioxidant Power (FRAP) analysis indicated nearly 50% lower FRAP antioxidant power of samples treated for 60 minutes (at all concentrations) compared to the control. Possible donation of electrons by the hydroxyl group of the phenolic compounds might be responsible for the loss in antioxidant power. The essential oil exhibited significantly lower antioxidant activity following ozonation, especially after 60-minute treatments compared to 30- and 90-minute ones. The loss of antioxidant power might be the result of ozone attacking carbon-carbon double bonds giving rise to new dicarbonyl compounds. Ozonation did not affect the phenolic profile and color of juniper berries.

Brodowska and Śmigielski (2013) applied ozone to cardamom seeds, juniper berries, white pepper drupes, dried blackcurrant berries, and dried onion flakes under the following conditions: room temperature (20 ± 1 °C), ozone concentrations of 150 and 160 g/m^3, flow rate 0.1 L/min, pressure 0.5–0.8 atm, and exposure time 10 minutes. The ozone treatment was not able to reduce the counts of total mesophilic bacteria in cardamom seeds, dried onion flakes, and white pepper drupes. However, ozonation was effective in the reduction of mesophilic bacteria populations (<10 CFU/g) in juniper and dried blackcurrant berries and total fungal count (<10 CFU/g) in cardamom seeds, dried blackcurrant berries, and white pepper drupes. Enterobacteriaceae were completely eliminated in all treatments. These results indicate that the effectiveness of ozone decontamination depends on the food matrix and its microflora.

The current literature demonstrates that although ozone is a potential decontaminant of herbs and spices, little is known about the mechanistic effects of ozone on microorganisms and other molecules (i.e., color, phenolic compounds). Different combinations of process parameters (especially time and ozone concentration) lead to quite different results, which may seem random without a deeper understanding of the underlying mechanisms of ozone sterilization. Additionally, the literature shows that different microorganisms exhibit a varied sensitivity to ozone. This means additional studies are needed to elucidate the mechanisms of microbial decontamination and the influence on quality parameters related to exposure of foods to ozone.

2.3 Irradiation

Ionizing radiation is recognized as safe by the World Health Organization (WHO 2013) and the European Commission (EC 1999a,b) for the treatment of spices and

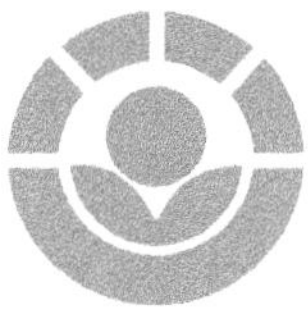

Figure 2.3 International icon for irradiated food required in EU and US food labels.

condiments. Three sources of radiation are approved for use on foods: gamma rays, X-rays, and electron beams or e-beams. Gamma rays are emitted from the radionuclides Cobalt 60 or Cesium 137; X-rays are produced by reflecting a high-energy stream of electrons off a target substance, usually a heavy metal; and electron beams are a stream of high-energy electrons propelled from an electron accelerator (WHO 2013). The application of ionizing radiation must comply with maximum doses of radiation absorbed by the food, generally set as <10 kGy (Farkas 2006; WHO 2013). Although irradiation of food products improves safety, extends shelf life, and does not compromise nutritional and sensory quality within certain radiation doses, it may adversely affect the composition of essential oils (Napoli et al. 2016; Brodowska et al. 2015). In addition, the removal of viruses and bacteria spores requires the use of high doses of radiation (10–50 kGy), which alters the chemical and sensory aspects of spices and herbs unfavorably. As the effect of radiation varies from matrix to matrix, even low doses of radiation (<1 kGy) can affect some products negatively, such as paprika (Yoon et al. 2014). Additionally, irradiated foods are often not approved by consumers, who tend to erroneously relate the mandatory label imposed by regulatory bodies (Figure 2.3) to radioactive or toxic food.

Song et al. (2014) investigated the effect of gamma irradiation against *E. coli* O157:H7 and *S. typhimurium* in black pepper (*Piper nigrum*) and red pepper (dried *Capsicum annuum*). Irradiation doses of 0, 1, 2, 3, and 5 kGy were tested and color change was evaluated. The initial population of these pathogens was below 1 log CFU/g in non-inoculated samples, and 10^5–10^6 CFU/g in inoculated ones. Although doses >1 kGy were more effective, higher irradiation doses within 2–5 kGy did not result in greater destruction rates in black pepper. For red pepper, the higher the irradiation dose, the lower were the final counts of pathogens. Reductions of *E. coli* and *S. typhimurium* for 5 kGy-irradiation ranged from 4.4 to 5.2 log CFU/g in black pepper and from 3.8 to 5.2 log CFU/g in red pepper. The decimal reduction dose (D-value) of the studied microorganisms was greater in red pepper, and *S. typhimurium* had larger D-values than those of *E. coli* for all treatments and pepper types. In general, the color coordinates L*, a*, and b* were not significantly different between 5 kGy-irradiated samples and the control. Additionally, color differences were not visually detected. As *Salmonella* spp. is the most resistant pathogen to irradiation within gram-negative bacteria, this work demonstrated that gamma irradiation is a valuable safety tool for black and red peppers.

Napoli et al. (2016) treated dried Sicilian oregano (*Origanum vulgare* ssp. *hirtum*) with gamma irradiation using different doses, 5 and 10 kGy. Irradiated and control samples were assessed for microbial load, essential oil profile, and sensory properties. The microbial counts of aerobic mesophilic bacteria, yeast and molds, and *Enterobacteriaceae* were significantly reduced even at the lowest irradiation dose (5 kGy), although the initial levels of untreated samples were already within safe levels. Total mesophilic bacteria, for instance, were reduced from 3.7–2.9 to <1 log CFU/g in all treatments, while yeasts and molds counts decreased from 2.0–2.9 to <1 log CFU/g. *Enterobacteriaceae* counts were reduced from <100 to <10 CFU/g at the same irradiation dose. The chemical profile of the essential oil comprised thymol and g-terpinene as main compounds, followed by p-cymene, a-terpinene, carvacrol and thymol methyl ethers, myrcene, and carvacrol. Irradiated oregano exhibited reduced levels of monoterpene hydrocarbons (55–65%) and an increase in oxygenated monoterpenes (30–150%), regardless of the irradiation dose. These results are attributed to irradiation-inducted oxidation of the hydrocarbon matrix in the essential oil components. Irradiated samples exhibited sensory differences in relation to color, odor, flavor, freshness, and overall acceptance scores compared to the control, except for bitter, pungent, astringent, and hay flavors.

Yoon et al. (2014) investigated the synergistic disinfection effect of gamma irradiation combined with sodium dichloroisocyanurate (NaDCC) on paprika fruits, aiming at reducing the irradiation dose necessary to lower the levels of gray mold (*Botrytis cinerea*). Preliminary experiments using paprika samples inoculated with *B. cinerea* (a mold that typically causes spoilage in paprika) revealed that their conidia were inactivated by 4 kGy-irradiation (D-value 0.99 kGy), and by the NaDCC treatment at 50 ppm. Combining irradiation and NaDCC, the D-value was significantly reduced by 1.06–0.58 kGy ($p < 0.05$) using different radiation doses up to 4 kGy. Fungal spoilage was significantly lowered compared to the isolated treatments. Although firmness and fracturability decreased following irradiation, no significant color changes were detected, which is important when processing paprika fruit into spice.

Molnár et al. (2018) tested different technologies for the microbial decontamination of spice paprika, including irradiation, steaming, microwave heating, microwave heating combined with re-wetting and intensive mixing, and radio-frequency heating. The samples were assessed for microbial load, bioactive components, color, and aroma. Steaming (108–125 °C/120 s) and irradiation (1, 5, and 10 kGy) were more effective than the other methods at reducing total mesophilic bacteria counts without impairing the product's chemical properties, except for color. At 1, 5 and 10 kGy doses, the aerobic mesophilic total count decreased from 6.84 log to 5.08, 4.71, and 2.91 log, respectively, and the mold count was reduced from 3.78 log to 3.54, 3.18, and 2.30 log, respectively. Even the lowest dose reduced the numbers of coliforms (3.71 log) and *Enterobacteriaceae* (3.28 log) to below the detection limit. The dominant bacilli microflora (*B. methylotrophicus, Bacillus pumilus*) decreased considerably following 1 and 5 kGy-irradiation – from 6.9×10^6 to 1.0×10^5 and 2.0×10^3 CFU/g, respectively – and disappeared completely at 10 kGy. The total carotenoid content was reduced by 54.8–62.7% depending on the radiation dose, while the total tocopherol content decreased by 23.1–39.8%. The reductions were proportional to the radiation dose. Vitamin C was less affected by irradiation, decreasing from 67.0 ± 7.0 to 63.9 ± 2.5, 66.9 ± 0.7, and 64.7 ± 1.2 mg/g, for respective radiation doses of 1, 5, and 10 kGy. Only the concentration of total carotenoids changed significantly. Color became considerably darker in all treatments.

Different microorganisms respond differently to gamma-irradiation, especially in varying matrices. In general, high inactivation rates are achieved in irradiated spices and herbs, although excessive doses may be required to destroy spores and fungi, leading to adverse sensory effects. Nevertheless, slight sensory differences can be accepted if substantial improvements in food safety and shelf life are achieved. Noteworthy is the importance of implementing education programs to consumers regarding irradiated foods, aiming at better social acceptance.

2.4 Pulsed Electric Field

Scientific studies on the use of pulsed electric field (PEF) for decontamination of condiments date back more than three decades (Keith et al. 1997). Nevertheless, most current industrial applications concern cold sterilization of liquid foods (Barba et al. 2015) due to their high thermal conductivity serving as a suitable transfer medium for electrical energy. PEF reduces microbial counts as a result of the rupture of microbial cells caused by pore formation and consequent destruction of the semipermeable barrier (Castro et al. 1993). In PEF treatments, high-intensity energy is discharged into the product in the form of pulses of different types (square wave, exponential decay, oscillatory, and bipolar) at electric strengths ranging from 20 to 80 kV/cm during very short periods (pulse width of 1–5 μs) and pulse frequency of 200–400 Hz (pulses/s). The energy consumption of pulsed light (PL) decontamination is lower compared to conventional thermal technologies, in addition to being a green method in terms of generation of toxic products, chemicals, and waste effluents (Barbosa-Canovas et al. 1998). The configuration of PEF systems changes according to the type of pulse (Figure 2.4), with square waves and exponential decay pulses generally used in food decontamination (Guerrero-Beltrán and Welti-Chanes 2016).

Although PEF is regarded as a non-thermal technology, fast and sudden temperature rises can result from PEF processing depending on the process conditions (i.e. electric field, processing time, flow rate, pulse width and shape, pulse-specific energy, frequency, refrigeration system), type of matrix (i.e. liquid or solid, porosity, moisture content, ionic compounds, pH, conductivity), and microorganism (type, population, growth phase). Electric field strength (kV/cm) is the distance between the electrodes of the treatment chamber and the voltage delivered. Specific energy of the pulse (kJ/kg), in turn, is a parameter that varies according to the geometry and conductivity of the food and is used to evaluate the process energy costs and to compare PEF efficiency with other technologies (Raso et al. 2014). Time is usually in the range of μs. Irreversible inactivation occurs with electric fields >2 kV/cm in microbial cells and >14 kV/cm in plant cells (Guerrero-Beltrán and Welti-Chanes 2016).

Different microorganisms have different resistance to PEF process parameters, as summarized in Table 2.1. In general, inactivation rates increase with time and the electric field strength, the latter over a threshold field strength called critical electric field strength (Ec), which varies according to different microorganisms but is generally >5 kV/cm. Generally, square wave pulses are more effective than exponential decay pulses due to the inefficacy of the long tail section caused by the slow decaying rate. In addition, higher frequencies and longer pulses seem to be more effective in PEF treatments of the same duration (Raso et al. 2014).

In general, PEF-treated foods maintain their sensory characteristics provided there is no significant temperature rise during processing. The content of functional compounds (i.e. phenolic compounds) may remain unchanged, decrease, or increase depending on the PEF-treatment conditions, but color, antioxidant activity, and vitamin C typically decrease (Guerrero-Beltrán and Welti-Chanes 2016). Studies assessing the potential of PEF in food decontamination comprise mainly liquid foods, such as fruit juice, milk, liquid egg, liquid egg yolk, liquid egg white, soy milk, and

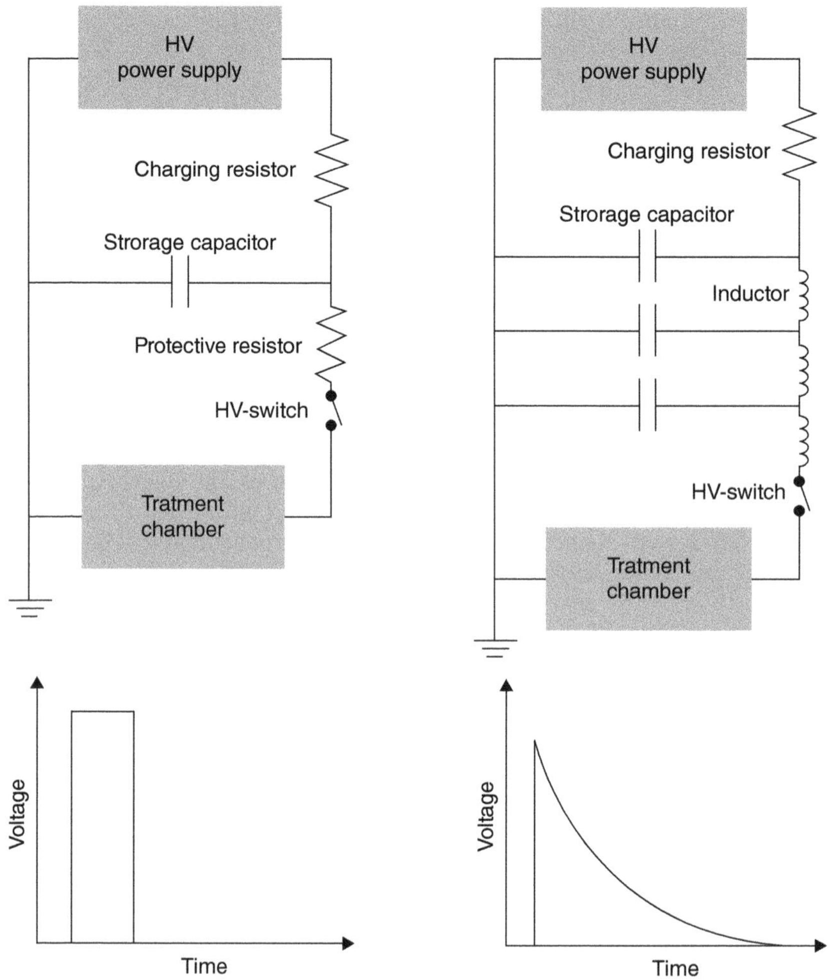

Figure 2.4 PEF system configuration for the production of exponential decay and square wave pulses. *Source:* Guerrero-Beltrán and Welti-Chanes 2016.

beer (Barba et al. 2015), for which typical reduction levels range from 1 to 6 log. Additional applications of PEF in the food industry are numerous. They include include enhancement of sugar yield in sugar beet, dewatering in krill, defatting of cattle bones, chicken by-products, and pig back rind, production of glue from hide shaving, manufacturing of gelatine from cattle bones, extraction of cod liver oil, defatting of cocoa nuts and palm fruits, improvement of fruit juice yield, and extraction of phenolics from spearmint (Sitzmann et al. 2016; Fincan 2015).

Keith et al. (1997) treated onion powder, dill, and basil with PEF under different conditions. Bipolar and reversal shaped-pulses with width of 1–10 μs, pulse number from 20 to 180, and electric field up to 100 kV/cm were tested. Aerobic bacteria (7.4×10^5–1.6×10^6 CFU/g), spores (1.1×10^5–1.13×10^6 CFU/g), total coliforms (<100 to 3.0×10^4 CFU/g), *E. coli* (<100 CFU/g), yeasts (<100 to 4.3×10^3 CFU/g), and mold

Table 2.1 Factors affecting microbial resistance to PEF

Process parameters		Microbial characteristics		Food parameters	
Electric field strength	***	Strain	***	Composition	***
Treatment time	***	Species	***	Conductivity	*
Pulsed width	*	*Growth conditions*		pH	***
Specific energy	***	Growth temperature	NMR	a_w	NMR
Frequency	*	Growth phase	**		
Temperature	***	*Recovery conditions*			
Pulse shape	*	Medium composition	***		
		Temperature	***		
		Recovery time	**		
		Oxygen concentration	NMR		

NMR = Needs More Research; *** Very significant; ** Significant; *Slightly significant.
Source: Raso et al. 2014.

(100–6000 CFU/g) were identified in the untreated samples. While the spices exhibited acceptable final microbial counts, limited 1 log-reduction levels were obtained following PEF treatment. The increase in pulse width from 1 to 10 μs resulted in slightly greater microbial reduction (improvement <0.3 log), but microbial levels decreased significantly with higher electric field strength. The microbial inactivation was slightly more effective using reversing polarity pulses (improvements up to 0.2 log). Equipment limitations prevented the investigation of wider ranges of the process parameters tested. Sensory and chemical characteristics of the PEF-treated spices were not evaluated.

Although lower inactivation rates were obtained by Keith et al. (1997) in PEF-treated spices compared to liquid foods, their results suggest that PEF has potential for spices and herbs provided the process parameters are further studied and optimized. Additionally, there is a gap in the literature concerning the actual molecular changes caused by PEF leading to microbial decontamination of foods and changes in chemical composition and sensory properties. Therefore, further research is required in order to establish PEF as a suitable decontamination method for herbs and spices.

2.5 Pulsed Light

Pulsed light is a non-thermal technology that inactivates pathogenic and food spoilage microorganisms through the use of intense, short-duration pulses of broad-spectrum light, including ultraviolet, visible, and infrared rays, but typically UV-light emitted by xenon lights. Photochemical and photothermal effects are likely responsible for the microbial inactivation. Although several high-intensity light flashes per second are able to destroy bacteria, yeasts, molds, and viruses rapidly, the inactivation may be limited to the superficial layers of the food due to the low penetration of light in solids (Elmnasser et al. 2007; Woodling and Moraru 2006). In fact, current industrial applications comprise disinfection of food contact surfaces and decontamination of beverages and liquid foods, such as sugar syrup and liquid egg (Koutchma 2016). UV light is an eco-friendly technology since it does not generate by-products, waste effluents, or toxic products. In addition, the system configuration is straightforward, comprising a power supply unit and a treatment chamber containing variable numbers of xenon lamps, which generate pulsed light at 200–1100 n with a pulse duration in the range of μs (Nicorescu et al. 2013). Typical process parameters are light frequency and wavelength, energy dose, voltage, energy emitted in each flash, and number and duration of light flashes. Bacterial reductions of 0.5–8 log have been reported depending on the process parameters, pulsed light system configuration (i.e. number of lamps, distance between lamps), target microorganisms, and the food matrix's characteristics (Hsu and Moraru 2011).

Just a few works have been published on pulsed light decontamination of spices. Nicorescu et al. (2013) used pulsed light to inactivate *Bacillus subtilis* in suspensions and spices. Inoculated and control samples of ground caraway, ground red pepper, and ground black pepper were placed in a circular plastic and then treated under circular stirring at 3000 V, 1 Hz with 10 F by using a three-lamp configuration giving an energy dose of 1 J/cm^2/flash. Each spice had different initial contamination levels, ranging from 10^3 to 10^5 CFU/g. There was a significant reduction of the microbial levels following the pulsed light treatment with 10 flashes (totaling 10 J/cm^2): 0.8 log for caraway and black pepper and 1 log for red pepper. Scanning Electron Microscopy (SEM) photographs revealed that the pulsed light treatment disrupted the microbial cells by collapsing and deforming their membranes with a consequent loss of cell content. Nevertheless, the log reduction was substantially lower than for liquid foods due to the shadowing effect caused by the absorption of light by the bacteria on the product's surface, hindering the inactivation of microorganisms in the inner layers. As a means of comparison, a liquid medium (0.9% saline solution) inoculated with 8.7 log of *B. subtilis* vegetative cells was treated with pulsed light. One single pulse at 0.6 J/cm^2 caused a complete reduction of the initial microbial population. However, SEM and DNA extraction analyses showed that differently from the spice samples, the bacterial cells in suspension were not disrupted, but instead exhibited changes in cell shape, expanded vacuoles, and cell membrane distortion.

Aflatoxins in spices and dried herbs are a major food safety issue as aflatoxin-producing fungi – mainly *Aspergillus parasiticus* and *Aspergillus flavus* – survive in low-moisture foods, and their toxins are very heat resistant. Aflatoxins (B1, B2, G1, and G2) are among the five most toxic mycotoxins and are inactivated at temperatures of 237–306 °C (Karlovsky et al. 2016; Rustom 1997). Pulsed light treatment has been proved effective by Wang et al. (2016) for aflatoxin degradation in rice. Rough rice and rice bran were treated with pulsed light at 0.52 J/cm^2/pulse for 80 and 15 seconds, respectively, exhibiting reductions in aflatoxin B1 and B2 of 39–75% and 86–90%.

These results show the potential of pulsed light decontamination in spices and other solid foods. Optimization of the pulsed light equipment via coupling of a fluidized bed or other stirring system aiming at efficient product exposure to light might be a way of achieving inactivation rates as high as for liquid foods.

2.6 Fumigation with Ethylene Dioxide

Ethylene dioxide (ETO) is a liquid at low temperatures but becomes a colorless flammable gas above 10.7 °C (OSHA 2002). ETO is an efficient non-thermal method to destroy bacteria (vegetative cells and spores), fungi, and even viruses. It is widely used to decontaminate herbs and spices in the US, New Zealand, and Australia. However, it has been phased out in several countries of the EU, in the UK, and in Japan due to the formation of carcinogenic substances (such as ethylene glycol and 2-chloroethanol) when in contact with the food components (Brodowska and Śmigielski 2014). The acute toxic effects related to the inhalation of ETO in humans and animals include respiratory tract and eye irritation, blurred vision, dizziness, headache, skin hypersensitivity accompanied by erythema and blisters, vomiting and diarrhea. Chronic exposure may result in impairment of the olfactory system. ETO inhalation is also linked to cancer, genetic damage, and spontaneous abortion (European Commission 2012; OSHA 2002). Based on these facts, the US Department of Labor (OSHA 2002) limits employee exposure to one part of ETO per million parts of air (1 ppm) in an eight-hour workday. At a concentration of 5 ppm, the exposure should not exceed 15-minute sampling periods.

A recent study reported that 35% of the global ETO demand is used for textile production (i.e. polyester), 25% for the manufacturing of soaps and detergents, and 10% or less for the production of pharmaceuticals, cosmetics, oilfield chemicals, and agricultural chemicals (Business Wire 2016). Over the last few years, ETO has been used for the cold sterilization of medical supplies and instruments, for reducing microbial counts in foodstuffs (including spices), and for controlling diseases in honeycombs (FAO 2014).

The fumigation of foods with ETO (including vegetables, spices, breads, meats, and beverages) was invented by Lloyd Hall in 1938 (patent US2107697A). The popularity of the ETO treatment decreased after the approval of irradiation for food sterilization in 1988 and the recent phase out as a food decontamination method in the EU. The safety of fumigated foods is controversial: while they are regarded as safe once the gas evaporates following fumigation, treated foods must be allowed to aerate for up to 24 hours after the treatment – a practice that is unlikely to be followed by all companies. The remaining ETO in the product can convert to toxic residues, such as ethylene chlorohydrin (ECH), ethylene glycol (EG), and ethylene bromohydrin (EBH) by the interaction of ETO with inorganic compounds of the food (FAO 2014). Studies from the US Environment Protection Agency (US EPA 2006) showed that ETO residual levels in spices are probably insignificant by the time of consumption as they decrease rapidly over the first few days following fumigation, reaching non-detectable levels ($\leq$0.1 ppm) after two months. However, Fowles et al. (2001) detected significant levels of ETO (>2 ppm) in 6.5% of retail spices samples imported into New Zealand. Additionally, Bononi et al. (2014) identified ECH in 29% of 63 samples of herbs, spices, and dried vegetables in amounts exceeding 0.3 mg/kg.

The efficiency of ETO fumigation toward microbial decontamination in spices has been proven in several studies, as reviewed by Schweiggert et al. (2007). Nonetheless, a slight alteration of color and taste, as well as loss of volatile compounds, have been observed in fumigated foods (Mayr and Suhr 1973; Farkas and Adrassy 1988). Additionally, their content of bioactive compounds (i.e. alkaloids, glycosides, and mucilage) may be significantly impaired (Brodowska and Śmigielski 2014). Toofanian and Stegeman (1988) compared the effects of ethylene oxide and gamma irradiation on the microbial counts and sensory quality of spices originally from China (ginger), Indonesia (cinnamon), and India (fennel and fenugreek) treated by a Dutch company. The first part of the spices was fumigated with ETO at a concentration of 1500/m^3 h for 8 hours, while the second part received gamma irradiation with Cobalt 60 at source activity of 40kCi and at different doses from 5 to 10 kGy. Both treatments were carried out at room temperature. The microbial inactivation rates were equivalent between fumigated and irradiated samples under the following radiation doses: 6 kGy for cinnamon and ginger, 6–10 kGy for fennel, and 6–8 kGy for fenugreek. The volatile oil content (VOC) of fumigated and irradiated cinnamon and fennel were equivalent; however, ginger lost 14% of the VOC following irradiation, while fumigated ginger exhibited the same VOC before and after treatment. The American Spice Trade Association (ASTA) estimated that ethylene oxide treatment is used for 40 to 85% of spices in the US (Food Safety News 2013), but they believe some companies may be choosing ETO fumigation over other methods because it does not need to be disclosed on the product label.

2.7 High Pressure CO_2 Coupled with Ultrasound

Ultrasound finds a wide range of applications in the food industry by aiding processes such as pasteurization, enzyme inactivation, extraction, cooking, freezing, drying, marinating, degassing, filtration, demolding, defoaming, gelation, emulsification, oxidation, and cutting (Majid et al. 2015; Knežević-Jugović et al. 2012; Chemat et al. 2011). The chemical effects of ultrasound are ascribed to cavitation, the collapse of microscopic bubbles in a liquid due to the negative pressure incurred during the rarefaction phase of the sound wave. Localized temperatures up to 500 °C and pressures as high as 1000 atm are produced for short periods (i.e. 400 μs) as a result of these implosions, with consequent bond breakage and generation of free radicals (Kuijpers et al. 2002; Luque-Garcı´ a and Luque de Castro 2003; Azmir et al. 2013). The mass transfer enhancement ascribed to cavitation results in higher energy and mass transfer rates, reduced thermal and concentration gradients, selective extraction, more effective mixing, and consequently shorter manufacturing processes, higher quality products, or both. Frequencies commonly applied in ultrasonic technology range from 20 kHz to 500 MHz (Majid et al. 2015; Chemat et al. 2011). Microorganisms destruction is attributed to the thinning of cell membranes, free radicals production, and localized heating. Ultrasound assisted-thermal treatments – such as pasteurization and sterilization – are accelerated, lessening the thermal damage and accordingly enhancing product quality (i.e., preservation of color, flavor, and nutritional value) and saving energy (Chemat et al. 2011).

High-pressure carbon dioxide (HPCD) has emerged in recent years as a novel non-thermal technology for food pasteurization. The food product is treated with either sub or supercritical pressurized CO_2 (which are non-toxic) in batches or continuous mode. Supercritical CO_2 is CO_2 at a temperature and pressure above its thermodynamical critical point ($T = 31.1\,°C$ and $P = 7.38\,MPa$). While supercritical CO_2 diffuses through solids like a gas and dissolves materials like a liquid, subcritical CO_2 (T and P below the critical point) is a gas or liquid acting in a single phase, depending on the temperature and pressure conditions. HPCD employs considerably lower pressures than the consolidated high-pressure processing (HPP): around 20 versus 300–600 MPa, respectively. HPCD has been already validated to inactivate bacteria, enzymes, and fungal and bacterial spores in several products, such as fruit juices, apple cider, milk, and tomato sauce (Garcia-Gonzalez et al. 2007). HPCD has been proven effective in the decontamination of chicken, pork, beef, fish, vegetables, seeds, cocoa powder, fruits, and also spices and herbs (i.e., paprika, mint, parsley, oregano, thyme, and chives) (Ferrentino and Spilimbergo 2011; Calvo and Torres 2010).

When combined with high-pressure CO_2, the effects of ultrasound are amplified. The use of dense-phase pressurized fluids, such as CO_2, in ultrasound-aided processes permits controlling the solubility and viscosity of substances, leading to high conversions in polymer precipitation and more efficient extractions (Kuijpers et al. 2002). These two processes combined were applied to the enzymatic hydrolysis of egg white proteins (Knežević-Jugović et al. 2012) and to the pasteurization of coconut water (Ferrentino and Spilimbergo 2015).

A research group from the Ainia Centro Tecnológico, in Spain, has been investigating a series of novel methods to decontaminate spices and herbs, including high-pressure CO_2 combined with ultrasound (HPCD + US), cold plasma, microwave, and infrared irradiation (GreenFooDec 2013). HPCD + US was applied to paprika, and the process conditions were optimized to achieve safe final microbial counts with minimum impairment of sensory properties. The optimum process conditions were set as 80 °C and 150 bar combined with ultrasound voltage of 75 V applied for 30 minutes to 180 g of paprika with an initial moisture content of 14%. Pressures higher than 200 bar did not result in further microbial destruction and additionally contributed to a partial extraction of capsaicinoids, which are responsible for the organoleptic properties of paprika. Also, treatments longer than 60 minutes did not further decrease the final microbial counts. The HPCD + US treatment resulted in a total reduction of molds and yeasts, enterobacteria, and pathogen microorganisms. Although spores and total viable counts were not eliminated – they were rather reduced to 0.5 log and 1 log CFU/g, respectively – there is no related legislation. Additionally, total viable counts were approximately equal to spore counts in most samples, meaning that most aerobes present in the sample were not in a viable form. As HPCD + US gave the best results in terms of color and final moisture compared to all other technologies tested on paprika, it was regarded as a viable alternative to moist-heat treatments and HPP processes for the decontamination of spices. Nevertheless, the research showed that terminal sterilization could not be guaranteed by HPCD + US alone; sterilization could be assured by adding other compounds to the CO_2 (such as H_2O_2, mixtures of H_2O_2, ethanol and water, peracetic, and trifluoroacetic acids), which would be unlikely to be unacceptable for use in foodstuffs, according to the study's authors.

2.8 Cold Plasma

Cold plasma is a non-thermal technology used for water treatment (pesticide degradation, dye degradation, and microbial decontamination), for polymer sterilization and surface modification, and in medicine for sterilization of equipment, wound healing, and treatment of diseases. Cold plasma has shown great potential for application in the food industry given the promising results reported in terms of microbial inactivation, toxin degradation, enzyme inactivation, and degradation of pesticide residues in foodstuffs (Pankaj and Keener 2017).

Plasma, the fourth state of matter, is an ionized gas into which sufficient energy is provided to free electrons from atoms or molecules and allow ions and electrons to coexist. Cold plasma can be generated by pumping ambient temperature gas with energy (i.e., radio frequency or microwave) under either atmospheric pressure or low-pressure conditions. The gas can be ambient or synthetic air, nitrogen, oxygen, helium, hydrogen, argon, and their mixtures. The plasma composition depends on the plasma source and the gas mixture. The antimicrobial effects of plasma are attributed to the different reactive species composing the plasma – excited oxygen, excited nitrogen, free radicals, charged particles, electrons, ions, reactive oxygen species, and UV photons. Reactive species within the plasma can damage the cell membranes, while UV photons can destroy the internal cellular components (Mošovská et al. 2018; Kim et al. 2017; Hertwig et al. 2015a; Hertwig et al. 2015b). Plasma equipment based on microwave-generated plasma and radio frequency-generated plasma are described in detail in Kim et al. (2017) and Brandenburg et al. (2009), respectively.

Hertwig et al. (2015a) treated three different types of herbs and spices (pepper seeds, crushed oregano, and paprika powder) with cold plasma for up to 90 minutes. The microflora and initial microbial load varied between products, with oregano being the sample with the lowest native microbial counts. Spores, vegetative bacteria, molds, and yeasts were destroyed at different rates in each product. The native microbial flora of the pepper seeds and the paprika powder were reduced by >3 log CFU/g after 60 minutes of plasma treatment. The mold and yeast counts and the total mesophilic aerobic counts of oregano were reduced by 1.6 log after 30 minutes and by 1.8 log CFU/g after 90 minutes, respectively. Although the treatment had a minor impact on the color (LAB) of black pepper seeds, dried oregano exhibited a slight reduction of greenness due to the destruction of chlorophyll, and the redness of paprika was significantly impaired after as little as 5 minutes of treatment. The plasma-treated paprika powder became lighter and yellowish, with total difference color values (ΔE) up to 46.9, indicating significant loss of carotenoids. The greater degradation of color in paprika was attributed to the fact that plasma is a surface treatment, and hence the interaction of plasma with the food itself rather than with the microorganisms on it is more pronounced in powders, which have a high surface-to-volume ratio.

Hertwig et al. (2015b) tested two different cold plasma systems for the decontamination of whole black pepper, one using a direct radio frequency-generated plasma jet and the other using a microwave-driven remote plasma. Naturally contaminated peppercorns and peppercorns inoculated with *B. subtilis* spores, *Bacillus atrophaeus* spores. and *S. enterica* were treated, and changes in the microbial counts, surface color, content of essential oils, and content of piperine were evaluated. After 30 minutes of remote microwave-generated plasma treatment, *S. enterica*, *B. subtilis* spores, and *B. atrophaeus* spores were reduced by 4.1, 2.4, and 2.8 log CFU/g, respectively. Direct plasma jet treatment resulted in significantly lower inactivation levels (0.6–2.7 log CFU/g), probably due to differences in the reactive species formed and accordingly, their different interactions with the product. Importantly, both plasma applications preserved the color, content of essential oils, and content of piperine of black pepper.

Mošovská et al. (2018) also tested cold plasma to decontaminate black pepper. Black peppercorns inoculated with *B. subtilis, E. coli, Salmonella enteritidis,* and *B. subtilis* endospores were treated by a low-temperature plasma produced by a Diffuse Coplanar Surface Barrier Discharge (DSCBD). The samples were treated for 60, 120, 180, 240, and 300 s at an input power of 400 W. The 300 s-treatment reduced the counts (in log CFU/g) of *B. subtilis* and *B. subtilis* spores from 7.36 to 2.30 and from 4.42 to 2.30, respectively. *E. coli* and *S. enteritidis* populations were reduced to below detection level (1.0 log CFU/g) from initial populations of 7.45 and 7.60 log CFU/g, respectively. The surface morphology and the chemical bonds were not altered by the plasma treatment, according to the SEM and the Attenuated Total

Reflectance – Fourier Transform Infrared Spectroscopy analyses. These results are evidence of the potential of cold plasma for the sterilization of heat-labile dry spices.

2.9 Conclusions

There is clearly no food technology alone that is capable of reducing microorganisms in herbs and spices to safe levels without impairing their nutritional and sensory properties to some extent. Chemical (ETO and ozone) and physical methods (radiation, PEF, PL, cold plasma) currently used all have advantages and drawbacks. In addition, some technologies that are highly efficient for liquid foods do not result in considerable microbial reduction levels in solid foods as herbs and spices; for instance, pulsed light. Nevertheless, these non-thermal technologies are less detrimental to product quality and, in general, are less energy demanding than conventional thermal methods, such as steaming and fumigation with ETO. Additionally, as spices and herbs vary considerably in terms of chemical composition, moisture content, physical form (dried leaves, powders, seeds, etc.), sensory characteristics, and manufacturing method, it is unlikely that one single technology can be regarded as the best one to assure microbial safety for spices and herbs in general. Novel decontamination technologies should rather be adapted to the specific product according to the purchaser demands, legislation requirements, and the spices/herbs manufacturer's budget.

References

Akbas, M.Y. and Ozdemir, M. (2008). Effect of gaseous ozone on microbial inactivation and sensory of flaked red peppers. *International Journal of Food Science and Technology* **43**: 1657–1662.

Almela, L., Nieto-Sandoval, J.M., and Fernández López, J.A. (2002). Microbial inactivation of paprika by a high-temperature short-X time treatment. Influence on color properties. *Journal of Agriculture and Food Chemistry* **50** (6): 1435–1440.

ASTA – American Spice Trade Association (2011). *Clean, Safe Spices: Guidance from the American Spice Trade Association*. Washington DC: American Spice Trade Association.

Azmir, J., Zaidul, I.S.M., Rahman, M.M. et al. (2013). Techniques for extraction of bioactive compounds from plant materials: a review. *Journal of Food Engineering* **117** (4): 426–436.

Barba, F.J., Parniakov, O., Pereira, S.A. et al. (2015). Current applications and new opportunities for the use of pulsed electric fields in food science and industry. *Food Research International* **77** (4): 773–798.

Barbosa-Canovas, G.V., Gongora-Nieto, M.M., and Swanson, B.G. (1998). Nonthermal electrical methods in food preservation. *Food Science and Technology International* **4**: 363–370.

Bi, X., Lim, J., and Henry, C.J. (2017). Spices in the management of diabetes mellitus. *Food Chemistry* **217**: 281–293.

Bononi, M., Quaglia, G., and Tateo, F. (2014). Identification of ethylene oxide in herbs, spices and other dried vegetables imported into Italy. *Food Additives & Contaminants: Part A* **31** (2): 271–275.

Brandenburg, R., Lange, H., von Woedtke, T. et al. (2009). Antimicrobial effects of UV and VUV radiation of nonthermal plasma jets. *IEEE Transactions on Plasma Science* **37** (6): 877–883.

Brodowska, A. and Śmigielski, K. (2013). Ozonation – an alternative decontamination method for raw plant materials. *Biotechnology and Food Sciences* **77** (1): 37–43.
Brodowska, A. and Śmigielski, K. (2014). Comparison of methods of herbs and spices decontamination. *Chemik* **68** (2): 97–102.
Brodowska, A.J., Śmigielski, K., Nowak, A. et al. (2015). The impact of ozone treatment in dynamic bed parameters on changes in biologically active substances of juniper berries. *PLoS One* **10** (12): e0144855.
Business Wire (2016). Ethylene Oxide (EO) Report: 2016 World Market Outlook and Forecast up to 2020 – Research and Markets. https://www.businesswire.com/news/home/20160408005347/en/Ethylene-Oxide-EO-Report-2016-World-Market (accessed 17 December 2019).
Calvo, L. and Torres, E. (2010). Microbial inactivation of paprika using high-pressure CO_2. *The Journal of Supercritical Fluids* **52** (1): 134–141.
Castro, J.A., Barbosa-Canovas, G.V., and Swanson, B.G. (1993). Microbial inactivation of foods by pulsed electric fields. *Journal of Food Processing and Preservation* **17**: 47–73.
Chemat, F., Huma, Z., and Khan, M.K. (2011). Applications of ultrasound in food technology: processing, preservation and extraction. *Ultrasonics Sonochemistry* **18** (4): 813–835.
Cullen, P.J., Tiwari, B.K., O'Donnell, C.P., and Muthukumarappan, K. (2009). Modelling approaches to ozone processing of liquid foods. *Trends in Food Science & Technology* **20** (3–4): 125–136.
Duncan, S.E., Moberg, K., Amin, K.N. et al. (2017). Processes to preserve spice and herb quality and sensory integrity during pathogen inactivation. *Journal of Food Science* **82** (5): 1208–1215.
Elmnasser, N., Guillou, S., Leroi, F. et al. (2007). Pulsed-light system as a novel food decontamination technology: a review. *Canadian Journal of Microbiology* **53**: 813–821.
Embuscado, M.E. (2015). Spices and herbs: natural sources of antioxidants – a mini review. *Journal of Functional Foods* **18**: 811–819.
European Commission (1999a). Directive 1999/2/EC of the European Parliament and of the Council of 22 February 1999 on the approximation of the laws of the Member States concerning foods and food ingredients treated with ionising radiation.
European Commission (1999b). Directive 1999/3/EC of the European Parliament and of the Council of 22 February 1999 on the establishment of a Community list of foods and food ingredients treated with ionising radiation.
European Commission (2004). European commission recommendation of 19 December 2003 concerning a coordinated programme for the official control of food stuffs for 2004 (2004/24/EC). *Official Journal of the European Union* **6** (2004): 29–37.
European Commission (2012). Recommendation from the scientific committee on occupational exposure limits for ethylene oxide. Employment, Social Affairs & Inclusion (SCOEL/SUM/160, June 2012)
European Food Safety Authority – EFSA (2016). The European Union summary report on trends and sources of zoonoses, zoonotic agents and food-borne outbreaks in 2016. European Centre for Disease Prevention and Control. Available at: https://www.ecdc.europa.eu/sites/default/files/documents/summary-report-zoonoses-foodborne-outbreaks-2016.pdf (accessed 17 December 2019).
FAO – Food and Agriculture Organization of the United Nations (2014). Manual of fumigation for insect control. Available at: http://www.fao.org/docrep/x5042e/x5042E0d.htm (accessed 10 April 2018).
FAO – Food and Agriculture Organization of the United Nations (2018). FAO statistics. Available at: http://www.fao.org/faostat (accessed 10 April 2018).
Farkas, J. (2006). Irradiation for better foods. *Trends in Food Science and Technology* **17**: 148–152.

Farkas, J. and Adrassy, E. (1988). Comparative analysis of spices decontaminated by ethylene oxide or gamma irradiation. *Acta Alimentaria* **17**: 77–94.

Ferrentino, G. and Spilimbergo, S. (2011). High pressure carbon dioxide pasteurization of solid foods: current knowledge and future outlooks. *Trends in Food Science & Technology* **22** (8): 427–441.

Ferrentino, G. and Spilimbergo, S. (2015). High power ultrasound assisted high pressure carbon dioxide pasteurization of fresh cut coconut. *Chemical Engineering Transactions* **44**: 1–6.

Fincan, M. (2015). Extractability of phenolics from spearmint treated with pulsed electric field. *Journal of Food Engineering* **162**: 31–37.

Fogele, B., Granta, R., Valciņa, O., and Bērziņš, A. (2018). Occurrence and diversity of Bacillus cereus and moulds in spices and herbs. *Food Control* **83**: 69–74.

Food Safety News (2013). Imports and exports: microbial-reduction techniques address the unique structures of spices (by Lydia Zuraw). Available at: http://www.foodsafetynews.com/2013/11/imports-microbial-reduction-techniques-address-the-unique-structures-of-spices/#.WsyvZIjwa70 (accessed 10 April 2018).

Fowles, J.R., Mitchell, J., and McGrath, H. (2001). Assessment of cancer risk from ethylene oxide residues in spices imported into New Zealand. *Food and Chemical Toxicology* **39**: 1055–1062.

Garcia-Gonzalez, L., Geeraerd, A.H., Spilimbergo, S. et al. (2007). High pressure carbon dioxide inactivation of microorganisms in foods: the past, the present and the future. *International Journal of Food Microbiology* **117** (1): 1–28.

GreenFooDec (2013). Development of novel and advanced decontamination sustainable technologies for the production of high quality dried herbs and spices. Ainia Centro Tecnológico, Valencia, Spain. Available at: http://www.greenfoodec.eu/index.htm (accessed 10 April 2018).

Guerrero-Beltrán, J.A. and Welti Chanes, J.S. (2016). Pulsed electric fields. In: *Encyclopedia of Food and Health* (eds. B. Caballero, P.M. Finglas and F. Toldrá), 561–565. Oxford: Academic Press/Elsevier https://doi.org/10.1016/B978-0-12-384947-2.00579-1.

Guzel-Seydim, Z.B., Greene, A.K., and Seydim, A.C. (2004). Use of ozone in the food industry. *LWT Food Science and Technology* **37**: 453–460.

Harris, G. (2013). Salmonella in spices prompts changes in farming. *The New York Times*. Available at: http://www.nytimes.com/2013/08/28/world/asia/farmers-change-over-spices-link-to-food-ills.html (accessed 5 February 2018).

Hertwig, C., Reineke, K., Ehlbeck, J. et al. (2015a). Impact of remote plasma treatment on natural microbial load and quality parameters of selected herbs and spices. *Journal of Food Engineering* **167** (A): 12–17.

Hertwig, C., Reineke, K., Ehlbeck, J. et al. (2015b). Decontamination of whole black pepper using different cold atmospheric pressure plasma applications. *Food Control* **55**: 221–229.

Hsu, L. and Moraru, C.I. (2011). Quantifying and mapping the spatial distribution of fluency inside a pulsed light treatment chamber and various liquid subtrates. *Journal of Food Engineering* **103**: 84–91.

Inan, F., Pala, M., and Doymaz, I. (2007). Use of ozone in detoxification of aflatoxin B1 in red pepper. *Journal of Stored Products Research* **43** (4): 425–429.

Kabak, B. and Dobson, A.D. (2017). Mycotoxins in spices and herbs - an update. *Critical Reviews in Food Science and Nutrition* **57** (1): 18–34.

Kaefer, C.M. and Milner, J.A. (2008). The role of herbs and spices in cancer prevention. *Journal of Nutritional Biochemistry* **19**: 347–361.

Karlovsky, P., Suman, M., Berthiller, F. et al. (2016). Impact of food processing and detoxification treatments on mycotoxin contamination. *Mycotoxin Research* **32**: 179–205.

Keith, W.D., Harris, L.J., Hudson, L., and Griffiths, M.W. (1997). Pulsed electric fields as a processing alternative for microbial reduction in spice. *Food Research International* **30** (3–4): 185–191.

Kim, J.G., Yousef, A.E., and Dave, S. (1999). Application of ozone for enhancing the microbiological safety and quality of foods: a review. *Journal of Food Protection* **62** (9): 1071–1087.

Kim, J.E., Oh, Y.J., Won, M.Y. et al. (2017). Microbial decontamination of onion powder using microwave-powered cold plasma treatments. *Food Microbiology* **62**: 112–123.

Knežević-Jugović, Z.D., Stefanović, A.B., Žuža, M.G. et al. (2012). Effects of sonication and high-pressure carbon dioxide processing on enzymatic hydrolysis of egg white proteins. *APTEFF – Acta Periodica Technologica* **43**: 1–342.

Koutchma, T. (2016). Ultraviolet light for decontamination and preservation of beverages, liquid foods, and ingredients. Reference Module in Food Science, Elsevier. Available at: https://doi.org/10.1016/B978-0-08-100596-5.21200-6.

Kuijpers, M.W.A., van Eck, D., Kemmere, M.F., and Keurentjes, J.T.F. (2002). Cavitation-induced reactions in high-pressure carbon dioxide. *Science* **298**: 1969–1970.

Luque-Garcı´ a, J.L. and Luque de Castro, M.D. (2003). Ultrasound: a powerful tool for leaching. *Trends in Analytical Chemistry* **22** (1): 41–47.

Majid, I., Nayik, G.A., and Nanda, V. (2015). Ultrasonication and food technology: a review. *Cogent Food & Agriculture* **1** (1): 1–11.

Mayr, G.E. and Suhr, H. (1973). Preservation and sterilization of pure and mixed spices. In: *Proceedings Conference on Spices*, 201–207. London: Tropical Products Institute.

McKee, L.H. (1995). Microbial contamination of spices and herbs: a review. *LWT Food Science and Technology* **28** (1): 1–11.

Molnár, H., Bata-Vidács, I., Baka, E. et al. (2018). The effect of different decontamination methods on the microbial load, bioactive components, aroma and colour of spice paprika. *Food Control* **83**: 131–140.

Mošovská, S., Medvecká, V., Halászová, N. et al. (2018). Cold atmospheric pressure ambient air plasma inhibition of pathogenic bacteria on the surface of black pepper. *Food Research International* **106**: 862–869.

Napoli, E., Mazzaglia, A., Restuccia, C. et al. (2016). The effect of γ-irradiation on chemical composition, microbial load and sensory properties of Sicilian oregano. *LWT Food Science and Technology* **72**: 566–572.

Nicorescu, I., Nguyen, B., Moreau-Ferret, M. et al. (2013). Pulsed light inactivation of Bacillus subtilis vegetative cells in suspensions and spices. *Food Control* **31** (1): 151–157.

Novak, J., Demirci, A., and Han, Y. (2008). Gas novel chemical processes: ozone, supercritical CO_2, electrolyzed oxidizing water, and chlorine dioxide. Food science and technology international. **14**: 437–441.

OSHA – US Occupational Safety and Health Administration (2002). Ethylene oxide – fact sheet. Available at: https://www.osha.gov/OshDoc/data_General_Facts/ethylene-oxide-factsheet.pdf (accessed 10 April 2018).

Ozonotech (2018). Food and hygiene ozone treatment. Available at: http://www.ozonetech.com/industries/food-and-beverage-ozone (accessed 8 February 2018).

Pankaj, S.K. and Keener, K.M. (2017). Cold plasma: background, applications and current trends. *Current Opinion in Food Science* **16**: 49–52.

Raso, J., Condón, S., and Álvarez, I. (2014). Non-thermal processing – pulsed electric field. In: *Encyclopedia of Food Microbiology*, 2e (eds. C.A. Batt and M.L. Tortorello), 966–973. Oxford: Academic Press.

Ribeiro-Santos, R., Andrade, M., Madella, D. et al. (2017a). Revisiting an ancient spice with medicinal purposes: cinnamon. *Trends in Food Science & Technology* **62**: 154–169.

Ribeiro-Santos, R., Andrade, M., and de Melo, N.R. (2017b). Use of essential oils in active food packaging: recent advances and future trends. *Trends in Food Science and Technology* **61**: 132–140.

Rustom, I.Y.S. (1997). Aflatoxin in food and feed: occurrence, legislation and inactivation by physical methods. *Food Chemistry* **59**: 57–67.

Sánchez-Camargo, A.P. and Herrero, M. (2017). Rosemary (*Rosmarinus officinalis*) as a functional ingredient: recent scientific evidence. *Current Opinion in Food Science* **14**: 13–19.

Schaarschmidt, S. (2016). Public and private standards for dried culinary herbs and spices – part I: standards defining the physical and chemical product quality and safety. *Food Control* **70**: 339–349.

Schweiggert, U., Carle, R., and Schieber, A. (2007). Conventional and alternative processes for spice production – a review. *Trends in Food Science & Technology* **18** (5): 260–268.

Sitzmann, W., Vorobiev, E., and Lebovka, N. (2016). Applications of electricity and specifically pulsed electric fields in food processing: historical backgrounds. *Innovative Food Science & Emerging Technologies* **37** (Part C): 302–311.

Song, W.-J., Sung, H.-J., Kim, S.-Y. et al. (2014). Inactivation of Escherichia coli O157:H7 and Salmonella Typhimurium in black pepper and red pepper by gamma irradiation. *International Journal of Food Microbiology* **172**: 125–129.

Sospedra, I., Soriano, J.M., and Mañes, J. (2010). Assessment of the microbiological safety of dried spices and herbs commercialized in Spain. *Plant Foods for Human Nutrition* **65** (4): 364–368.

Souza, L.P.d., Faroni, L.R.D., Heleno, F.F. et al. (2018). Effects of ozone treatment on postharvest carrot quality. *LWT Food Science and Technology* **90**: 53–60.

Srinivasan, K. (2017). Ginger rhizomes (*Zingiber officinale*): a spice with multiple health beneficial potentials. *Pharma Nutrition* **5** (1): 18–28.

Srivastav, S., Fatima, M., and Mondal, A.C. (2017). Important medicinal herbs in Parkinson's disease pharmacotherapy. *Biomedicine & Pharmacotherapy* **92**: 856–863.

Tiwari, B.K.; Rice, C.R.G. (2012). Regulatory and legislative issues. In: O'Donnell, C., Tiwari, B.K., Cullen, P.J., Rice, C.R.G. (Eds.), *Ozone in Food Processing*. Wiley, Oxford, pp. 7–17.

Toofanian, F. and Stegeman, H. (1988). Comparative effect of ethylene oxide and gamma irradiation on the chemical sensory and microbial quality of ginger, cinnamon, fennel and fenugreek. *Acta Alimentaria* **17**: 271–281.

Torlak, E., Sert, D., and Ulca, P. (2013). Efficacy of gaseous ozone against salmonella and microbial population on dried oregano. *International Journal of Food Microbiology* **165** (3): 276–280.

US EPA – Unites States Environment Protection Agency (2006). Report of the Food Quality Protection Act (FQPA) – Tolerance Reassessment and Risk Management Decision (TRED) for ethylene oxide. Available at: https://nepis.epa.gov (accessed 10 April 2018).

US Food and Drug Administration – FDA (2001). Secondary direct food additives permitted in food for human consumption. *Federal Register* **66** (123): 33829–33830.

Van Doren, J.M., Kleinmeier, D., Hammack, T.S., and Westerman, A. (2013). Prevalence, serotype diversity, and antimicrobial resistance of salmonella in imported shipments of spice offered for entry to the United States, FY2007–FY2009. *Food Microbiology* **34** (2): 239–251.

Wang, B., Mahoney, N.E., Pan, Z. et al. (2016). Effectiveness of pulsed light treatment for degradation and detoxification of aflatoxin B1 and B2 in rough rice and rice bran. *Food Control* **59**: 461–467.

Woodling, S.E. and Moraru, C.I. (2006). Effect of spectral range in surface inactivation of listeria innocua using broad-spectrum pulsed light. *Journal of Protection* **70**: 909–916.

World Health Organization – WHO (2013). General standard for irradiated foods. Codex Alimentarius, 106–1983, Rev.1–2003.

Yoon, M., Jung, K., Lee, K.-Y. et al. (2014). Synergistic effect of the combined treatment with gamma irradiation and sodium dichloroisocyanurate to control gray mold (Botrytis cinerea) on paprika. *Radiation Physics and Chemistry* **98**: 103–108.

3

Recent Developments in High-Quality Drying of Herbs and Spices

Wei Jin[1,2], Min Zhang[1], Weifeng Shi[2], and Arun S. Mujumdar[3]

[1]*State Key Laboratory of Food Science and Technology, Jiangnan University, 214122 Wuxi, Jiangsu, China*

[2]*Nestlé R&D Centre Shanghai Ltd., 201812 Shanghai, China*

[3]*Department of Chemical and Biochemical Engineering, Western University, London, Ontario, Canada*

3.1 Introduction

Herbs and spices are natural products that are especially valued for their distinctive flavor, aroma, color, and preservative effect as well as pharmaceutical and nutritional properties (Srinivasan 2005; Kivilompolo and Hyötyläinen 2007; Parveen et al. 2014). Proper processing should be carried out on such fresh produce before being used to flavor and/or preserve food, cure illness, or enhance cosmetics (Chanchal and Swarnlata 2008; Kaefer and Milner 2008; Iriti et al. 2010). Fresh harvested herbs and spices have high inherent moisture content and often a high load of microorganisms; immediate processing should be implemented to prevent biological deterioration after harvesting since they have a tendency to perish rapidly. Among the processes applied for post-harvest food preservation, drying/dehydration is regarded as the most common and cost-effective way to avoid losses of these raw materials (Muller et al. 1989). It is also necessary to eliminate the potential safety risk owing to the formation of toxic substances (Parto 2015; Xie et al. 2016).

Drying is one of the foremost and most often used methods for food processing and it is an indispensable preservative approach in the food industry. It aims at reducing moisture content and hence the water activity to a safe level which extends product shelf life, reduces the complexity of packaging, shipment, and storage, and provides a diverse range of products for consumers (Doymaz 2005; Hamrouni-Sellami et al. 2011; Hamrouni-Sellami et al. 2013). Thus, this technology is widely utilized for drying foodstuffs such as grains (Zhou et al. 2018), vegetables (Wang et al. 2013), fruits

Herbs, Spices and Medicinal Plants: Processing, Health Benefits and Safety, First Edition.
Edited by Mohammad B. Hossain, Nigel P. Brunton, and Dilip K. Rai.

(Nathakaranakule et al. 2010), spices (Balasubramanian et al. 2016), herbs (Balasubramanian et al. 2016), and other food products (Sa-adchom et al. 2011).

Surprisingly, there is an increasing demand from consumers for dried products with most of the original characteristics of the fresh products. In order to address this consumer need, considerations must be given to drying in order to retain the taste, aroma, color, nutrients, and texture of the plants to the maximum possible extent (Crivelli et al. 2002). Apart from quality concerns, drying efficiency is another important factor for assessing drying performance, which includes total energy consumption, drying duration, drying rate, and so on.

The drying process involves an external and internal heat and mass transfer to remove moisture and/or other volatile substances by vaporization from a solid, semi-solid, or liquid feedstock (Mujumdar 2007). However, drying mechanisms are hard to precisely describe and model since they involve simultaneous heat, mass, and momentum transfer through the processed substance along with phase changes and with/without chemical and/or biochemical transformations (Mujumdar and Huang 2007). Drying is recognized as the most energy-intensive unit operation for most industrial processes (Raghavan et al. 2005; Zhang and Jiang 2014; Onwude et al. 2016a,b); certain reports state that drying operations consume from 10% to 15% of national industrial energy in several developed countries (Klemeš et al. 2008; Satimehin 2014; Onwude et al. 2016a,b), and approximately 30–40% in some developing countries (Karim and Hawlader 2005).

Many traditional drying methods have been utilized in the production of herbs and spices, such as solar drying (Özcan et al. 2005), hot air drying (Demiray and Tulek 2014), vacuum drying (Wang et al. 2018), as well as microwave drying (MD) (Arslan et al. 2010). However, almost all these techniques require long drying duration and high energy consumption, thus resulting in processed samples of inferior quality (Moses et al. 2014; Karam et al. 2016). It is necessary to process them under suitable drying conditions because herbs and spices are highly heat sensitive. A single drying method is rarely capable of achieving both a premium product quality and high drying efficiency; various novel drying methods have been designed, fabricated, and adopted to enhance drying efficiency as well as to obtain well-desired quality products.

The aim of this chapter is to present an overview of the recent progress made in the high quality and efficient drying of herbs and spices. The relative advantages of some selected innovative drying methods (mainly combined drying methods) in offering high-quality drying with high efficiency. Additionally, recommendations and future research trends on the drying of herbs and spices are also suggested.

3.2 Novel Combined Drying Methods

Conventional "single" drying methods (e.g. solar drying, hot air drying, microwave drying, etc.) rarely produce dried herbs and spices of good quality with high drying efficiency (Buchaillot et al. 2009; Mohamed et al. 2012; Argyropoulos and Müller 2014). The combination of two or more different drying methods can provide a synergistic effect, resulting in the fewest changes of most quality properties while minimizing energy consumption and processing time (Raso and Barbosa-Cánovas 2003; Huang et al. 2012).

Particular attention has been drawn to developing innovative combined drying methods for herbs and spices, to further improve the drying performance and enhance product quality. Here, recent combined drying methods are summarized, categorized, and presented.

3.2.1 Solar-Related Combined Drying Methods

Solar energy is most commonly used renewable source for the drying of fruits (Kaveh et al. 2015), vegetables (Yaldız and Ertekin 2001), herbs and spices (Janjai et al. 2008; Jin et al. 2018a,b), and other foodstuffs (Basunia and Abe 2001). Solar drying is a sustainable and economical friendly process for agricultural products (Mustayen et al. 2014). However, this technique has several drawbacks and limitations, such as inferior quality, an inefficient and uncontrollable drying process, intensive labor, insect infestation, and a large area requirement (Deshmukh et al. 2014; Rabha et al. 2017a,b; Yahya et al. 2017).

Based on solar energy utilization, solar drying can be grouped into three major types: (Aghaei et al. 2019) direct solar drying where raw materials are directly exposed to the sunlight; (Amer et al. 2018) indirect solar drying or convective solar drying; and (Antal et al. 2011) hybrid or mixed-mode solar drying. Meanwhile, two basic types of convective solar dryers are available: the natural and forced type. In addition, classification of solar dryers according to structural aspects places them into three general groups: (Aghaei et al. 2019) the greenhouse type, (Amer et al. 2018) the collector type, and (Antal et al. 2011) the heat pump (HP)-assisted type. Table 3.1 shows herbs and spices that are subjected to solar-related combined drying and the methods used, and details are presented in the following sections.

Forced convection solar dryers are convenient to handle large amounts of post-harvested agricultural products (Belessiotis and Delyannis 2011). Rabha et al. (2017a,b) designed and fabricated an indirect-type forced convection solar tunnel dryer for drying of thin layer ghost chili pepper. The drying system consists of a semi-continuous-type tunnel dryer, two double-pass Solar Air Heaters (SAHs), a shell and tube heat exchanger, and a blower. Figure 3.1a presents a schematic layout and Figure 3.1b shows the cross-sectional profile of this SAH. They found that the drying time required to reduce the moisture ratio of ghost chili pepper from 589.6% dry basis, (db) to 12% (db) was 123 hours in solar tunnel dryer, compared to 193 hours for direct solar drying. Direct solar drying had not only a longer drying duration, but also negative effects on the color, texture, and quality of dried products. El-Sebaii and Shalaby (2013) studied the mathematical models of thin layer drying to specify a suitable model for describing the drying behavior of thyme and mint in an indirect-mode forced convection solar dryer. According to the results, Midilli and Kucuk model ($MR = 0.9891 \exp(-0.0568t^{3.0459}) + 0.029t$) was suitable for describing the thin layer solar drying of mint. However, for drying of thyme, the Page model ($MR = \exp(-6.2032 \times 10^{-8} t^{4.9107})$) and another model derived from the Page model ($MR = \exp(-(0.0341t)^{4.9107})$) gave the best result. The cost of drying mint and thyme in the indirect-mode forced convection solar dryer was 0.025 and 0.087 €/kg, respectively. Bhardwaj et al. (2019) designed and developed an indirect forced convection solar dryer equipped with sensible heat storage material (SHSM) and phase change material (PCM) for drying of *Valeriana jatamansi*. Results showed that solar drying using SHSM and PCM had the highest value (0.051 kg/hr), followed

Table 3.1 Applications of solar-related hybrid drying for herbs and spices

Herbs and spices	Drying facilities	References
Ghost chili pepper	Forced convection solar tunnel dryer Direct solar radiation	Rabha et al. (2017a,b)
Thymus	Forced convection solar dryer	El-Sebaii and Shalaby (2013)
Valeriana Jatamansi	Forced convection solar dryer coupled with sensible heat storage material and phase change material	Bhardwaj et al. (2019)
Peppermint	Forced convection solar tunnel greenhouse dryer	Morad et al. (2017)
Java tea leaf and sabah snake grass leaf	Solar greenhouse dryer with integrated a heat pump (HP)	Tham et al. (2017)
Roselle	Forced convection solar air heating collector system assisted with granite Solar greenhouse dryer Solar greenhouse dryer integrated with intermittent HP Hot air dryer HP dryer	Tham et al. (2018) Kareem et al. (2017)
Habanero chili	Fluidized bed dryer coupled with a low temperature solar collector Direct solar radiation	Rodríguez et al. (2013)
Mint	Forced convection solar dryer Solar-assisted fluidized bed dryer integrated with a HP Solar collector dryer HP dryer Solar-assisted HP dryer	El-Sebaii and Shalaby (2013) Ceylan and Gürel (2016) Şevik (2014)
Parsley	Solar collector dryer HP dryer Solar-assisted HP dryer	Şevik (2014)
Rosemary	Forced convection solar dryer with a solar air collector and an auxiliary heater	Mghazli et al. (2017)
Chamomile	Solar collector dryer with heat exchanger and heat storage unit	Amer et al. (2018)
Saffron	Photovoltaic–thermal solar dryer equipped with a HP	Mortezapour et al. (2012)
Misai Kucing	Solar-assisted HP dryer	Gan et al. (2017)

by solar drying without using thermal storage mediums (0.028 kg/hr) and traditional shade drying (0.018 kg/hr). In terms of drying duration to reduce moisture content from 89% to 9%, solar drying using SHSM and PCM had the shortest drying time of 120 hours, solar drying without using thermal storage materials required a drying time of 216 hours, while the 336 hours for shade drying was the longest time. The

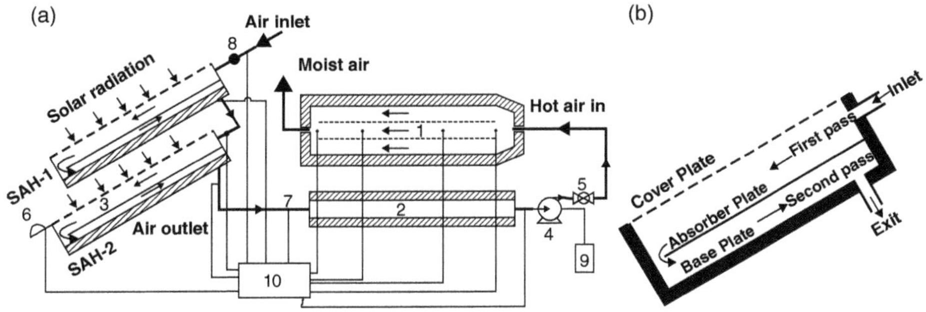

Figure 3.1 (a) Schematic layout of a solar tunnel dryer: 1. Tunnel dryer, 2. Shell and tube heat exchanger for energy storage, 3. Solar air heater, 4. Air blower, 5. Ball valve, 6. Pyranometer, 7. Thermocouple, 8. Flow meter, 9. Energy meter, 10. Data acquisition system. (b) cross-sectional profile of a solar air heater.

comparison also showed that the solar dryer without SHSM had an average energy and exergy efficiency of 9.8% and 0.14%, respectively, whereas an energy and exergy efficiency of 26.10% and 0.81% was obtained when SHSM was applied to solar drying.

Greenhouse solar dryers utilize a regular greenhouse structure to store solar energy during the daytime or to transfer excess thermal energy from inside the greenhouse to a heat storage zone (Morad et al. 2017). Normally, this type of solar dryer uses transparent plastic covers as air heaters. Morad et al. (2017) fabricated three identical solar tunnel greenhouse dryers and then experimented by drying peppermint plants and leaves. This dryer also used two suction air fans to increase the air speed inside the drying system. Drying rate, drying efficiency, drying cost, and product quality under different operational conditions were examined and the experimental results showed that the drying rate was accelerated by 22.78% for whole plants under the continuous fan operating mode, and 24.8% for leaves with the periodical fan operating mode. Operating the solar tunnel greenhouse under the continuously fan operating mode resulted in the highest volatile oil retention for plants (0.83%) and leaves (1.52%), with 0.77%, and 1.33% under periodical fan operating mode. Meanwhile, with the periodical operating mode for peppermint plants, the operational costs were reduced by 6.95% compared to that of the continuously fan operating mode. Tham et al. (2017) conducted comparative experiments to study the drying characteristics of herbs using an industrial scale solar greenhouse dryer (SGD) assisted with a HP unit. The results of their study showed that SGD integrated with a HP unit successfully reduced the room relative humidity (RH) by 10–15%. Also, a HP unit can help to maintain room RH at a maximum value of 65% throughout the drying process, therefore mitigating the product rehydration issue. The drying rate of Java tea was improved three to fourfold from 0.004–0.008 gH_2O/g dry matter (dm) min to 0.018–0.025 g H_2O/g dm min, whereas 10% drying time was reduced for both Java tea leaf and Sabah snake grass leaf with the enhancement from a HP unit. Meanwhile, the supply of dry air from the HP unit with a magnitude of 0.25–0.50 m/s helps to improve the drying rate of the herbs as well as minimize the non-uniformity of drying temperature and RH inside the SGD. The same authors also examined the effects of four different drying methods: HA drying, HP drying, SGD, and solar greenhouse with intermittent heat pump (SGIHP) drying on the drying kinetics and quality properties of Roselle (Tham et al. 2018). In terms of drying rate, HP drying had the highest drying rate at a range from 0.054 to 0.212 g H_2O/g dm min, while SGD had the lowest drying rate at 0.042 g H_2O/g dm min. The color analysis showed that the total color change of HA dried (both 35 and 40 °C) calyx was slightly higher than solar (SGD and SGIHP) dried calyx, whereas HA dried petals had a lower color change at 40 and 45 °C. Meanwhile, the HP dried Roselle exhibited consistent color among all the selected drying methods. The significant retention of principle component analysis (PCA) was observed in SGD and SGIHP dried Roselle samples (p <0.05), while a higher content of catechin acid was obtained in HP dried samples (p <0.05).

Solar air collectors can be categorized into three types: (Aghaei et al. 2019) single-pass, (Amer et al. 2018) double-pass, and (Antal et al. 2011) multi-pass collectors. A fluidized bed dryer assisted by a low temperature solar collector was developed by Rodríguez et al. (2013), and the drying process conducted in two systems: (Aghaei et al. 2019) an open-air sun dryer; (Amer et al. 2018) and a pilot fluidized bed dryer coupled with a low-temperature solar collector for air heating. The moisture content of Habanero chili was reduced to 5% from 90% after a drying time of 10.3 hours, with good product quality. Experimental results showed that the reduction in drying time reached an average value of 50%, and an energy reduction of 2.6 kW for every dried chili. Ceylan and Gürel (2016) conducted comparative experiments to investigate the drying characteristics of the solar air collector assisted fluidized bed dryer for drying of mint leaves. Their drying system consisted of a solar air collector, a parabolic trough collector, and a HP unit. During the daytime, the solar air collector provided the required heat energy for the drying process, and heated water in the parabolic trough collector was stored in the depot, which would be used in the drying process during the night. The air temperatures for the solar air collector, the parabolic trough collector, and the HP operating modes were controlled with accuracies of ±0.35, ±0.444, and ± 0.478 °C, respectively. Their results showed this drying system had energy and exergy efficiency of 50% and 26%, respectively. They concluded that this kind of solar drying system can be used with temperature control for different applications, such as heating greenhouses and preheating in air conditioning systems. A new dryer with a solar air collector was designed, constructed, and tested on drying mint and parsley (Şevik 2014). The main components of this system were a Double-Pass Solar Air Collector (DPSAC), drying chamber, HP unit, photovoltaic (PV) unit, and a control and measurement unit (Figure 3.2). Additionally, a proportional-integral-derivative (PID) control unit was installed in order to keep a constant air temperature during the drying process. The coefficient performance of the dryer for drying mint and parsley was calculated as 2.28 and 2.17, respectively. The energy utilization ratios of the dryer for drying mint and parsley were calculated as 0.18–0.25 and 0.2–0.26, respectively. On the other hand, experimental results also indicated that the DPSAC, HP unit, PV unit, and PID control unit could work in coordination with each unit and the dried products had good physical properties, such as color, shrinkage, and taste. The performance of a forced convective multi-pass solar air heating collector (MPSAHC) drying system enhanced with granite for drying Roselle was investigated by Kareem et al. (2017). The experiments were performed under the daily average RH, solar radiation, and ambient temperature and wind speed of 64.5%, 635.49 W/m^2, 32.24 °C and 0.81 m/s, respectively. An average drying rate of 33.57 g/kgm^{2}h was achieved, while a system optical efficiency, collector efficiency, drying efficiency, and moisture pickup efficiency

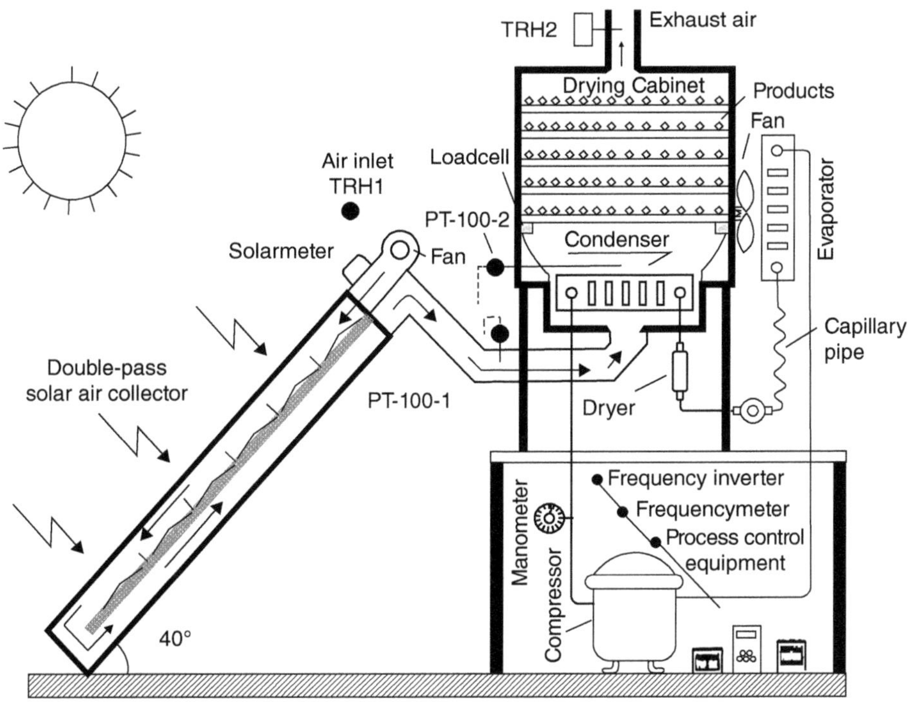

Figure 3.2 Schematic of PID-controlled double pass solar air collector-heat pump drying system.

of 70.53%, 64.08%, 36.22%, and 66.95% were obtained, respectively. The MPSAHC dryer was 21 hours faster with fair color retention, comparing to the open-air solar drying approach which was conducted under the same weather conditions. The techno economic analysis indicated that the payback period of this drying system was 2.14 years. Mghazli et al. (2017) studied the drying kinetics of rosemary in an indirect active solar dryer with a separate solar collector and a drying unit. Drying experiments were carried out at four different air temperatures (50, 60, 70, and 80 °C) and also two air speeds (300 and 150 m^3/h) with the ambient temperature in the range of 26–37 °C. Results showed that the drying time could be reduced by an increase of air temperature. Midilli and Kucuk model ($MR = 0.9969 \exp(-0.0381t^{1.2702}) - 0.0022\,t$, under air temperature: 80 °C and air flow rate: 150 m^3/h) showed the best fit to the experimental drying data. In the covered ranges, the effective moisture diffusivity values (D_{eff}) ranged from 9.74×10^{-11} to 1.48×10^{-10} m^2/s based on Fick's diffusion model. The Arrhenius relation with an activation energy value of 54.37 kJ/mol expressed an effect of temperature on the diffusivity. As shown in Figure 3.3, Amer et al. (2018) developed a hybrid dryer consisting of a solar collector, a heat exchanger, two drying chambers (main and second), a reflector, plus a supplementary electrical heater immersed in a water tank. Around 32–35 and 10–12 kg of fresh chamomile can be processed in the main and second drying chamber, respectively. A temperature controller was installed in order to maintain the air temperature inside of drying chamber. The moisture content on a wet basis was reduced from an initial value

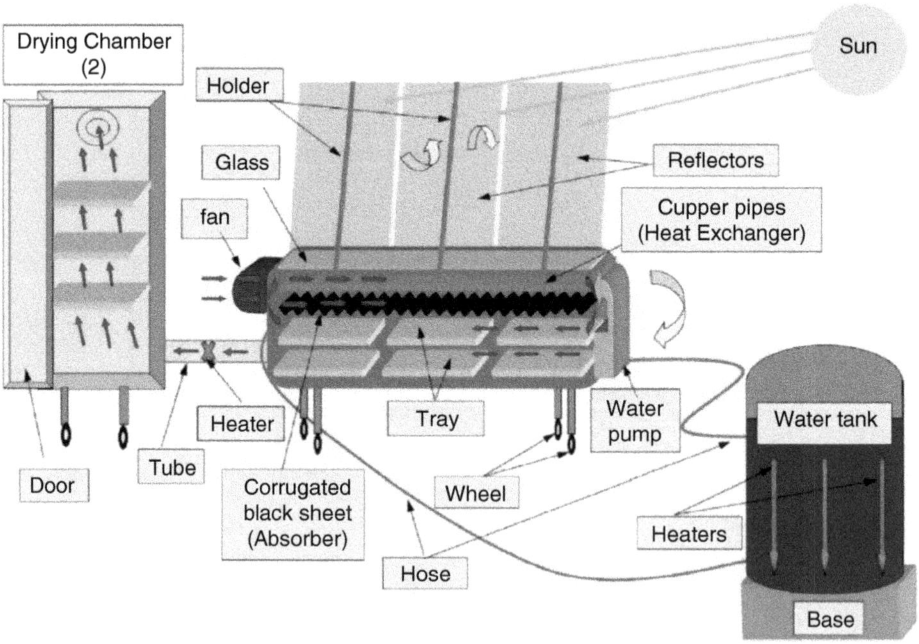

Figure 3.3 Schematic of an integrated solar drying system.

of 72–75% to 6% by using this integrated dryer, compared to 60 hours to reduce it to 9–10% by open sun drying. Meanwhile, nine mathematical models of thin layer drying were verified to determine the most suitable model for describing the drying kinetics of chamomile, and the Midili model proved best.

By recovering waste thermal energy in HP systems, they enable drying at lower temperatures and a lower cost and thereby provide efficient and eco-friendly techniques (Mortezapour et al. 2012). Hence, solar dryers equipped with HP units have been widely developed and implemented. For example, Mortezapour et al. (2012) reported on a HP-assisted hybrid photovoltaic–thermal solar drying system for drying of saffron (Figure 3.4). The effects of air mass flow rate at three levels (0.008, 0.012, and 0.016 kg/s), drying air temperature at three levels (40, 50, and 60 °C), and two different drying modes (with and without the HP unit) on the operating parameters of the dryer were investigated. They showed that energy consumption and total drying time reduced as the air mass flow rate and drying air temperature increased. By applying the HP unit, the electrical efficiency of the solar collector was increased, whereas the total energy consumption and drying time were decreased. The highest values for thermal and electrical efficiency of this solar collector were found to be 28% and 10.8%, respectively. The maximum dryer efficiency of 72% and the highest specific moisture extraction rate of 1.16 were obtained at an air mass flow rate of 0.016 kg/s and an air temperature of 60 °C with the enhancement of the HP unit. Gan et al. (2017) investigated the effects of different drying conditions by solar enhanced HP drying on drying characteristics and product quality of Misai Kucing. Experimental results showed that the drying rates by solar assisted HP drying in all trials were higher than solar drying. They also showed that during the initial and later stages of drying, the effect of RH

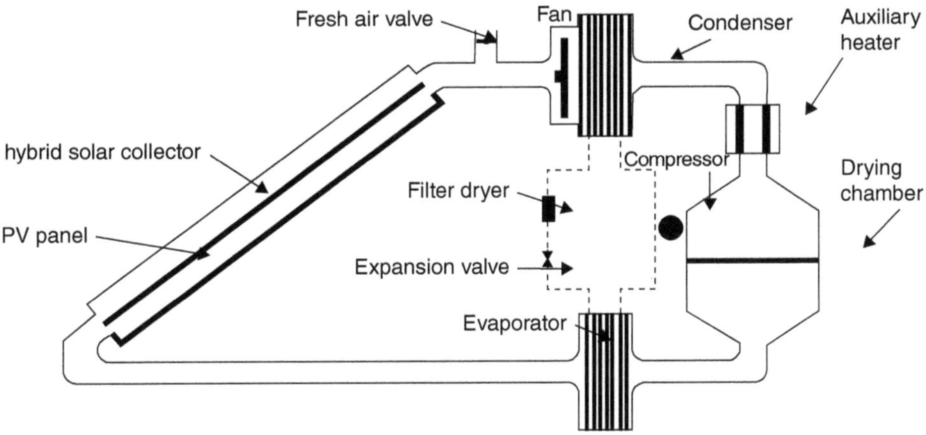

Figure 3.4 Schematic of solar dryer equipped with a heat pump system.

and air velocity on the drying rate is significant. In addition to the lengthy time process, solar dried samples had the greatest total color change as compared to solar assisted HP dried ones. Additionally, a significant difference has been found between the content of sinensetin (SEN) in fresh samples and solar dried samples ($p < 0.05$). Among all the dried samples, solar assisted HP dried samples obtained the highest SEN and rosmarinic acid (RA) retention of 83.07% in leaves and of 92.54% in flowers, respectively. For solar assisted HP dried samples, there were no significant differences ($p > 0.05$) in the retention of SEN and RA as compared to fresh samples.

3.2.2 Microwave-Related Combined Drying Methods

The microwave is a form of electromagnetic energy generated by magnetrons under the combination of electrical and magnetic fields, with wavelengths ranging from 100 to 0.1 cm and magnetic frequencies between 300 MHz (100 cm) and 300 GHz (0.1 cm) (Pozar 2005; Sorrentino and Bianchi 2010). Two commonly used microwave frequencies in the industrial food processing bands are 915 and 2450 MHz. Water is a typical bipolar molecule, it is repeatedly rotated, which is influenced by the rapidly changing polarity of electromagnetic field, and heat is volumetrically generated throughout the material due to friction between the molecules, so water is rapidly vaporized and transported to the exterior of material (Vadivambal and Jayas 2010).

Compared to conventional drying techniques, microwave drying has many merits including fast drying rate (Wray and Ramaswamy 2015), short processing duration (Wang et al. 2004), rapid and precise control (Li et al. 2006), clean drying process, and low operational cost (Rattanadecho and Makul 2016; Ekezie et al. 2017). However, solo microwave drying has some drawbacks that include uneven heating, possible structural damage, and limited penetration depth of the microwave field into the products (Zhang et al. 2006). Therefore, this technology is often integrated with other techniques to overcome the limitations of just microwave drying. Table 3.2 lists the recent applications of microwave-related combined drying for herbs and spices which are introduced in detail in the following sections.

Table 3.2 Applications of microwave-related hybrid drying for herbs and spices

Herbs and spices	Drying methods	References
Green pepper	Convective (CV) drying Convective-microwave-ultrasound drying	Szadzińska et al. (2017)
	CV drying Convective drying enhanced with microwave (CVMW) CVMW drying and periodically with infrared radiation CV drying enhanced periodically with microwave and infrared radiation CV drying enhanced periodically with infrared radiation	Łechtańska et al. (2015)
Ginger	Air drying Freeze drying Infrared drying Microwave drying	An et al. (2016)
	Intermittent microwave combined with convective drying Microwave fluidized bed drying	Lv et al. (2016)
Nutmeg mace	Pulsed microwave assisted hot air drying	Meetha et al. (2016)
Rosemary	Microwave-vacuum (MV) drying	Calín-Sánchez et al. (2011)
Sweet basil, marjoram, and true lavender	CV drying MV drying CV pre-drying and MV finish-drying	Calín-Sánchez et al. (2012); Calín-Sánchez et al. (2015); Łyczko et al. (2019)
Strobilanthes crispus	CV drying Freeze drying MV drying CV pre-drying and MV finish-drying	Chua et al. (2019)

Szadzińska et al. (2017) reported on drying of green pepper with a convective-assisted microwave-ultrasound (CVMU) dryer and convective (CV) dryer. The drying rate, total energy consumption, and quality attributes of the dried products were examined. A schematic view of the CVMU drying system is displayed in Figure 3.5; this combined drying system allows CV drying with microwave and ultrasound enhancement separately as well as in different combinations. The drying time achieved the highest reduction of 88% in microwave enhanced CV drying, and only 39% in ultrasound enhanced CV drying. The microwave enhanced CV drying process had the lowest energy consumption value (1.26 kWh), approximately 84% of energy was saved compared to the energy consumption of the CV drying process, which amounted to 7.97 kWh. From the nutritional aspect, ultrasound enhanced CV drying was demonstrated to retain most of the vitamin C and up to 70%. In terms of color, the best-dried biological samples were obtained by utilizing convection, microwave, and ultrasound simultaneously. Moreover, the CVMU dried green pepper had low water activity and better rehydration ability.

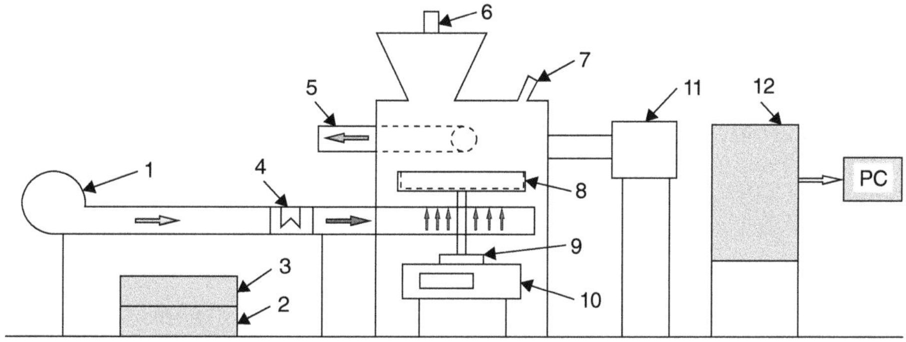

Figure 3.5 Scheme of a hybrid dryer: 1. Fan, 2. Airborne Ultrasound System (AUS), 3. Ultrasound feeder, 4. Electric heater, 5. Air outlet, 6. Ultrasound transducer AUS, 7. Pyrometer, 8. Rotating sample pan, 9. Drive sample pan, 10. Balance, 11. Microwave generator, 12. Control cupboard.

Table 3.3 Five different drying methods and their performances for green pepper

Drying methods	Drying time (min)	Total energy consumption (kWh)	Water activity in the dried sample (aw)	Retention of vitamin C (%)
CV	1127 ± 28	6.5 ± 0.1	0.560 ± 0.03	46.54
CVMW	364 ± 9	3.3 ± 0.1	0.445 ± 0.03	63.91
$CVMW + IR_{per}$	274 ± 6	4.8 ± 0.1	0.412 ± 0.04	24.91
$CV + MW_{per} + IR_{per}$	345 ± 8	3.8 ± 0.1	0.419 ± 0.04	42.97
$CV + IR_{per}$	699 ± 19	6.9 ± 0.1	0.398 ± 0.03	16.86

CV: pure convective drying throughout the whole process, CVMW: convective drying enhanced with microwaves throughout the whole process, $CVMW + IR_{per}$: convective drying enhanced with microwaves throughout the whole process and periodically with infrared radiation, $CV + MW_{per} + IR_{per}$: convective drying enhanced periodically with microwave and infrared radiation, $CV + IR_{per}$: convective drying enhanced periodically with infrared radiation.

As showed in Table 3.3, Łechtańska et al. (2015) compared the effects of five different drying methods with different applications of microwave and infrared (IR) radiation on drying kinetics, energy consumption, and quality aspects of green pepper. The results of their study showed that enhancement of CV drying by both microwave and IR energy ($CVMW + IR_{per}$ or $CV + MW_{per} + IR_{per}$) significantly reduced the drying time, which was up to 76% as compared to pure CV drying. The CVMW drying method led to the highest vitamin C retention (63.91%) compared to that of CV drying (46.54%). Meanwhile, CVMW drying had the lowest energy consumption of 3.3 ± 0.1 kWh, $CV + IR_{per}$ drying had the highest energy consumption of 6.9 ± 0.1 kWh, the lowest vitamin C retention of 16.86%, and the worst visual appearance and color. Their study revealed that CV drying enhanced with both microwave and/or IR could significantly reduce the drying time and energy consumption, improve the color of finish products, as well as enable better vitamin C retention compared to pure CV drying.

An et al. (2016) evaluated air drying (AD), freeze drying (FD), IR drying, and microwave drying (MD), as well as intermittent microwave combined with convective drying (IM&CD), on ginger slices. The quality properties of the dried samples were compared on total phenolic content (TPC), total flavonoid contents (TFCs), and pharmacologically active compounds (6-, 8-, 10-gingerols and 6-shogaol). Experimental results (Table 3.4 and Figure 3.6) showed that FD, IR, and IM&CD had a higher retention of TPC and TFC, than AD and MD process. However, FD and IR had a relatively higher energy consumption and longer drying duration, especially freeze

Table 3.4 Drying time, energy consumption, and extraction yield for different dried gingers

Drying methods	Fresh	AD	IR	FD	MD	IM&CD
Drying time (h)	N.A.	12.0 ± 0.5	6.0 ± 0.7	44.5 ± 2.0	1.8 ± 0.3	1.5 ± 0.2
Energy consumption (kW h/g H_2O)	N.A.	3.30 ± 0.08	12.23 ± 0.24	33.7 ± 0.53	2.7 ± 0.12	3.21 ± 0.1
TPC (mg GAE/g dw)	11.97 ± 0.33	9.69 ± 0.54	11.35 ± 0.66	13.83 ± 0.31	8.41 ± 0.35	11.28 ± 0.40
TFC (mg Rutin/g dw)	13.49 ± 0.36	12.08 ± 1.17	14.52 ± 0.23	13.32 ± 0.52	12.55 ± 0.74	15.42 ± 0.87

AD: hot air drying, IR: infrared drying, FD: freeze drying, MD: microwave drying, IM&CD: intermittent microwave-convection drying, TPC: total phenolic, GAE: gallic acid equivalents, TFC: total flavonoids content.

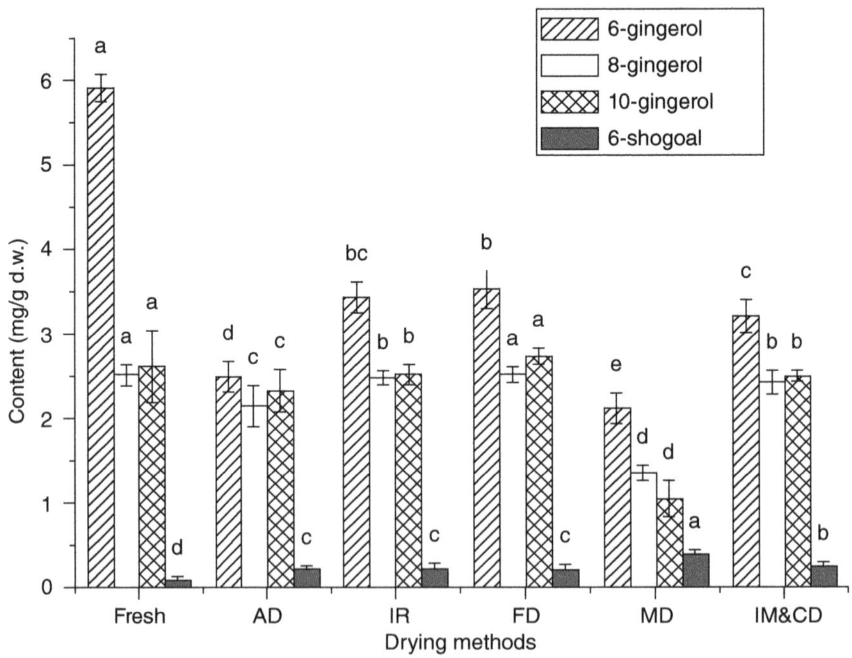

Figure 3.6 Changes of 6-, 8-, 10-gingerol, and 6-shogaol content of ginger extract during AD, IR, FD, CM, and IM&CD drying processes. AD: hot air drying, IR: infrared drying, FD: freeze drying, MD: microwave drying, IM&CD: intermittent microwave-convection drying. For each column, values followed by the same letter (a–c) are not statistically different at $p < 0.05$ as measured by Duncan's test.

drying. Therefore, concerning both the drying efficiency and quality aspects of dried products, IM&CD would be the best option for heat-sensitive material owing to its greater efficiency, better quality retention, and lower cost, and has a broad market prospect for industrial-scale application.

Lv et al. (2016) investigated the feasibility of using a new microwave fluidized bed drying (MFBD) method for ginger slices. The schematic diagram of this MFBD system is presented in Figure 3.7. The material tray and vibration frame are fixed together inside the dryer and connected with a vibration motor through a damping spring. When the vibration motor works, the raw materials in the tray start rolling and are in a suspended state. Six magnetrons are evenly located at the top of the drying chamber independently. The problem of local overheating can be solved through the even arrangement of magnetrons and the fluidization system of raw materials. For MFBD at microwave power 2.0–0.4 W/g, the browning issue caused by localized overheating was eliminated effectively. Meanwhile, low nuclear magnetic resonance was used to detect the products in different drying stages in order to better understand the water flow characteristics of ginger slices in MFBD. The state of water can be classified as free water (FW), immobilized water (IW), and bonded water (BW). FW was the main water state in fresh samples and converted to the IW quickly at the initial stage, and

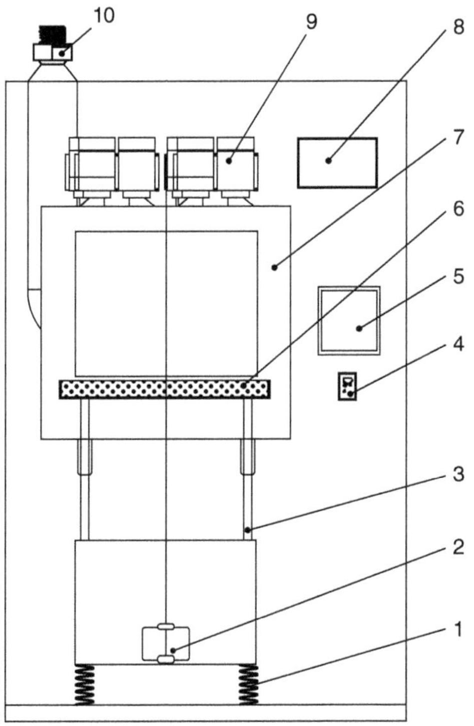

Figure 3.7 Schematic diagram of a MFBD equipment; 1. Damping spring, 2. Vibration motor, 3. Vibration frame, 4. Frequency converter, 5. Touch screen, 6. Material tray, 7. MFD chamber, 8. Monitor, 9. Magnetron, 10. Induced draft fan.

both FW and IW decreased until the final stage was reached. Finally, the content of BW increased to a certain level, and then the dried ginger slices could be stored safely.

Meetha et al. (2016) studied the influence of pulsed-microwave enhanced hot air drying (PMHAD) on color retention of nutmeg mace. Experiments were performed at an air temperature of 45 °C with three different microwave power intensities (0.5, 1, and 1.445 kW) with 30 seconds pulsation, and the color values of dried nutmeg mace were compared to market samples using a colorimeter. The preferred color of dried nutmeg mace is usually darker, more reddish, and less yellowish. Among the PMHAD dried samples, the power intensity of 1.445 kW gave darker, 1 kW gave more reddish, and 0.5 kW gave less yellowish colors, while the market samples were lighter and yellowish. This proved that the PMHAD method delivered more color retention compared to market samples.

Microwave-Vacuum Drying (MVD) eliminates some of the difficulties and disadvantages of both microwave drying and vacuum drying, which helps to improve energy efficiency and product quality (Cui et al. 2004; Giri and Prasad 2007). Calín-Sánchez et al. (2011) studied the aroma components and sensory quality of rosemary at different vacuum levels and microwave power intensities. The required time to dry rosemary was shortened by the increment of vacuum level and microwave power intensity. Experimental results showed that the higher the vacuum level inside the dryer at a specific microwave power, and/or the higher the microwave power, the lower the total quantity of volatiles. However, the higher vacuum level and microwave power intensity led to shorter drying times. The optimum conditions to dry the samples were 72–74 kPa and 360 W for 39 minutes and 240 W and 0 kPa (56 minutes were required), compared to almost 180 minutes required for drying rosemary using pure CV drying. This study also revealed that MVD could be applied for drying of very sensitive materials, such as rosemary, and for this purpose very high vacuum levels with low microwave power intensity should be applied. Calín-Sánchez et al. (2015) evaluated the influences of drying method on the quality of marjoram. CV drying, MVD, and a combination of convective pre-drying and Microwave-Vacuum Finish-Drying (CVPD + MVFD) were carried out on marjoram. Volatile compounds from marjoram samples were extracted by hydro distillation and analyzed by gas chromatography (GC). Thirty-three compounds were tentatively identified and quantified, among them *cis*-sabinene hydrate (229 mg/100 g, db) and terpinen-4-ol (169 mg/100 g, db) being the major components. The results showed significant differences in the aroma quality of marjoram dried by different methods. The total quantity of volatiles of fresh marjoram (825 mg/100 g, db) was considerably reduced by most of the drying methods, except for the MVD at 240 and 360 W. The MVD method at 240 W was the optimal condition, followed by the combined method with 50 °C and 240 or 360 W. The drying time was relatively short (≈162 and 158 minutes, respectively), and good aroma quality was observed through sensory analysis (high scores for fresh and vegetable odor). The same researchers also examined the effects of drying methods on the aroma compounds of sweet basil with the same drying methods mentioned before (Calín-Sánchez et al. 2012). The total quantity of volatiles was considerably reduced from 32.1 g/kg of fresh sweet basil to 14.4 g/kg of dried sweet basil by employing both CV drying and MVD. CVPD at 40 °C and then MVFD at 360 W was the optimal process for drying sweet basil, the time required was relatively short (≈250 minutes), with a relatively high quantity of volatile compounds (16.7 g/kg) and good aroma quality. In another study, the effects of drying methods (CV drying, MVD, CVPD+MVFD) on the degree of volatile constituents of true lavender leaves was studied by Łyczko et al. (2019). The volatile components of dried lavender were extracted and identified by headspace solid-phase micro extraction coupled with the gas chromatography mass spectrometry technique (GC–MS), and total essential oil (EO) content was also verified using hydrodistillation extraction method. The major constituents were two p-cymen-8-ol (4.09%), a mixture of borneol and lavandulol (4.66%), o-cymene (4.81%), bornyl acetate (5.57%), (E)-caryophyllene (6.11%), eucalyptol (7.28%), and γ-cadinene (10.53%). It was also observed that CV drying at 60 °C was the most optimal method to retain flavoring properties, while the highest EO retention was obtained by MVD at 480 W. Chua et al. (2019) examined the antioxidant activity and yield of phytosterols and essential oil volatiles of *Strobilanthes crispus* samples dried by four different drying techniques: FD; CV drying at 40, 50, and 60 °C; MVD at 6, 9, and 12 W/g; and CVPD+MVFD at 50 °C and 9 W/g. Experimental results showed that 33 volatile components were detected by GC–MS, and the major constituents were 2-hexen-1-ol, 2-hexenal, 1-octen-3-ol, linalool, and benzaldehyde. FD dried samples had the lowest water activity and better color preservation. A suitable microwave power and air temperature led to higher antioxidant activities: CV drying at 40 °C and MVD at 9 W/g had the highest antioxidant activity. In terms of phenolic content, CV drying at 60 °C led to the highest value. The highest phytosterol content and total volatile components were obtained with MVD at 9 W/g and CV drying at 50 °C, respectively. On the other hand, the drying kinetics of *Strobilanthes crispus* for CV drying, MVD, and CVPD+MVFD were expressed as a good fit to the exponential equation or the modified Page model. MVD consumed the lowest energy among all the drying methods because it had the shortest drying duration owing to use of microwaves throughout the drying process.

3.2.3 Other Energy Sources-Related Combined Drying Methods

Apart from energy sources of solar and microwave, many conventional drying methods associated with other energy sources have been established and adopted for the drying of herbs and spices.

As seen from Figure 3.8, Mihindukulasuriya and Jayasuriya (2015) constructed and tested a lab scale mixed-mode rotary drying equipment for chili drying. This dryer can operate in three different modes: hot air (HA) mode, IR mode, and IR assisted with hot air (IRHA) mode. At 70 °C, the HA mode consumed the highest power, which was 60.4% more than IR mode as well as 33.5% more than the IRHA mode. For color, it was found that in IR mode, the redness of the dried samples was decreased by 30% compared to those of the HA mode and IRHA mode at 70 °C. And for loss of capsaicin content, IR mode led to 2% and 22% greater than HA mode and IRHA mode at 70 °C, respectively. Between HA mode and IRHA mode at a temperature range from 65 to 70 °C, the quality properties regarding capsaicin content and color were very similar. A positive correlation was identified between drying time and energy consumption for both HA and IRHA mode, whereas a negative correlation was found in IR mode. Considering overall performance indicators (color, capsaicin content, energy consumption, and drying time), the optimum operation condition

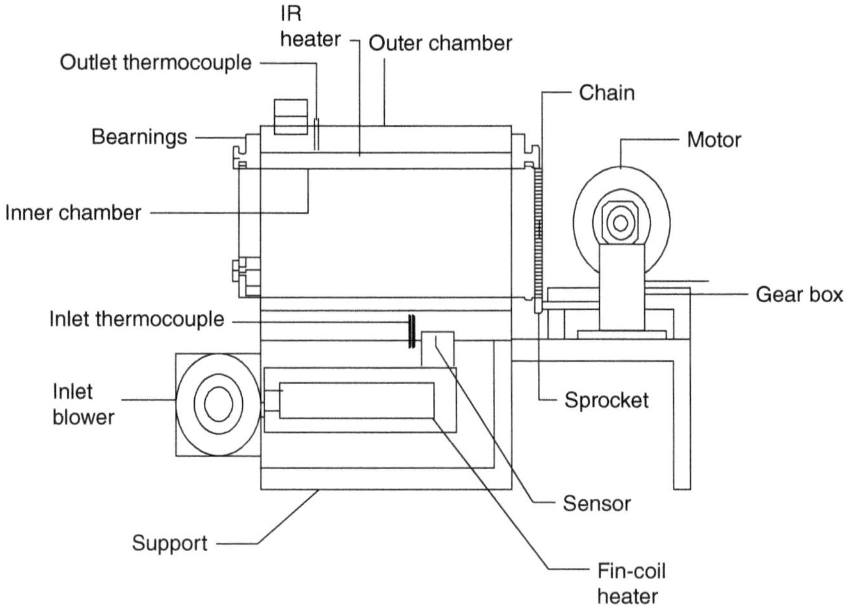

Figure 3.8 Schematic illustration of a combined IR and hot air rotary dryer.

for drying chili was performed at 70, 65, and 50 °C in HA, IRHA, and IR mode, respectively.

Naidu et al. (2015) compared the effects of HA drying (50 °C) with 58–63% RH, low humidity air (LHA) drying (50 °C with 28–30% RH), and radiofrequency (RF) drying (50 °C with 56–60% RH) on the quality aspects of dill greens (*Anethum graveolens*). The results showed that the drying time of HA and RF was longer (around 22%) compared to that of HA. Lightness, greenness, and yellowness of the LHA-dried sample were higher than those of the RF- and HA-dried ones. Extracts from LHA-dried samples had good free radical scavenging activities from 5% to 88%. Further, methanolic extracts of LHA-dried samples had a perceptible impact on scavenging free radicals. According to consumer acceptance studies, around 70% and 80% of the consumers selected the "Like Very Much" rating to a snack food, "Vada," made from fresh and dried dill greens, respectively.

Antal et al. (2011) investigated the effects of vacuum freeze drying (VFD) and HA drying on the essential oil composition and rehydration ability of spearmint leaves, and VFD was performed at high (150–250 Pa) and low pressure (10–30 Pa) in the experiment. It was found that drying time and essential oil content were strongly affected by vacuum pressure. Higher pressure increased the drying time but preserved the major volatile compounds of dried samples. In terms of dried product quality, VFD-dried spearmint leaves had better quality compared to hot air-dried ones. At the same time, VFD-dried samples also had higher rehydration rates (0.5 minutes) than hot air-dried ones (5 minutes) at a water temperature of 75 °C. It was recommended that the drying of spearmint leaves should be performed by VFD and the pressure in the drying chamber should not be too low.

3.3 Other Innovative Drying Methods

More recently, some alternative innovative techniques such as refractance-window (RW) drying, ultrasound (US) technology, pulsed electric field (PEF) treatment prior to drying, CO_2 drying, and osmotic dehydration (OD), have offered opportunities to enhance both product quality and drying efficiency.

RW drying is a suitable method for heat-sensitive products. It operates under comparatively lower temperatures (usually below 70 °C) and atmospheric pressure, and requires a short drying duration (Ochoa-Martínez et al. 2012; Rostami et al. 2018). Aghaei et al. (2019) studied the effects of traditional drying, oven drying, and RW drying methods on saffron; RW and oven drying at three temperatures of 60, 70, and 80 °C, and traditional drying at room temperature (20–25 °C), were used to treat the samples. The results showed that RW drying with 200 μm Mylar membrane and oven drying were the most efficient methods in terms of short drying duration of 25.28 and 22.28 minutes, respectively. RW drying with Pyrex glass led to the highest bioactive compounds including picrocrocin (112.83 $E^{1\%}_{257nm}$), safranal (51.79 $E^{1\%}_{330nm}$), and crocin (274.76 $E^{1\%}_{440nm}$). RW drying at 70 °C is the most suitable method for drying saffron and it can be recommended as an improved method for obtaining the most favored dried samples.

US is a very promising technology for food processing, and comprises a series of mechanisms such as heating, cavitation, structural effects, and rectified diffusion (Jambrak et al. 2007). The application of ultrasound can improve internal and/or external mass transfer at low temperatures, destroy microorganisms, and minimize degradation of thermolabile components, and hence ultimately improve the quality characteristics of food products (Pereira and Vicente 2010; Rodríguez et al. 2014). Rodríguez et al. (2014) investigated the effects when different US power levels (0, 6.2, 12.3, and 18.5 kW/m^3) were tested during a convective drying (air temperatures: 40, 50, 60, 70, and 80 ± 1.2 °C; air speed: 1, 2, and 3 m/s) in a high-void bed of thyme leaves. The results showed that the drying time could be reduced by 30% at the air speed of 1 m/s at 40 or 50 °C when US was used. For different US power intensities applied in experiments, they observed the influence on the external resistance to the mass transfer was significantly higher than its influence on the internal resistance ($p < 0.05$). Nevertheless, the influence of US application on mass transfer was only found at an applied air speed of 3 m/s and air temperatures below 70 °C.

Bušić et al. (2014) compared the effects of three different drying methods (HA drying, freeze drying, and CO_2 drying) on the degree of native bioactive and sensory attributes of basil (*Ocimum basilicum* L.). It was reported that freeze drying was the best method for retaining the color, essential oils, bioactive components, and antioxidant capacity of basil. CO_2 drying requires a longer drying time, therefore the essential oil content of the dried sample was decreased from 0.21% to 0.96% as the drying time was increased. Phenolic acids were identified by high performance liquid chromatography (HPLC), and rosmarinic, chicoric, caftaric, and caffeic, and rosmarinic acid were the most abundant components in all samples. It was also shown that the longer CO_2 drying time (four hours) was the most important factor which significantly affected polyphenolics retention and the antioxidant capacity of dried products. CO_2-dried samples obtained higher scores in terms of taste and appearance compared to those dried by HA drying, but there was a need to optimize CO_2 drying to further improve aroma retention. They concluded that shorter CO_2 drying duration (2 or 3 hours) and pressures of 80–100 bar at 40 °C might be the most suitable condition for drying of basil.

Pretreatment is usually performed prior to drying in order to obtain certain benefits in physical and/or chemical changes of processed products. Pretreatment can also contribute to an enhanced dehydration rate, reduced energy consumption, and preserved product quality (Mard et al. 2012). The effects of PEF pretreatment on the drying behavour of red pepper were investigated by Won et al. (2015). PEF treatment was performed at an electric field strength of 1.0–2.5 kV/cm using a fixed pulse width of 30 μs at a pulse frequency of 100 Hz, and PEF treatment duration was set at three different levels: 1, 2, and 4 s. PEF-pretreated (2.5 kV/cm, 100 Hz, 4 s) samples achieved the target moisture content of 15% after 3.2 hours of drying, against 4.9 hours for untreated samples to reach the same moisture content, which corresponds to a decrease in the drying time of up to 34.7%. It took 3.9 hours to reach the target moisture level when the shortest PEF pretreatment (2.5 kV/cm, 100 Hz, 1 s) was applied, indicating a 20.4% reduction in drying time. The reduced drying time suggests that PEF treatment induced cell membrane damage, which might positively affect the drying kinetics by facilitating the transport of water and solute. From a quality perspective, the reduction in drying time by PEF treatment led to higher retention of carotenoid pigments. According to some preliminary reports, it has been shown that OD is an effective method to achieve a high efficiency of dehydration and enhance taste (Changrue et al. 2008; Figiel and Michalska 2017). Boggia et al. (2013) studied both the process variables and mixture composition of the OD process for dehydrating Protected Designation of Origin (PDO) Genovese basil. They found the optimized condition to obtain the best appearance and aroma of dried leaves was 67.5 °C with a dipping time of 55 s in a brine containing 65% water, 20% sorbitol, and 15% NaCl. However, they did not find a significant improvement of the quality of the final product through the use of trehalose.

3.4 Conclusion and Suggestions for Future Research

Production and consumption of processed herbs and spices is increasing as they play a vital role in seasoning and/or preserving foods, and also for perfuming, coloring, and pharmaceutical purposes. Innovative techniques of food drying are a response to the increasing consumer demand for high-quality processed products, that are also economically and environmentally sustainable. The latest developments of solar-related, microwave-related, and other energy source-enhanced combined drying techniques, as well as other emerging innovative drying methods in respect of drying of herbs and spices, have been introduced in this chapter.

Future research challenges and trends for drying of herbs and spices include the following:

- Developing flexible, cost-effective, multiuse drying methods, especially for thermal-sensitive herbs and spices.
- Applying suitable pretreatment and/or post-treatment methods to improve the quality of dried products.
- Using process analytical tools or in-line measurement techniques to track the drying process and dynamically/adequately regulate critical process parameters.

- Establishing reliable mathematical models (especially in complicated drying systems) through the model-based (MB) approach, fuzzy logic (FL) approach, and neural nets (NNs) approach, as well as computational fluid dynamic (CFD) simulation.
- Fabricating eco-friendly dryers by utilizing pollution-free or renewable energy sources.
- Devising automatic, intelligent, and continuous drying systems to simplify operation, improve efficiency, and minimize cost.

Acknowledgments

We acknowledge the financial support from the National Natural Science Foundation Program of China (Contract No. 31671864), China Key Research Program (Contract No. 2016YFD0400704-5), Jiangsu Province (China) "Collaborative Innovation Center for Food Safety and Quality Control" Industry Development Program, Jiangsu Province (China) Infrastructure Project (Contract No. BM2014051) all of which enabled us to carry out this study.

References

Aghaei, Z., Jafari, S.M., and Dehnad, D. (2019). Effect of different drying methods on the physicochemical properties and bioactive components of saffron powder. *Plant Foods for Human Nutrition* **74**: 171–178.

Amer, B.M.A., Gottschalk, K., and Hossain, M.A. (2018). Integrated hybrid solar drying system and its drying kinetics of chamomile. *Renewable Energy* **121**: 539–547.

An, K., Zhao, D., Wang, Z. et al. (2016). Comparison of different drying methods on Chinese ginger (*Zingiber officinale Roscoe*): changes in volatiles, chemical profile, antioxidant properties, and microstructure. *Food Chemistry* **197**: 1292–1300.

Antal, T., Figiel, A., Kerekes, B., and Sikolya, L. (2011). Effect of drying methods on the quality of the essential oil of spearmint leaves (*Mentha spicata L.*). *Drying Technology* **29**: 1836–1844.

Argyropoulos, D. and Müller, J. (2014). Changes of essential oil content and composition during convective drying of lemon balm (*Melissa officinalis L.*). *Industrial Crops and Products* **52**: 118–124.

Arslan, D., Özcan, M.M., and Mengeş, H.O. (2010). Evaluation of drying methods with respect to drying parameters, some nutritional and colour characteristics of peppermint *(Mentha x piperita L.)*. *Energy Conversion and Management* **51**: 2769–2775.

Balasubramanian, S., Roselin, P., Singh, K.K. et al. (2016). Postharvest processing and benefits of black pepper, coriander, cinnamon, fenugreek, and turmeric. *Critical Reviews in Food Science and Nutrition* **56**: 1585–1607.

Basunia, M.A. and Abe, T. (2001). Thin-layer solar drying characteristics of rough rice under natural convection. *Journal of Food Engineering* **47**: 295–301.

Belessiotis, V. and Delyannis, E. (2011). Solar drying. *Solar Energy* **85**: 1665–1691.

Bhardwaj, A.K., Kumar, R., and Chauhan, R. (2019). Experimental investigation of the performance of a novel solar dryer for drying medicinal plants in Western Himalayan region. *Solar Energy* **177**: 395–407.

Boggia, R., Leardi, R., Zunin, P. et al. (2013). Dehydration of PDO genovese basil leaves (*Ocimum basilicum maximum L. cv genovese gigante*) by direct osmosis. *Journal of Food Processing and Preservation* **37**: 621–629.

Buchaillot, A., Caffin, N., and Bhandari, B. (2009). Drying of lemon myrtle (*Backhousia citriodora*) leaves: retention of volatiles and color. *Drying Technology* **27**: 445–450.

Bušić, A., Vojvodić, A., Komes, D. et al. (2014). Comparative evaluation of CO_2 drying as an alternative drying technique of basil (*Ocimum basilicum L.*) – the effect on bioactive and sensory properties. *Food Research International* **64**: 34–42.

Calín-Sánchez, Á., Szumny, A., Figiel, A. et al. (2011). Effects of vacuum level and microwave power on rosemary volatile composition during vacuum–microwave drying. *Journal of Food Engineering* **103**: 219–227.

Calín-Sánchez, Á., Lech, K., Szumny, A. et al. (2012). Volatile composition of sweet basil essential oil (*Ocimum basilicum L.*) as affected by drying method. *Food Research International* **48**: 217–225.

Calín-Sánchez, Á., Figiel, A., Lech, K. et al. (2015). Dying methods affect the aroma of Origanum majorana L. analyzed by GC-MS and descriptive sensory analysis. *Industrial Crops and Products* **74**: 218–227.

Ceylan, İ. and Gürel, A.E. (2016). Solar-assisted fluidized bed dryer integrated with a heat pump for mint leaves. *Applied Thermal Engineering* **106**: 899–905.

Chanchal, D. and Swarnlata, S. (2008). Novel approaches in herbal cosmetics. *Journal of Cosmetic Dermatology* **7**: 89–95.

Changrue, V., Orsat, V., and Raghavan, G.S.V. (2008). Osmotically dehydrated microwave vacuum drying of strawberries. *Journal of Food Processing and Preservation* **32**: 798–816.

Chua, L.Y.W., Chua, B.L., Figiel, A. et al. (2019). Antioxidant activity, and volatile and phytosterol contents of strobilanthes crispus dehydrated using conventional and vacuum microwave drying methods. *Molecules* **24**: 1397.

Crivelli, G., Nani, R.C., and Di Cesare, L.F. (2002). Influence of processing on the quality of dried herbs. *Atti VI Giornate Scientifiche SOI* **2**: 463–464.

Cui, Z.W., Xu, S.Y., and Sun, D.W. (2004). Effect of microwave-vacuum drying on the carotenoids retention of carrot slices and chlorophyll retention of chinese chive leaves. *Drying Technology* **22**: 563–575.

Demiray, E. and Tulek, Y. (2014). Drying characteristics of garlic (*Allium sativum L*) slices in a convective hot air dryer. *Heat and Mass Transfer* **50**: 779–786.

Deshmukh, W., Varma, M.N., Chang, K.Y., and Wasewarm, K.L. (2014). Investigation of solar drying of ginger (*zingiber officinale*): emprical modelling, drying characteristics, and quality study. *Chinese Journal of Engineering* https://doi.org/10.1155/2014/305823.

Doymaz, I. (2005). Drying characteristics and kinetics of okra. *Journal of Food Engineering* **69**: 275–279.

Ekezie, F.C., Sun, D.W., Han, Z., and Cheng, J.H. (2017). Microwave-assisted food processing technologies for enhancing product quality and process efficiency: a review of recent developments. *Trends in Food Science & Technology* **67**: 58–69.

El-Sebaii, A.A. and Shalaby, S.M. (2013). Experimental investigation of an indirect-mode forced convection solar dryer for drying thymus and mint. *Energy Conversion and Management* **74**: 109–116.

Figiel, A. and Michalska, A. (2017). Overall quality of fruits and vegetables products affected by the drying processes with the assistance of vacuum-microwaves. *International Journal of Molecular Sciences* **18**: 71.

Gan, S.H., Chua, L.S., Aziz, R. et al. (2017). Drying characteristics of *Orthosiphon stamineus* Benth by solar assisted heat pump drying. *Drying Technology* **35**: 1755–1764.

Giri, S.K. and Prasad, S. (2007). Drying kinetics and rehydration characteristics of microwave-vacuum and convective hot-air dried mushrooms. *Journal of Food Engineering* **78**: 512–521.

Hamrouni-Sellami, I., Wannes, W.A., Bettaieb, I. et al. (2011). Qualitative and quantitative changes in the essential oil of *Laurus nobilis L.* leaves as affected by different drying methods. *Food Chemistry* **126**: 691–769.

Hamrouni-Sellami, I., Rahali, F.Z., Rebey, I.B. et al. (2013). Total phenolics, flavonoids, and antioxidant activity of sage (*Salvia officinalis L.*) plants as affected by different drying methods. *Food and Bioprocess Technology* **6**: 806–817.

Huang, L., Zhang, M., Wang, L. et al. (2012). Influence of combination drying methods on composition, texture, aroma and microstructure of apple slices. *LWT - Food Science and Technology* **47**: 183–188.

Iriti, M., Vitalini, S., Fico, G., and Faoro, F. (2010). Neuroprotective herbs and foods from different traditional medicines and diets. *Molecules* **15**: 3517–3555.

Jambrak, A.R., Mason, T.J., Paniwnyk, L., and Lelas, V. (2007). Accelerated drying of button mushrooms, Brussels sprouts and cauliflower by applying power ultrasound and its rehydration properties. *Journal of Food Engineering* **81**: 88–97.

Janjai, S., Srisittipokakun, N., and Bala, B.K. (2008). Experimental and modelling performances of a roof-integrated solar drying system for drying herbs and spices. *Energy* **33**: 91–103.

Jin, W., Mujumdar, A.S., Zhang, M., and Shi, W.F. (2018a). Novel drying techniques for spices and herbs: a review. *Food Engineering Reviews* **10**: 34–45.

Jin, W., Zhang, M., and Shi, W.F. (2018b). Evaluation of ultrasound pretreatment and drying methods on selected quality attributes of bitter melon (*Momordica charantia l.*). *Drying Technology* **37**: 387–396.

Kaefer, C.M. and Milner, J.A. (2008). The role of herbs and spices in cancer prevention. *The Journal of Nutritional Biochemistry* **19**: 347–361.

Karam, M.C., Petit, J., Zimmer, D. et al. (2016). Effects of drying and grinding in production of fruit and vegetable powders: a review. *Journal of Food Engineering* **188**: 32–49.

Kareem, M.W., Habib, K., Ruslan, M.H., and Saha, B.B. (2017). Thermal performance study of a multi-pass solar air heating collector system for drying of Roselle (*Hibiscus sabdariffa*). *Renewable Energy* **113**: 281–292.

Karim, M.A. and Hawlader, M.N.A. (2005). Drying characteristics of banana: theoretical modelling and experimental validation. *Journal of Food Engineering* **70**: 35–45.

Kaveh, M., Chayjan, A.R., and Esna-Ashari, M. (2015). Thermal and physical properties modelling of terebinth fruit (*Pistacia atlantica L.*) under solar drying. *Research in Agricultural Engineering* **61**: 150–161.

Kivilompolo, M. and Hyötyläinen, T. (2007). Comprehensive two-dimensional liquid chromatography in analysis of Lamiaceae herbs: characterisation and quantification of antioxidant phenolic acids. *Journal of Chromatography A* **1145**: 155–164.

Klemeš, J., Smith, R., and Kim, J.K. (2008). *Handbook of Water and Energy Management in Food Processing*. Cambridge: Woodhead Publishing.

Łechtańska, J.M., Szadzińska, J., and Kowalski, S.J. (2015). Microwave- and infrared-assisted convective drying of green pepper: quality and energy considerations. *Chemical Engineering and Processing: Process Intensification* **98**: 155–164.

Li, Z., Wang, N., Raghavan, G.S.V., and Cheng, W. (2006). A microcontroller-based, feedback power control system for microwave drying processes. *Applied Engineering in Agriculture* **22**: 309–314.

Lv, W.Q., Li, S., Han, Q. et al. (2016). Study of the drying process of ginger (*Zingiber officinale Roscoe*) slices in microwave fluidized bed dryer. *Drying Technology* **34**: 1690–1699.

Łyczko, J., Jałoszyński, K., Surma, M. et al. (2019). HS-SPME analysis of true lavender (*Lavandula angustifolia Mill.*) leaves treated by various drying methods. *Molecules* **24**: 764.

Mard, N.D., Boudhrioua, N., Kechaou, N. et al. (2012). Influence of air drying temperature on kinetics, physicochemical properties, total phenolic content and ascorbic acid of pears. *Food and Bioproducts Processing* **90**: 433–441.

Meetha, J.N., Muhammadali, P., Joy, M.I. et al. (2016). Pulsed microwave assisted hot air drying of nutmeg mace for better colour retention. *Journal of Spices and Aromatic Crops* **25**: 84–87.

Mghazli, S., Ouhammou, M., Hidar, N. et al. (2017). Drying characteristics and kinetics solar drying of Moroccan rosemary leaves. *Renewable Energy* **108**: 303–310.

Mihindukulasuriya, S.D.F. and Jayasuriya, H.P.W. (2015). Drying of chilli in a combined infrared and hot air rotary dryer. *Journal of Food Science and Technology* **52**: 4895–4904.

Mohamed, H.A.R., Sallam, Y.I., El-Leithy, A.S., and Aly, S.E. (2012). Lemongrass (*Cymbopogon citratus*) essential oil as affected by drying methods. *Annals of Agricultural Science* **57**: 113–116.

Morad, M.M., El-Shazly, M.A., Wasfy, K.I., and El-Maghawry, H.A.M. (2017). Thermal analysis and performance evaluation of a solar tunnel greenhouse dryer for drying peppermint plant. *Renewable Energy* **101**: 992–1004.

Mortezapour, H., Ghobadian, B., Minaei, S., and Khoshtaghaza, M.H. (2012). Saffron drying with a heat pump–assisted hybrid photovoltaic–thermal solar dryer. *Drying Technology* **30**: 560–566.

Moses, J.A., Norton, T., Alagusundaram, K., and Tiwari, B.K. (2014). Novel drying techniques for the food industry. *Food Engineering Reviews* **6**: 43–55.

Mujumdar, A.S. (2007). *Handbook of Industrial Drying*. Philadelphia: Taylor & Francis.

Mujumdar, A.S. and Huang, L.X. (2007). Global R&D needs in drying. *Drying Technology* **25**: 647–658.

Muller, J., Reisinger, G., and Muhlbauer, W. (1989). Drying of medicinal and aromatic plants in a greenhouse solar dryer. *Landtechnik* **2**: 58–65.

Mustayen, A.G.M.B., Mekhilef, S., and Saidur, R. (2014). Performance study of different solar dryers: a review. *Renewable and Sustainable Energy Reviews* **34**: 463–470.

Naidu, M.M., Vedhashree, M., Satapathy, P. et al. (2015). Effect of drying methods on the quality characteristics of dill (*Anethum graveolens*) greens. *Food Chemistry* **192**: 849–856.

Nathakaranakule, A., Jaiboon, P., and Soponronnarit, S. (2010). Far-infrared radiation assisted drying of longan fruit. *Journal of Food Engineering* **100**: 662–668.

Ochoa-Martínez, C.I., Quintero, P.T., Ayala, A.A., and Ortiz, M.J. (2012). Drying characteristics of mango slices using the Refractance window^{TM} technique. *Journal of Food Engineering* **109**: 69–75.

Onwude, D.I., Hashim, N., and Chen, G. (2016a). Recent advances of novel thermal combined hot air drying of agricultural crops. *Trends in Food Science & Technology* **57**: 132–145.

Onwude, D.I., Hashim, N., Janius, R.B. et al. (2016b). Modeling the thin-layer drying of fruits and vegetables: a review. *Comprehensive Reviews in Food Science and Food Safety* **15**: 599–618.

Özcan, M., Arslan, D., and Ünver, A. (2005). Effect of drying methods on the mineral content of basil (*Ocimum basilicum L.*). *Journal of Food Engineering* **69**: 375–379.

Parto, N. (2015). *Case Study: Pathogens and Spices*. Toronto: Queen's Printer for Ontario.

Parveen, S., Das, S., Begum, A. et al. (2014). Microbiological quality assessment of three selected spices in Bangladesh. *International Food Research Journal* **21**: 1327–1330.

Pereira, R.N. and Vicente, A.A. (2010). Environmental impact of novel thermal and non-thermal technologies in food processing. *Food Research International* **43**: 1936–1943.

Pozar, D.M. (2005). *Microwave Engineering*. New Jersey: Wiley.

Rabha, D.K., Muthukumar, P., and Somayaji, C. (2017a). Energy and exergy analyses of the solar drying processes of ghost chilli pepper and ginger. *Renewable Energy* **105**: 764–773.

Rabha, D.K., Muthukumar, P., and Somayaji, C. (2017b). Experimental investigation of thin layer drying kinetics of ghost chilli pepper (*Capsicum Chinense Jacq.*) dried in a forced convection solar tunnel dryer. *Renewable Energy* **105**: 583–589.

Raghavan, G.S.V., Rennie, T.J., Sunjka, P.S. et al. (2005). Overview of new techniques for drying biological materials with emphasis on energy aspects. *Brazilian Journal of Chemical Engineering* **22**: 195–201.

Raso, J. and Barbosa-Cánovas, G.V. (2003). Nonthermal preservation of foods using combined processing techniques. *Critical Reviews in Food Science and Nutrition* **43**: 265–285.

Rattanadecho, P. and Makul, N. (2016). Microwave-assisted drying: a review of the state-of-the-art. *Drying Technology* **34**: 1–38.

Rodríguez, E.C., Fiueroa, I.P., and Mercado, C.A.R. (2013). Feasibility analysis of drying process habanero chili using a hybrid-solar-fluidized bed dryer in Yucatan Mexico. *Journal of Energy and Power Engineering* **7**: 1898–1908.

Rodríguez, J., Mulet, A., and Bon, J. (2014). Influence of high-intensity ultrasound on drying kinetics in fixed beds of high porosity. *Journal of Food Engineering* **127**: 93–102.

Rostami, H., Dehnad, D., Jafari, S.M., and Tavakoli, H.R. (2018). Evaluation of physical, rheological, microbial, and organoleptic properties of meat powder produced by Refractance window drying. *Drying Technology* **36**: 1076–1085.

Sa-adchom, P., Swasdisevi, T., Nathakaranakule, A., and Soponronnarit, S. (2011). Drying kinetics using superheated steam and quality attributes of dried pork slices for different thickness, seasoning and fibers distribution. *Journal of Food Engineering* **104**: 105–113.

Satimehin, A.A. (2014). A mathematical model for deep bed drying of gelatinized white yam (*Dioscorea rotundata, Poir*). *International Journal of Energy Engineering* **4**: 33–39.

Şevik, S. (2014). Experimental investigation of a new design solar-heat pump dryer under the different climatic conditions and drying behavior of selected products. *Solar Energy* **105**: 190–205.

Sorrentino, R. and Bianchi, G. (2010). *Microwave and RF Engineering*. New York, NY: Wiley.

Srinivasan, K. (2005). Spices as influencers of body metabolism: an overview of three decades of research. *Food Research International* **38**: 77–86.

Szadzińska, J., Łechtańska, J., Kowalski, S.J., and Stasiak, M. (2017). The effect of high power airborne ultrasound and microwaves on convective drying effectiveness and quality of green pepper. *Ultrasonics Sonochemistry* **34**: 531–539.

Tham, T.C., Ng, M.X., Gan, S.H. et al. (2017). Effect of ambient conditions on drying of herbs in solar greenhouse dryer with integrated heat pump. *Drying Technology* **35**: 1721–1732.

Tham, T.C., Ng, M.X., Gan, S.H. et al. (2018). Impacts of different drying strategies on drying characteristics, the retention of bio-active ingredient and colour changes of dried Roselle. *Chinese Journal of Chemical Engineering* **26**: 303–316.

Vadivambal, R. and Jayas, D.S. (2010). Non-uniform temperature distribution during microwave heating of food materials–a review. *Food and Bioprocess Technology* **3**: 161–171.

Wang, J., Xi, Y.S., and Yu, Y. (2004). Microwave drying characteristics of potato and the effect of different microwave powers on the dried quality of potato. *European Food Research and Technology* **219**: 500–506.

Wang, Y., Zhang, M., Mujumdar, A.S., and Mothibe, K.J. (2013). Microwave-assisted pulse-spouted bed freeze-drying of stem lettuce slices – effect on product quality. *Food and Bioprocess Technology* **6**: 3530–3543.

Wang, J., Chung-Lim Law, C.L., Nema, P.K. et al. (2018). Pulsed vacuum drying enhances drying kinetics and quality of lemon slices. *Journal of Food Engineering* **224**: 129–138.

Won, Y.C., Min, S.C., and Lee, D.U. (2015). Accelerated drying and improved color properties of red pepper by pretreatment of pulsed electric fields. *Drying Technology* **33**: 926–932.

Wray, D. and Ramaswamy, H.S. (2015). Novel concepts in microwave drying of foods. *Drying Technology* **33**: 769–783.

Xie, L., Mujumdar, A.S., Xiao, H.W., and Gao, Z.J. (2016). Recent technologies and trends in medicinal herb drying. In: *Drying Technologies for Foods: Fundamentals & Applications (Part II)* (eds. P.K. Nema, B.P. Kaur and A.S. Mujumdar). New Delhi: New India Publishing Agency.

Yahya, M., Fudholi, A., and Sopian, K. (2017). Energy and exergy analyses of solar-assisted fluidized bed drying integrated with biomass furnace. *Renewable Energy* **105**: 22–29.

Yaldız, O. and Ertekin, C. (2001). Thin layer solar drying of some different vegetables. *Drying Technology* **19**: 583–596.

Zhang, M. and Jiang, H. (2014). Recent food drying R&D at Jiangnan University: an overview. *Drying Technology* **32**: 1743–1750.

Zhang, M., Tang, J., Mujumdar, A.S., and Wang, S. (2006). Trends in microwave-related drying of fruits and vegetables. *Trends in Food Science & Technology* **17**: 524–534.

Zhou, X., Liu, L., Fu, P. et al. (2018). Effects of infrared radiation drying and heat pump drying combined with tempering on the quality of long-grain paddy rice. *International Journal of Food Science and Technology* **53**: 2448–2456.

4
Conventional Extraction Techniques for Bioactive Compounds from Herbs and Spices

Md Abu Bakar Siddique[1], Katerina Tzima[1,2], Dilip K. Rai[2], and Nigel Brunton[1]
[1]*School of Agriculture and Food Science, University College Dublin, Dublin, D04V1W8-4, Ireland*
[2]*Department of Food BioSciences, Teagasc Food Research Centre Ashtown, Dublin, D15 KN3K, Ireland*

4.1 Introduction

Herbs and spices are a recognized source of bioactive compounds of many different chemical classes and with many real and potential applications in foods and medicines. This fact has been recognized for millennia and thus there is a long history of the use of techniques to concentrate the substances responsible for the beneficial effects. The first record of the use of herbs for medicine can be found in Sumerian clay tablets from 4000 years ago, which include descriptions of the use of thyme (*Thymus* spp.) and licorice (*Glycyrrhiza glabra*) for medical applications. This practice then evolved toward the use of concentrates derived from medicinal herbs and some of the earliest techniques used were infusion and decoction; other techniques have evolved from these practices as practitioners recognized that extraction techniques could be designed to target particular groups of medicinal compounds. As outlined in other chapters in this book, extraction techniques have now evolved to the point where recovery of the compound is not only targeted at a particular group of compounds, but also designed to be as efficient as possible through recovering the highest yield while minimizing energy and the use of toxic solvents. Notwithstanding this, the basic principles of a targeted extraction remain the same. First of all, the source material is usually pretreated to physically facilitate release of the target compound from its intracellular location. This step can range from simple maceration to the use of high-voltage electric fields to puncture cell walls. The next step involves choice of a suitable solvent

Herbs, Spices and Medicinal Plants: Processing, Health Benefits and Safety, First Edition.
Edited by Mohammad B. Hossain, Nigel P. Brunton, and Dilip K. Rai.

into which the target compound can partition. This is a crucial step and the choice will not only be dictated by the polarity of the target compound but also by its intended application. For example, the widespread use of food-friendly ethanol for functional food applications. Once an appropriate solvent has been chosen, the next step involves maximizing opportunities for the target compound to partition into it. This can be maximized by ensuring that the solvent penetrates into the solid, dissolves the target compound effectively, and transports it into the solvent. The principles behind this process are described in detail in this chapter in Section 4.2.1; however, in essence, choice of the correct solvent, time for extraction to occur, and extraction temperature are the parameters that most effect yields at this point. The final step involves further concentrating the extract by, for example, partitioning it into another solvent (liquid–liquid extraction, LLE) or absorbing the target compound onto a solid matrix and then releasing it using a smaller volume of suitable solvent (solid phase extraction). The present chapter will concentrate on the first two steps of the extraction process described above and will elucidate some of the fundamental principles which apply.

4.2 Principles of Extraction

Extraction from herbs and spices for their medicinal and flavor-adding value has long been practiced, where the aim is to selectively separate bioactive compounds while maintaining optimum quality and quantity. Selection of the extraction process should be carried out in a manner that allows the extraction of bioactive compounds with maximum efficiency but also with specificity and selectivity to simplify the subsequent separation steps.

The principle of extraction lies in the distribution of a component into two immiscible phases, which further enable the separation and recovery of these compounds. The analyte will be distributed between the two phases according to the distribution constant, temperature, and the relative volumes of the phases. However, the extraction rates are based on the migration kinetics and hence are governed by the temperature and diffusion rate in the two phases (Smith 2003). This book details novel methods for the extraction of bioactives from herbs and spices. These methods have some advantages over conventional techniques in terms of energy efficiency and yields; however, in many cases there are issues with upscaling, capital investment costs, and the technical expertise required to carry them out. Therefore, this chapter examines the use of conventional extraction techniques which benefit from relatively low capital costs, the availability of off-the-shelf systems, and are simple to carry out. Based on the physical state of herbs and spices, conventional extraction processes can be divided into liquid–liquid and solid–liquid extraction (SLE).

4.2.1 Solid–Liquid Extraction

SLE is one of the most widely used methods to extract bioactive compounds from herbs and spices. In this type of extraction, the bioactive compounds physically or chemically bound to the solid matrices must be transferred to the solvent phase by dissolution or desorption. The solute/solvent mixture then diffuses to the solid surface and moves across the interface around the particle to the bulk-liquid phase (Ziaedini

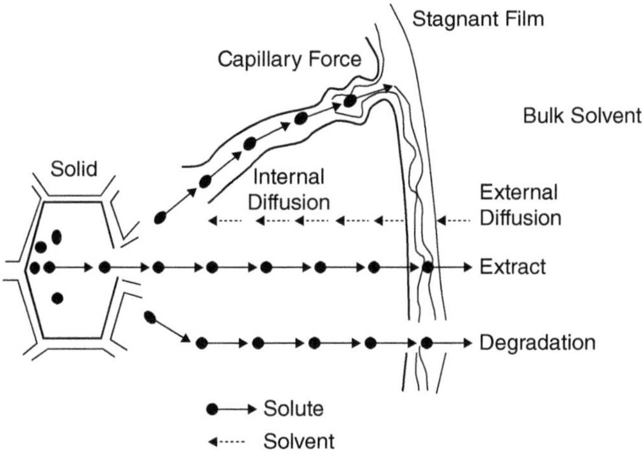

Figure 4.1 Extraction of solute particles from solid matrices by using liquid solvent. *Source:* taken from Aguilera (2003).

et al. 2010). If the extracting solvent is uniformly present on the solid matrix, the material near the surface will be dissolved into the solvent first leaving a porous structure on the solid residue. The solvent then starts to penetrate to the outer layer to reach more deeply bound solutes and the operation becomes progressively more difficult. When the solutes are strongly adsorbed onto the solid matrix, the energy of interaction between the compounds and the solid must be overcome. When the solutes are retained in the plant organic cells, extraction conditions must be severe enough to disrupt the cell to facilitate the extraction process (Camel 2014). Generally, a series of phenomenological steps can occur during the interaction of the solid-containing particle and the solvent (Figure 4.1). Such as:

1. transferring the solvent from the bulk of the solution into the solid matrix;
2. penetration or diffusion of the solvent into the solid surface;
3. dissolution of the solvent into the solute;
4. transport of the solute from the solid matrix to the surface;
5. transferring of the extract from the surface into the bulk solution;
6. separation and discharge of the extract and solid (Aguilera 2003).

According to Raynie (2000), the time progression of the extraction process can be depicted as illustrated in Figure 4.2, where the relationship between extraction yield and progress of extraction (such as solvent volume, time, equilibrium stages, etc.) can be represented by three phases. (i) The initial, steep region, where the phenomena of solute partitioning and solubilization occurs. (ii) This equilibrium phase is then followed by a period where mass transfer resistance begins to operate in the solid–liquid interface; during this period the mass transfer by convection and diffusion is the major phenomenon occurring. (iii) In the last phase, the solute must enter the extracting solvent by overcoming the interaction that binds it to the solid matrices.

The time taken by the bioactive compounds to reach equilibrium is determined by the rate of mass transfer of the solute into the extracting solvent. Transportation

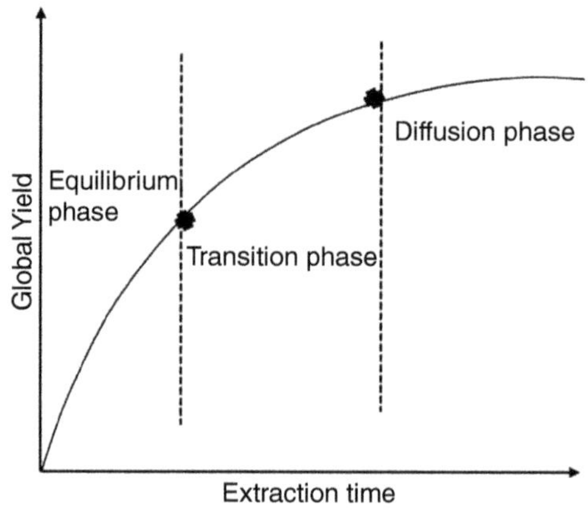

Figure 4.2 Schematic presentation of yield versus time in a model extraction processes. *Source:* adapted from Raynie (2000).

of the solute inside the solid matrix occurs due to the concentration gradient at the solid–liquid interface and can be described by the diffusion Eq. (4.1) below:

$$\frac{N_c}{A_T} = -D\,\frac{dC_c}{dz} \tag{4.1}$$

where N_C is the rate of dissolution of the solute C in the solution (kg/sec), A_T is the area of the solid–liquid interface (m^2), D is the diffusion coefficient (m^2/sec), C_C is the concentration of solute C in the solution (kg/m^3), and z is the distance inside the porous of the solid matrix (m).

The negative sign of the relationship indicates that particle flow occurs from regions of higher concentration to the lower concentrations. Since the mass transfer process in the solid is strongly depend on the size, shape, and presence of pores, the diffusion coefficient (D) is expressed as effective diffusivity D_{eff} (Aguilera 2003; Takeuchi et al. 2008), which is defined as:

$$D_{eff} = \frac{\varepsilon}{\tau}D \tag{4.2}$$

where, ε is the void fraction or porosity of the solid and τ is the tortuosity of the pores. Eq. (4.2) describes the diffusion of the bioactive compounds and solvent mixture occurring inside the solid surface and, finally, the movement of the bioactive particles surrounded by stagnant film to the bulk-liquid phase. However, changes in the concentration and the concentration gradient with time occur in several practical cases. In these situations, Fick's second law can describe how diffusion causes the concentration to change with respect to time. Assuming no change in diffusivity with solute concentration, the rate of diffusion can be described as in Eq. (4.3)

$$\frac{\partial C}{\partial t} = \nabla(D_{eff} - \cdot \nabla C) \tag{4.3}$$

where, C is the concentration of the solute, t is time (s), and D_{eff} is the effective diffusion coefficient or diffusivity, m^2 s^{-1}.

Considering that particles have a spherical shape and concentration differences will only be relevant in one radial (z) direction, the diffusion can be derived as Eq. (4.4):

$$\frac{\partial C}{\partial t} = D_{eff}\frac{\partial^2 C}{\partial z^2} \tag{4.4}$$

SLE can be applied in many different manners and over the decades many subclasses of the technique have been used, including Soxhlet extraction, maceration, infusion or decoction, percolation, and steam distillation or hydro-distillation. The proceeding sections describe some of these techniques and their advantages and disadvantages with respect to extraction of bioactive compounds from herbs and spices. Selection of the specific technique normally depends on the type of materials, desired quality of valuable compounds, expected time to finish the extraction process, and sometimes the viability of the solvents.

4.2.1.1 Soxhlet Extraction The Soxhlet extraction technique is based on the use of the Soxhlet apparatus, which comprises a porous cellulose cell (the thimble), a flask containing the organic solvent, and a reflux condenser on the top of the extractor. When the organic solvent is heated up, the vapor travels through a distillation arm and drips down to the thimble containing the solid sample. Once the extractor is flooded with the condensed solvent, a siphon removes the solvent back to the flask at the bottom. The main feature of this method is the recirculation of the extracting solvent, avoiding possible saturation of the solvent during the maceration step. The technique could be described as a discontinuous solvent infusion and static extraction from the solid materials when the liquid fills the thimble (Camel 2014). The main advantage of this method is its requirement for less quantity of solvent to extract from several plant materials. However, the extraction system requires longer processing and may lack selectivity and induce thermal degradation of targeted molecules. Selection of solvent is another important parameter that should be considered, since optimal extraction of targeted molecules depends on the polarity of solvents. Sometimes, a co-solvent is used to match the polarity of the targeted compounds, which, however, can increase the processing cost. The separation of solvent from the extracted compound is another expensive step and is considered harmful for the environment. Despite these drawbacks, the Soxhlet extraction technique is still frequently used in laboratories due to its simplicity, ability to be used for multiple extractions, and lack of requirement for a filtration step.

4.2.1.2 Maceration Maceration is a very old process where the whole or previously ground plant materials are kept in contact with an appropriate solvent, named as menstruum, for a specified amount of time, from several hours to days for equilibration under ambient temperature. This mixture is frequently agitated until the soluble matter dissolves; afterwards, the marc (damp solid material) is pressed, and finally, the combined liquids are clarified by filtration or decantation after standing. Generally, the purpose of this process is to soften and break plant materials and thereby enhance the solubility of the target phytochemicals in the solid material. Although this process is often considered to be an inefficient process due to the longer time requirement, maceration has found application for extraction of phenolic compounds and antioxidants from plant materials, using solvents such as dichloromethane, ethanol, methanol, water/methanol mixture, and, recently, cyclotides have been extracted using hydrochloric solution (Li et al. 2007; Teixeira and da Costa 2005; Yeshak et al. 2012). Digestion is another type of maceration where gentle heat is applied during the process of extraction.

4.2.1.3 Infusion or Decoction Infusion and decoction adhere to the same extraction principle as maceration; in both techniques the plant material is soaked in cold or boiled water. In comparison to infusion and maceration, the applications of the decoction process lie in extracting heat stable compounds from hard plant materials such as roots and barks, and usually results in oil-soluble compounds (Azwanida 2015). A specified amount of cold or boiling water is added to the milled sample material for short period of time during infusion; while in decoction, the sample is boiled in water for 15–30 minutes.

These techniques are used for several extraction processes, such as the extraction of medicinal compounds from herbs or tea. Li et al. (2007) also reported that the traditional decoction process could be effectively used for the extraction of antioxidants from plant matrices.

4.2.1.4 Percolation Percolation is a process that uses a percolator where the solvent is added slowly onto the powdered solid matrices. The solvent absorbs the soluble compounds and drips out through the filtered bottom of the container. The percolation process is normally continued at moderate rate (e.g. six drops per minute) until the extraction is completed and later evaporation is used to concentrate the extracts (Azwanida 2015; Rathi et al. 2006). The main advantage of percolation is the shorter processing time, greater flexibility, and in some cases exhaustive extraction of the compounds. However, this process is not considered a feasible one for some herbs.

4.2.1.5 Hydro-distillation and Steam Distillation The hydro-distillation process uses water as a solvent. The mechanism of hydro-distillation is similar to the Soxhlet extraction, where the mixture of sample material and water is placed in a retort and heat is applied to vaporize the mixture. This process is normally used to separate volatile and non-volatile molecules, such as essential oils, from aromatic plants. Hot water facilitates the movement of compounds from the plant material by rupturing the plant tissues. The mixture is then condensed and after separating substances in a separator, the water is reused. This process has the advantage of using no expensive solvents (only water); however, its use is limited due to the longer time requirement leading to thermal degradation of some valuable compounds. On the other hand, the technique of steam distillation employs the passing of steam through the plant materials directly. A combination of heated steam and gentle pressure allows the essential oils to be released from the plant matrices. Different combinations of time, temperature, and pressure are used depending on the plant materials.

4.2.2 Liquid–Liquid Extraction

The LLE technique is commonly applied to partition a target analyte from a liquid phase to another liquid phase. The technique can be useful because of its operational simplicity and the availability of a wide range of suitable organic solvents. The principle of LLE is that the compound to be extracted partitions between two immiscible phases (Figure 4.3). One phase is normally aqueous and the other phase is an organic

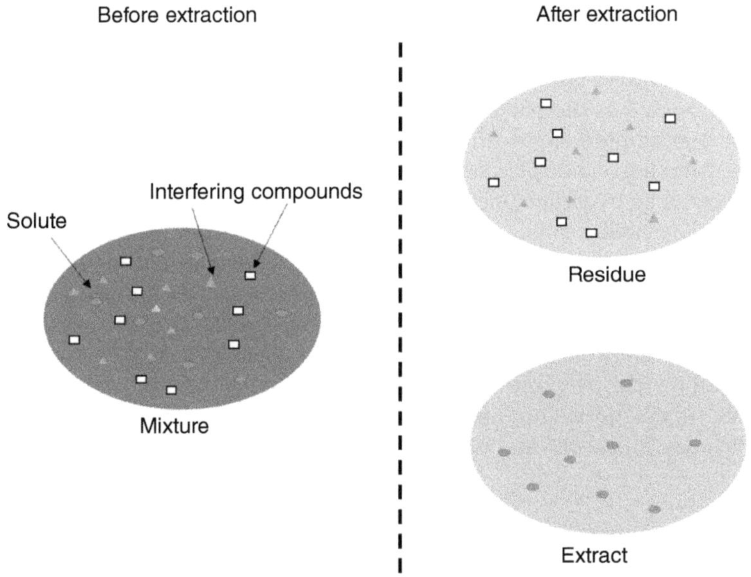

Figure 4.3 Schematic diagram of liquid–liquid extraction technique.

solvent, in which the sample and matrix have different solubilities. The basic steps of LLE are as follows.

1. Uniform mixing of two immiscible phases.
2. Making contact between the feed and the extraction solvent.
3. Performing a selective transfer of the desired compound from one phase to other.
4. Allowing the separation of the two resulting phases.
5. Recovery of the solvent from each phase (Mandal et al. 2015).

The movement of a particular compound from one phase to another is generally governed and driven by the thermodynamic forces or electrochemical potential for an ionic species. The distribution coefficient or partition coefficient and the distribution ratio are two parameters normally used to describe the distribution of a component between two immiscible solvents.

The movement of the chemical species continues until equilibrium is reached, where the ratio of the concentration of a component (i) in the organic phase (C_{i0}) to that in the aqueous phase (C_{ia}) is given by equilibrium distribution coefficient (K_i) as,

$$K_i = C_{i0}/C_{ia} \tag{4.5}$$

On the other hand, the distribution ratio of the target compounds between the solvents is defined as the ratio of the total analytical concentration of the substance in the organic layer to its total analytical concentration in the aqueous phase.

Since herbs and spices are solids, LLE is not used for the initial extraction of target molecules from these matrices. Rather, the technique has found application for concentration target molecules following an initial SLE; for example, to partition compounds with low polarity into an organic solvent from an aqueous extract.

4.3 Factors Affecting Extraction

Section 4.2 describes in detail the fundamental principles which operate when attempting to extract a target compound using a variety of techniques. These underlying principles have served as the basis for a very large number of studies over many decades which have attempted to identify the best conditions for the recovery of a particular bioactive from herb and spice sources. Therefore, the aim of the present section is to give the reader an overview of recent studies which have identified optimal conditions for isolating particular bioactives using conventional techniques. The information will not only be of use to readers interested in using conventional methods for isolating bioactives from herbs and spices, but also to those with an interest in methods which use cell disruption techniques to facilitate release of intracellular compounds, as these require a subsequent step in which the principles of conventional extraction determine the extraction yield. The following sections divide conventional extraction techniques into three subcategories and outline, describe, and critically evaluate recent studies which have identified optimal condition for the recovery of particular bioactives.

4.3.1 Solid–Liquid Extraction

SLE is one of the most widely used methods to extract valuable compounds from herbs and spices. This process is commonly used in the food, medicinal, and aromatic industries to obtain important substances such as carotenoids or flavonoids. A great number of studies have been carried out to optimize extraction of pure compounds or standardized extracts followed by analysis of these extracts for their bioactive properties, which are suitable for applications in the food and pharmaceutical industries. Yields of target compounds are unsurprisingly a factor of the type of herb or spice on which the extraction was carried out. For example, Hinneburg et al. (2006) determined the total phenolic and antioxidant activities of hydro-distilled extracts from basil, laurel, parsley, juniper, aniseed, cumin, cardamom, and ginger. These authors found the highest antioxidant activities from the extract of basil and laurel, while the total phenols expressed as gallic acid equivalents were found in the order: basil > laurel > cumin > fennel. Wojdylo et al. (2007) carried out a similar study on the ground dried plant material from 32 herbs of 21 botanical families grown in Poland and showed that highest level of phenolics was found in *Echinacea purpurea,* while the lowest was in *Carum carvi.* These authors also reported that total phenolic contents of the six spices decreased in the following order: balm > sage > horehound > rosemary > thyme > oregano. High-performance liquid chromatography (HPLC) determination showed that the highest levels of the most abundant phenolic compounds (mainly caffeic acid and neochlorogenic acid) were found in the leaves of *Tanacetum vulgare* (1700 mg/100 g dw), *Melissa officinalis* (969 mg/100 g dw), *Lithospermum. officinale* (630 mg/100 g dw), and *Thymus vulgaris* (607 mg/100 g dw). It has been reported that differences in the quantities of phenolic compounds were likely due to genotypic and environmental differences (namely, climate, location, temperature, fertility, diseases, and pest exposure) within species, choice of parts tested, time of taking samples, and determination methods (Kim and Lee 2004; Shan et al. 2005).

Furthermore, the phenolic and antioxidant activities of an aqueous extract of dried powder of garlic, ginger, and cayenne pepper were evaluated by Otunola and Afolayan (2013). Results demonstrated that all the extracts from the spices possessed a high content of phenolics, flavonoids, flavanols, and proanthocyanidins, with the pepper extract having higher amounts of each polyphenol investigated. In another study, Howard et al. (2000) reported that the methanolic extract (50%) of the pepper fruit contained a high level of L-ascorbic acid and carotenoids including carotenoids such as β-cryptoxanthin, α-carotene, β-carotene, capsanthin, and zeaxanthin at maturity. On the other hand, the hot water extracts of 13 different spices used in meat processing showed clove having the highest phenolic content (108.28 μg catechin equivalent/g), while the total flavonoids varied from 324.08 μg quercetin equivalent/g for thyme to 3.38 μg quercetin equivalent/g for coriander. The antioxidant properties of the abovementioned polyphenols are assumed due to their redox properties, which allows them to act as a reducing agents, hydrogen donors, metal chelators, and single oxygen quenchers. Many of the beneficial activities – such as anti-inflammatory, antiallergenic, antiviral, antithrombotic, anticarcinogenic, and antimicrobial effects – of polyphenols from herbs and spice extracts are believed to be due their free radical scavenging and antioxidant activity (Soobrattee et al. 2005). For example, the ethanolic (80–96%, v/v) extracts of a range of finely ground spice powders extracted for 1 to 4 days at 10 °C to room temperature were assayed for their antimicrobial activities against *Escherichia coli, Klebsiella pneumoniae, Pseudomonas aeruginosa, Staphylococcus aureus, Bacillus subtilis, Pseudomonas fluorescens, Salmonella typhi,* and fungal strains of *Candida albicans* and *Rhizopus zygospores* (Baljeet et al. 2015; Siddhartha et al. 2017). Results showed that extracts from cinnamon, garlic, tamarind, and clove displayed significant antimicrobial activity (80–94%); however, the severity of the effect against bacteria varied depending on the types of extract used (Siddhartha et al. 2017). The impact of spice and herb extracts on microbial activity not only depended on the types of extracts but also the types of microbials used in the analysis. In this context, while the research work done by Chan et al. (2018) described the higher susceptibility of gram positive bacteria (*Bacillus cereus* and *S. aureus*) to applied extracts than that of the gram negative bacteria (*E. coli* and *Salmonella typhimurium*), contradictory results asserting that gram negative bacteria were more sensitive than gram positive were reported by Baljeet et al. (2015).

Many factors, such as extraction time, temperature, solid material to solvent ratio, type of solvent, pH, and particle size of herb and spice materials can influence the extraction yields as well as their bioactive potentiality. Akkol et al. (2008) reported that the values of total phenolic contents of sage varied from 2830 to 21 230 mg per 100 g of extracts, depending on the types of solvent used, where the highest amount of phenolic compounds was observed in 50% methanol extracts, followed by pure methanol, ethyl acetate, and *n*-hexane extracts, respectively. Working with commonly used herbs and spices, Do et al. (2014) showed that extraction yields of phytochemicals decreased in the following order: 50% aqueous acetone >50% aqueous ethanol >75% aqueous methanol >50% aqueous methanol >75% aqueous acetone >75% aqueous ethanol >100% methanol > RO water >100% ethanol >100% acetone. It has also been reported that the extraction yield of pure methanol is higher than that of pure ethanol (and pure acetone, showing the increase of extraction yield of *Limnophila aromatica* with increasing polarity of the solvent used in extraction). Similarly, Dent et al. (2013) reported that binary solvent systems are more efficient in extracting polyphenols from sage than mono-solvent systems. However, these authors have reported a comparable yield between the extractions carried out with 30% ethanol or acetone with that of the distilled water at a higher temperature and longer extraction period. Moreover, solvents such as acetone (80%), ethanol (80%), methanol (80%), and distilled water were used to extract phenolic compounds from ground powders of rhizome of turmeric, inflorescence of torch ginger, leaves of lemon grass, and leaves of curry leaf (Sepahpour et al. 2018). While 80% acetone was shown to be the most efficient solvent for the extraction of total phenolic compounds from turmeric, torch ginger, and lemon grass (221.68, 98.10, and 28.19 mg GA/g dw, respectively), for the recovery of phenolic compounds from curry leaf (92.23 mg GA/g dw), 80% ethanol was the most appropriate solvent. Furthermore, the extraction yield from the solid materials can also vary depending on the liquid to solid ratio. Maintaining a suitable liquid to solid ratio is important, since a lower ratio can produce extracts with reduced bioactive compounds, while a higher ratio can result in a loss of valuable solvents. Mohamad et al. (2010) found an increase of solvent to raw material ratio beyond 5 : 1 did not have any significant impact on the yield of *Eurycoma longifolia*. Similarly, Fan et al. (2015) reported that total flavonoids and total phenolic contents extracted from asparagus residues (*Asparagus officinalis* L.) were firstly increased with the increasing liquid to solid ratio and then decreased. Since the mass transfer was primarily related to the solid interior, greater volumes of solvent could hardly increase the amount of extraction. However, the increased yield at the beginning could be due to the enhanced mass transfer of the solutes to the bulk solvent.

Although high temperature is assumed to increase the global extraction yield from herbs and spices, extreme conditions are normally avoided to circumvent any harmful effect on the biological activity of the extracts. For example, Chen et al. (1985) found that high temperature (100 °C and 20 minutes) completely removed the antimicrobial activities of extracts obtained from the core and the outer layers of onion, the white and the green parts of green onion, garlic bulb, ginger, ginger root, sweet pepper, chili pepper, brown pepper, and mustard. Other evidence of lowering antioxidant activity of garlic bulbs from 60 to 100 °C has been mentioned by Yin and Cheng (1998). Moreover, it has been observed that the content of total polyphenol-rich extract from wild sage (*Salvia officinalis* L.) obtained at 60 °C and 90 °C with 30% and 50% ethanol decreased during a longer period of extraction. According to Fick's second law, after a certain period of extraction a final equilibrium between the solute concentration in the solid material and in the bulk solution is reached and after this point a longer period of time is not considered to be a useful parameter for increasing the production yield. Ziaedini et al. (2010) investigated the effects of temperature (50, 60, 70, 80, 90 °C) and time (5, 10, 20, 40, 80 minutes) on catechins and caffeine solubility in water from Iranian green tea. The best combinations of temperature and time extraction with water were 20–40 minutes and 80 °C for epigallocatechin, epicatechin, and caffeine; and 80 minutes and 90 °C for catechin, epicatechin gallate, and epigallocatechin gallate. Particle size can also influence the amount of bioactive extraction from herbs and spices. In this context, Borhan et al. (2013) reported water extraction from the dried and grinded powder in nanoparticles of *Centella asiatica* L. had almost a 50% higher extraction yield with 7.09 mg/g as compared to the microparticles. Similarly, Durling et al. (2007) mentioned that the bioactive compound extraction from sage decreased with increasing particle size from 1 to 3 mm due to the decreasing diffusion of hydroalcoholic solvent into the solid particle, and the limitation of solvent–solute diffusion out of the particles. These authors also recommended a moderate temperature (up to 40 °C) and extraction time (no longer than 3 hours) to avoid the vaporization of volatile essential oil components and potential loss of solvent by vaporization. Ereifej et al. (2016) determined the extract from 10 different spices from the local market of Jordan (*Syzygium aromaticum* L., *Coriandrum sativum* L., *Cuminum cyminum* L., *Zingiber officinale* Rosc., *Elettaria cardamomum, Curcuma longa, Rhus coriaria* L., *Cinnamomum zeylanicum* Blume, *Foeniculum vulgare* Mill, and *Laurus nobilis* L.) by using ethanol, methanol, and acetone at various temperatures such as 20, 40, and 60 °C. The results showed that at 60 °C the highest amount of total phenolics was obtained from cloves using all three solvents (Table 4.1).

4.3.2 Liquid–Liquid Extraction

In LLE different solvents are used depending on the types of bioactive compound to be separated especially from the crude extracts of herbs and spices. Alcohols, acetone, and ethyl acetate are common solvents for extracting polar compounds. Fewer polar compounds can be extracted by mixtures of alcohol–water as well as non-polar solvents such as chloroform or hexane. LLE is generally used to selectively isolate and purify the bioactive compounds obtained from crude liquid extracts of solid herbs and spices. For instance, Kumaran and Karunakaran (2007) used LLE with ethyl acetate, hexane, or aqueous fractions to identify the 2,2-diphenyl-1-picrylhydrazyl (DPPH) free radical scavenging components from the defatted crude SLE extract of *Coleus aromaticus*. Strong DPPH radical-scavenging activity (*in vitro*) was shown only by the ethyl acetate phase, when compared with water and hexane phases. Being the major polyphenol in *C. aromaticus,* rosmarinic acid was most likely to be responsible for most of the observed antioxidant activity. Similarly, methanolic extracts from the aerial parts of *Ballota nigra, Lamium maculatum, Leonurus cardiaca, Marrubium vulgare,* and *Galeopsis tetrahit* were subsequently partitioned by LLE between petroleum ether, dichloromethane, ethyl acetate, or *n*-butanol (Matkowski et al. 2008). These authors mentioned that LLE with polar solvents such as ethyl acetate or *n*-butanol can significantly improve the antioxidant potential in some cases and therefore can provide hints for using certain solvents for herbal preparations. The phenolic and non-phenolic fraction of a chloroform extract of pulverized oregano were separated using LLE methods. Oregano extract and fractions were tested for antioxidant activity as well as antimicrobial activity on *E. coli, S. aureus,* and *B. cereus*. Fractions with intermediate polarity showed the highest antimicrobial effect, while the antimicrobial effect decreased with the increasing polarity of the fraction. In one study, Gherman et al. (2000) studied the qualitative analysis of main bioactive volatile compounds such as menthol, menthone, isomenthone, 1,8-cineole, menthyl acetate, limonene, β-myrcene, and carvone by using gas chromatography in the extracts prepared by the liquid–liquid method from seven different peppermint samples. Furthermore, Wang et al. (2013) used LLE to isolate and purify resveratrol from an aqueous suspension of *Polygonum cuspidatum* using four different solvents systems, namely: ethyl acetate, ethyl acetate : petroleum ether (1 : 1), petroleum ether, and methyl tert-butyl ether. Methyl tert-butyl ether showed the highest extraction of resveratrol (92.6% ± 9.2%) followed by ethyl acetate : petroleum ether (91.7% ± 6.5%), ethyl acetate (81.8% ± 7.3%), and petroleum ether (10.6% ± 4.3%). To obtain volatile extracts from the distillate (steam distilled at 55 °C for 3 hours, 95 mm Hg) of thyme, basil, rosemary, chamomile, lavender, cinnamon, and clove, Lee and Shibamoto (2001, 2002) used a continuous LLE system. Results showed that all the extracts demonstrated dose-dependent inhibitory activity between the

Table 4.1 Bioactive compounds extracted from herbs and spices by using solid–liquid extraction techniques

Herbs and spices	Extraction method and types of solvents	Mentioned bioactive compounds	Biological Activities	Reference
Mexican oregano	Hydro-distillation, maceration and separated by liquid–liquid extraction by Ethanol and Ethyl acetate.	Methylmaleic anhydride, thymoquinone, thymol, carvacrol, thymol acetate, carvacrol acetate, and phenolic acids	Antimicrobial and antioxidant activities	Cid-Perez et al. (2019)
Turmeric, curry leaf, torch ginger, and lemon grass extracts	Solid-liquid extraction with 80% acetone, 80% ethanol, 80% methanol	Phenolic compounds	Antioxidant activity	Sepahpour et al. (2018)
Oregano	Solid extraction by 80% methanol	Polyphenols	Cellular antioxidant activity and *in vitro* inhibition of α-glucosidase, α-amylase and pancreatic lipase	Gutierrez-Grijalva et al. (2019)
Ocimum gratissimum leaves	Extraction from dried leaves with water and ethanol	Polyphenolic extract	Anticolitis effects	Alabi et al. (2018)
Matricaria chamomilla	Hydro distillation, maceration (aqueous ethanolic solution) and Soxhlet extraction (*n*-hexane)	Umbelliferone and herniarin	Antioxidant activity	Molnar et al. (2017)
Ginger (*Zingiber officinale*)	Extraction from the powder by distilled water, 70% ethanol, diethyl ether, ethyl acetate, and n-butanol	6-gingerol, 6-shogaol, and 6-paradol	Antioxidant, anti-inflammatory, and xanthine oxidase inhibitory activities	S. H. Nile and Park (2015)

Cumin, ginger, garlic	Ethanolic extracts	—	Antimicrobial activity	Baljeet et al. (2015)
Garlic (*Allium sativum*), pepper (*Piper nigrum*), and bird chili (*Capsicum frutescens*)	Extraction with hot water, ethanol	Phenolic and flavonoid components	Antioxidant and antimicrobial activities	Kittisakulnam et al. (2017)
Garlic, ginger, and cayenne pepper	Aqueous extraction	Phenolics, flavonoids, flavonols, and proanthocyanidins	Antioxidant activities	Otunola and Afolayan (2013)
Oregano, lavender, curly leaved parsley, fennel, paprika	Extraction form areal dried parts with acetone	—	Anticancer activity	Berrington and Lall (2012)
Fenugreek, mustard, and henna	Aqueous extraction	—	Antimicrobial activity tested on gram-negative and gram-positive bacteria	Das et al. (2012)
Rosmarinus officinalis L.	Steam distillation	Essential oils	Antimicrobial and anticancer activity	Wang et al. (2012)
Dried clove buds	Steam distillation	Eugenol, eugenyl acetate, and benzyl alcohol	Antioxidant property	Lee and Shibamoto (2001)

concentrations (10–500 μg/ml) and antioxidant activity. The inhibitory effect of the extracts on formation of hexanoic acid was in the following descending order: thyme > basil > rosemary > chamomile > lavender and cinnamon.

Analysis of the impact of different solvents on isolating and purifying resveratrol from an aqueous suspension of *P. cuspidatum* was carried out by using four different solvents: ethyl acetate, ethyl acetate : petroleum ether (1 : 1), petroleum ether, and methyl tert-butyl ether. Methyl tert-butyl ether showed the highest extraction of resveratrol (92.6% ± 9.2%) followed by ethyl acetate : petroleum ether (91.7% ± 6.5%), ethyl acetate (81.8% ± 7.3%), and petroleum ether (10.6 ± 4.3%) (Wang and Lin 2013). The recovery of organic acids from the black liquor of *Typha latifolia* pulp prior to the bioethanol fermentation process showed that a lower pH and temperature gave the highest yield for the LLE (Kim et al. 2016). Experimental results and fitted models showed the optimum extraction conditions of LLE were at pH 1 and 25 °C, while the reaction time had no effect on the extraction.

4.3.3 Soxhlet Extraction

Soxhlet extraction of bioactive compounds from herbs and spices is a long established practice, which is useful to apply when the bioactive compounds from a material have limited solubility into a particular solvent. Although this method needs a large volume of organic solvent and a long extraction time, Soxhlet extraction is frequently used for extracting valuable compounds from plant material due to its reputation for providing complete extraction in comparison with the other conventional techniques. However, this reputation is not always deserved as the longer exhaustive extraction times frequently do not result in higher yields of the target compounds than other conventional methods. For example, Molnar et al. (2017) reported that extraction yields obtained from *Matricaria chamomilla* with supercritical CO_2 (1.57 ± 0.11 g/100 g) were more comparable to the yield obtained with *n*-hexane in Soxhlet apparatus (4.6 ± 0.24 g/100 g); however, maceration using 50% ethanol, provided a much higher extraction yield (20.85 ± 0.44 g/100 g) of the desired compounds. The extracts prepared using Soxhlet methods also demonstrated lower antioxidant activity than those of the supercritical CO_2. Similarly, Bimakr et al. (2011) compared conventional Soxhlet extraction from dried and ground spearmint leaves with the supercritical CO_2 extraction and showed that Soxhlet extraction has a higher crude extraction yield (257.67 mg/g) than the other (60.57 mg/g). However, the supercritical CO_2 extract was found to contain more representatives of the main flavonoid compounds (seven bioactive flavonoids) at high concentrations compared to the 70% ethanol Soxhlet extraction (five bioactive flavonoids). Comparing the results with four different solvents, the authors pointed out that the highest extraction yield (267.3 mg/g) was found with methanol extraction followed closely by ethanol 70% extraction (257.6 mg/g). The lowest extraction yield was obtained by using petroleum ether (30.4 mg/g). Sagun et al. (2006) also investigated the antimicrobial activity of Soxhlet extracts from some herbs in methanol, ethanol, *n*-hexane, and water against *Listeria monocytogenes* Serovars and found that the methanolic extracts demonstrated higher antimicrobial activity than ethanol and *n*-hexane extracts. Similar to the solvent type, in Soxhlet-type extractions solvent volume can also influence the amount of extraction yield. For instance, Chuichulcherm et al. (2013) stated that the amount of capsaicinoids increased (6.6%) when the ethanol volume increased (50%). Furthermore, Jaiswal and Naik (2018) reported that traditional Soxhlet extraction of the antioxidant compound 6-gingerol from *Z. officinale* resulted in a higher yield (3.85%) than supercritical CO_2 based extraction (2.41%). Although the compound 6-gingerol was found to be higher (389 mg/g) in supercritical CO_2 than in Soxhlet, extracts from *Z. officinale* exhibited higher amounts of total phenol and flavonoid contents. Soxhlet extraction of cinnamon by methanol displayed remarkable inhibition (*in vitro*) on both yeast and mammalian α-glucosidase suggesting the presence of potential enzyme inhibiting compounds in the extract (Shihabudeen et al. 2011). Wong et al. (2014), on the other hand, reported lower amounts (62–73%) of cinnamaldehyde in essential oil from Soxhlet extracts of *C. zeylanicum* than that from steam distillation (90%). Several other authors have reported the antimicrobial activity of extracts from clove, ajowan, cinnamon, *Allium vineale, Chaerophyllum macropodum, Prangos ferulacea, Schisandra chinensis* Baill. seeds, cumin (*C. cyminum*), fenugreek (*Trigonella foenum-graecum*), cloves (*S. aromaticum*), cardamom (*E. cardamomum* Maton), and black pepper (*Piper nigrum*) against different bacterial strains such as *L. monocytogenes* serovars, *E. coli, S. aureus, S. typhi, B. cereus 882,* and enterococci using Soxhlet extraction with solvents such as ethanol, *n*-hexane, methanol, and acetone (Mohamad et al. 2010; Revati et al. 2015; Sagun et al. 2006; Teng and Lee 2014). These studies revealed the highest antimicrobial effect of ethanolic extracts from cinnamon and garlic against enterococcal strains, methanolic extracts of *A. vineale* against *L. monocytogenes*, while the lowest or no antimicrobial effect was found from ethanol extracts of fenugreek, cardamom, and the water extracts of selected Turkish herbs (*A. vineale, C. macropodum,* and *P. ferulacea*) against the selected microbial strains.

Similar to other extraction methods, the extraction yield in Soxhlet extraction also varies depending on the extraction time, temperature, and the size of the sample materials. For instance, Umamaheshwari and Reddy (2016) obtained a maximum oil yield of 51% at 100 °C for an extraction time of 150 minutes using 15 g of dried bitter gourd seeds and 50 ml of *n*-hexane. On the other hand, Alara et al. (2018) reported that the highest yield of extract (10.01% ± 0.85% w/w), total phenolic content (53.96 ± 1.45 mg GAE/g dw), and total flavonoid content (30.09 ± 0.44 mg QE/g dw) were achieved from *Veronica cinerea* leaves using an extraction time of two hours, solid-to-solvent of 1 : 20 g/ml, and ethanol concentration of 60% v/v. Optimal conditions for extraction of ginger oil from fresh ginger using acetone in Soxhlet extraction were reported to be 80 °C for 60 minutes (Kanadea and Bhatkhandeb 2016). While using ethanol as a solvent, Azian et al. (2014) showed that during the first two hours the concentrations of ginger bioactive compounds extracts (6-, 8-, 10-gingerols and 6-shogaol) were relatively low once the ginger matrix was saturated with the solvent; the amount of bioactive compounds for the next six hours increased, with the highest concentrations discernible at eight hours. It has been assumed that higher temperatures and finer particle sizes of the sample materials enhance the extraction yield. Although the finer particle sizes offer a greater surface area for mass transfer, Baldosano et al. (2015) stated that similar to the larger particle size, the finer particles also could hinder the extraction process of *Spondias purpurea* bark due to the formation of agglomerates. Therefore, a suitable particle size was recommended that can enhance the mass transfer of the bioactive compounds and yet prevents agglomeration (Table 4.2).

Table 4.2 Recent examples of using conventional Soxhlet extraction technique for extracting bioactive compounds from herbs and spices and their biological activities

Herbs and spices	Extraction method and types of solvents	Mentioned bio-active compounds	Biological Activities	Reference
Moringa peregrina	Soxhlet extraction using *n*-hexane	Phenolic compounds	Antioxidant activity	Mohammadpour et al. (2019)
Capparis spinosa L. from Lipari Island	Soxhlet extraction with 60% methanol in water	Phenolic and flavonoid compounds	Radical scavenging and reductive activities	Mollica et al. (2019)
Leaves of *Vernonia amygdalina* (VA) and *Ocimum gratissimum* (OG)	Soxhlet extraction and cold maceration with 80% methanol	—	Anti-diabetic efficiencies	Okoduwa et al. (2016)
Paprika oleoresins	Conventional Soxhlet extraction with hexane	Paprika pigments and α-tocopherol	Anticancer activity and free radical scavenging	Saponjac et al. (2014)
Japanese pepper, cardamom, and fennel seeds	Conventional Soxhlet extraction by ethanol	Hydrocarbon, Alcohol, Carbonyl compounds, acid, ester, ketone	Antiradical efficiencies	Leblebici et al. (2012)
Cinnamon bark	Soxhlet extraction with methanol	Tannins, flavonoids, glycosides, terpenoids, coumarins, and anthraquinones	Inhibitory activity against yeast α-glucosidase and rat-intestinal α-glucosidase	Shihabudeen et al. (2011)
Cinnamomum tamala	Soxhlet extraction with petroleum ether	eugenol and α-caryophyllene	antitumor and anti-angiogenic activity	Thanekar et al. (2016)
Ximenia americana	Soxhlet extraction with chloroform, ethyl acetate, methanol, ethanol, and water.	phenolic compounds, flavonoids, tannins, and glycosides	*in vitro* antioxidant and anti-inflammatory activities	Shettar et al. (2015)
Indian medicinal and aromatic plant	Extraction with ethanol	—	Antitumor, and enzyme inhibitory activity	Nile et al. (2017)

4.4 Optimized Extraction Techniques for Herbs and Spices

In recent years, a limited number of studies have been focused on the optimization of extraction techniques (conventional and subcritical water extraction [SWE]) from different herbs and spices as summarized in Table 4.3. In many studies, the Box–Behnken experimental design and/or the response surface methodology (RSM) constituted the model for optimizing the different extraction techniques (Majeed et al. 2016; Ramírez-Godínez et al. 2017; Pavlić et al. 2016; Zeković et al. 2016; Ahmadian-Kouchaksaraie et al. 2016).

Majeed et al. (2016) have optimized phenolic extraction from oregano (*Origanum vulgare*) leaves through a conventional SLE process aided by RSM (Table 4.3). Their results revealed that the antioxidant yield of antioxidant extract was significantly influenced by parameters such as time, solute-to-solvent ratio, and solvent consistency. Ramírez-Godínez et al. (2017) optimized conventional solid–liquid of antioxidant from ginger (*Z. officinale*), where temperature was shown to be the critical parameter for the extraction of antioxidant compounds, unlike sample amount and time.

Studies have shown that SWE is both an environmentally friendly and efficient method for the recovery of phenolic compounds from the byproducts of herbs and spices (Ahmadian-Kouchaksaraie et al. 2016; Pavlić et al. 2016). The results from these studies have shown that SWE leads to significant benefits regarding polyphenolic yield and in a considerably shorter time when compared to maceration. The same extraction technique was also applied by Vladić et al. (2017) and optimized for the polyphenol extraction from winter savory (*Satureja montana* L.). The authors have also concluded that SWE resulted in significant improvement of the extract based on the increased levels of total phenols, total flavonoids, and their antioxidant capacity (Table 4.3). Zeković et al. (2016) have extracted polyphenols and EO of coriander (*C. sativum* L.) seed simultaneously using SWE with improved total extraction yield and polyphenols. In this case, the optimization of the total volatile content through RSM was not possible based on the dissimilarity among the observed results and the second-order polynomial model. Therefore, it was established that the total volatile fraction and polyphenols could be co-extracted at the optimal conditions for polyphenols (100.5 °C, 87.6 bar, 10 minutes), as the maximum content of EO was attained at 100 °C, 60 bar, and 10 minutes.

4.5 Conclusion

Due to the long history of the use of herbs and spices in medicinal and culinary applications a huge repository of information on this topic is available in peer-reviewed sources. The present chapter has attempted to describe in a ground up manner the basic scientific principles which govern the conventional extraction process, while also giving an overview of recent work in the area. This information is of value not only to readers interested in using conventional methods but also those interested in techniques which are essentially a hybrid of conventional and novel methods. In the process of compiling this chapter it has become apparent to the authors that in many cases other authors have failed to take into account some of the fundamental principles governing extraction of target compounds from herbs and spices and have thus been

Table 4.3 Estimated optimal conventional extraction parameters for maximum (poly)phenol recovery from herbs and spices

Herbs species	Conditions tested	Activity determination	Optimal conditions	Reference
Origanum vulgare L.	**Solvent**: Methanol : Water **Solvent ratio**: 90 : 10, 80 : 20, 70 : 30 (ml/ml) **Solute** : **Solvent ratio**: 1 : 5, 1 : 12.5, 1 : 20 (g/ml) **Time**: 4,10,16 (h) **Particle Size**: 20, 65, 110 (μm)	Total phenolics (TP) 2,2-Diphenyl-1-picrylhydrazyl Free Radical Assay (DPPH)	**Solvent ratio**: 70 : 30 ml/ml **Solute** : **Solvent**: 1 : 20 g/ml **Extraction time**: 16 h **Solute particle size**: 20 μm	Majeed et al. (2016)
Zingiber officinale	**Solvent**: Water *Box-Behnken experimental design* **Temperature**: 20, 55, 90 (°C) **Time**: 5, 15, 25 (min) **Sample quantity**: 2, 6, 10 (g/100 ml)	TP DPPH Ferric Reducing Antioxidant Power Assay (FRAP)	**Temperature**: 90 °C **Time**: 15 min **Sample quantity**: 2 g/100 ml	Ramírez-Godínez et al. (2017)
Subcritical water extraction (SWE) on *Salvia officinalis* L. by-products	**Solvent**: HCl: Water *Box–Behnken experimental design* **Solvent ratio**: 0 : 100, 0.75 : 99.25, 1.50 : 98.5 (ml/ml) **Temperature**: 120, 170, 220 (°C) **Time**: 10, 20, 30 (min)	TP Total flavonoids (TF) DPPH Trolox equivalent antioxidant capacity Assay (TEAC) Reducing Power Assay	**Solvent concentration**: 0% **Temperature**: 201.5 °C **Time**: 15.8 min	Pavlić et al. (2016)

SWE on *Coriandrum sativum* L.	**Solvent**: Water *Box–Behnken experimental design* **Temperature**: 100, 150, 200 (°C) **Pressure**: 30, 60, 90 (bar) **Extraction time**: 10, 20, 30 (min)	TP Total extraction yield (Y) Total volatile compounds (TVCs)	*For TP*: **Temperature**: 100.5 °C **Pressure**: 87.6 bar **Extraction time**: 10 min *For Y*: **Temperature**: 180.5 °C **Pressure**: 35.1 bar **Extraction time**: 10.8 min *For TVC*: **Temperature**: 100 °C **Pressure**: 60 bar **Extraction time**: 10 min	Zeković et al. (2016)
SWE on *Crocus sativus* petals of saffron industry residues	**Solvent:** Water *Box–Behnken experimental design* **Water-to-solid ratio**: 20, 40, 60 (ml/g) **Temperature**: 120, 140, 160 (°C) **Time**: 20, 40, 60 (min)	TP TF DPPH FRAP	**Water to solid (W/S) ratio**: 36 ml/g **Temperature**: 159 °C **Time**: 54 min	Ahmadian-Kouchaksaraie et al. (2016)
SWE on *Satureja montana* L.	**Solvent:** Water *Box–Behnken experimental design* **Temperature**: 79.15, 100, 150, 200, 220.5 (°C) **Time**: 5.9, 10, 20, 30, 34.1 (min)	TP DPPH	**Temperature**: 200 °C **Time**: 20.8 min	Vladić et al. (2017)

unable to recommend the best conditions to extract them. Thus, readers are counseled to always be mindful of underlying factors governing an extraction process they are attempting to develop.

References

Aguilera, J.M. (2003). Solid-liquid extraction. In: *Extraction Optimization in Food Engineering* (eds. C. Tzia and G. Liadakis), 51–70. New York, NY: CRC Press.

Ahmadian-Kouchaksaraie, Z., Niazmand, R., and Najafi, M.N. (2016). Optimization of the subcritical water extraction of phenolic antioxidants from *Crocus sativus* petals of saffron industry residues: Box-Behnken design and principal component analysis. *Innovative Food Science & Emerging Technologies* **36**: 234–244.

Akkol, E.K., Goger, F., Kosar, M., and Baser, K.H.C. (2008). Phenolic composition and biological activities of Salvia halophila and Salvia virgata from Turkey. *Food Chemistry* **108** (3): 942–949. https://doi.org/10.1016/j.foodchem.2007.11.071.

Alabi, Q.K., Akomolafe, R.O., Omole, J.G. et al. (2018). Polyphenol-rich extract of *Ocimum gratissimum* leaves ameliorates colitis via attenuating colonic mucosa injury and regulating pro-inflammatory cytokines production and oxidative stress. *Biomedicine & Pharmacotherapy* **103**: 812–822. https://doi.org/10.1016/j.biopha.2018.04.071.

Alara, O.R., Abdurahman, N.H., and Ukaegbu, C.I. (2018). Soxhlet extraction of phenolic compounds from Vernonia cinerea leaves and its antioxidant activity. *Journal of Applied Research on Medicinal and Aromatic Plants* **11**: 12–17. https://doi.org/10.1016/j.jarmap.2018.07.003.

Azian, M., Anisa, A.I., and Iwai, Y. (2014). Mechanisms of ginger bioactive compounds extract using Soxhlet and accelerated water extraction. *World Academy of Science, Engineering and Technology* **8** (5): 438–442.

Azwanida, N.N. (2015). A review on the extraction methods use in medicinal plants, principle, strength and limitation. *Medicinal and Aromatic Plants* **4**: 1–6.

Baldosano, H.Y., Castillo, M.B.M.G., Elloran, C.D.H., and Bacani, F.T. (2015). Effect of particle size, solvent and extraction time on tannin extract from Spondias purpurea bark through soxhlet extraction. Paper presented at DLSU Research Congress, De La Salle University, Manilla, The Phillipines.

Baljeet, S.Y., Simmy, G., Ritika, Y., and Roshanlal, Y. (2015). Antimicrobial activity of individual and combined extracts of selected spices against some pathogenic and food spoilage microorganisms. *International Food Research Journal* **22** (6): 2594–2600.

Berrington, D. and Lall, N. (2012). Anticancer activity of certain herbs and spices on the cervical epithelial carcinoma (HeLa) cell line. *South African Journal of Botany* **79**: 178–178.

Bimakr, M., Rahman, R.A., Taip, F.S. et al. (2011). Comparison of different extraction methods for the extraction of major bioactive flavonoid compounds from spearmint (Mentha spicata L.) leaves. *Food and Bioproducts Processing* **89** (1): 67–72.

Borhan, M.Z., Ahmad, R., Rusop, M., and Abdullah, S. (2013). Green extraction: enhanced extraction yield of Asiatic acid from *Centella asiatica* (L.) Nanopowders. *Journal of Applied Chemistry* **2013**: 7. https://doi.org/10.1155/2013/460168.

Camel, V. (2014). Extraction methodologies: general introduction. In: *Handbook of Chemical and Biological Plant Analytical Methods* (ed. K. Hostettmann), 17–41. Unitd Kingdom: Wiley.

Chan, C.L., Gan, R.Y., Shah, N.P., and Corke, H. (2018). Polyphenols from selected dietary spices and medicinal herbs differentially affect common food-borne pathogenic bacteria and lactic acid bacteria. *Food Control* **92**: 437–443. https://doi.org/10.1016/j.foodcont.2018.05.032.

Chen, H., Chang, M., and Chang, T. (1985). Antibacterial properties of some spice plants before and after heat treatment. *Zhonghua Minguo wei sheng wu ji mian yi xue za zhi= Chinese journal of microbiology and immunology* **18** (3): 190–195.

Chuichulcherm, S., Prommakort, S., Srinophakun, P., and Thanapimmetha, A. (2013). Optimization of capsaicin purification from *Capsicum frutescens* Linn. With column chromatography using Taguchi design. *Industrial Crops and Products* **44**: 473–479. https://doi.org/10.1016/j.indcrop.2012.10.007.

Cid-Perez, T.S., Avila-Sosa, R., Ochoa-Velasco, C.E. et al. (2019). Antioxidant and antimicrobial activity of Mexican oregano (Poliomintha longiflora) essential oil, hydrosol and extracts from waste solid residues. *Plants-Basel* **8** (1): 22. https://doi.org/10.3390/plants8010022.

Das, S., Anjeza, C., and Mandal, S. (2012). Synergistic or additive antimicrobial activities of Indian spice and herbal extracts against pathogenic, probiotic and food-spoiler micro-organisms. *International Food Research Journal* **19** (3): 1185–1191.

Dent, M., Dragovic-Uzelac, V., Penic, M. et al. (2013). The effect of extraction solvents, temperature and time on the composition and mass fraction of polyphenols in Dalmatian wild sage (*Salvia officinalis* L.) extracts. *Food Technology and Biotechnology* **51** (1): 84.

Do, Q.D., Angkawijaya, A.E., Tran-Nguyen, P.L. et al. (2014). Effect of extraction solvent on total phenol content, total flavonoid content, and antioxidant activity of *Limnophila aromatica*. *Journal of Food and Drug Analysis* **22** (3): 296–302.

Durling, N.E., Catchpole, O.J., Grey, J.B. et al. (2007). Extraction of phenolics and essential oil from dried sage (*Salvia officinalis*) using ethanol–water mixtures. *Food Chemistry* **101** (4): 1417–1424.

Ereifej, K.I., Feng, H., Rababah, T.M. et al. (2016). Effect of extractant and temperature on phenolic compounds and antioxidant activity of selected spices. *Food and Nutrition Sciences* **7** (05): 362.

Fan, R., Yuan, F., Wang, N. et al. (2015). Extraction and analysis of antioxidant compounds from the residues of *Asparagus officinalis* L. *Journal of Food Science and Technology-Mysore* **52** (5): 2690–2700. https://doi.org/10.1007/s13197-014-1360-4.

Gherman, C., Culea, M., and Cozar, O. (2000). Comparative analysis of some active principles of herb plants by GC/MS. *Talanta* **53** (1): 253–262. https://doi.org/10.1016/S0039-9140(00)00458-6.

Gutierrez-Grijalva, E.P., Antunes-Ricardo, M., Acosta-Estrada, B.A. et al. (2019). Cellular antioxidant activity and in vitro inhibition of alpha-glucosidase, alpha-amylase and pancreatic lipase of oregano polyphenols under simulated gastrointestinal digestion. *Food Research International* **116**: 676–686. https://doi.org/10.1016/j.foodres.2018.08.096.

Hinneburg, I., Dorman, H.J.D., and Hiltunen, R. (2006). Antioxidant activities of extracts from selected culinary herbs and spices. *Food Chemistry* **97** (1): 122–129. https://doi.org/10.1016/j.foodchem.2005.03.028.

Howard, L.R., Talcott, S.T., Brenes, C.H., and Villalon, B. (2000). Changes in phytochemical and antioxidant activity of selected pepper cultivars (capsicum species) as influenced by maturity. *Journal of Agricultural and Food Chemistry* **48** (5): 1713–1720. https://doi.org/10.1021/jf990916t.

Jaiswal, S.G. and Naik, S. (2018). Contribution of agricultural produce spice *Zingiber officinale* to a sustainable food system: green extraction and stability study of antioxidant compounds. *Open Agriculture* **3** (1): 326–338.

Kanadea, R. and Bhatkhandeb, D. (2016). Extraction of ginger oil using different methods and effect of solvents, time, temperature to maximize yield. *International Journal of Advances in Science Engineering and Technology* **4**: 241–422.

Kim, D.O. and Lee, C.Y. (2004). Comprehensive study an vitamin C equivalent antioxidant capacity (VCEAC) of various polyphenolics in scavenging a free radical and its structural relationship. *Critical Reviews in Food Science and Nutrition* **44** (4): 253–273. https://doi.org/10.1080/10408690490464960.

Kim, G.-H., Park, S.-J., and Um, B.-H. (2016). Response surface methodology for optimization of solvent extraction to recovery of acetic acid from black liquor derived from *Typha latifolia* pulping process. *Industrial Crops and Products* **89**: 34–44.

Kittisakulnam, S., Saetae, D., and Suntornsuk, W. (2017). Antioxidant and antibacterial activities of spices traditionally used in fermented meat products. *Journal of Food Processing and Preservation* **41** (4): e13004.

Kumaran, A. and Karunakaran, R.J. (2007). Activity-guided isolation and identification of free radical-scavenging components from an aqueous extract of *Coleus aromaticus*. *Food Chemistry* **100** (1): 356–361. https://doi.org/10.1016/j.foodchem.2005.09.051.

Leblebici, M.E., Machmudah, S., Sasaki, M., and Goto, M. (2012). Antiradical efficiency of essential oils from plant seeds obtained by supercritical CO_2, Soxhlet extraction, and hydrodistillation. *Separation Science and Technology* **48** (2): 328–337. https://doi.org/10.1080/01496395.2012.690810.

Lee, K.-G. and Shibamoto, T. (2001). Antioxidant property of aroma extract isolated from clove buds [*Syzygium aromaticum* (L.) Merr. Et Perry]. *Food Chemistry* **74** (4): 443–448.

Lee, K.-G. and Shibamoto, T. (2002). Determination of antioxidant potential of volatile extracts isolated from various herbs and spices. *Journal of Agricultural and Food Chemistry* **50** (17): 4947–4952.

Li, H.-B., Jiang, Y., Wong, C.-C. et al. (2007). Evaluation of two methods for the extraction of antioxidants from medicinal plants. *Analytical and Bioanalytical Chemistry* **388** (2): 483–488.

Majeed, M., Hussain, A.I., Chatha, S.A. et al. (2016). Optimization protocol for the extraction of antioxidant components from *Origanum vulgare* leaves using response surface methodology. *Saudi Journal of Biological Sciences* **23**: 389–396.

Mandal, S.C., Mandal, V., and Das, A.K. (2015). *Essentials of Botanical Extraction: Principles and Applications*. Academic Press.

Matkowski, A., Tasarz, P., and Szypula, E. (2008). Antioxidant activity of herb extracts from five medicinal plants from Lamiaceae, subfamily Lamioideae. *Journal of Medicinal Plant Research* **2** (11): 321–330.

Mohamad, M., Ali, M., and Ahmad, A. (2010). Modelling for extraction of major phytochemical components from *Eurycoma longifolia*. *Journal of Applied Sciences* **10** (21): 2572–2577.

Mohammadpour, H., Sadrameli, S.M., Eslami, F., and Asoodeh, A. (2019). Optimization of ultrasound-assisted extraction of Moringa peregrina oil with response surface methodology and comparison with Soxhlet method. *Industrial Crops and Products* **131**: 106–116. https://doi.org/10.1016/j.indcrop.2019.01.030.

Mollica, A., Stefanucci, A., Macedonio, G. et al. (2019). Chemical composition and biological activity of *Capparis spinosa* L. from Lipari Island. *South African Journal of Botany* **120**: 135–140. https://doi.org/10.1016/j.sajb.2018.02.397.

Molnar, M., Mendesevic, N., Subaric, D. et al. (2017). Comparison of various techniques for the extraction of umbelliferone and herniarin in *Matricaria chamomilla* processing fractions. *Chemistry Central Journal* **11**: 78. https://doi.org/10.1186/s13065-017-0308-y.

Nile, S.H. and Park, S.W. (2015). Chromatographic analysis, antioxidant, anti-inflammatory, and xanthine oxidase inhibitory activities of ginger extracts and its reference compounds. *Industrial Crops and Products* **70**: 238–244. https://doi.org/10.1016/j.indcrop.2015.03.033.

Nile, S.H., Nile, A.S., and Keum, Y.-S. (2017). Total phenolics, antioxidant, antitumor, and enzyme inhibitory activity of Indian medicinal and aromatic plants extracted with different extraction methods. *3 Biotech* **7** (1): 76.

Okoduwa, S.I.R., Umar, I.A., James, D.B. et al. (2016). Evaluation of extraction protocols for anti-diabetic phytochemical substances from medicinal plants. *World Journal of Diabetes* **7** (20): 605–614. https://doi.org/10.4239/wjd.v7.i20.605.

Otunola, G.A. and Afolayan, A.J. (2013). Evaluation of the polyphenolic contents and some antioxidant properties of aqueous extracts of garlic, ginger, Cayenne pepper and their mixture. *Journal of Applied Botany and Food Quality* **86**: 66–70. https://doi.org/10.5073/Jabfq.2013.086.010.

Pavlić, B., Vidović, S., Vladić, J. et al. (2016). Subcritical water extraction of sage (*Salvia Officinalis* L.) by-products-process optimization by response surface methodology. *The Journal of Supercritical Fluids* **116**: 36–45.

Ramírez-Godínez, J., Jaimez-Ordaz, J., Castañeda-Ovando, A. et al. (2017). Optimization of physical conditions for the aqueous extraction of antioxidant compounds from ginger (*Zingiber officinale*) applying a box-Behnken design. *Plant Foods for Human Nutrition* **72**: 34–40.

Rathi, B.S., Bodhankar, S.L., and Baheti, A.M. (2006). Evaluation of aqueous leaves extract of Moringa oleifera Linn for wound healing in albino rats. *Indian Journal of Experimental Biology* **44** (11): 898–901.

Raynie, D.E. (2000). Extraction. In: *Encyclopedia of Separation Science* (ed. I.D. Wilson), 118–128. Oxford: Academic Press.

Revati, S., Bipin, C., Chitra, P., and Minakshi, B. (2015). In vitro antibacterial activity of seven Indian spices against high level gentamicin resistant strains of enterococci. *Archives of Medical Science* **11** (4): 863–868. https://doi.org/10.5114/aoms.2015.53307.

Sagun, E., Durmaz, H., Tarakci, Z., and Sagdic, O. (2006). Antibacterial activities of the extracts of some herbs used in Turkish herby cheese against *listeria monocytogenes* serovars. *International Journal of Food Properties* **9** (2): 255–260.

Saponjac, V.T., Cetojevic-Simin, D., Cetkovic, G. et al. (2014). Effect of extraction conditions of paprika oleoresins on their free radical scavenging and anticancer activity. *Central European Journal of Chemistry* **12** (3): 377–385. https://doi.org/10.2478/s11532-013-0378-1.

Sepahpour, S., Selamat, J., Manap, M.Y.A. et al. (2018). Comparative analysis of chemical composition, antioxidant activity and quantitative characterization of some phenolic compounds in selected herbs and spices in different solvent extraction systems. *Molecules* **23** (2): 402. https://doi.org/10.3390/molecules23020402.

Shan, B., Cai, Y.Z., Sun, M., and Corke, H. (2005). Antioxidant capacity of 26 spice extracts and characterization of their phenolic constituents. *Journal of Agricultural and Food Chemistry* **53** (20): 7749–7759. https://doi.org/10.1021/jf051513y.

Shettar, A.K., Kotresha, K., Kaliwal, B.B., and Vedamurthy, A.B. (2015). Evaluation of in vitro antioxidant and anti-inflammatory activities of *Ximenia americana* extracts. *Asian Pacific Journal of Tropical Disease* **5** (11): 918–923.

Shihabudeen, H.M.S., Priscilla, D.H., and Thirumurugan, K. (2011). Cinnamon extract inhibits alpha-glucosidase activity and dampens postprandial glucose excursion in diabetic rats. *Nutrition and Metabolism* **8**: 46. https://doi.org/10.1186/1743-7075-8-46.

Siddhartha, E., Sarojamma, V., and Ramakrishna, V. (2017). Bioactive compound rich Indian spices suppresses the growth of beta-lactamase produced multidrug resistant bacteria. *Journal of Krishna Institute of Medical Sciences University* **6** (1): 10–24.

Smith, R.M. (2003). Before the injection—modern methods of sample preparation for separation techniques. *Journal of Chromatography A* **1000** (1–2): 3–27.

Soobrattee, M.A., Neergheen, V.S., Luximon-Ramma, A. et al. (2005). Phenolics as potential antioxidant therapeutic agents: mechanism and actions. *Mutation Research, Fundamental and Molecular Mechanisms of Mutagenesis* **579** (1–2): 200–213. https://doi.org/10.1016/j.mrfmmm.2005.03.023.

Takeuchi, T.M., Leal, P.F., Favareto, R. et al. (2008). Study of the phase equilibrium formed inside the flash tank used at the separation step of a supercritical fluid extraction unit. *The Journal of Supercritical Fluids* **43** (3): 447–459. https://doi.org/10.1016/j.supflu.2007.08.002.

Teixeira, D.M. and da Costa, C.T. (2005). Novel methods to extract flavanones and xanthones from the root bark of Maclura pomifera. *Journal of Chromatography. A* **1062** (2): 175–181.

Teng, H. and Lee, W.Y. (2014). Antibacterial and antioxidant activities and chemical compositions of volatile oils extracted from *Schisandra chinensis* Baill. Seeds using simultaneous distillation extraction method, and comparison with Soxhlet and microwave-assisted extraction. *Bioscience, Biotechnology, and Biochemistry* **78** (1): 79–85.

Thanekar, D., Dhodi, J., Gawali, N. et al. (2016). Evaluation of antitumor and anti-angiogenic activity of bioactive compounds from *Cinnamomum tamala*: in vitro, in vivo and in silico approach. *South African Journal of Botany* **104**: 6–14.

Umamaheshwari, P. and Reddy, P.D.S. (2016). Effect of operating parameters on extraction of oil from bitter gourd seeds: a kinetic and thermodynamic study. *International Journal of Science & Research* **5** (2): 1243–1246.

Vladić, J., Canli, O., Pavlić, B. et al. (2017). Optimization of *Satureja montana* subcritical water extraction process and chemical characterization of volatile fraction of extracts. *The Journal of Supercritical Fluids* **120**: 86–94.

Wang, X. and Lin, T. (2013). *Needleless Electrospinning of Nanofibers: Technology and Applications*. Pan Stanford.

Wang, W., Li, N., Luo, M. et al. (2012). Antibacterial activity and anticancer activity of *Rosmarinus officinalis* L. essential oil compared to that of its main components. *Molecules* **17** (3): 2704–2713. https://doi.org/10.3390/molecules17032704.

Wang, D.-G., Liu, W.-Y., and Chen, G.-T. (2013). A simple method for the isolation and purification of resveratrol from *Polygonum cuspidatum*. *Journal of Pharmaceutical Analysis* **3** (4): 241–247.

Wojdylo, A., Oszmianski, J., and Czemerys, R. (2007). Antioxidant activity and phenolic compounds in 32 selected herbs. *Food Chemistry* **105** (3): 940–949. https://doi.org/10.1016/j.foodchem.2007.04.038.

Wong, Y., Ahmad-Mudzaqqir, M., and Wan-Nurdiyana, W. (2014). Extraction of essential oil from cinnamon (*Cinnamomum zeylanicum*). *Oriental Journal of Chemistry* **30** (1): 37–47.

Yeshak, M.Y., Burman, R., Eriksson, C., and Goransson, U. (2012). Optimization of cyclotide extraction parameters. *Phytochemistry Letters* **5** (4): 776–781. https://doi.org/10.1016/j.phytol.2012.09.001.

Yin, M.-c. and Cheng, W.-s. (1998). Antioxidant activity of several allium members. *Journal of Agricultural and Food Chemistry* **46** (10): 4097–4101.

Zeković, Z., Kaplan, M., Pavlić, B. et al. (2016). Chemical characterization of polyphenols and volatile fraction of coriander (*Coriandrum sativum* L.) extracts obtained by subcriticalwater extraction. *Industrial Crops and Products* **87**: 54–63.

Ziaedini, A., Jafari, A., and Zakeri, A. (2010). Extraction of antioxidants and caffeine from green tea (Camelia sinensis) leaves: kinetics and Modeling. *Food Science and Technology International* **16** (6): 505–510. https://doi.org/10.1177/1082013210367567.

5
Novel Extraction Techniques for Bioactive Compounds from Herbs and Spices

Andrea P. Sánchez-Camargo[1], Lidia Montero[2,3], Jose A. Mendiola[4], M. Herrero[4], and E. Ibáñez[4]

[1]*Food Chemistry Research Group, High Pressure Laboratory, Departamento de Química, Facultad de Ciencias Universidad Nacional de Colombia, Carrera 30 No. 45-03, 111321, Bogotá D.C., Colombia*
[2]*University of Duisburg-Essen, Applied Analytical Chemistry, Universitaetsstr. 5, 45141 Essen, Germany*
[3]*Teaching and Research Center for Separation (TRC), University of Duisburg-Essen, Universitaetsstr. 5, 45141 Essen, Germany*
[4]*Laboratory of Foodomics, Bioactivity and Food Analysis Department, Institute of Food Science Research (CIAL-CSIC), Nicolás Cabrera 9, 28049 Madrid, Spain*

5.1 Introduction

Currently, there is enormous interest in searching for bioactive compounds of natural origin. The increasing number of publications demonstrating the efficacy of such compounds in promoting human health has undoubtedly raised the interest of researchers and companies. Among the different sources of bioactive compounds, the most widely known are plants, herbs and spices, and agricultural by-products; although marine sources have also shown great potential (Ibañez et al. 2012).

However, not only is it important to select the right natural source of a specific bioactive compound or product, but also the processes involved in their production should be carefully optimized to improve the efficiency of the process and to minimize both loss of bioactivity and harm to the environment.

Developed societies are becoming increasingly concerned about the environment and its preservation. Since the early 1990s, the Green Chemistry movement has led the change toward a more sustainable and environmentally benign chemistry industry and has explored new ways to reduce or eliminate the use or generation of hazardous

Herbs, Spices and Medicinal Plants: Processing, Health Benefits and Safety, First Edition.
Edited by Mohammad B. Hossain, Nigel P. Brunton, and Dilip K. Rai.

substances from chemical products and processes and to improve all types of chemical products and processes by reducing their impact on human health and environment. As defined by Anastas and Warner (1998) "Green Chemistry is the use of chemistry techniques and methodologies that reduce or eliminate the use or generation of feedstocks, products, by-products, solvents, reagents, etc. that are hazardous to human health or the environment." Green Chemistry technologies involve all types of chemical processes and focus on three main aspects that dominate the principles of Green Chemistry: waste, hazard (health, environmental, and safety), and energy (Anastas and Warner 1998).

Under this framework, it is easy to understand the need for development of new and advanced extraction techniques able to resolve important drawbacks associated with the use of conventional techniques. Characteristics of traditional extraction processes usually employed to extract bioactives (mainly solid–liquid extraction) involve the extensive use of toxic organic solvents and exhibit high energy usage while providing low selectivity and low extraction yields. These deficiencies can be partially or completely overcome by using newly developed advanced extraction techniques which are faster, more selective, and more environmentally friendly.

In this chapter, an overview of the principles and applications of advanced extraction techniques, such as supercritical fluid extraction (SFE), pressurized liquid extraction (PLE), ultrasound-assisted extraction (UAE), microwave-assisted extraction (MAE), enzyme-assisted extraction (EAE), and combinations thereof are presented, focused on the extraction of bioactives from herbs and spices. It is our goal to show the huge potential of these techniques for the extraction of high added-value compounds (with improved bioactivity) while complying with the Green Chemistry goals.

5.2 Pressurized Liquid Extraction (PLE)

5.2.1 Description of the Technique

PLE is based on the use of pressurized solvents at high temperatures (always below their critical points), under conditions in which the solvents are maintained in liquid state during the extraction process. Under these conditions, solvents acquire different properties compared to ambient pressure, which incurs several advantages. This technique is also commonly known as pressurized fluid extraction (PFE), pressurized hot solvent extraction (PHSE), or accelerated solvent extraction (ASE). A great variety of solvents can be employed for the extraction, although, nowadays, the use of the environmentally greenest possible solvent is always sought. Among these, water attracts special attention due to the modification of its physicochemical properties when submitted to high temperatures and pressures. In this instance, the technique is renamed subcritical water extraction (SWE), superheated water extraction (SHWE), or pressurized hot water extraction (PHWE). In any case, the main principles and instrumental requirements are the same regardless of the solvent employed.

The basic instrumental requirements for performing PLE are not too complicated. The main instruments are: pump, extraction cell, pressure valves, oven, and a collection vessel. The pump is needed to introduce the solvent inside the extraction cell, as well as to push the extract out once the extraction is finished. This pump should be able to achieve the desired pressure (normally between 35 and 200 bar) in the extraction cell. The solvents employed for extraction should be oxygen free in order to avoid oxidation of the bioactives, as well as to prevent cavitation in the pump. To achieve this, degassing by ultrasound or a helium purge are commonly employed. The extraction cell should have two on/off valves in order to keep conditions stable regarding the pressure set for the extraction. Usually, the extraction cell is made of stainless steel and is suitable for very high pressures. The extraction cell is placed inside an oven, which controls the applied temperature. The maximum working temperature in most instruments is around 200 °C. Lastly, a collection vessel is required. Despite these basic instrumental requirements, the equipment employed can be more sophisticated. For instance, if dynamic extraction instead of a static process is desired, more accurate pumps might be needed in order to maintain a precise flow rate during the whole extraction procedure. In this case, a heating coil should be included inside the oven so that the solvent reaches the extraction cell at the expected temperature. A device to vent the whole system is also common in most PLE instruments; a nitrogen circuit can also be included allowing complete purging after extraction as well as ensuring that all the extracting solvent reaches the collection vial once the extraction is finished. While there exist several commercial options, lab-made instruments are also quite common. Further information on how to build a PLE extraction system may be found in Turner and Ibañez (2011).

The main advantages related to PLE come from the particular extraction conditions employed; that is, high temperature and pressures. The main requirement of any PLE extractor is to ensure an extraction pressure high enough to keep the solvents in liquid state despite the very high temperatures that may be used. Under these conditions, the mass transfer rate is greatly favored due to the increase in solubility of the analytes in the sample matrix as well as due to a decrease in the viscosity and surface tension of the solvent that further enhances mass transfer. Thus, faster extraction processes with lower volumes of solvents are required. When extraction takes place using water as solvent, the same phenomena occurs. However, in this latter case other physical changes are produced. These changes are related to the water dielectric constant. The dielectric constant (ε) can be used as a measure of the polarity of a solvent. This parameter is very significantly affected by temperature when the water is maintained in liquid state. In fact, although the dielectric constant of water at room temperature is around 80, being by far the most polar solvent, this value decreases to $\varepsilon = 25$–30 (at ca. 200–250 °C) when the temperature is increased; that is, similar to that presented by some organic solvents, such as ethanol or methanol. Thus, the change in this property when using water implies that superheated water may acquire new physical and solvent properties that might be very interesting for developing new extraction processes for medium to low polarity compounds, avoiding the use of organic solvents. Thus, the use of SWE can be suggested as a useful green alternative to the employment of organic solvents in some applications. Indeed, although not feasible for every application, the use of SWE can be therefore seen as the "greenest" one within the PLEs.

In PLE, the solvent is the most critical factor since it will directly influence the type of extractable compounds. Solvent selection depends on the particular aim of the extraction process; the most adequate solvent considering the nature and characteristics of the target analytes should be selected, generally considering that like dissolves like. Moreover, environmental considerations have a great influence on this selection as the greenest possible solvent should be always employed.

Once the solvent or solvent mixture is selected, the temperature is the most influential parameter in any PLE process. As a general rule, when extracting natural matrices, higher extraction temperatures provide higher extraction yields. It has been repeatedly observed how the use of very high temperatures is not always detrimental to the recovery of bioactives from natural matrices. However, due to the nature of those components and their lability, it has to be considered that too high extraction temperatures could potentially lead to the degradation of compounds. For this reason, the use of experimental designs to optimize the extraction temperature is always recommended, while monitoring as a response variable the presence of bioactives in the extracts.

Extraction pressure may also have an important impact on the process. However, research has shown that once the pressure is enough to maintain the solvent liquid, its effect is quite limited. For this reason, pressures of 50–100 bar are usually employed. These values are enough to keep the liquid state at the usually employed temperatures. Moreover, theoretically, the pressure might exert a rupture effect on the sample being extracted, further increasing the mass transfer rates. As regards the extraction time, this variable, even though important, has a smaller influence. Extraction time refers to the time in which the solvent is effectively in contact with the sample being extracted at the set temperature and pressure. It is also called static extraction time. This latter term refers to static extractions in which a given volume of solvent is left in contact with the sample at the desired extraction conditions for a specific period of time. In general, relatively short static extraction times (5–20 minutes) are applied for the extraction of bioactives from natural matrices. Longer times do not generally produce better results as an equilibrium between sample components and solvent is reached. Another possibility is to run dynamic extractions in which the solvent flows through the sample at fixed extraction conditions and at a fixed flow rate (Saldaña and Valdivieso-Ramírez 2015). Most common commercial instruments only work in static mode, meaning that most dynamic extraction applications are based on the use of lab-made equipment.

Other variables that should also be considered include the possibility of running more than one static extraction cycle in order to further exhaust the sample. This approach is also common for the extraction of bioactives from plant materials (Luthria 2008; Howard and Pandjaitan 2008). A variation of this multiple extraction process using the same sample is the employment of sequential extractions, which are based on repetitive extractions in which the temperature is raised gradually from one step to the next, so that different extract compositions are obtained.

Other considerations, common to other extraction processes, deal with the sample size, moisture content, or dispersing agent employed, among others, and should be optimized appropriately for each particular application.

5.2.2 Applications of PLE to Herbs and Spices

PLE has been used to extract a wide range of different compounds from herbs and spices, such as phenolic compounds, essential oils, anthraquinones, alkaloids, or even pesticides.

As mentioned, in order to obtain the best extraction efficiency, many of the applications carry out an optimization of the main PLE parameters that affect the extraction process. Besides the extraction parameters of the PLE process, the type, chemical structure, and stability of the target compounds should be carefully studied.

5.2.2.1 Phenolic Compounds PLE has been used for the extraction of phenolic compounds from a huge number of vegetable matrices. The extraction conditions selected depend on the content and type of the phenolic compounds present in the sample.

As mentioned above, temperature is the most important parameter affecting both the extraction yield and stability of the compounds. Even if the extraction yield increases with a rise in temperature, however, many of the phenolic compounds are thermolabile, and this fact should be carefully considered. For example, coumarins from *Cnidii fructus* or *Heracleum leskowii* degrade above 150 °C (Gao et al. 2013; Skalicka-Woźniak and Głowniak 2012). Therefore, the temperature should be selected to balance the extraction efficiency and the stability of the compounds of interest (Skalicka-Woźniak and Głowniak 2012). Temperatures from 50 to 100 °C usually allow an increase in the extraction yield, while when temperatures rise above 100 °C, the recovery of analytes is generally limited (Runnqvist et al. 2010).

Other than temperature, extraction time and static cycles are parameters that are commonly studied to improve the extraction efficiency. For example, Gao et al. studied the effect of the extraction temperature, extraction time, and static cycles for the isolation of bioactive constituents (coumarins) from *C. fructus* (Gao et al. 2013). The optimization of the extraction parameters was carried out by response surface methodology (RSM); degradation of coumarins, as mentioned, was observed at temperatures above 150 °C. Extraction conditions selected as the best compromise between maximum yield and maximum recovery of bioactive coumarins were: 122 °C, five minutes, and two extraction cycles.

Another key factor that always has to be optimized is the selection of the extraction solvent employed to extract the phenolic compounds from the matrix. The use of a solvent with a high affinity and specificity for the target compounds may provide a more effective and selective extraction, avoiding the co-extraction of unwanted compounds present on the matrix (Skalicka-Woźniak and Głowniak 2012).

The most used solvents in PLE extraction of herbal phenolic compounds are methanol, ethanol, and their mixtures with water. The selection of these solvents depends mainly on the range of polarities of the phenolic compounds, their chemical structure, and stability.

A study of the solvent effect on hydroxyanthraquinone extraction from *Rumex crispus* was developed by Wianowska (2014a). In this plant, hydroxyanthraquinones are found mainly in glycoside form, while the aglycone form represents only a small proportion of the total phenolic content. Due to the presence of sugar units in the glycoside forms, these kinds of compound are expected to be more soluble in water than the aglycone forms; therefore, the extracting solvent selected should be a methanol/water mixture rich in water (aglycones are better extracted with methanol due to their less polar nature). However, in this study, mixtures with a high water content gave rise to extracts with a high aglycone concentration. This result might be due to the hydrolytical degradation of the glycosides into their aglycone form, enhanced by the high temperatures employed in the PLE process. Hence, in this case, to obtain an extract without degradation, methanol was employed as the extracting solvent.

Ionic liquids (ILs) have been also suggested as environmentally friendly solvents with interesting properties for the extraction of bioactive compounds from herbs and spices; their main features are their thermal stability and their capacity to solubilize compounds of a wide range of polarities (Zhang et al. 2006). Although the use of ILs in

PLE is very recent and there have only been a few publications, this approach seems to be very successful. One example is the use of the ionic liquid-based pressurized liquid extraction (ILs-PLE) of rutin and quercetin from different herbs (*Flos sophorae* Immaturus, *Crateagus pinnatifida* Bunge, *Hypericum japonicum* Thunb, and *Folium mor*) (Wu et al. 2012). The optimized ILs-PLE provided higher extraction yields than traditional extraction processes.

5.2.2.2 Essential Oils The extraction of essential oils from herbal materials by PLE has been successfully applied with advantages over traditional extraction methods such as distillation, ultrasound extraction, or Soxhlet extraction (Chienthavorn et al. 2011). In general, temperatures between 60 and 100 °C, and extraction times from 5 to 30 minutes, seem to be the more convenient for PLE extraction of essential oils (Nur Ain et al. 2012; Wianowska 2014b; Kukula-Koch et al. 2014; Liu et al. 2012a; Eikani et al. 2013; Pouralinazar et al. 2012).

In some cases, essential oils obtained by PLE can contain compounds that are not extracted by conventional extraction techniques. For instance, PLE extract of *Iris dichotoma* Pall contains a significant quantity of long-chained fatty acids esters, while the same extracts obtained by hydro-distillation contain mainly simple terpenes (Kukula-Koch et al. 2014).

Considering that the composition of essential oils is very complex and includes lipophilic and hydrophilic components, it is expected that the composition of PLE extracts will mainly depend on solvent polarity (Miron et al. 2011). Frequently, mixtures of ethanol/water are used in order to include the whole range of polarities of the essential oil components, being the extraction of lipophilic compounds that is enhanced when an hydroalcoholic solvent rich in ethanol is employed; on the other hand, extracts rich in hydrophilic analytes are achieved when higher amounts of water are present in the extracting solvent mixture (Cho et al. 2007). Although other organic solvents, such as *n*-hexane, acetonitrile, ethyl acetate, or dichloromethane, have been studied for essential oil extraction by PLE (Cho et al. 2007; Wianowska 2014b), as mentioned previously, the use of ethanol and water as extracting solvents have the key advantages of being green, GRAS (generally recognized as safe), and food-grade solvents.

5.2.2.3 Alkaloids The main compounds responsible not only for the characteristic pungency of the pepper but also for its bioactive effects are alkaloids such as piperine, chavicine, piperidine, and piperetine (Butt et al. 2013; Liu et al. 2015).

PLE has been employed for the extraction of piperine and piperidine from commercial peppers as a way of evaluating their quality (De Mey et al. 2014). Considering that piperine and piperidine have a completely different solubility in water, a selective extraction of each compound is possible by employing dichloromethane at 70 °C for the extraction of piperine, and water at 50 °C for the complete recovery of piperidine. The effect of the physical state of the sample (powder, cracked peppercorns, or peppercorns) was also studied. The recovery of piperine from whole peppercorns was much lower than with the grinded sample; it seems clear that non-treated material did not allow enough contact with the solvent and, therefore, lower yields were achieved.

5.3 Supercritical Fluid Extraction (SFE)

5.3.1 Description of the Technique

SFE is based on the use of solvents at temperatures and pressures above their critical points. The term "critical point" was coined by Thomas Andrews, who further elucidated the meaning of Cagniard de la Tour's *état particulier* (Berche et al. 2009).

The physical properties of supercritical fluids are between a gas and a liquid. For instance, the density of a supercritical fluid is similar to a liquid while its viscosity is similar to a gas and its diffusivity is between gas and liquid. Thermal conductivities are relatively high in supercritical fluids and have large values near the critical point. Surface tension is close to zero at the critical point, being similar to gases and much smaller than for liquids. Many other physical properties, such as relative permittivity and solvent strength, etc., highly related to density, show large gradients with pressure above the critical point. Changes in these properties are crucial when dealing with extraction since they are related to changes in solubility and mass transfer ratios.

One of the most valuable characteristics of SFE is the greatly reduced (often to zero) employment of toxic organic solvents. In this sense, SFE using green solvents has been suggested as a clean alternative to hazardous processes and, thus, SFE has found a growing niche. Here, carbon dioxide is the solvent most commonly used to extract bioactives from natural sources. In fact, CO_2 has a series of interesting properties for bioactive extraction:

- It is cheap.
- Its critical conditions are easily attainable (30.9 °C and 7.38 MPa).
- It is an environmentally friendly solvent that is also considered GRAS for its use in the food/pharma industry.

At supercritical conditions, CO_2 presents a high diffusivity, whereas its solvent strength and density can be easily modified by tuning the temperature and pressure applied. Another important characteristic of this technique, when using supercritical CO_2, is the possibility of attaining solvent-free extracts. Once the extraction procedure is finished, the depressurization of the system allows CO_2 to turn into gas and leave the matrix while the compounds extracted from the matrix, and solubilized in the CO_2 at high pressures, remain in the collection vessel. These properties are responsible for the extended use of supercritical CO_2 for extraction of bioactive compounds

Although the discovery of the critical phenomena is attributed to Charles Cagniard de la Tour in 1822 (Berche et al. 2009), SFE was first introduced as an alternative extraction method in 1879 by Hannay and Hogarth. However, it was not until around 1960 that this extraction method started to be thoroughly investigated as an alternative to conventional extraction methods, such as Solid-Liquid Extraction (SLE) and Liquid-Liquid Extraction (LLE), requiring large amounts of hazardous chemicals such as chlorinated solvents. This technique has been already employed to extract a wide variety of interesting compounds from very different herbal materials (Herrero et al. 2013; Mendiola et al. 2007). The widest application of supercritical fluids is in the extraction field, especially when using carbon dioxide. The first patent dealing with SFE was by Messmore in 1943 (Messmore 1943), although the first industrial application was developed by Zosel in 1978 (Zosel 1978).

The main drawback of $SCCO_2$ is its low polarity, a problem that can be overcome by employing polar modifiers (co-solvents) to change the polarity of the supercritical fluid and to increase its solvating power toward the analyte of interest. For example, the addition of relatively small percentages (1–10%) of methanol to carbon dioxide expands its extraction range to include more polar analytes. The modifiers can also reduce the analyte–matrix interactions, improving their quantitative extraction (Björklund et al. 2005). Despite some other solvents being proposed for SFE (namely: propane, butane, dimethyl ether, etc.) none of them fulfill the principles of Green Chemistry and Green Engineering as well as CO_2 (Anastas and Zimmerman 2003).

Along with SFE, Gas Expanded Liquid Extraction (GXL) has been recently proposed as a clean alternative for obtaining bioactive compounds from vegetal matrixes. A GXL is a mixed solvent composed of a compressible gas (such as CO_2) dissolved in an organic solvent (Scurto et al. 2009). In some cases, the gas solubility enhancement in GXLs is up to two orders of magnitude relative to the same organic solvent at ambient conditions. Basically, GXL extraction consists of $SCCO_2$ mixed with a high amount (50–90%) of solvent (i.e. ethanol) at a low pressure and temperature to avoid one single supercritical phase formation. Moreover, GXLs have the advantage of requiring mild working pressures, reducing the energy consumption and hence the cost of the process. Similar to supercritical fluids, GXLs have been shown to improve mass transfer by decreasing interfacial tension, reducing viscosity, and increasing diffusivity (Akien and Poliakoff 2009; Reyes et al. 2014). When using compressed CO_2 to expand less volatile liquid phases, the vapor–liquid equilibrium is such that the vapor phase is dominated by CO_2. The presence of CO_2 in the vapor phase provides safety benefits in the case of oxygen-based oxidation reactions by reducing the tendency to form explosive hydrocarbon/O_2 mixtures in the vapor phase. As drawback of GXL, it should be noted that GXL do not completely eliminate the organic solvent, as SFE using neat CO_2 does (Scurto et al. 2009).

Several parameters are involved in the extraction of bioactives from herbal sources by SFE. Among them, it is necessary to precisely control the effect of the extraction temperature, pressure, percentage, type of modifier addition, and amount of sample to be extracted, as well as its particle size and use of dispersing agents. The first parameters are more related to the solubility of the target compounds in the supercritical fluid, since changes in the extraction temperature and pressure will have a strong influence on the solvent properties, such as density. Although supercritical solvents have diffusivity in the matrix that is higher than liquids, a decrease in the sample particle size generally produces an increase in the extraction yield obtained, mainly due to the increase in the surface contact between sample and solvent, thus increasing mass transfer. Nevertheless, in some applications the use of dispersing agents (e.g. sea sand, glass beads, diatomaceous earth) or hydromatrix to absorb liquid from the sample can be useful.

SFE can be performed in solid and liquid matrices: for solid samples, the equipment comprises an extraction vessel of a given internal volume; for liquid samples (oils, juices, etc.), the extraction plant uses an extraction column in which the extraction is performed in countercurrent mode. Countercurrent extraction is performed by introducing the sample in the system from the top of the column and the pressurized solvent from the bottom; in this process, the components distribute between the solvent and the liquid sample, which flows countercurrent through the separation column. Depending on the separation factor between the components to be extracted, the desired contact time between the solvent and the sample can be varied by adjusting the height of the sample introduction into the extraction column or modifying the performance of the separation column, in terms of height and diameter, or of the packing material (structured/random, packing dimensions, surface area, etc.) (Brunner 1994; Brunner 2005).

For a more detailed description of the equipment used for SFE, readers are referred to Herrero et al. (2006).

5.3.2 Applications of SFE to Herbs and Spices

SFE has been widely studied for the recovery of bioactive compounds from herbs and spices and several recent reviews can be found dealing with this application (Herrero et al. 2013; De Melo et al. 2014; Fornari et al. 2012).

Among the type of matrices that have been extracted from herbs and spices, roots, rhizomes, leaves, bark, flowers, fruits, and seeds have been studied (De Melo et al. 2014); their content and composition in bioactive compounds being variable and dependent on factors such as location, harvesting time, cultivation practice, soil nutrients, and climatic conditions (Pereira et al. 2008). Considering the nature and the physical properties of $SCCO_2$, SFE has been mainly used to extract non-polar bioactive compounds, such as fatty acids, triglycerides, phytosterols, terpenoids, tocopherols, and carotenoids, among others (De Melo et al. 2014). Table 5.1 summarizes some remarkable studies published over five years (2010–2014) for the SFE of bioactive compounds from herbs and spices.

5.3.2.1 Phenolic Compounds Herbs and spices have been widely used as a source of phenolic compounds, due to their functional properties that have been extensively used in pharmaceutical formulations or as additives in food products (Embuscado 2015). SFE of phenolic compounds usually requires the addition of ethanol and methanol as modifiers of the polarity of $SCCO_2$ due to their inherent polar nature. Usually, quantities of up to 20% (Ansari and Goodarznia 2012; Santoyo et al. 2014; Camila et al. 2010) are employed, although percentages as low as 2–5% have been shown to be useful to extract, for instance, polyphenols and terpenoids (Kraujalis and Venskutonis 2013). Some studies have demonstrated that spices and herbs, such as rosemary, oregano, sage, hyssop, and thyme, extracted with SFE possess a high content of phenolic compounds with an antioxidant activity comparable to the activity of BHA (butyl hydroxy anisol) (Babovic et al. 2010). Although so far antioxidant activity is the most studied feature of these extracts, other biological properties such as anti-inflammatory, antiviral, antibacterial, cytotoxicity, and antiproliferative against cancer cells are beginning to be explored (Cheah et al. 2010; Ocaña-Fuentes et al. 2010; Valdés et al. 2013; Santoyo et al. 2014). Valdés et al. 2013, studied the effect of rosemary extracts rich in polyphenols (rosmarinic acid, carnosol, carnosic acid), obtained using PLE and SFE, on gene expression of human SW480 and HT29 colon cancer cells. The study demonstrated that carnosol/carnosic acid-enriched extracts showed the strongest effect on the proliferation of both cell lines. Meanwhile, Santoyo et al. (2014) evaluated the antiviral properties of supercritical CO_2 extracts obtained from thyme species (*Thymus vulgaris*, *Thymus hyemalis*, and *Thymus zygis*) against the herpes simplex virus type 1 (HSV-1) at different stages of the virus infection. Results indicated that when cells were pretreated with the thyme extracts, an important reduction in virus infectivity was achieved, with the *T. zygis* extract being more effective than other thyme species.

Table 5.1 Some remarkable recent published works (2010–2014) dealing with the use of SFE for the extraction of bioactive components from herbs and spices

Source	Bioactive compound of interest	Extraction conditions			Related functional bioactivities	Reference
		Solvent	P (MPa)/T (°C)	Extraction time (min)/Mode		
Ginger (*Zingiber officinale* R.)	Phenolic compounds	CO_2 Propane	CO_2: 25/60 Propane: 10/60	180/dynamic	Antioxidant activity	1
Green Tea Leaves	Caffeine	CO_2 + ethanol (1–3% w/w)	23/65	120/dynamic	Stimulant	2
Magnolia officinalis	Honokiol and Magnolo	CO_2	40/80	60 + 40/ static + dynamic/	antioxidant, anti-inflammatory activities	3
Oregano Leaves (*Origanum vulgare*)	Essential oil	CO_2	30/40.	NI/dynamic	Anti-inflammatory activity	4
Rosemary (*Rosmarinus officinalis*)	Phenolic compounds	CO_2	30/40	300/dynamic	Antioxidant activity	5
Rosemary (*Rosmarinus officinalis*)	Carnosic acid, Carnosol, Rosmarinic acid	CO_2 + ethanol (7% w/w)	150/40	300/dynamic	Antiproliferative colon cancer cells activity	6
Rosemary (*Rosmarinus officinalis*)	Volatil compounds, carnosic, and carnosol	CO_2 + ethanol (5–10% w/w)	15/40	180/dynamic	Antioxidant activity for use in edible oils	7
Rosemary + spinach leaves (50%)	Phenolic diterpenes and carotenoids	CO_2	30/40	300/dynamic	Antioxidant activity	8
Spearmint (*Mentha spicata* L.)	Essential oil	CO_2	9/35	30/static	Antioxidant activity	9
Thyme (*Thymus vulgaris, Thymus hyemalis, Thymus zygis*)	Thymol, carvacrol, borneol, linalool	CO_2	30/40	480 min/dynamic	Antiviral activity	10

NI, No indicated.

5.3.2.2 Essential Oils SFE of essential oils from herbs and spices has increasing importance considering their wide application in the manufacture of foodstuffs, cosmetics, cleaning products, fragrances, herbicides and insecticides, and the advantages that SFE can provide (Fornari et al. 2012).

Nowadays, research involving SFE of essential oils from herbs and spices is based on three different approaches: (i) the use of $SCCO_2$ as an alternative replacement for steam distillation and *n*-hexane as extraction agents, in order to improve extraction yields and avoid environment and health hazards (Shao et al. 2014; Przygoda and Wejnerowska 2015; Pavlić et al. 2015; Bagheri et al. 2014); (ii) enhancement of the concentration of the compound(s) responsible for the bioactivity and/or for the organoleptic properties by developing integrated SFE processes that include additional steps (e.g. sample pretreatment or fractionation) (Arranz et al. 2015; Gañán and Brignole 2013; De Oliveira et al. 2014; Santoyo et al. 2014; Gañán et al. 2015; Sánchez-Camargo et al. 2014); and (iii) the exploration of new bioactive compounds from distinctive herb species and testing of their bioactivity (Maran and Priya 2015). In many of the aforementioned studies, the use of experimental design has been a great help in minimizing the number of experiments required to determine the optimum extraction conditions.

Considering the great variation among bioactive compounds and the huge number of plant species, recently Azmir et al. (2013) adapted a strategy from Farnsworth et al. (1985) to build up a standard and integrated approach to screen out these compounds. Selection of plant spices, evaluation of toxicity, sample preparation and extraction, elemental analysis, biological testing, isolation of active compounds and *in vivo* analysis are among the steps proposed before marketing of bioactive compounds.

5.4 Ultrasound-Assisted Extraction (UAE)

5.4.1 Description of the Technique

UAE uses acoustic cavitation to cause disruption of cell walls, reduction of the particle size, and enhancement of contact between the solvent and the target compound. It is very versatile, due to the possibility of using several solvents of different polarities. Moreover, it allows fast extraction, which crucially avoids degradation of labile compounds. It also uses low amounts of solvents and is cost effective; therefore, the development of UAE methods could represent a key point in sustainable development (Picó 2013).

In UAE, only a small portion of the ultrasound spectrum is used; namely, power ultrasounds. Power ultrasounds, having frequencies between 20 kHz and 100 MHz, are well known to have significant effects on the rate of various physical and chemical processes such as cleaning, degassing, solubilization, homogenization, emulsification, sieving, filtration, and crystallization. Power ultrasound involves the mechanical and chemical effects of cavitation. When a liquid is irradiated by ultrasound, micro-bubbles form, grow, and oscillate extremely fast – and eventually collapse powerfully if the acoustic pressure is high enough. These collapses, occurring near a solid surface, generate micro-jets and shock waves that result in cleaning, erosion, and fragmentation of the surface. Micro-discharges due to high electrical fields generated by deformation and fragmentation of the bubbles and the formation of radicals could be responsible for the observed chemical effects (Ötles 2009). The uses of ultrasound are broadly distinguished into two groups: high and low intensity. Low-intensity ultrasound is involved in non-destructive analysis to provide information on physicochemical properties (e.g. in fruits it is used to study firmness, ripeness, sugar content, and acidity). Conversely, high-intensity ultrasound – low frequency (16–100 kHz) high power (typically 10–1000 W/cm^2) – can modify food properties physically or chemically. High-intensity ultrasound is used, among other applications, to speed up and improve extraction efficiency (Picó 2013).

Selection of the best extraction solvent for UAE depends on its physical properties (surface tension, viscosity, and vapor pressure) which may affect the cavitation intensity in a liquid phase. The cavitation intensity increases for solvents with low vapor pressure, high viscosity, and high surface tension, although the cavities are more easily formed with a solvent that has a high vapor pressure, low viscosity, and low surface tension. Thus, solvents with high surface tensions, densities, and viscosities generally have a higher threshold for cavitation but more harsh conditions once cavitation begins (Vardanega et al. 2014).

The use of ultrasound in extraction processes has two main requirements: a liquid medium (at least 5% of the overall medium) and a source of high-energy vibrations (ultrasounds) (Vardanega et al. 2014). The vibrational energy source is called a transducer, which transfers the vibration (after amplification) to the so-called sonotrode or ultrasonic probe, which is in direct or indirect contact with the processing medium. The two pieces of ultrasound apparatus most commonly used for extraction are the ultrasonic cleaning bath and the more powerful probe system. For small extraction volumes, an ultrasound horn with the tip submerged in the fluid can be sufficient. Large volumes of fluids have to be in an ultrasound bath or in continuous or recycled-flow sonoreactors (Ötles 2009). While most of the research effort in UAE has concentrated on ultrasound itself, some studies have also examined the coupling between ultrasound and other techniques; examples will be provided in Section 5.7 of this chapter.

UAE of bioactive compounds is increasingly efficient at directly transferring knowledge into technology for commercial development. This novel process can extract analytes under a concentrated form (low volumes of solvent) and free from any contaminants or artifacts. The new systems developed so far clearly demonstrate the advantages of UAE in terms of yield, selectivity, operating time, energy input, and even preservation of thermolabile compounds (Ötles 2009).

5.4.2 Applications of UAE to Herbs and Spices

As mentioned, ultrasound has been recognized for its potential industrial application in the phyto-pharmaceutical extraction industry for a wide range of herbal extracts. The mechanical effects of ultrasound together with the disruption of biological cell walls to release their content provide important benefits to extractive processes (Vilkhu et al. 2008). Due to these advantages, UAE has been used in many applications in food research.

5.4.2.1 Phenolic Compounds Among bioactive compounds, phenolics have been the target of numerous applications using UAE (Rathod and Rathod 2014; Both et al. 2014; Xia et al. 2006; Hossain et al. 2012; Chemat et al. 2011).

Several studies have demonstrated that the extraction yield of phenolic compounds depends strongly on the extraction technique, solvent polarity, and temperature (Sultana et al. 2009; Lapornik et al. 2005). For this reason, the optimization of the variables involved in UAE by RSM has gained interest in order to reduce the number of experimental runs, cost, and time. Barbero et al. (2008) studied the effect of the ultrasound-assisted variables type of solvent, extraction temperature, extraction time, amount of sample, and solvent volume on the extraction of capsaicinoids from hot cayenne pepper. The authors found that at the optimal conditions (methanol, 50 °C, and 10 minutes of extraction time), 100% of the capsaicinoids were recovered and the amount of sample and the solvent volume were not relevant parameters (Barbero et al. (2008)). Ghasemzadeh et al. (2014) also found that ultrasonic power (80–150 W), methanol percentage in the solvent mixture (40–80%), and extraction temperature (40–80 °C) significantly affected the extraction yield of catechin, naringin, and quercetin from curry leaves (Ghasemzadeh et al. 2014). Optimal conditions were obtained using an ultrasonic power of 145.52 W at 55.9 °C with 80% methanol; extracts achieved showed important anticancer and antioxidant activities. UAE was also employed to extract phenolic compounds (coumaric and 2-hidroxycinnamic acid, among others) from bay leaves (*Laurus nobilis* L.). The effects of several experimental factors, such as sonication time (20–60 minutes), solid/liquid ratio (1 : 4–1 : 8 g/ml), and concentration of ethanol in the solvent (0–70%) on extraction of phenolic compounds were evaluated through a randomized complete factorial design (3^3). The optimal extraction conditions were solid/liquid ratio 1 : 12 (g/ml), and time of sonication 40 minutes, with an ethanol concentration of 35%.

5.4.2.2 Essential Oils Some herbs and spices, like artemisia (Da Porto et al. 2009), peppermint (Shotipruk et al. 2001), laurel (*Laurus nobilis* L.), rosemary (*Rosmarinus officinalis* L.), thyme (*Thymus vulgaris* L.), and oregano leaves (*Oreganum majorana*), have been submitted to UAE to improve essential oil extraction (Roldán-Gutiérrez et al. 2008). Roldán-Gutiérrez et al. (2008) stated that UAE is more effective than steam distillation and SHWE for aroma compound extraction. UAE provides extracts with an aroma closer to the natural, due to the higher concentration of the most volatile fraction. Morsy (2015) studied the influence of UAE followed by hydro-distillation of *Elettaria cardamomum* L. seeds. The authors concluded that sonication power and sonication time highly influenced the yield and quality (high-terpinyl acetate/1, 8-cineole ratio) of the obtained essential oil. The optimal operating conditions include water-to-dried seeds ratio of 12, sonication at 10% of the maximal power (30 W), and a sonication time of 30 minutes prior to hydro-distillation for another 30 minutes; the process is considerably shorter (30 minutes vs. 6 hours) than the traditional hydro-distillation employed for full extraction of essential oil from cardamom seeds. Moreover, UAE has been coupled to vacuum distillation to obtain flavor compounds from spearmint leaves (Da Porto et al. 2009). Results showed that the combination of these processes provided extracts with higher flavoring strength due to the increased concentration of desirable oxygenated compounds (from 5 to 8 times) compared to hydro-distillation. Extraction yields of flavor volatiles increased from 0.01–0.02% by hydro-distillation to 0.04–0.13% by ultrasound coupled to vacuum distillation.

5.5 Microwave-Assisted Extraction (MAE)

5.5.1 Description of the Technique

MAE uses microwave radiation that causes motion of polar molecules and rotation of dipoles to heat solvents to promote the transfer of target compounds from the sample matrix into the solvent (Ötles 2009). Just like UAE, MAE allows fast extractions with a small amount of extraction solvent; avoiding degradation of thermolabile compounds and providing green extracts from herbal resources.

Microwaves are non-ionizing electromagnetic waves located within the frequency band of 300 MHz–300 GHz (between the radio-frequency range and the infrared at the higher frequency) in the electromagnetic spectrum; 2450 MHz frequency is generally used in domestic microwave ovens and for extraction purposes (Routray and Orsat 2012). In MAE, the sample is heated using microwaves, at typical powers of 700 W for a short time. Compared to traditional extraction techniques, the use of microwaves allows a decrease in extraction times, significantly limiting the amount of solvent needed.

MAE was first described in 1986 (Ganzler et al. 1986); in this work, a domestic microwave was used as sample preparation technique prior to chromatography. A variety of compounds from seeds, foods, and feeds were extracted; the process was found to be more efficient than classical Soxhlet or LLE. The application of microwave irradiation to the extraction of compounds from biological samples has been a more recent development.

A microwave system consists normally of three basic parts (Routray and Orsat 2012):

- *Magnetron*. The microwave source. This consists of a vacuum tube with a central electron-emitting cathode of highly negative potential surrounded by a structured anode that forms cavities, which are coupled by the fringing fields and have the intended microwave resonant frequency.
- *Wave guide*. Transmission lines and wave guides can be used for guiding the electromagnetic waves. In the food industry and domestic oven applications, the most common are standing wave devices, where the microwaves irradiate by slot arrays (that cut the wall currents) or horn antennas (specially formed open ends) of waveguides.
- Applicator or oven.

The solvent is one of the most important factors in MAE extraction. In general, the higher the dielectric constant of the solvent, the higher its capacity to absorb microwave energy, which can lead to faster rate of heating of the solvent with respect to the herbal material (Routray and Orsat 2012). A combination of solvents leads to varying selectivity and microwave heating capacity. For extraction of thermolabile compounds, a solvent combination with relatively low dielectric properties can be used to ensure that the solvent temperature will remain lower to cool-off the solutes once they are liberated into the solvent. In this case, the microwave energy interacts preferentially with the plant matrix (Kaufmann and Christen 2002). Even ionic liquids can be used as potential solvents for MAE of vegetable compounds. The anions and cations of ionic liquids have been described as having an influence on the extraction of polyphenolic compounds, and the ionic liquids with electron-rich aromatic π-system were found to enhance the extraction yield (Du et al. 2009).

In general, samples for MAE are homogenized and mixed with a solvent and the suspension irradiated at a frequency greater than 2000 MHz for short periods of time. Heating is usually repeated several times with periods of cooling in between to prevent boiling. Efficiencies seen with this technique approach those of classical Soxhlet extraction but it can be performed much more rapidly. Further modifications of the technique mimic sweep co-distillation or steam distillation with air sweeping the surface of the heated sample and being collected by a condenser that protrudes through the oven housing (Worsfold et al. 2005). MAE techniques have also been developed using closed-system microwave heating that implies an increase of pressure due to the heating at temperatures higher than the boiling point of the solvent; thus, extraction takes place in a similar condition as PLE.

There are two approaches to applying microwave energy, namely, the mere bulk heating of a mixture through the use of absorbing containers and solvents (oven-type apparatus with samples in closed-vessel conditions), and the more refined, although demanding, selective heating of the target materials. These two approaches have led to the development of two main types of laboratory extraction instruments.

By using selective heating, it is possible to operate safely and much more efficiently under open-vessel conditions (i.e. atmospheric pressure); under these conditions, operating temperatures remain low. Once fitted with an appropriate reflux column, the system is auto-controlled in terms of temperature. A technology combining microwave and Soxhlet extraction was designed in 1998 (Garcia-Ayuso et al. 1998). This extraction technique, called microwave-assisted Soxhlet extraction, uses two sources of energy, namely microwaves applied on the extraction chamber of a modified Soxhlet apparatus, and electrical heating applied on the distillation flask.

5.5.2 Applications of MAE to Herbs and Spices

Over the last years, MAE has been increasingly employed for the extraction of bioactive compounds in herbs and species due to the quality of the final extracts (Heng et al. 2013). The most interesting bioactive compounds susceptible to being extracted with MAE are phenolic compounds, essential oils, alkaloids, and saponins.

5.5.2.1 Phenolic Compounds The recovery of phenolic compounds by MAE is being widely studied nowadays, due to the high extraction yields that this technique is able to provide. Indeed, yields obtained by MAE usually are as high as those achieved using conventional processes, but with shorter extraction times (Flórez et al. 2015).

The main objective in MAE extraction of phenolic compounds is to obtain high extraction yields without affecting the stability of bioactive compounds. Thus, it is important to optimize all the parameters affecting the extraction process; that is, extraction solvent, extraction temperature, microwave power, irradiation time, liquid to solid ratio, extract cycle, and, in some cases, extraction pressure (Fang et al. 2015).

As in all extraction processes, extraction of target compounds is greatly affected by the type of solvent; methanol, ethanol, and their mixtures with water in different proportions have been described as optimal solvents for MAE recovery of phenolic compounds from different herbs. Additionally, the material to solvent ratio is another parameter to study in order to obtain a complete extraction of the target compounds while employing the minimum quantity of solvent possible (Liu et al. 2012b). This ratio may vary between 5 and 30 ml/g for the recovery of phenolic compounds of different herbs.

For the extraction of phenolic compounds such as flavonols, flavones, flavanones, or phenolic acids, usually moderate temperatures (between 50 and 80 °C) are employed to preserve the stability of the bioactive (Fang et al. 2015; Ruan et al. 2014; Bekdeşer et al. 2014; Liu et al. 2012b).

In terms of extraction time, as a general rule, recoveries increase with an increase in the extraction time. But exposing the phenolic compounds to microwaves and heat for long time periods can degrade the bioactive compounds, and, therefore, most of the applications of MAE for the extraction of phenolic compounds use extraction times between 2 and 25 minutes. These extraction times are far shorter than the times required for conventional extraction techniques.

Another important factor in MAE is the microwave power. By increasing power, it is possible to enhance the yield; however, as occurs with the temperature, high power can give rise to a degradation of some compounds. For this reason, relatively low powers (180–600 W) are used to achieve an herbal extract with intact phenolic compounds (Liu et al. 2012b).

5.5.2.2 Essential Oils MAE is considered one of the best options for the extraction of herbal plants' essential oils due to the high extraction efficiency and good quality of the obtained essential oil (Costa et al. 2014). In fact, essential oil extraction is the widest MAE application for herbs and spices.

In this particular application, it is worth mentioning the technique known as solvent-free microwave extraction (SFME). SFME consists of the extraction of the compounds of interest from a fresh sample locked into a microwave reactor without the addition of any solvent or water. This technique decreases the hydrolysis, transesterification, and oxidation reactions during the extraction. Therefore, the oxygenated compounds, responsible for the odoriferous quality of the essential oils, are not affected by the process and they appear in the extract in higher quantities, giving rise to an extract with better quality and properties (Orio et al. 2012).

Filly et al. (2014) conducted a scaling up of a SFME method, from laboratory to pilot scale, for the extraction of essential oils from rosemary. Optimum conditions selected were: irradiation power of 3 kW, 30 minutes at 100 °C, 75 l pilot microwave reactor. The results revealed extraction yields and quantity of oxygenated compounds (0.50% and 36.2%, respectively) comparable to laboratory scale experiments (0.54% and 32%, respectively). Furthermore, reduction in costs compared to conventional hydro-distillation (HD) was proved, since the expended energy and time were greatly reduced (4.5 kWh/g of essential oil and 120 minutes for HD and 0.25 kWh/g of essential oil and 30 minutes for SFME). These data may open up good perspectives for application of this method at industrial scale.

Microwave-assisted hydro-distillation technique (MAHD) is another technique derived from MAE; it is carried out by employing water as the exclusive solvent for extraction. This technique has been widely employed for the extraction of essential oils from herbs and spices such as *Bunium persicum* Boiss (Mazidi et al. 2012), *Pimenta dioica* (Jiang et al. 2013), *Mentha piperita* L. (Gavahian et al. 2015), *Coriandrum sativum* L. (Sourmaghi et al. 2015), *Curcuma longa* L., and *Carum carvi* (Akloul et al. 2014), or several Lamiaceae family herbs (*Origanum majorana* L., *Mentha pulegium* L., and *Melissa officinalis* L.) (Petrakis et al. 2014).

5.5.2.3 Alkaloids Compared to conventional methods for alkaloid extraction (heat reflux extraction [HRE], infusion extraction [IE], or UAE), MAE has demonstrated important advantages in terms of yield and extraction time. Liang et al. (2014) evaluated all the parameters that affect the extraction of alkaloids from *Portulaca oleracea* by MAE, concluding that temperature was the main factor influencing the process. In general, the recovery of alkaloids improves with an increase in temperature (Zhou et al. 2012).

Due to the basic nature of alkaloids, in some cases the solvent selection includes the addition of acidified solutions to the extracting solvent in order to enhance their selective recovery (Jiang et al. 2009). For example, Zhou et al. (2012) tested the addition of different proportions of hydrochloric acid in a mixture of methanol/water (90 : 10, *v/v*) for the extraction of alkaloids from *Chelidonium majus* L. The addition of the optimized quantity of acid (0.5% HCl) provided an enhanced extraction of the target compounds.

MAE extraction of alkaloids from herbs and species has not only been focused on bioactive alkaloids (Liang et al. 2014; Zhou et al. 2012), but also on toxic alkaloids like yucanotine and related aconite alkaloids (Song et al. 2012).

5.5.2.4 Saponins Different studies have been conducted on the extraction of saponins using MAE. Examples are the MAE extraction of steroid saponins from the medical herb *Paris polyphylla,* for which optimal conditions were: an irradiation power of 300 W, liquid to solid ratio of 20 ml/g using a mixture of ethanol/water, 70 : 30 (v/v), 50 °C and 15 minutes (Xiao et al. 2014). MAE conditions for the extraction of triterpene saponins from *Pulsatilla turczaninovii* were 500 W of microwave power at 80 °C for 3 minutes, employing the same extraction solvent and the same solid to liquid ratio. As can be seen, the main differences relate to extraction temperature and time. Although the extraction of saponins is enhanced at high temperatures, the percentage of saponins extracted starts to decrease when a high temperature is maintained for a long time due to the thermal degradation of the compounds. In the abovementioned applications, the conditions employed are different but compatible with the thermal stability of saponins since one of them employs a moderate temperature (50 °C) over a longer time (15 minutes) while the other carries out the extraction at a high temperature (80 °C) but over a short time (3 minutes). Both strategies protect the bioactive compounds allowing their efficient extraction.

The temperature employed during extraction not only depends on the thermal stability of the compounds, but also on the boiling point of the solvent. In this sense, vacuum microwave-assisted extraction (VMAE) can decrease the extraction system pressure, and therefore the boiling temperature of the extraction solvent can be lower, thus allowing the extraction process to be performed at more milder temperatures. As an example, Hiranvarachat et al. (2015) studied the extraction kinetic of saponins from the herbaceous plant *Centella asiatica,* comparing MAE and VMAE extractions. The solvent selected was ethanol. VMAE carried out at 60 kPa obtained a higher quantity of saponins thanks to the effect of the vacuum pressure, which reduced the boiling point of ethanol from 78 °C, at atmospheric pressure, to 65 °C at 60 kPa. However, the lower pressures (40 and 20 kPa) showed lower extraction efficiencies related to a lower diffusivity of the saponins with the decrease of the solvent boiling point. A schematic diagram of the system employed in this study is shown in Figure 5.1.

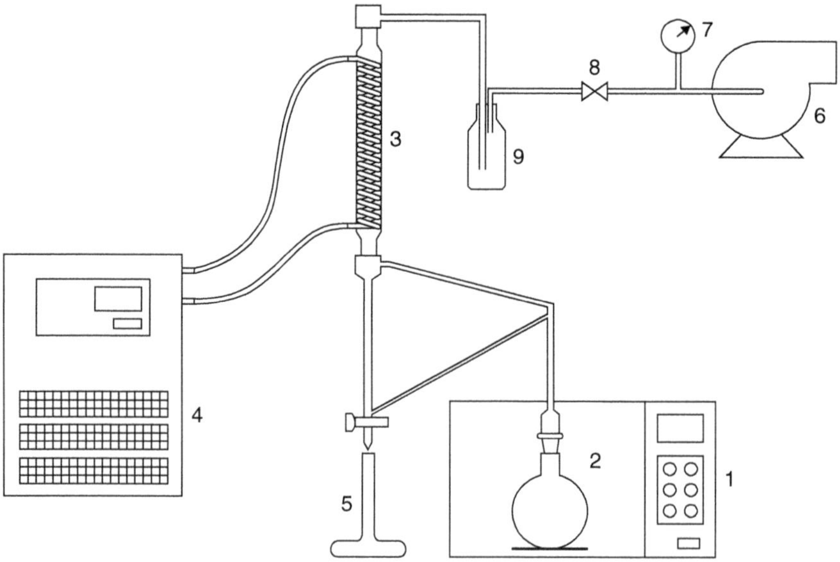

Figure 5.1 Schematic diagram of the vacuum microwave-assisted extraction (VMAE) and associated units. 1: domestic microwave oven; 2: round-bottom flask; 3: external condenser; 4: cooling water system; 5: graduated cylinder; 6: vacuum pump; 7: pressure gauge; 8: pressure-control valve; 9: vapor trap. *Source:* Reprinted from Hiranvarachat et al. 2015, with permission from John Wiley and Sons.

5.6 Enzyme-Assisted Extraction (EAE)

5.6.1 Description of the Technique

Given the ever-increasing demand for new, environmentally friendly, advanced extraction methods, due to the particular nature of plant materials, the use of enzymes to assist in the extraction of bioactives is gaining attention. Plant cells possess a strong cell wall that is usually structured in a three-dimensional matrix formed by polysaccharides and glycoproteins. Among the variety of cell wall constituents, cellulose, hemicellulose, pectin, and lignin are the most common groups. These structures provide a physical barrier that hinders or makes difficult the extraction of linked components. For this reason, the use of enzymes to effectively weaken cell wall structures is useful, also in combination with other extraction techniques, as will be described below.

Enzymes catalyze hydrolysis reactions of the cell wall components with a huge degree of specificity, regioselectivity, and usually under mild reaction conditions, which further favors the recovery of bioactive compounds. Thus, depending on the material to be extracted, cellulases, hemicellulases, pectinases, or mixtures thereof are employed. As a result, the cell walls are effectively weakened and their porosity is increased, thus facilitating the extraction of the target components.

Consequently, in order to develop effective EAE processes, the first information that should be obtained is the composition of the cell wall of the plant material to be extracted. This knowledge will allow the precise selection of the most appropriate enzymes. Once the enzyme, or enzyme cocktail, is selected, different parameters should be considered, including enzyme charge, reaction temperature, reaction time, pH of the reaction medium, as well as other considerations related to the physical state of the sample. In general, a reduced particle size will help to increase the efficiency of the enzyme treatment, increasing surface contact. Regarding the rest of the parameters, these will be strongly related to the enzyme or enzymes to be used, as each enzyme usually possesses narrow working ranges in terms of temperature and pH. Thus, if a mixture of enzymes is to be used, compromise values should be selected in order to ensure all the reactions working. Reaction time is also an important parameter; since not all the enzymes possess fast hydrolysis rates, long reaction times are common. In fact, a two-hour treatment may be regarded as quite short, while it is normally lengthy for other extraction techniques.

Once the reaction is finished, the solid matter is separated from the solution by centrifugation. Other processes may require enzyme inactivation, generally by increasing the temperature. Although there are applications for the use of enzymes alone in the extraction of bioactives, this technique is more convenient if coupled to other advanced extraction techniques, such as PLE or SFE, as the damage caused to the cells definitely helps increase the penetration of the solvents into the matrix, thus enhancing the mass transfer rate and favoring the recovery of the target compounds.

5.6.2 Applications of EAE to Herbs and Spices

EAE has been mainly applied to herbs and spices to obtain oleoresins, essential oils, spice emulsion, spice essence, encapsulated spices, powders, etc., due to the high yield and quality of the products obtained (Chandran et al. 2012).

Although, as mentioned in this chapter, many different extraction processes are currently used for essential oil and oleoresin recovery from spices, recently application of enzymes during the extraction process has gained attention due to its advantages in terms of yield and greenness. As mentioned, enzymes must be selected based on their action on the cell wall components and the chemical composition of the spice material (Chandran et al. 2012). Considering the composition of the primary cell wall of plants (Jordan et al. 2012), cellulases, hemicelullases, and pectinases have been commonly used (Miron et al. 2013; Azmir et al. 2013). Besides the type of enzyme selected, other factors such as pH, reaction time, spice/enzyme ratio, and temperature should be adjusted to find the optimal reaction conditions (Sowbhagya et al. 2011). Table 5.2 presents some recent applications of EAE for essential oils and oleoresins from herbs and spices. Chandran et al. (2012) reported the use of a mixture of cellulase, β-glucananse, pectinase, and xylamase to increase the yield of essential oil from 0.9% to 1.8% in black pepper and 1.9% to 2.5% in cardamom (Chandran et al. 2012). Also, application of enzymes during the extraction of ginger has been reported to increase the yield of essential oil and gingerol recovery to 5% and 90%, respectively (Nagendra chari et al. 2013). Similarly, Naidu et al. (2012) concluded that the use of EAE is very useful for obtaining a higher yield of vanilla extract and a superior quality of vanilla flavor, avoiding the traditional laborious and time-consuming curing process (Naidu et al. 2012). Mixtures of enzymes have been also employed to enhance the extraction yield and biological activities of essential oils; for instance, *Thymus capitatus* and *Rosmarinus officinalis* leaves were submitted to an enzymatic pretreatment to isolate the essential oils by hydro-distillation. Results showed that the combination of cellulase and hemicellulase promoted a 109% and 20% increase in the

Table 5.2 Some remarkable recent published works dealing with the use of EAE of bioactive components from herbs and spices

Source	Bioactive compound of interest	Pre-treatment enzyme	Extraction technique	Reference
Vanilla planifolia	Vanilla extract (Vanillin)	Viscozyme®, Tea leaf enzyme extract (TLEE)	S-L Extraction (Ethanol)	1
Black pepper	Essential oil	Cellulase, β-glucanase, pectinase, and xylanase	Steam distillation	2
Cardamom	Essential oil	Cellulase, β-glucanase, pectinase, and xylanase	Steam distillation	2
Cumin seeds (*Cuminum cyminum*)	Essential oil	Cellulase, Hemicellulase, Protease, Pectinase Viscozyme®	Steam distillation Hydrodistillation	3
Ginger (*Zingiber officinale* R.)	Oleoresin (Gingerol)	α-amylase, viscozyme, cellulase, pectinase	S-L Extraction (Ethanol, Acetone)	4
Lemon balm (*Melissa officinalis*)	Phenolic compounds	Cellulase, endo-1,4-β-xylanase, pectinase	Pressurized Liquid Extraction (PLE)	5
Turmeric	Oleoresin Curcuminoid Volatile oil	α-Amylase, Glucoamylase, Xylanase + Cellulase	S-L Extraction (Acetone)	6
	Essential oil	Cellulase, hemicellulose	Hydrodistillation	7
Thyme (*Thymus capitatus* L.)				
Rosemary (*Rosmarinus officinalis* L.)	Essential oil	Cellulase, hemicellulase,	Hydrodistillation	7
Bay leaves (*Laurus nobilis* L.)	Volatile oil Hydrodistilled leaf residues extracts	Cellulase, hemi-cellulase, xylanase	Hydrodistillation S-L Extraction	8

S–L, Solid–Liquid.

essential oil yields for *T. capitatus* and *R. officinalis*, respectively. The combination of both enzymes also induced an increase of 38% in the amount of carvacrol, the main component in *T. capitatus*. In terms of associated bioactivity, essential oils obtained from the hemicellulase-treated samples were the most effective (Hosni et al. 2013).

5.7 Integration of Different Extraction Techniques

As mentioned in the introduction, nowadays the idea of obtaining valuable products of high quality and bioactivity, while improving the efficiency of the process and reducing operation costs and impact on human health and environment, is of outmost importance. Although the different extraction techniques that have been discussed throughout this chapter can each be considered a good approach, the possibility of integrating some of them in the same process can be even more effective in achieving the mentioned goals of effectiveness, greenness, and sustainability. Thus, by using this approach, purification of valuable components from different raw materials and sequential extraction of different compounds from the same sample can be achieved (Boyadzhiev et al. 2006).

Below, some of the most important integrated novel extraction processes that have been developed since 2012 for the extraction of compounds of interest from herbs and spices are presented.

5.7.1 Ultrasound–Microwave-Assisted Extraction (UMAE)

Ultrasound–microwave-assisted extraction (UMAE), also named ultrasonic–microwave synergistic extraction (UMSE), is a new technique that combines ultrasound and microwaves and, thus, the mechanisms of action of both techniques: the vibration-cavitation of UAE and the high energy of MAE (Zeng et al. 2015). As a result, an enhancement of the mass transfer mechanism is observed, caused by a high momentum and energy that induce the rupture of the plant cell and faster release of the compounds of interest from the matrix to the extraction solvent (Chan et al. 2011). This combined technique has been described as a powerful and efficient technique achieving high yields and purities with short extraction times and low solvent consumption (Lianfu and Zelong 2008; Chen et al. 2010). Consequently, UMAE accelerates the extraction procedure and, besides, improves the selectivity and simplifies the extraction operation (Xiao et al. 2012).

Since 2012, UMAE methodology has been successfully applied to the extraction of bioactive compounds from herbs; for example, Xiao et al. (2012) developed a new UMAE method for the extraction of alkaloids from *Picrasma quassioides*. A study and optimization of all the parameters affecting extraction yield during UMAE extraction (extraction temperature and time, liquid/solid ratio, and ultrasonic power) was carried out. They concluded that the correct selection of the solvent is crucial to obtain an optimal extraction process. Additionally, the solvent/solid ratio and the extraction time also had an important effect on the extraction yield. Optimal conditions in terms of process efficiency were as follows: water/methanol (90 : 10, *v/v*) as extracting solvent, 21 ml/g of liquid/solid ratio, 13 minutes extraction time.

Ionic liquids have also been applied in UMAE technology under the name of ionic liquid-based ultrasonic/microwave-assisted extraction (IL-UMAE) for the efficient extraction of bioactive compounds in herbs. Particularly, IL-UMAE has been successfully used for the extraction of steroid saponins from *Dioscorea zingiberensis* C. H. Wright (Wang et al. 2014). When ILs are involved in the extraction, their characteristics should also be optimized; that is, type of IL, length of alkyl chains, and IL concentration. In this work, several ILs were tested according to the characteristics of the target compounds. The length of the alkyl chain has an influence on the extraction since the increase in the carbon chain decreases the extraction rate, whereas the extraction yield of saponins increases with the concentration of IL. However, at a certain point, further increasing the IL concentration leads to a slight decreasing tendency on the yield due, probably, to the fact that a higher concentration could be translated in a higher viscosity, and therefore the penetration ability of the solution in the matrix is reduced. Finally, the optimum parameters were set at the use of 1-ethyl-3-methylimidazolium tetrafluoroborate ([EMIm]BF4) solution at a concentration of 0.5 mol/l, with a solvent to material ratio of 15 ml/g, 500 W of microwave irradiation, and 8 minutes of extraction time.

5.7.2 Enzyme-Based–Ultrasound–Microwave-Assisted Extraction (EUMAE)

The combination of EAE and UMAE as an integrated extraction process that is still not very common; however, some pioneer works have been published very recently dealing with the use of this integrated process for the extraction of, for example, the phenolic compound oricinol glucoside from the rhizomes of the herb *Curculigo orchioides* Gaertn (Liu et al. 2014). The first step in this process consists of the incubation of the powdered sample with the enzyme solution. Cellulase (3 ml) was the enzyme selected to hydrolyze and degrade the plant cell wall; incubation was carried out for 10 hours at 45 °C. For the next step, the factors involved in the UMAE extraction process were optimized; the process selected was as follows: the residue obtained after enzyme incubation was redissolved in a mixture of ethanol/water (70 : 30, *v/v*) with a solvent to material ratio of 8 ml/g. The extraction was carried out at 50 °C for 15 minutes at 400 W of irradiation.

Extraction time and temperature were the most influential factors on the extraction yield, with time being the most important parameter; for instance, a small change in the extraction time provided significant changes on the orcinol glucoside extraction. Compared to other new and classical extraction methods, such as hot water extraction, Soxhlet, MAE, UAE, or even UMAE, enzyme-based–ultrasound–microwave-assisted extraction (EUMAE) under optimum conditions achieved a better yield of the target compounds.

5.7.3 Supercritical Fluid Extraction–Pressurized Fluid Extraction (SFE–PLE)

Considering that SFE and PLE are two of the most important novel extraction techniques for bioactive isolation; their combination in a sequential or *in situ* extraction configuration has an interesting future applicability.

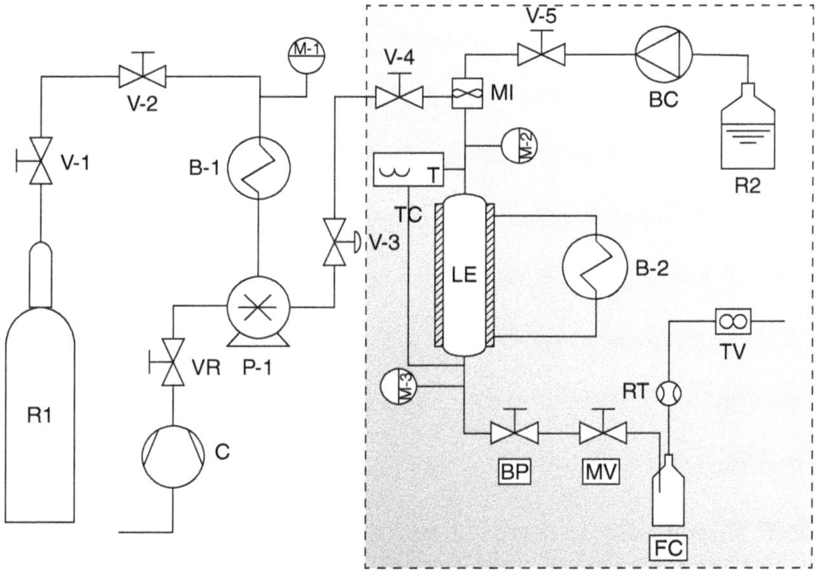

Figure 5.2 Schematic diagram of the home-built equipment designed to perform SFE–PLE to deflavor and recover curcuminoids from turmeric. R1: CO_2 reservoir; R2: extracting solvent reservoir; P-1: CO_2 pump; C: compressor; BC: HPLC pump; B-1: thermostatic bath; B-2: heating bath; LE: extraction cell; TC: temperature controllers; FC: collector flask; M: manometers; RT: glass float rotameter; TV: flow totalizer; V: blocking valves; MV: micrometric valve with a heating system; BP: back pressure regulator. *Source:* Reprinted from Osorio-Tobón et al. 2014, with permission from Elsevier.

Osorio-Tobón et al. (2014) developed home-built equipment that could be employed for both SFE and PLE (Figure 5.2). They used this equipment for the sequential extraction of curcuminoids from the rhizomes of *Curcuma longa* L. The integration of both processes consisted of a first deflavoration of the rhizomes with SFE and, in the same vessel, the extraction of the residue by PLE. To optimize the PLE process, the parameters tested were: temperature (between 60 and 80 °C) and pressure (between 10 and 35 MPa). Results showed that although, as expected, temperature had the main impact on the process, the combined effect of temperature and pressure was also important. The authors described that between 60 and 70 °C, an increase in pressure caused a negative effect on the curcuminoid extraction. This fact could be due to a decrease of the active surface of the raw material at higher pressures that could lead to a smaller surface contact between the solvent and the target compounds by the effect of the compacted material. Nevertheless, when the temperature was raised to 80 °C, the effect of the temperature and pressure on the yield was complex and variable, and a final increase on the extraction yield was observed due to the high mass transfer rate induced by the high temperature. Finally, the operation conditions were set at 60 °C and 10 MPa, allowing a reduction in the extraction time of 2 or 2.5 times compared to conventional extractions. The economic study also revealed that this SFE–PLE methodology is an attractive and economically feasible process.

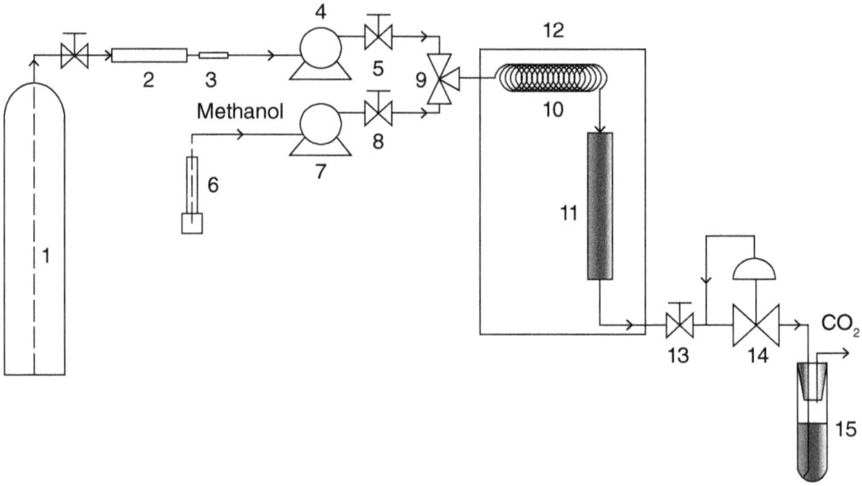

Figure 5.3 Schematic diagram of PLE system: 1: CO_2 tank; 2: molecular sieve filter; 3: ss 2 μm pore size filter; 4: carbon dioxide transfer pump; 5, 8, 13: two-way needle valves; 6: water vessel; 7: high-pressure piston pump; 9: three ways valve; 10: preheating coil; 11: extraction cell; 12: thermostated oven; 14: back-pressure regulator; 15: sample collection vessel. *Source:* Reprinted from Golmakani et al. 2014, with permission from Elsevier.

A different use of the PLE–SFE combination was carried out by Golmakani et al. (2014). In this application, a PLE extraction of the antioxidant compounds of *Scutellaria pinnatifida* followed by a SFE clean-up was developed. For this purpose, the authors used a modified SFE apparatus to develop a PLE process; the introduction of a switching valve after the pump allowed the changing of the solvent alternately in the different extraction steps (Figure 5.3). Hence, the implemented process started with PLE extraction with methanol, followed by a rinse of the PLE system (residual solvent, cell, tubing, and back pressure regulator) with supercritical CO_2 at the end of each extraction. Conditions of temperature, pressure, static, and dynamic extraction time and flow rate of this combined process were optimized in order to obtain the maximum extraction yield, total phenolic, total flavonoid, and antioxidant activity.

5.7.4 Supercritical Fluid Extraction Assisted by Ultrasound (SFE–UAE)

In order to evaluate the benefits of this integrated process, the extraction of capsaicinoids and phenolic compounds from *Capsicum frutescens* L. was tested (Santos et al. 2015). The extraction of capasaicinoids and phenolic compounds was carried out combining both processes on an ultrasound-assisted SFE unit (Figure 5.4).

In this work, the authors studied the global yield and the SFE kinetic of the extraction in order to compare the use of SFE–UAE with a SFE extraction without ultrasound irradiation. Two parameters affect the global yield: the US power and the application time of US. Results showed that at short times (60 minutes) and low US power (200 W) there are no statistically significant differences in the extraction yield

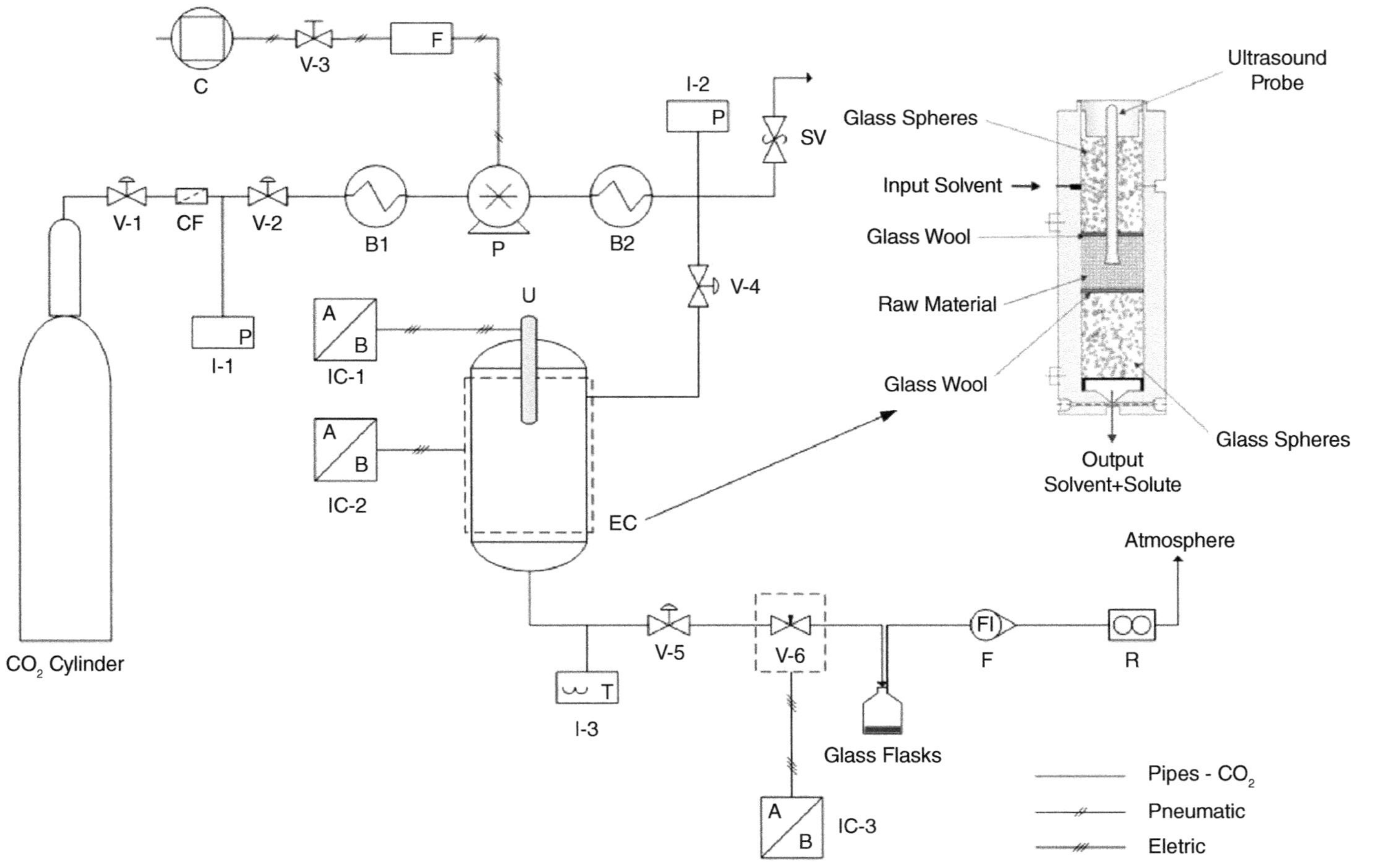

Figure 5.4 Diagram of the SFE + US unit: V-1, V-2, V-3, V-4 and V-5: control valves; V-6: micrometer valve; SV: safety valve; C: compressor; F: compressed air filter; CF: CO_2 filter; B1: cooling bath; P: pump; B2: heating bath; I-1 and I-2: pressure indicators; I-3: temperature indicator; IC-1, IC-2 and IC-3: indicators and controllers of ultrasound power, temperature of extraction column, and temperature of micrometer valve, respectively; U: ultrasound probe; R: flow totalizer; F: flow meter; EC: extraction column and internal configuration of the extraction bed of 295 ml for SFE + US used in the kinetic experiments. *Source:* Reprinted from Santos et al. 2015, with permission from Elsevier.

between both techniques. However, a positive effect on the extraction yield of the SFE–UAE was achieved when higher power was applied (360 W). Accordingly, the irradiation time and the ultrasound power used in both processes were statistically significant for the extraction yield. Once optimized, parameters for the SFE–UAE were set at 360 W and 60 minutes.

Regarding kinetics, the authors demonstrated that the application of ultrasound to the SFE had a positive effect, since at the end of the process the extraction yield obtained by SFE–UAE was 35% higher than the yield achieved by SFE alone. This increase was related to the application of ultrasound irradiation that promoted the rupture of the cells, and therefore the accessibility of the solvent to the inner structures of the matrix, as well as the acoustic streaming and mechanic vibration produced by the ultrasonic irradiation. Consequently, the extraction rates and efficiency of extraction were greatly improved. At this point, it is worth mentioning that the main phenomenon involved in UAE, cavitation, cannot be considered when ultrasounds are applied together with SFE because the formation of bubbles is not possible in the absence of phase boundaries.

Besides applications in which SFE and UAE extraction take place at the same time, some works integrate both techniques sequentially. This is the case in the fragmentation extraction of non-polar and polar compounds from *Coriandrum sativum* L. seeds (Zeković et al. 2015). The objective of this strategy was to carry out three sequential extractions consisting of a first SFE extraction step for obtaining essential oils, followed by an UAE with a mixture ethanol/water (70 : 30, *v/v*) for the recovery of moderately polar polyphenols, and ending with another UAE with water for the extraction of the more polar fraction. Conditions selected for the essential oil extraction by SFE were the following: 100 bar of pressure at 100 °C with a CO_2 flow rate of 0.194 kg/h, for four hours, setting 15 bar and 23 °C at the separator. For the UAE, the selected conditions were: a solvent to sample ratio of 10 ml/g, a frequency of 40 kHz, and 140 W of ultrasound power carried out at 30 °C. Here, the particle size of the sample had a huge influence on the extraction yield. It was demonstrated that a smaller particle size give rise to an increment on the extraction yield of essential oils on the SFE extraction, and to a linear increment of total phenol content and total flavonoid content during UAE.

5.8 Conclusions and Future Outlook

In this chapter, we have tried to demonstrate the usefulness of novel techniques for extracting valuable compounds, with important biological activities, from different herbs and spices. The advantages of these new technologies (PLE, SFE, UAE, MAE, EAE, and combined processes) have been underlined, mainly focusing on the Green Chemistry perspective, as sustainable and viable procedures to substitute for more conventional extraction techniques. For all of them, a description of the technology, the main parameters involved in the process, and the latest applications in the field of bioactives (mainly centered on phenolics, essential oils, and alkaloids) have been presented and discussed.

Although all these novel processes have been recognized as advantageous from an environmental point of view, the sustainability and eco-friendliness of a particular process is a goal that has to be approached through the application of analysis tools, such as life-cycle analysis (LCA). Real measures of the environmental impact and costs associated with these technologies would allow the selection of the best processes to be implemented at large scale.

Other interesting fields of research that can help improve the abovementioned processes even further have also been suggested in this chapter. The use of new solvents, such as ILs, and integrated processes open the door to the development of more efficient, cost-effective, clean, and sustainable processes. In this sense, the combination of ILs with supercritical fluids can allow us to integrate reaction and extraction processes into the same system; that is, carrying out a reaction in the most favorable phase (the ionic liquid) while the reaction products can later be extracted into the supercritical phase. This is just an example, as many others suggested in this chapter, of the possibilities offered by the combination of novel processes using green solvents (supercritical carbon dioxide, water, ethanol, ILs, GXLs, etc.) in which multiple operation conditions can be optimized and performed in the same platform, thus minimizing production costs. Operations that can be integrated include raw material pretreatment, reactions (biocatalysis, transesterification), extraction, biofuel conversion, and biorefinery of raw materials into their main and valuable constituents. To do this, a combination of processes, including use of enzymes, disruption methods such as US, and intensification methods like US applied to SFE, can provide new solutions for the sustainable production of, for instance, bioactives from herbs and spices.

Acknowledgments

A.P.S.C. thanks to the Administrative Department of Science, Technology and Innovation COLCIENCIAS (Colombia) for her Ph.D. Scholarship. M.H. would like to thank MICINN for his "Ramón y Cajal" research contract. The authors would also like to thank Projects AGL2011-29857-C03-01 (MINECO, Spain) and ALIBIRD-CM, S2013/ABI-2728 (Comunidad de Madrid), for their financial support.

References

Akien, G.R. and Poliakoff, M. (2009). A critical look at reactions in class I and II gas-expanded liquids using CO_2 and other gases. *Green Chemistry* **11** (8): 1083–1100.

Akloul, R., Benkaci-Ali, F., and Eppe, G. (2014). Kinetic study of volatile oil of *Curcuma longa* L. rhizome and *Carum carvi* L. fruits extracted by microwave-assisted techniques using the cryogrinding. *Journal of Essential Oil Research* **26** (6): 473–485.

Anastas, P.T. and Warner, J.C. (1998). *Green Chemistry: Theory and Practice*. New York: Oxford University Press.

Anastas, P.T. and Zimmerman, J.B. (2003). Peer reviewed: design through the 12 principles of green engineering. *Environmental Science & Technology* **37** (5): 94–101.

Ansari, K. and Goodarznia, I. (2012). Optimization of supercritical carbon dioxide extraction of essential oil from spearmint (*Mentha spicata* L.) leaves by using Taguchi methodology. *The Journal of Supercritical Fluids* **67**: 123–130.

Arranz, E., Jaime, L., de las Hazas, M.L. et al. (2015). Supercritical fluid extraction as an alternative process to obtain essential oils with anti-inflammatory properties from marjoram and sweet basil. *Industrial Crops and Products* **67**: 121–129.

Azmir, J., Zaidul, I.S.M., Rahman, M.M. et al. (2013). Techniques for extraction of bioactive compounds from plant materials: a review. *Journal of Food Engineering* **117** (4): 426–436.

Babovic, N., Djilas, S., Jadranin, M. et al. (2010). Supercritical carbon dioxide extraction of antioxidant fractions from selected Lamiaceae herbs and their antioxidant capacity. *Innovative Food Science & Emerging Technologies* **11** (1): 98–107.

Bagheri, H., Manap, M.Y.B.A., and Solati, Z. (2014). Antioxidant activity of *Piper nigrum* L. essential oil extracted by supercritical CO_2 extraction and hydro-distillation. *Talanta* **121**: 220–228.

Barbero, G.F., Liazid, A., Palma, M., and Barroso, C.G. (2008). Ultrasound-assisted extraction of capsaicinoids from peppers. *Talanta* **75** (5): 1332–1337.

Bekdeşer, B., Durusoy, N., Özyürek, M. et al. (2014). Optimization of microwave-assisted extraction of polyphenols from herbal teas and evaluation of their in vitro hypochlorous acid scavenging activity. *Journal of Agricultural and Food Chemistry* **62** (46): 11109–11115.

Berche, B., Henkel, M., and Kenna, R. (2009). Critical phenomena: 150 years since Cagniard de la tour. *Revista Brasileira de Ensino de Física* **31**: 2602–2610.

Björklund, E., Sparr-Eskilsson, C., Paul, W. et al. (2005). Extraction. supercritical fluid extraction. In: *Encyclopedia of Analytical Science* (eds. P. Worsfold, A. Townshend and C. Poole), 597–604. Oxford: Elsevier.

Both, S., Chemat, F., and Strube, J. (2014). Extraction of polyphenols from black tea–conventional and ultrasound assisted extraction. *Ultrasonics Sonochemistry* **21** (3): 1030–1034.

Boyadzhiev, L., Dimitrov, K., and Metcheva, D. (2006). Integration of solvent extraction and liquid membrane separation: an efficient tool for recovery of bio-active substances from botanicals. *Chemical Engineering Science* **61** (12): 4126–4128.

Brunner, G. (1994). *Gas Extraction: An Introduction to Fundamentals of Supercritical Fluids and the Application to Separation Processes*. Darmstadt: Springer.

Brunner, G. (2005). Supercritical fluids: technology and application to food processing. *Journal of Food Engineering* **67** (1): 21–33.

Butt, M.S., Pasha, I., Sultan, M.T. et al. (2013). Black pepper and health claims: a comprehensive treatise. *Critical Reviews in Food Science and Nutrition* **53** (9): 875–886.

Camila, G., Pereira, C.G., and Meireles, M.A.A. (2010). Supercritical fluid extraction of bioactive compounds: fundamentals, applications and economic perspectives. *Food and Bioprocess Technology* **3** (3): 340–372.

Chan, C.H., Yusoff, R., Ngoh, G.C., and Kung, F.W.L. (2011). Microwave-assisted extractions of active ingredients from plants. *Journal of Chromatography A* **1218** (37): 6213–6225.

Chandran, J., Amma, K.P.P., Menon, N. et al. (2012). Effect of enzyme assisted extraction on quality and yield of volatile oil from black pepper and cardamom. *Food Science and Biotechnology* **21** (6): 1611–1617.

Cheah, E.L., Heng, P.W., and Chan, L.W. (2010). Optimization of supercritical fluid extraction and pressurized liquid extraction of active principles from *Magnolia officinalis* using the Taguchi design. *Separation and Purification Technology* **71** (3): 293–301.

Chemat, F., Humma, Z., and Khan, M.K. (2011). Applications of ultrasound in food technology: processing, preservation and extraction. *Ultrasonics Sonochemistry* **18** (4): 813–835.

Chen, Y., Gu, X., Huang, S.Q. et al. (2010). Optimization of ultrasonic/microwave assisted extraction (UMAE) of polysaccharides from *Inonotus obliquus* and evaluation of its anti-tumor activities. *International Journal of Biological Macromolecules* **46** (4): 429–435.

Chienthavorn, O., Poonsukcharoen, T., and Pathrakorn, T. (2011). Pressurized liquid and superheated water extraction of active constituents from *Zingiber cassumunar roxb.* Rhizome. *Separation Science and Technology* **46** (4): 616–624.

Cho, S.K., El-Aty, A.A., Choi, J.H. et al. (2007). Optimized conditions for the extraction of secondary volatile metabolites in *Angelica* roots by accelerated solvent extraction. *Journal of Pharmaceutical and Biomedical Analysis* **44** (5): 1154–1158.

Costa, S.S., Gariepy, Y., Rocha, S.C., and Raghavan, V. (2014). Microwave extraction of mint essential oil–temperature calibration for the oven. *Journal of Food Engineering* **126**: 1–6.

Da Porto, C., Decorti, D., and Kikic, I. (2009). Flavour compounds of *Lavandula angustifolia* L. to use in food manufacturing: comparison of three different extraction methods. *Food Chemistry* **112** (4): 1072–1078.

De Melo, M.M.R., Silvestre, A.J.D., and Silva, C.M. (2014). Supercritical fluid extraction of vegetable matrices: applications, trends and future perspectives of a convincing green technology. *The Journal of Supercritical Fluids* **92**: 115–176.

De Mey, E., De Maere, H., Dewulf, L. et al. (2014). Assessment of the N-nitrosopiperidine formation risk from piperine and piperidine contained in spices used as meat product additives. *European Food Research and Technology* **238** (3): 477–484.

De Oliveira, P.M.A., de Almeida, R.H., de Oliveira, N.A. et al. (2014). Enrichment of diterpenes in green coffee oil using supercritical fluid extraction–characterization and comparison with green coffee oil from pressing. *The Journal of Supercritical Fluids* **95**: 137–145.

Du, F.Y., Xiao, X.H., Luo, X.J., and Li, G.K. (2009). Application of ionic liquids in the microwave-assisted extraction of polyphenolic compounds from medicinal plants. *Talanta* **78** (3): 1177–1184.

Eikani, M.H., Golmohammad, F., Amoli, H.S., and Sadr, Z.B. (2013). An experimental design approach for pressurized liquid extraction from cardamom seeds. *Separation Science and Technology* **48** (8): 1194–1200.

Embuscado, M.E. (2015). Spices and herbs: natural sources of antioxidants–a mini review. *Journal of Functional Foods* https://doi.org/10.1016/j.jff.2015.03.005.

Fang, X., Wang, J., Hao, J. et al. (2015). Simultaneous extraction, identification and quantification of phenolic compounds in *Eclipta prostrata* using microwave-assisted extraction combined with HPLC–DAD–ESI–MS/MS. *Food Chemistry* **188**: 527–536.

Farnsworth, N.R., Akerele, O., Bingel, A.S. et al. (1985). Medicinal plants in therapy. *Bulletin of the World Health Organization* **63** (6): 965–981.

Filly, A., Fernandez, X., Minuti, M. et al. (2014). Solvent-free microwave extraction of essential oil from aromatic herbs: from laboratory to pilot and industrial scale. *Food Chemistry* **150**: 193–198.

Flórez, N., Conde, E., and Domínguez, H. (2015). Microwave assisted water extraction of plant compounds. *Journal of Chemical Technology and Biotechnology* **90** (4): 590–607.

Fornari, T., Vicente, G., Vázquez, E. et al. (2012). Isolation of essential oil from different plants and herbs by supercritical fluid extraction. *Journal of Chromatography A* **1250**: 34–48.

Gañán, N. and Brignole, E.A. (2013). Supercritical carbon dioxide fractionation of *T. minuta* and *S. officinalis* essential oils: experiments and process analysis. *The Journal of Supercritical Fluids* **78**: 12–20.

Gañán, N.A., Dambolena, J.S., Martini, R.E., and Bottini, S.B. (2015). Supercritical carbon dioxide fractionation of peppermint oil with low menthol content–experimental study and simulation analysis for the recovery of piperitenone. *The Journal of Supercritical Fluids* **98**: 1–11.

Ganzler, K., Salgo, A., and Valkó, K. (1986). Microwave extraction: a novel sample preparation method for chromatography. *Journal of Chromatography A* **371**: 299–306.

Gao, F., Hu, Y., Ye, X. et al. (2013). Optimal extraction and fingerprint analysis of *Cnidii fructus* by accelerated solvent extraction and high performance liquid chromatographic analysis with photodiode array and mass spectrometry detections. *Food Chemistry* **141** (3): 1962–1971.

Garcia-Ayuso, L.E., Sanchez, M., Fernandez de Alba, A., and Luque de Castro, M.D. (1998). Focused microwave-assisted soxhlet: an advantageous tool for sample extraction. *Analytical Chemistry* **70** (11): 2426–2431.

Gavahian, M., Farahnaky, A., Farhoosh, R. et al. (2015). Extraction of essential oils from *Mentha piperita* using advanced techniques: microwave versus ohmic assisted hydrodistillation. *Food and Bioproducts Processing* **94**: 50–58.

Ghasemzadeh, A., Jaafar, H.Z., Karimi, E., and Rahmat, A. (2014). Optimization of ultrasound-assisted extraction of flavonoid compounds and their pharmaceutical activity from curry leaf (*Murraya koenigii* L.) using response surface methodology. *BMC Complementary and Alternative Medicine* **14** (1): 318.

Golmakani, E., Mohammadi, A., Sani, T.A., and Kamali, H. (2014). Phenolic and flavonoid content and antioxidants capacity of pressurized liquid extraction and perculation method from roots of *Scutellaria pinnatifida* A. Hamilt. subsp *alpina* (Bornm) Rech. f. *The Journal of Supercritical Fluids* **95**: 318–324.

Heng, M.Y., Tan, S.N., Yong, J.W.H., and Ong, E.S. (2013). Emerging green technologies for the chemical standardization of botanicals and herbal preparations. *TrAC Trends in Analytical Chemistry* **50**: 1–10.

Herrero, M., Cifuentes, A., and Ibanez, E. (2006). Sub-and supercritical fluid extraction of functional ingredients from different natural sources: plants, food-by-products, algae and microalgae: a review. *Food Chemistry* **98** (1): 136–148.

Herrero, M., Castro-Puyana, M., Mendiola, J.A., and Ibañez, E. (2013). Compressed fluids for the extraction of bioactive compounds. *TrAC Trends in Analytical Chemistry* **43**: 67–83.

Hiranvarachat, B., Devahastin, S., and Soponronnarit, S. (2015). Comparative evaluation of atmospheric and vacuum microwave-assisted extraction of bioactive compounds from fresh and dried *Centella asiatica* L. leaves. *International Journal of Food Science & Technology* **50** (3): 750–757.

Hosni, K., Hassen, I., Chaâbane, H. et al. (2013). Enzyme-assisted extraction of essential oils from thyme (*Thymus capitatus* L.) and rosemary (*Rosmarinus officinalis* L.): impact on yield, chemical composition and antimicrobial activity. *Industrial Crops and Products* **47**: 291–299.

Hossain, M.B., Brunton, N.P., Patras, A. et al. (2012). Optimization of ultrasound assisted extraction of antioxidant compounds from marjoram (*Origanum majorana* L.) using response surface methodology. *Ultrasonics Sonochemistry* **19** (3): 582–590.

Howard, L. and Pandjaitan, N. (2008). Pressurized liquid extraction of flavonoids from spinach. *Journal of Food Science* **73** (3): 151–157.

Ibañez, E., Herrero, M., Mendiola, J.A., and Castro-Puyana, M. (2012). Extraction and characterization of bioactive compounds with health benefits from marine resources: macro and micro algae, cyanobacteria, and invertebrates. In: *Marine Bioactive Compounds: Sources, Characterization and Applications* (ed. M. Hayes), 585–598. New York: Springer US.

Jiang, Z., Liu, F., Goh, J.J.L. et al. (2009). Determination of senkirkine and senecionine in *Tussilago farfara* using microwave-assisted extraction and pressurized hot water extraction with liquid chromatography tandem mass spectrometry. *Talanta* **79** (2): 539–546.

Jiang, Z.T., Feng, X., Li, R., and Wang, Y. (2013). Composition comparison of essential oils extracted by classical hydro distillation and microwave-assisted hydrodistillation from *Pimenta dioica*. *Journal of Essential Oil Bearing Plants* **16** (1): 45–50.

Jordan, D.B., Bowman, M.J., Braker, J.D. et al. (2012). Plant cell walls to ethanol. *Biochemical Journal* **442**: 241–252.

Kaufmann, B. and Christen, P. (2002). Recent extraction techniques for natural products: microwave-assisted extraction and pressurized solvent extraction. *Phytochemical Analysis* **13** (2): 105–113.

Kraujalis, P. and Venskutonis, P.R. (2013). Supercritical carbon dioxide extraction of squalene and tocopherols from amaranth and assessment of extracts antioxidant activity. *The Journal of Supercritical Fluids* **80**: 78–85.

Kukula-Koch, W., Skalicka-Wozniak, K., Sieniawska, E. et al. (2014). Comparative study on the volatiles'composition of *Iris dichotoma pall.* Rhizome extracts. *Farmácia* **62** (5): 874–881.

Lapornik, B., Prošek, M., and Wondra, A.G. (2005). Comparison of extracts prepared from plant by-products using different solvents and extraction time. *Journal of Food Engineering* **71** (2): 214–222.

Lianfu, Z. and Zelong, L. (2008). Optimization and comparison of ultrasound/microwave assisted extraction (UMAE) and ultrasonic assisted extraction (UAE) of lycopene from tomatoes. *Ultrasonics Sonochemistry* **15** (5): 731–737.

Liang, X., Tian, J., Li, L. et al. (2014). Rapid determination of eight bioactive alkaloids in *Portulaca oleracea* L. by the optimal microwave extraction combined with positive–negative conversion multiple reaction monitor (+/– MRM) technology. *Talanta* **120**: 167–172.

Liu, X., Abd El-Aty, A.M., Cho, S.K. et al. (2012a). Characterization of secondary volatile profiles in *Nigella sativa* seeds from two different origins using accelerated solvent extraction and gas chromatography-mass spectrometry. *Biomedical Chromatography* **26** (10): 1157–1162.

Liu, Y., Yang, L., Zu, Y. et al. (2012b). Development of an ionic liquid-based microwave-assisted method for simultaneous extraction and distillation for determination of proanthocyanidins and essential oil in *Cortex cinnamomi*. *Food Chemistry* **135** (4): 2514–2521.

Liu, X., Hu, Y., and Wei, D. (2014). Optimization of enzyme-based ultrasonic/microwave-assisted extraction and evaluation of antioxidant activity of orcinol glucoside from the rhizomes of *Curculigo orchioides Gaertn*. *Medicinal Chemistry Research* **23** (5): 2360–2367.

Liu, H.L., Luo, R., Chen, X.Q. et al. (2015). Identification and simultaneous quantification of five alkaloids in *Piper longum* L. by HPLC–ESI-MS n and UFLC–ESI-MS/MS and their application to *Piper nigrum* L. *Food Chemistry* **177**: 191–196.

Luthria, D.L. (2008). Influence of experimental conditions on the extraction of phenolic compounds from parsley (*Petroselinum crispum*) flakes using a pressurized liquid extractor. *Food Chemistry* **107** (2): 745–752.

Maran, J.P. and Priya, B. (2015). Supercritical fluid extraction of oil from muskmelon (*Cucumis melo*) seeds. *Journal of the Taiwan Institute of Chemical Engineers* **47**: 71–78.

Mazidi, S., Rezaei, K., Golmakani, M.T. et al. (2012). Antioxidant activity of essential oil from black Zira (*Bunium persicum Boiss.*) obtained by microwave-assisted hydrodistillation. *Journal of Agricultural Science and Technology* **14** (5): 1013–1022.

Mendiola, J.A., Herrero, M., Cifuentes, A., and Ibañez, E. (2007). Use of compressed fluids for sample preparation: food applications. *Journal of Chromatography A* **1152** (1): 234–246.

Messmore, H.E. (1943). Process for producing asphaltic materials. United States Patent 2420185 (Priority number: US19430471299 19430104).

Miron, T.L., Plaza, M., Bahrim, G. et al. (2011). Chemical composition of bioactive pressurized extracts of Romanian aromatic plants. *Journal of Chromatography A* **1218** (30): 4918–4927.

Miron, T.L., Herrero, M., and Ibáñez, E. (2013). Enrichment of antioxidant compounds from lemon balm (*Melissa officinalis*) by pressurized liquid extraction and enzyme-assisted extraction. *Journal of Chromatography A* **1288**: 1–9.

Morsy, N.F. (2015). A short extraction time of high quality hydrodistilled cardamom (*Elettaria cardamomum* L. *Maton*) essential oil using ultrasound as a pretreatment. *Industrial Crops and Products* **65**: 287–292.

Nagendra chari, K.L., Manasa, D., Srinivas, P., and Sowbhagya, H.B. (2013). Enzyme-assisted extraction of bioactive compounds from ginger (*Zingiber officinale Roscoe*). *Food Chemistry* **139** (1): 509–514.

Naidu, M.M., Kumar, P.S., Shyamala, B.N. et al. (2012). Enzyme-assisted process for production of superior quality vanilla extracts from green vanilla pods using tea leaf enzymes. *Food and Bioprocess Technology* **5** (2): 527–532.

Nur Ain, N.A., Zaibunnisa, A.H., Zahrah, H., and Norashikin, S. (2012). An experimental design approach for the extraction of lemongrass (*Cymbopogon citratus*) oleoresin using pressurised liquid extraction (PLE). *International Food Research Journal* **20** (1): 451–455.

Ocaña-Fuentes, A., Arranz-Gutiérrez, E., Senorans, F.J., and Reglero, G. (2010). Supercritical fluid extraction of oregano (*Origanum vulgare*) essentials oils: anti-inflammatory properties based on cytokine response on THP-1 macrophages. *Food and Chemical Toxicology* **48** (6): 1568–1575.

Orio, L., Cravotto, G., Binello, A. et al. (2012). Hydrodistillation and in situ microwave-generated hydrodistillation of fresh and dried mint leaves: a comparison study. *Journal of the Science of Food and Agriculture* **92** (15): 3085–3090.

Osorio-Tobón, J.F., Carvalho, P.I., Rostagno, M.A. et al. (2014). Extraction of curcuminoids from deflavored turmeric (*Curcuma longa* L.) using pressurized liquids: process integration and economic evaluation. *The Journal of Supercritical Fluids* **95**: 167–174.

Ötles, S. (2009). *Handbook of Food Analysis Instruments*. Boca Raton: CRC Press Taylor & Francis Group.

Pavlić, B., Vidović, S., Vladić, J. et al. (2015). Isolation of coriander (*Coriandrum sativum* L.) essential oil by green extractions versus traditional techniques. *The Journal of Supercritical Fluids* **99**: 23–28.

Pereira, C.G., Gualtieri, I.P., Maia, N.B., and Meireles, M.A.A. (2008). Supercritical extraction to obtain vetiver (*Vetiveria zizanioides* L. *Nash*) extracts from roots cultivated hydroponically. *Journal of Agricultural Science and Technology* **35** (2): 44–50.

Petrakis, E.A., Kimbaris, A.C., Perdikis, D.C. et al. (2014). Responses of Myzus persicae (Sulzer) to three Lamiaceae essential oils obtained by microwave-assisted and conventional hydrodistillation. *Industrial Crops and Products* **62**: 272–279.

Picó, Y. (2013). Ultrasound-assisted extraction for food and environmental samples. *TrAC Trends in Analytical Chemistry* **43**: 84–99.

Pouralinazar, F., Yunus, M.A.C., and Zahedi, G. (2012). Pressurized liquid extraction of *Orthosiphon stamineus* oil: experimental and modeling studies. *The Journal of Supercritical Fluids* **62**: 88–95.

Przygoda, K. and Wejnerowska, G. (2015). Extraction of tocopherol-enriched oils from Quinoa seeds by supercritical fluid extraction. *Industrial Crops and Products* **63**: 41–47.

Rathod, S.S. and Rathod, V.K. (2014). Extraction of piperine from *Piper longum* using ultrasound. *Industrial Crops and Products* **58**: 259–264.

Reyes, F.A., Mendiola, J.A., Ibanez, E., and del Valle, J.M. (2014). Astaxanthin extraction from *Haematococcus pluvialis* using CO_2-expanded ethanol. *The Journal of Supercritical Fluids* **92**: 75–83.

Roldán-Gutiérrez, J.M., Ruiz-Jiménez, J., and de Castro, M.L. (2008). Ultrasound-assisted dynamic extraction of valuable compounds from aromatic plants and flowers as compared with steam distillation and superheated liquid extraction. *Talanta* **75** (5): 1369–1375.

Routray, W. and Orsat, V. (2012). Microwave-assisted extraction of flavonoids: a review. *Food and Bioprocess Technology* **5** (2): 409–424.

Ruan, C., Xiao, X.H., and Li, G.K. (2014). Microwave-assisted extraction coupled with countercurrent chromatography for the rapid preparation of flavonoids from *Scutellaria barbata D. Don. Journal of Separation Science* **37** (11): 1364–1369.

Runnqvist, H., Bak, S.A., Hansen, M. et al. (2010). Determination of pharmaceuticals in environmental and biological matrices using pressurised liquid extraction—Are we developing sound extraction methods? *Journal of Chromatography A* **1217** (16): 2447–2470.

Saldaña, M.D. and Valdivieso-Ramírez, C.S. (2015). Pressurized fluid systems: phytochemical production from biomass. *The Journal of Supercritical Fluids* **96**: 228–244.

Sánchez-Camargo, A.P., Valdés, A., Sullini, G. et al. (2014). Two-step sequential supercritical fluid extracts from rosemary with enhanced anti-proliferative activity. *Journal of Functional Foods* **11**: 293–303.

Santos, P., Aguiar, A.C., Barbero, G.F. et al. (2015). Supercritical carbon dioxide extraction of capsaicinoids from malagueta pepper (*Capsicum frutescens* L.) assisted by ultrasound. *Ultrasonics Sonochemistry* **22**: 78–88.

Santoyo, S., Jaime, L., García-Risco, M.R. et al. (2014). Supercritical fluid extraction as an alternative process to obtain antiviral agents from thyme species. *Industrial Crops and Products* **52**: 475–480.

Scurto, A.M., Hutchenson, K., and Subramaniam, B. (2009). Gas-expanded liquids: fundamentals and applications. In: *Gas-Expanded Liquids and near-Critical Media: Green Chemistry and Engineering* (eds. A.M. Scurto, K. Hutchenson and B. Subramaniam), 3–37. Washington, DC: American Chemical Society Symposium Series.

Shao, Q., Deng, Y., Liu, H. et al. (2014). Essential oils extraction from *Anoectochilus roxburghii* using supercritical carbon dioxide and their antioxidant activity. *Industrial Crops and Products* **60**: 104–112.

Shotipruk, A., Kaufman, P.B., and Wang, H.Y. (2001). Feasibility study of repeated harvesting of menthol from biologically viable menthaxpiperata using ultrasonic extraction. *Biotechnology Progress* **17** (5): 924–928.

Skalicka-Woźniak, K. and Głowniak, K. (2012). Pressurized liquid extraction of coumarins from fruits of *Heracleum leskowii* with application of solvents with different polarity under increasing temperature. *Molecules* **17** (4): 4133–4141.

Song, L., Zhang, H., Liu, X. et al. (2012). Rapid determination of yunaconitine and related alkaloids in aconites and aconite-containing drugs by ultra high-performance liquid chromatography–tandem mass spectrometry. *Biomedical Chromatography* **26** (12): 1567–1574.

Sourmaghi, M.H.M., Kiaee, G., Golfakhrabadi, F. et al. (2015). Comparison of essential oil composition and antimicrobial activity of *Coriandrum sativum* L. extracted by hydrodistillation and microwave-assisted hydrodistillation. *Journal of Food Science and Technology* **52** (4): 2452–2457.

Sowbhagya, H.B., Srinivas, P., Purnima, K.T., and Krishnamurthy, N. (2011). Enzyme-assisted extraction of volatiles from cumin (*Cuminum cyminum* L.) seeds. *Food Chemistry* **127** (4): 1856–1861.

Sultana, B., Anwar, F., and Ashraf, M. (2009). Effect of extraction solvent/technique on the antioxidant activity of selected medicinal plant extracts. *Molecules* **14** (6): 2167–2180.

Turner, C. and Ibañez, E. (2011). Pressurized hot water extraction and processing. In: *Enhancing Extraction Processes in the Food Industry-Contemporary Food Engineering* (eds. N. Lebovka, E. Vorobiev and F. Chemat), 223–255. Boca Raton: CRC press.

Valdés, A., García-Cañas, V., Rocamora-Reverte, L. et al. (2013). Effect of rosemary polyphenols on human colon cancer cells: transcriptomic profiling and functional enrichment analysis. *Genes & Nutrition* **8** (1): 43–60.

Vardanega, R., Santos, D.T., and Meireles, M.A.A. (2014). Intensification of bioactive compounds extraction from medicinal plants using ultrasonic irradiation. *Pharmacognosy Reviews* **8** (16): 88.

Vilkhu, K., Mawson, R., Simons, L., and Bates, D. (2008). Applications and opportunities for ultrasound assisted extraction in the food industry: a review. *Innovative Food Science & Emerging Technologies* **9** (2): 161–169.

Wang, P., Ma, C., Chen, S. et al. (2014). Ionic liquid-based ultrasonic/microwave-assisted extraction of steroidal Saponins from *Dioscorea zingiberensis* CH Wright. *Tropical Journal of Pharmaceutical Research* **13** (8): 1339–1345.

Wianowska, D. (2014a). Hydrolytical instability of hydroxyanthraquinone glycosides in pressurized liquid extraction. *Analytical and Bioanalytical Chemistry* **406** (13): 3219–3227.

Wianowska, D. (2014b). The influence of purge times on the yields of essential oil components extracted from plants by pressurized liquid extraction. *Journal of AOAC International* **97** (5): 1310–1316.

Worsfold, P., Townshend, A., and Poole, C.F. (2005). *Encyclopedia of Analytical Science*. Boston: Elsevier.

Wu, H., Chen, M., Fan, Y. et al. (2012). Determination of rutin and quercetin in Chinese herbal medicine by ionic liquid-based pressurized liquid extraction–liquid chromatography–chemiluminescence detection. *Talanta* **88**: 222–229.

Xia, T., Shi, S., and Wan, X. (2006). Impact of ultrasonic-assisted extraction on the chemical and sensory quality of tea infusion. *Journal of Food Engineering* **74** (4): 557–560.

Xiao, X., Si, X., Tong, X., and Li, G. (2012). Ultrasonic microwave-assisted extraction coupled with high-speed counter-current chromatography for the preparation of nigakinones from *Picrasma quassioides (D. Don) Benn. Phytochemical Analysis* **23** (5): 540–546.

Xiao, X.H., Yuan, Z.Q., and Li, G.K. (2014). Separation and purification of steroidal saponins from *Paris polyphylla* by microwave-assisted extraction coupled with countercurrent chromatography using evaporative light scattering detection. *Journal of Separation Science* **37** (6): 635–641.

Zeković, Z., Bušić, A., Komes, D. et al. (2015). Coriander seeds processing: sequential extraction of non-polar and polar fractions using supercritical carbon dioxide extraction and ultrasound-assisted extraction. *Food and Bioproducts Processing* **95**: 218–227.

Zeng, H., Zhang, Y., Lin, S. et al. (2015). Ultrasonic–microwave synergistic extraction (UMSE) and molecular weight distribution of polysaccharides from *Fortunella margarita* (Lour.) Swingle. *Separation and Purification Technology* **144**: 97–106.

Zhang, S., Sun, N., He, X. et al. (2006). Physical properties of ionic liquids: database and evaluation. *Journal of Physical and Chemical Reference Data* **35** (4): 1475–1517.

Zhou, Q., Liu, Y., Wang, X., and Di, X. (2012). Microwave-assisted extraction in combination with capillary electrophoresis for rapid determination of isoquinoline alkaloids in *Chelidonium majus* L. *Talanta* **99**: 932–938.

Zosel, K. (1978). Separation with supercritical gases: practical applications. *Angewandte Chemie International Edition* **71**: 702–709.

6
Approaches to Analytical Techniques – Characterizing Phytochemicals in *Verbascum* spp.

Anna-Maria Keaveney[1,3], Ambrose Furey[2,3], and Brigid Lucey[1]

[1]*Department of Biological Sciences, Cork Institute of Technology, Bishopstown, Cork, T12 P928, Ireland*

[2]*Mass Spectrometry Research Group, Department of Physical Sciences, Cork Institute of Technology, Bishopstown, Cork, T12 P928, Ireland*

[3]*Centre for Research in Advanced Therapeutic Engineering and BioExplore, Cork Institute of Technology, Rossa Avenue, Bishopstown, T12 P928, Ireland*

6.1 Introduction

There is a global interest in the use of botanicals,[1] whether as medicines, cosmetics, novel foods, or food ingredients (Newman and Cragg 2012; Pferschy-Wenzig and Bauer 2015), with a market of approximately 83 billion dollars. Botanicals still command a role in drug discovery, with over half of the new drugs (characterized as small biomolecules) approved between 1981 and 2010 based on naturally derived compounds; only 36% of new drug targets were of synthetic origin (Pferschy-Wenzig and Bauer 2015). It has also been estimated that 25% of modern drugs and 60% of anticancer medicines are derived from natural compounds (Pferschy-Wenzig and Bauer 2015).

Antimicrobials, and specifically antibiotics, were, and in most cases still are, used diversely and extensively from the food industry to the medical and healthcare sectors.

[1] Botanicals are also defined as herbs, plants, or phytomedicines. Herbal drugs are defined as whole or plant parts, algae, fungi, or lichens in unprocessed or crude state, usually in dried form but sometimes fresh (Gautam et al. 2010).

Herbs, Spices and Medicinal Plants: Processing, Health Benefits and Safety, First Edition.
Edited by Mohammad B. Hossain, Nigel P. Brunton, and Dilip K. Rai.

The rise of antibiotic resistance and the removal of antibiotics from much of the food chain necessitates alternative antimicrobial approaches. Serious conditions such as TB and, for example, the infectious exacerbations of cystic fibrosis are becoming more challenging to treat effectively because of increasing antibiotic resistance among the associated pathogens. Biofilm formation by pathogenic microbes adds another layer of risk to vulnerable consumers within a wide range of sectors (Xia et al. 2013). In response, botanicals, essential oils, and plant-derived compounds are being investigated for antimicrobial efficacy (Wagner and Ulrich-Merzenich 2009; Palaniappan and Holley 2010).

There is also a resurgence of interest in the use of traditional medicines based on whole or crude extract of plants (WHO 2005, 2013; Wiesner and Knöss 2014) which are used to treat conditions such as cardiovascular disease (Furey and Tassell 2008; Tachjian et al. 2010; Tassell et al. 2010), anxiety (McIntyre et al. 2016), cancer (Yin et al. 2013), and psychiatric disorders (Sarris 2018), among others. The increased use of herbal medicines (mainly for mild to moderate illnesses) was found to be associated with a number of factors, including dissatisfaction with conventional treatment, previous good experiences with the use of herbal medicines, positive aspects associated with herbal medicine, as well as family traditions (Welz et al. 2018).

More and more research is being conducted to support this broad range of botanical applications (Atanasov et al. 2015). A search on the PubMed database using typical search terms such as "plant," "plant pharmacology," "plant chemistry," is illustrated in Figure 6.1 below and shows, from a low base, a year on year increase in the number of publications with a phytochemical/traditional medicinal focus, with a peak of over 55 000 in 2014. It is considered that appropriate regulation of botanicals (product and process) should provide a significant stimulus to research (Bilia 2014; Bouin and Wierer 2014; Knöss et al. 2014; Pelkmans and Renda 2014; Atanasov et al. 2015).

Analysis of botanicals is increasingly conducted within a regulatory and research-focused framework (Kroes 2014; Sharma 2015; Wagner et al. 2016). From a regulatory point of view, this is due mainly to concerns from the regulatory authorities that untested or unregulated products were being used as medicines (WHO 2005, 2013; Yadav et al. 2011; Rivera et al. 2013; Knöss et al. 2014; Wiesner and Knöss 2014; Palhares et al. 2015; Pferschy-Wenzig and Bauer 2015; Sharma 2015). The Traditional Medicine Strategy 2014–2023 is the latest report from the World Health Organization (WHO 2013) and follows on from its earlier Traditional Medicine Strategy Report (2003–2005) (WHO 2005) and The World Traditional Medicines Situation (WHO 2011) in which it sets out strategies to assist countries in developing the role played by both traditional medicines and traditional practitioners in public health. The latest strategy report was developed in response to the World Health Assembly Resolution on Traditional Medicine (Searo.who.int 2019) who requested further developments in this area, including the establishment of pharmaceutical research in developing countries, increased training of practitioners, and increased financial support for research and product development.

Although this increase in research reflects the increased interest in this area, it also acknowledges the need for robust analysis of botanicals so as to address quality and safety issues such as: (i) growth and collection; (ii) authentication (adulteration); (iii) processing (extraction, stability); (iv) standard and validated analysis; and finally (v) clinical safety and (vi) efficacy, in order to provide consistency both in composition and bioactivity (generally referred to as standardization and pharmaco-equivalence) (WHO 2005; WHO 2013; Govindaraghavana and Sucher 2015). There is also an

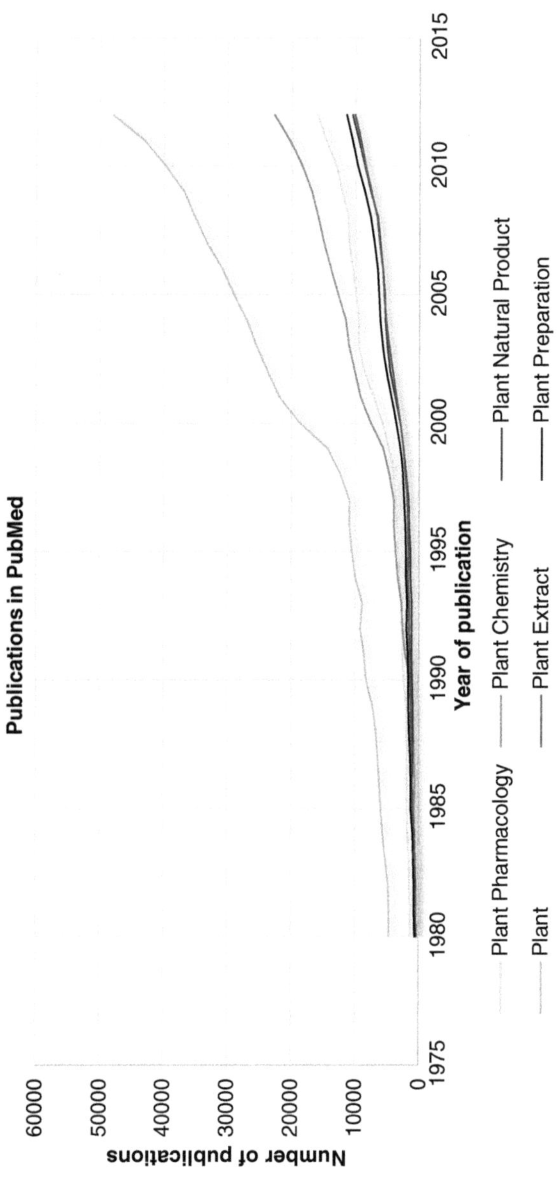

Figure 6.1 PubMed publication numbers based on key words, Plant, Plant Pharmacology, Plant Chemistry, Plant Extract, Plant preparation, and Plant Natural Product over the period 1980 to 2012. *Source:* The data was generated from MEDSUM: an online MEDLINE summary tool by Galsworthy, MJ. Hosted by the Institute of Biomedical Informatics (IBMI), Faculty of Medicine, University of Ljubljana, Slovenia. URL: www.medsum.info.

increasing awareness of the unique challenges that botanicals pose in trying to address these factors (Mosihuzzaman and Choudhary 2008; Rivera et al. 2013; Bilia 2014; Wiesner and Knöss 2014; Palhares et al. 2015; Pferschy-Wenzig and Bauer 2015).

Figure 6.2 outlines the range of issues that need to be considered in terms of both the research and the manufacturing of botanicals. These issues are not as a whole unique to each process category, but most tend to overlap; for example, many of the quality issues of authentication, adulteration, and stability are equally important in the area of research and manufacturing as they are the processing steps. A good example of this can been seen in the review article by Beer and Neff (2013) where they use an evidence-based medicine approach (i.e. clinical efficacy) to argue for the lack of pharmaco-equivalence (not all the extracts followed the same extraction procedure). The authors note that two extracts – for example, the isopropanolic extraction procedure and ethanolic extraction procedure BNO1055 of *Cimicifuga racemose* or black cohosh – were effective (in this case for climacteric complaints as determined by Oxford Levels of Evidence (LOE) and Grades of Recommendation (GR)), while other extraction solvent systems were not. By combining all the different extracts (using different extraction procedures) together and assuming they were the same, the results were being skewed. There is a need to recognize that although each extract originated from the same herb, not all extracts contain the same constituent profile and so the efficacy of each extract may be different.

All these developments require continuing improvements in analytical techniques to ensure quality control and adherence to good manufacturing practice (GMP) (Yadav et al. 2011; Knöss et al. 2014; Palhares et al. 2015; Sharma 2015). However, while there has been progress in terms of individual techniques and practices (discussed throughout this chapter), the response to the development of an overarching model or framework has been somewhat problematic due to the lack of harmonization across national regulations, including quality requirements and health claims (Govindaraghavana and Sucher 2015). While not claiming to offer a comprehensive cover of quality assurance/management systems, the following should give an outline to some of the main approaches proposed.

The International Council for Harmonization (ICH) offers guidance to assist pharmaceutical manufacturers on quality management systems (QMSs). These systems are based on International Organization for Standardization (ISO) quality concepts. Under EU legislation Directive 2004/24/EC, herbal medicinal products are included. Interestingly, Bilia et al. (2001, 2002) commented that ICH guidelines (for stability issues in this case) might need more than mere transposing onto botanicals, indicating that the process may be more complicated than was originally understood. Another model (from the food sector) is that of Total Management Systems (TMSs) (Early 1995). TMS forms a tertiary layer (of quality management) built around Quality Assurance (QA) and QMSs. While QA looks at the strategic development of a quality system, including policies, systems, and maintaining quality (plus Quality Control [QC] aimed at implementing the QA and GMP), QMS seeks to develop the QA system in a more structured and formal way. QMS strategies can assist in the development of QA policies, develop strategic plants, and document the QA system.

Kamil (2013) and Govindaraghavana and Sucher (2015) both proposed a quality assurance procedure throughout all aspects of the supply chain (herbal/botanical material) from farm to product, including the implementation of GMPs, safety, cultivation, handling, processing, and production. The aim is to ensure phytochemical consistency (and thus efficacy) by focusing on authenticity and homogeneity of the

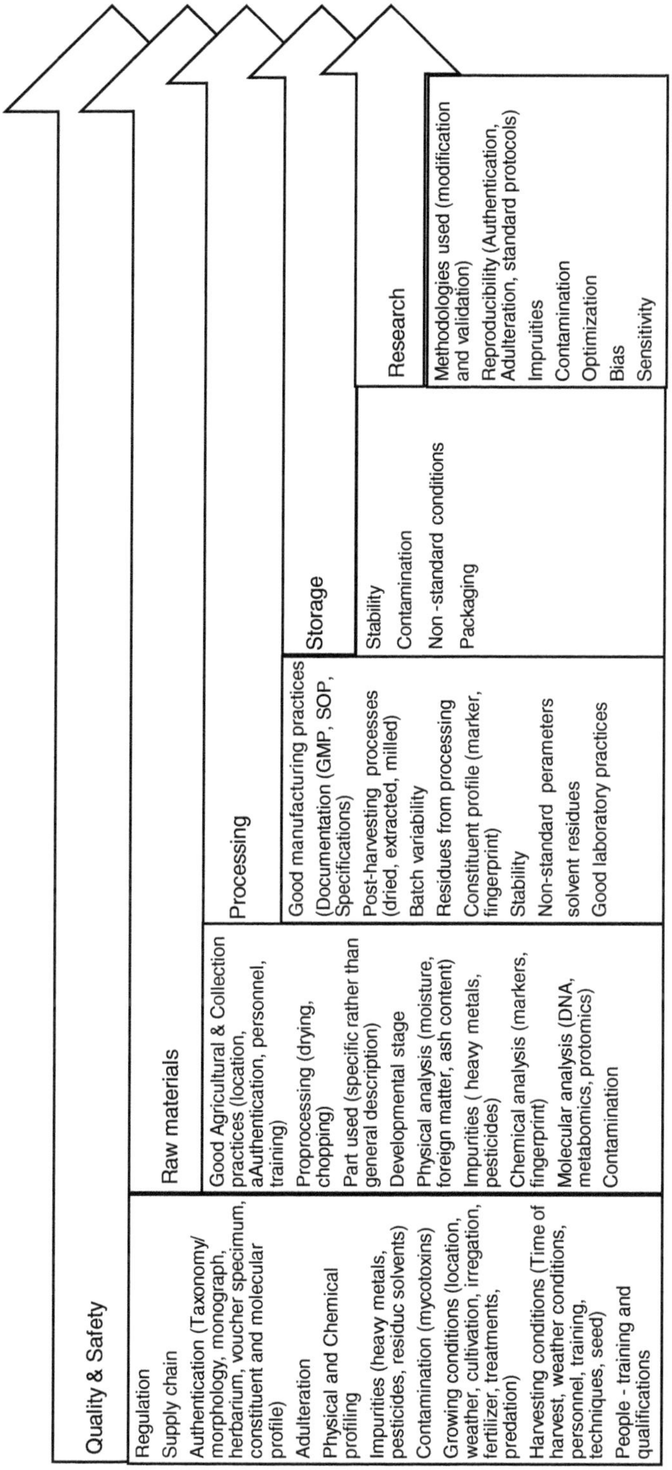

Figure 6.2 Outline of potential considerations that need to be considered in research and manufacture of complex botanicals.

herbs together with manufacturing processes strictly following current GMP. Thus, the quality assurance model should include good agricultural and collection practice (GA&CP), good plant authentication and identification practice (GPAIP), and GMP implemented together with validated analytical methods.

Govindaraghavana and Sucher's (2015) proposal in relation to the supply chain is an interesting starting point. Based on the field to product concept, i.e. the supply chain, it could form the cohesive element required. If that supply chain stretched from GA&CP (WHO 2003) to GMP to Good Laboratory practice and onwards it could link all the elements that are currently non-standardized. It would not matter at what point on the supply chain you entered, provided you stayed cognizant of the fact that there is always an upstream and downstream component to be considered. There are also critical points in any production or process that need to be considered and these critical points act as control or stop points. These critical control points act at critical junctions in the procedure or process to evaluate what is needed in terms of the overall process or procedure. Finally, the supply chain and critical control points are underpinned by validated methods and quality assurance/quality control/risk analysis documentation. Figure 6.3 provides an illustration of how the model could function.

Therefore, a Total QMS is required to ensure dependable results, based on:

a. Field to product (botanicals as part of the supply chain).
b. Critical control points for each step in the process or procedure.
c. Quality assurance/quality control/risk analysis and validated methods.
d. Multidisciplinary team involvement.

The critical control points can be viewed similarly to HACCP (Hazard and Critical Control Points) (https://www.fsai.ie/food_businesses/haccp/haccp.html) used in the food industry and it is envisioned that they would function in the same way. Identification of critical control points should be centered around, for example, GMP or GPAIP to provide a basis on which to ensure that crucial elements are not missed and that the overall quality and safety of botanical products is maintained. The judgment of these critical points will be influenced by the relevant regulation and legislation required.

Finally, botanicals, of necessity given their complexity, lend themselves to a multidisciplinary approach. Bringing together appropriately diverse skilled personnel assists the overall process by providing multiple perspectives and helping to ensure that all appropriate aspects are included and considered.

6.2 The Challenge of Complexity

Much of the difficulty described above arises because botanicals contain a mixture of active, partially active, and inactive substances and these combined characteristics exhibit a level of complexity that makes analysis difficult (ensuring consistency and reproducibility), methods are therefore time consuming (multiple compounds take time to separate and analyze), and expensive (cost of equipment, instrumentation, personnel, and consumables). Most importantly, this inherent complexity is coupled with significant variability; thus, one of the corner stones of scientific research, consistency and therefore reproducibility, is significantly compromised. Heinrich (2010) put this most eloquently in referring to the challenges inherent in the determination of

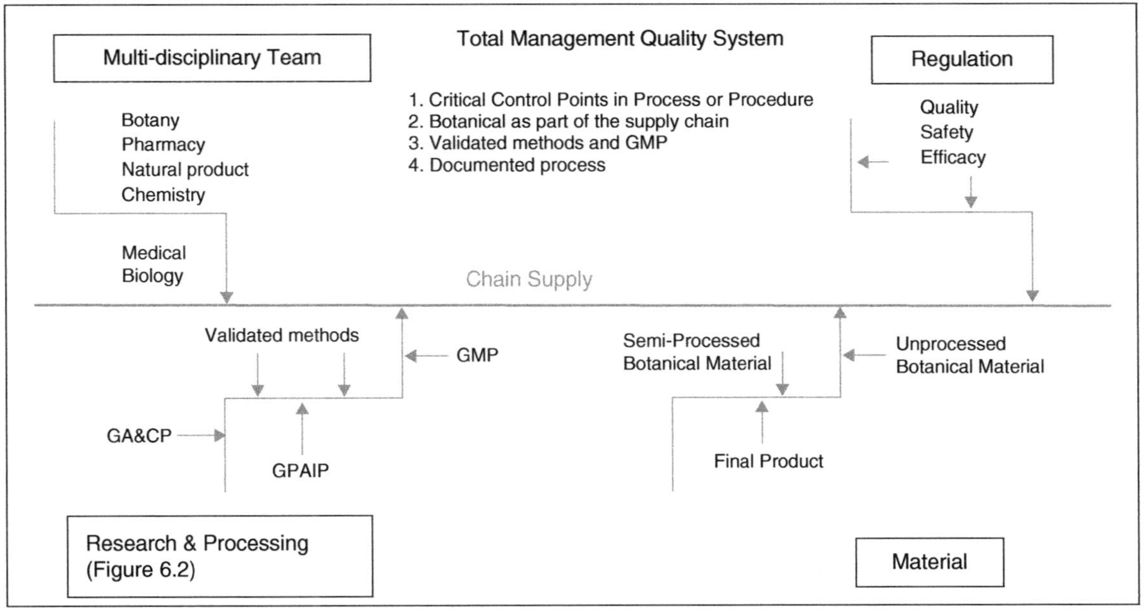

Figure 6.3 Total Management Quality System for processes and procedures related to botanicals. GPAIP – Good Plant Authentication and Identification Practice, GMP – Good Manufacturing Practice, GA&CP – Good Agriculture and Collecting Practice. *Source:* Adapted elements from Govindaraghavana and Sucher (2015).

multiple compounds in samples with complex matrices. Additionally, because of the complexity (of the botanical), the compounds can vary both qualitatively and quantitatively depending on diverse factors such as plant nutrition, growth conditions, etc. and therefore the pharmacological effect may not be consistent or reproducible. However, there are also unique opportunities as their complexity also provides a unique and bountiful supply of structurally diverse natural compounds (Li and Vederas 2009; Heinrich 2010; Henrich and Beutler 2013).

These difficulties echo those previously encountered in other areas of chemical analysis such as environmental monitoring of toxins, residues, and contaminants (De Brabander et al. 2009; Dévier et al. 2011), which grappled with the challenges inherent in the chemical analysis of complex systems. Effect-directed analysis (EDA) is a good example of an approach used to address the analytical challenges (in environmental monitoring), due to the complexity of environmental pollutants but also the increased demands because of enhanced monitoring of environmental systems following the growth in regulation/legislation in this sector. EDA is an approach which links biotesting, together with sequential fractionation (of the complex environmental sample) and chemical analysis, to ultimately identify the effect-causing compound(s). Only the active fractions were further analyzed, not the inactive fractions, thus reducing the analytical workload. EDA also has the advantage that prior knowledge of expected chemical(s) is not needed during analysis (Dévier et al. 2011).

Nevertheless, significant challenges remain across all stages of the process. These include transformational reactions that lead to more toxic compounds, potential additive, antagonistic, and synergistic reactions, multiple compounds and a lack of reference standards, and lowering of detection/quantification limits due to more stringent regulation and standards. The presence of multiple compounds and polar metabolites (within botanicals) have been identified as two of the major analytical challenges.

Despite all the challenges outlined above, advances in analytical chemistry have provided greater opportunities to identify and measure toxins and contaminants in the environment. Mass spectroscopy (MS) (generally used in combination with chromatography techniques such as gas chromatography [GC] or liquid chromatography [LC]) enables complex organic mixtures to be separated and analyzed. One example is the use of multiple tandem electrospray MS as the basis for a novel method which was developed to study azaspiracid (plus hydroxyl analog) contamination in shellfish (James et al. 2002, 2003; Furey et al. 2010).

Therefore, although this chapter will focus on challenges specific to research on plants, it should not be taken as indicating that all these issues are new and unique to plants. These are common issues that are common problems to many complex and dynamic biological systems.

This chapter presents an examination of the current challenges when studying and analyzing botanicals. As an illustration of how these challenges impact on the phytochemical analysis of botanicals, a case study approach using *Verbascum* spp. (mullein) is presented.

The European Pharmacopeia specifies *Verbascum* as the dried flowers, reduced to the corolla and the androecium, of *Verbascum thapsus* L., *Verbascum densiflorum* Bertol. (*Verbascum thapsiforme* Schrad), and *Verbascum phlomoides* L. (EMA 2008, 2018). The dried leaf and stem of great mullein (*V. thapsus*) is mentioned in the British Herbal Pharmacopeia (BHP 1983). The British Herbal Pharmacopeia (1996) includes a monograph, consisting of the dried leaves of *V. thapsus* L., *V. densiflorum* Bertol. (*V. thapsiforme* Schrad), and *V. phlomoides* L. (mullein leaf) (Bradley 2006). The root is mentioned in some references (Grieve 1974 reported in EMA 2008, 2018). The seed appears to be mainly used to kill fish (EMA 2008, 2018). Unfortunately, not many of the research papers include any reference to the respective monographs, although Światek et al. (1982) referred to using the flowers (petals and stamens) of *V. thapsiforme* consistent with pharmacopeia. Georgiev et al. (2011a) also referred to the European Pharmacopeia and that the plant material could be drawn from the flowers of *V. densiflorum, V. phlomoides,* and *V. thapsus*. However, it was noted that the flowers of *V. thapsus* were not now generally used in studies (Klimek et al. 2010). Turker et al. (2004) referred to the manual of the vascular flora of Carolinas and identified herbaria specimens which were used to assist in the identification of the wildcrafted specimens used in the research. On a more positive note, nearly all the papers, especially where the herb was wildcrafted, mentioned a botanical authentication and most noted the qualifications of the person who identified the plant and/or the distinguishing features on which identification was made (Muazaz et al. 2014).

The starting point to any analytical approach on botanicals is authentication and identification of the plant material. This could be based primarily on taxonomic and morphological data supported by chemical marker or fingerprinting data; however, metabolic and/or molecular and DNA barcoding may provide additional information (EMA 2008; Karaveliogullari and Aytaç 2008; Bucar et al. 2013; Nybom et al. 2014; Srivastava and Saggoo 2014; Mishra et al. 2016; EMA 2018). Basic information such as verifying botanical identification (Gross and Warner 1978; Rose 2006), parts used (described in appropriate botanical terms), checking for adulteration, sampling issues, documentation, and storage are needed so that published reports and comparisons between published results can be properly evaluated. These issues are further discussed in the following papers including reference to voucher specimens (Hildreth et al. 2007), IUPAC technical report (Mosihuzzaman and Choudhary 2008), on botanical nomenclature and taxonomy (Bennett and Balick 2014), pharmacognosy in research (Pferschy-Wenzig and Bauer 2015), phytochemical variation (Dhami and Mishra 2015), and quality assessment (Govindaraghavana and Sucher 2015).

6.3 Extraction Processes

Because of the complex nature of botanicals, the initial steps of sample preparation and purification are particularly important to ensure that the constituents, and most importantly potential active constituents, are not lost, distorted, or destroyed during any of the preprocessing (prewashing, drying, or grinding) and extraction stages (Sander et al. 2006; Sasidharan et al. 2011).

Extraction is typically a first step in the process of isolation and characterization of constituents; therefore, larger (g/kg) batch sizes are recommended to ensure sufficient material remains following aliquot sampling for testing in the various downstream chemical and biological assays (Weller 2012). Additionally, as the constituents are held in a complex matrix within the plant, it is not possible to extract all the constituents or constituent groups; therefore, some will remain in the plant after the extraction process. It is important to stress that the amount of constituent/constituent group extracted reflects what is recoverable in contrast to what is present in the original plant (Sander et al. 2006).

In general terms, the preparation of a plant extract can be relatively straightforward, starting with an initial bulk extract (aqueous/methanol or ethanol) or alternatively multiple cycles of extractions or fractionations with different solvents, typically of increasing polarity (e.g. *n*-hexane, dichloromethane/ethyl acetate, methanol, and water) (Heinrich 2010). The exact requirements will depend on the constituents concerned; however, if the constituent profile is unknown, a broad spectrum of different polarity solvents needs to be considered and solvent gradient fractionation employed.

The process typically starts with a maceration step to provide a crude extract, but more technical extraction processes can also be used, including Soxhlet, sonication, turbo-extraction, microwave-assisted, pressurized fluid extraction, supercritical fluid, agitation, digestion, and reflux. It is recommended that the techniques should be form-appropriate. For example, in comparing the contents of a product by phytochemical assays, the methods used to solubilize solid preparations may require exhaustive Soxhlet extraction of the herbs in contrast to sonification required merely to dissolve solid extracts. (Bucar et al. 2013; Atanasov et al. 2015). The sample clean-up can differ depending on the specific requirements of the methods being used, whether it is simply to remove particulate matter (filtration or centrifugation) or, in contrast, where the extraction may need to be concentrated (liquid–liquid extraction, evaporation or solvent exchange, solid-phase extraction [SPE]). Thermolabile compounds need to be considered with any heating step (Sasidharan et al. 2011) and with solvent evaporation steps.

The efficiency of the extraction process can be affected by factors such as the type of solvent, temperature, pressure, extraction time, solvent pH, and the number of extraction cycles (Sander et al. 2006). Bucar et al. (2013) mentions that the polarity and stability of the compounds to be extracted, the toxicity, volatility, viscosity, and purity of the solvent, probability of artifacts, and finally the amount of bulk material to be extracted are some of the considerations that require attention when extracting compounds in a non-soluble matrix such as plants.

It is also imperative, when researching plants used in traditional medicine, that the same or equivalent traditional extraction processes should be used (Heinrich 2010) as standard. Traditionally, herbs were used fresh or dried and could be processed in a variety of ways (Grieve 1974, 1981). Crude extracts using between 25% and 90% ethanol as solvent or, alternatively, water have been usual, although wine, brandy, or whiskey (as alternative alcohols) with addition of glycerine, vinegar, or sugar can also be used as the solvent for internal use (Green 2000). The extraction process typically has included maceration, percolation, and reflux methods, although many traditional processes can include heating and cooling steps or non-standard solvents, thereby significantly complicating the process (Grieve 1974; Dar et al. 2018).

Additionally, as the solvent used will determine the chemical content of the extract, this can have a significant effect on the bioactivity of the resulting extract (Sasidharan et al. 2011). For hydrophilic (water soluble) compounds, polar solvents such as water, methanol, ethanol, and ethyl-acetate or miscible combinations of such solvents (pH adjustment may be necessary) are applicable, while for more lipophilic (fat-soluble) compounds, dichloromethane or mixtures thereof with methanol can be used. Hexane and chloroform can be used to remove chlorophyll. The removal of chlorophyll can be advantageous as it can (along with highly apolar compounds such as fatty acids and polar compounds such as polyphenols [tannins]) be problematic and interfere with bioassays. Chlorophyll can interact with fatty acids and exhibit antioxidant activity (reported in Atanasov et al. 2015). Additionally, chloroform suffers from several deficiencies including restrictions on use due to its classification as "reasonably anticipated to be a human carcinogen" based on animal experimentation. It is listed as a potential occupational carcinogen (NTP 2016). Dichloromethane can be used as a toxicologically safer solvent to chloroform.

Thus, the determination of constituents in botanicals represents a significant challenge for the analyst. These mainly center round the complexity of plants, the matrix within which the constituents are found, and any variability in solubility between constituents. The main steps and methods used from extraction to analysis are outlined in Table 6.1. Extraction methods are also described in more detail in the publications of Sasidharan et al. (2011) and Bucar et al. (2013).

Table 6.2 outlines the extraction processes noted in published (and referenced throughout this review) research on *Verbascum*, and it illustrates certain gaps in current knowledge of the phytochemistry of this genus, which are discussed throughout the remainder of the chapter.

In terms of processing, dried and ground (to a powder) samples of different species of *Verbascum* are mainly used (Tatli et al. 2004a). Drying was mainly in air at room temperature (Georgiev et al. 2011b; Khan et al. 2011) although oven drying at 40 °C has also been employed (Dulger et al. 2015).

In terms of the extraction processes, crude maceration of the air dried samples was mainly used as a first stage (Barbour et al. 2004; Tatli et al. 2007; Talib and Mahasneh 2010; Georgiev et al. 2011b; Khan et al. 2011), although the Soxhlet extraction was also fairly prominently mentioned as an extraction method (Dulger and Gonuz 2004; Turker et al. 2004; Dulger and Ugurlu 2005; Dulger 2006; Mothana et al. 2008; Dulger et al. 2015). The reflux method was also mentioned (Tatli et al. 2004a). There were also papers which omitted to specify the specific extraction method used (Dülger et al. 2002).

Traditionally, the flowers were also boiled in milk before being applied externally or boiled and the vapors used externally, in addition to decoction or a water extract (Quinlan 1883; Grieve 1974; McCarthy and O'Mahony 2010). Except for the water extract, this is not reflected in any of the papers.

Table 6.1 Steps in the extraction of botanical material

Extraction	Extraction parameters	Sample clean-up
Maceration/percolation	Solvent, ionic solvents	Filtration
Soxhlet extraction	Temperature	Centrifugation
Sonication extraction	Pressure	Solid-phase extraction (SPE)
Pressurized fluid extraction	Time	Liquid–liquid extraction
Agitation	pH	Semi-preparative liquid chromatography (LC)
Reflux (hydrolysis)	Number of extractions	
Digestion	Compounds	
Turbo-extraction	Artifacts	
Microwave-assisted		
Supercritical fluid		
Extraction on solid-phases		

Source: Adapted from Sander et al. (2006) and Bucar et al. (2013).

Table 6.2 Extraction processes reported in research of *Verbascum* spp

Process	Action
Plant (flowers, leaves, stem, roots)	Freshly picked, location, voucher, and authentication mentioned
Dried	Mainly air dried but reference to freeze drying. Occasional mention of drying at room temp. or 40 °C
Initial solvent	Methanol mainly but also ethanol and water. Very occasionally acetone, butanol, chloroform or dichloromethane
Temperature, pressure, pH, time, and number of extractions	Rarely mentioned
Extraction process	Maceration, occasionally Soxhlet apparatus or reflux. Solid-phase extraction was used as a step prior to HPLC
Clean-up	Evaporation of methanol, purification steps, removal of chlorophyll, centrifugation
Part of herb used	Mentioned but often only in general terms not specific parts

The solvent used for initial bulk extractions of polar and semi-polar compounds has mainly been methanol (Barbour et al. 2004; Khan et al. 2011), although ethanol (Kumar et al. 2010) and water (Barbour et al. 2004) have also been used. Very occasionally, chloroform (Turker et al. 2004), acetone (Zhao et al. 2011; Boğa et al. 2016), butanol (Armatu et al. 2011), and dichloromethane (reported in Tatli and Akdemir 2006) have been used when non-polar compounds are being extracted. However, although pressure, temperature, time, pH, and number of extractions are all noted in some reports as variables in the extraction process, they have rarely been discussed critically. In reports where this information has been disclosed, extraction temperatures have usually been conducted at room temperature or, less frequently, at 40, 50 or 70 °C (Tatli et al. 2006).

Many extraction processes included the removal of chlorophyll and other lipophilic compounds with chloroform (Tatli et al. 2006; Akdemir et al. 2011). These researchers reported that flash evaporation was used to remove methanol and that purification was conducted using Merck Lobar columns (RP-8 and RP-18), with analytes eluted with a water–methanol gradient.

Finally, although most of the papers have referred to the traditional use of this herb and the fact that this was the stimulus for the research, there has been little evidence to date that the ethnomedical interest extends to the processing of the herb beyond the use of water or alcohol solvents for extraction (Turker and Camper 2002).

6.4 Separation and Detection

The work for this review has highlighted that the research on botanicals is at a remarkably early stage. In particular, it has demonstrated a great need for the use of more robust and validated analytical techniques. The reference standards for many constituents of interest are sometimes difficult to obtain or are not commercially available. Current methods, whether analytical or bioassay, tend to require some form of modification to take account of, for example, the complex nature of botanicals and selectivity or sensitivity issues (Bucar et al. 2013). Validated methods of analysis are only slowly being developed, although that movement appears to be occurring more quickly in terms of analytical methods (Klimek et al. 2010; Cieśla et al. 2011; Bucar et al. 2013). However, there are encouraging moves to assist this process; for example, the increasing development of standard reference materials (SRMs) by the National Institute of Standards and Technology (NIST) will provide certified values (measure of certainty of the standard) for organic constituents and selected trace elements, which can be used in characterizing dietary supplements for potency, authenticity, and contamination or adulteration (Sander et al. 2006).

Thin layer chromatography (TLC), high-performance liquid chromatography (HPLC), together with mass spectrometry (MS), are the recommended separation and detection methods for botanical research (EMA 2008, 2018; Wagner and Ulrich-Merzenich 2013). Because of the polar nature of many botanical constituents, they are very suited to liquid chromatography as a form of analysis to determine qualitative and quantitative information on the constituent composition.

Table 6.3 outlines the reported advantages and disadvantages of various techniques used in the separation and detection of phytochemicals, which are also outlined in more detail (with references) in the surrounding text.

The separation techniques typically involve one or more steps of column chromatography (HPLC, HPTLC, and GC). They can also be coupled with tandem mass spectrometers (e.g. quadrupole ion trap MS, linear ion trap MS, triple quadrupole MS) to confirm compound identity while the structure and chirality of isolated compounds can only be conclusively determined by nuclear magnetic resonance spectroscopy (NMR) (Atanasov et al. 2015; Caixach et al. 2016).

This methodology is used in the separation of fractions and identification of constituents of *Verbascum* spp. For example, using a bioactivity mediated approach, Akdemir et al. (2011) employed a polyamide column high-resolution electrospray ionization mass spectrometry (HR-ESIMS) (ICN, vacuum liquid chromatography [VLC]) (of the lyophilized water phase) eluted with water H_2O, followed by increasing concentration of methanol. This resulted in six fractions (A to F) which were analyzed for activity. The most active fraction (D) was further fractioned using LiChroprep C_{18} (Merck, C-18, Sepralyte 40 μm, VLC). Water plus increasing amounts of methanol (0–100%) was employed resulting in the isolation of ajugol, aucubin, catalpol, and four additional fractions D_{1-4}. Again, the most active fractions were rechromatographed (D_3) on LiChroprep C18 (medium pressure liquid chromatography [MPLC]) with water and gradients of 30–70% methanol. This yielded lasianthoside I, ilwensisaponin A and ilwensisaponin C. Fraction D4 was purified by silica gel column chromatography (Merck, 230–400 mesh) using a chloroform : methanol solvent solution from 70 : 30 to 60 : 40. This yielded verbascoside. The structure of the isolated compounds was investigated using UV, IR, 1D-, and 2DNMR and mass spectroscopy (HR-ESIMS) (Akdemir et al. 2011)

For any given technique, the specific method needs to be developed, optimized, and validated (Tistaert et al. 2011). A "design of experiments" provides a multivariate approach to optimizing the analytical method under investigation. This model typically analyses all factors which have a potential to influence the experimental outcome simultaneously in order to assess their impact. For chromatography, these

Table 6.3 Advantages and disadvantages in the methods used for chemical characterization of botanicals

Method	Advantages	Disadvantages
TLC	Flexibility to optimize operational parameters	Low reproducibility
	Readily available	Low resolution
	Easy to use	High compound concentration required
	Economical	Estimate of quantitative information
		Control (sample spotting, vapor, detection reagents)
HPTLC	Increased reproducibility, resolution, and sensitivity	
	Smaller particle size (5 μm)	
	Speed	
	Smaller amounts of solvents	
	Minimum sample clean-up	
	unlike HPLC, can use mobile phases of pH 8 and above	
ME - TLC	Increased separation efficiency and sensitivity	Estimate of quantitative information
	Increased signal enhancement over TLC and HPTLC	Vapor phase needs to be controlled
	Reduced detection limits	
	Easier to operate than standard TLC	
Densitometric TLC	Improved qualitative analysis	
2-Dimensional Chromatography/TLC	Increased peak capacity	Long analysis time
Graft - TLC	Increased separation capacity	Long analysis time
HPLC	Easy to operate	Expensive equipment
	Fully automated	Noxious chemicals
	High resolution, sensitivity, and selectivity	Detection of co-elution compounds
	Can be coupled to different detectors, e.g. UV, UV-diode array, FLD, MS	Silica based columns are vulnerable to relatively acidic and basic mobile phases and high temperatures
		Limited modification
UHPLC	Superior to HPLC in terms of resolution and separation	Increased back pressure
	Shorter column, therefore less solvent used	Availability of stable stationary phases
	Significantly shorter analysis time (factor of 8)	

(continued)

Table 6.3 (*continued*)

Method	Advantages	Disadvantages
HILIC	Good retention and separation of hydrophilic compounds	
	Uses more environmentally friendly solvents	
GC	Coupled with detectors with increased sensitivity and efficiency	Potential for degradation of thermos-labile compounds
	GC-MS reduced analysis time	Limited to volatile compounds
CE	Low solvent consumption	Overlapping peaks
	Decreased operational costs	Non-reproducible migration times
	Less environmental impact	Limited sample volume
	High resolution	Additional sample preparation (concentration)
CEC	High resolution with selectivity and reproducibility	Bubble formation and Joule heating
pCEC	Increased speed and reproducibility	Some loss of efficiency
		Additional work on accuracy, repeatability, and detection limit needed

TLC, Thin Layer Chromatography; *HPTLC*, High-Performance Thin Layer Chromatography; *M-E TLC*, Microemulsion Thin Layer Chromatography; *Densitometric TLC*, Densitometric Thin Layer Chromatography; *Two-Dimensional TLC*, Two-Dimensional Thin Layer Chromatography; *Graft-TLC*, Coupled-layer Planar Chromatography; *HPLC*, High-Performance Liquid Chromatography; *UHPLC*, Ultra-High Performance Liquid Chromatography; *HILIC*, Hydrophilic Interaction Chromatography; *GC*, Gas Chromatography; *MS*, Mass Spectrometry; *CE*, Capillary Electrophoresis; *CEC*, Capillary Electro-chromatography; *pCEC*, Pressurized Capillary Electro-chromatography.
Source: Chopra et al. (2006); Tistaert et al. (2011).

factors include the composition of the mobile phase, buffer concentration and pH, detection wavelength, column temperature, injection volume, sample concentration, and column type.

6.4.1 Thin Layer Chromatography (TLC) and High-Performance Thin Layer Chromatography (HPTLC)

TLC and HPTLC, together with a suitable detection system, are used to identify and differentiate between botanical constituents; for example, to authenticate an herb or to identify an adulterant (Chopra et al. 2006; Tian et al. 2009).

Although TLC is still used and accepted regarding characterization and pharmacopeia standards (i.e. Monographs, Quality control standards, current Good Manufacturing Practice (cGMP) and botanical reference materials (BMRs)), it is increasingly being supplanted by other more effective chromatographic methods, such as HPTLC, HPLC, and NMR amongst others, because of TLC's poor reproducibility, low resolution, and imprecise quantitative measurement (Tistaert et al. 2011). Furthermore, sample spotting, the vapor saturation inside the development chamber, and unstable coloration from detection reagents are difficult variables to control. Nevertheless, it still retains advantages in terms of relative cost, versatility, and flexibility in optimization (Marchand et al. 2007).

Wagner and Bladt (1996) recommend a chloroform–methanol–water (60 : 40 : 4) system as the mobile phase to detect iridoid glycosides from a methanol extract of *V. densiflorum* flower. The iridoid glycosides catalpol (T1) and aucubin (T2) and derivatives (e.g. veronicoside and aucubin-ayloside) migrate into the R_f range 0.45–0.75 and are detected with anisaldehyde sulfuric acid reagent as gray, blue, and violet zones in visible light. Enrichment by *n*-butanol extraction is recommended where the concentration of iridoid glycosides is low. Catalpol (T1) and aucubin (T2) show up as gray zones (R_f 0.4 to 0.5) and a prominent blue zone at R_f 0.4 (verbascosaponine). Wagner and Bladt (1996), using a solvent system of ethyl acetate-formic acid-glacial acetic acid-water (100 : 11 : 11 : 26), detected three zones with a similar depth of colour, using natural products/polyethylene glycol reagent (NP/PEG No. 28) under UV light, 365 nm, at R_f 0.4, 0.5, and 0.6. These colored zones are indicative of flavonoid glycosides. The reference compounds were rutin (R_f ~ 0.4), chlorogenic acid (R_f ~ 0.5), and hyperoside (R_f ~ 0.6). Apigenin (R_f 0.6) and luteolin glucoside (R_f 0.75) were also detected and a green zone (hesperidin) at R_f ~ 0.45 was detected using natural products reagent (NP No. 28) in UV light, 365 nm.

TLC analysis using recoated silica gel 60 F254 aluminum sheets was more recently reported (in the investigation of iridoid glycosides and neolignin glycosides) and a similar solvent system of chloroform : methanol : water (61 : 32 : 7 v/v/v) was employed. UV fluorescence was also used together with a vanillin, H_2SO_4 reagent heated to 105 °C for one to two minutes (reported in Emam 2010).

Some of the earlier constituent analysis (iridoid glycosides) of *Verbascum* spp. employed TLC as the sole analytical method (Grabias and Swiatek (1987), referenced by Alipieva et al. (2014)). Additionally, a 2010 study of ethanol fractions from *Verbascum sinaiticum* flower was examined for constituents using TLC and eluted with serial gradients of chloroform and methanol (from 0% to 100%). Flavonoids and terpenoids were visualized with *p*-anisaldehyde/sulfuric acid reagent and heated at 105 °C. The plates were sprayed with iodoplatinic acid and dried in the fume hood to detect alkaloids (Talib and Mahasneh 2010).

HPTLC as a method is more accurate and has increased reproducibility compared to standard TLC. It is, therefore, increasingly being used across the whole range of industry standards, and elsewhere, to show conformity with GMP, monograph identity standards, and adulterating species. Chopra et al. (2006) developed and validated International Conference on Harmonization (ICH) guidelines for precision, recovery, robustness, and ruggedness for a HPTLC method to determine the presence of trigonelline in herbal extracts using TLC aluminum plates precoated with silica gel 60F-254 (20 cm × 10 cm) as the stationary phase. Six-mm bands (of sample) were applied as spotting using a Camag microliter syringe. Additional parameters employed included: a constant application rate of 150 nl/s, space between bands of 10 mm, slit dimensions remain at 5 mm × 0.45 mm, and scanning speed of 20 mm/s. Trigonelline hydrochloride from Sigma–Aldrich was used as the standard. The mobile phase consisted of *n*-propanol–methanol–water (4 : 1 : 4, v/v/v). A twin-trough glass chamber saturated with the mobile phase was used for the linear ascending development, with an optimized chamber saturation time of 30 minutes at room temperature

(25 ± 2 °C) and relative humidity of 55% ± 5%. The chromatogram run was 80 mm. A Camag TLC scanner III was used for spectrodensitometric scanning (CAMAG 2018) and analysis in absorbance mode at 269 nm. Detection and quantification limits were determined and sensitivity and selectivity were verified by statistical analysis.

Increased separation efficiency and signal enhancement were obtained with microemulsion TLC leading to a reduction in detection limits and improved sensitivity (Tistaert et al. 2011). Microemulsion TLC is considered to provide a rapid fingerprinting method of analysis suitable for the authentication and quality assessment of herbs (Cui et al. 2005).

Microemulsions comprise macroscopically homogeneous, optically transparent fluids which have only been used in TLC since 2000. They are extracted in methanol and do not require the additional clean-up stages often required for conventional TLC due to the higher solubilizing ability and lower interfacial tension of the microemulsion system. They further differ from conventional TLC in that the vapor phase remains relatedly constant, because the main component of the solvent is water, thereby substantially improving reproducibility. Additionally, humidity (30–90%) and temperature (17–28%) were in this case also found not to affect separation (Cui et al. 2005). Substantial signal enhancement was observed for the microemulsion TLC which is thought to be due to the restricted space (resulting from the microemulsion process) affecting its optical reading, including its UV–Vis absorption, fluorescence, chemiluminescence, phosphorescence, circular dichroism, or NMR spectra. Cui et al. (2005) found that the separation (of licorice compounds) was clearer and sharper with more concentrated spots and less tailing (enhanced sensitivity and lower detection limits).

Other improvements in TLC-based analytical methods include densitometric TLC (Gabriëls and Plaizier-Vercammen 2003), and two-dimensional TLC, which increase separation capacity and coupled-layer planar chromatography.

Cieśla et al. (2011) used a 2D TLC method to resolve compounds from the polar fraction from the flower of selected species of *Verbascum*. Here, silica gel plates were used with AcOEt-MeOH-H_2O- 25% aqueous NH_3 in the ratio of (55 : 35 : 9 : 1, w/v/v/v) as the first mobile phase followed by MeOH-AcOEt-H_2O-HCOOH (10 : 90 : 26 : 22, v/v/v/v). The visualizing reagent was vanillin–sulfuric acid. The resulting chromatograms were scanned using the CAMAG TLC Reprostar 3 device with videostore and processed using the Image J image-processing program. It is important to note that this was perhaps the only paper to include details on variables that can affect extraction and processing (as mentioned above in Section 6.3 [Sander et al. 2006; Sasidharan et al. 2011]). The 2D TLC method was validated (using a referenced method) for specificity, precision (reproducibility and intermediate precision), and robustness. The authors reported that only changes in temperature and heating time may affect the intensity of some spots.

The authors (Cieśla et al. 2011) argued that the separation of polar compounds can be challenging with HPLC or GC methods due to the inherent non-volatility of compounds such as iridoid glycosides (present in *Verbascum* spp.) and lack of or weak chromophores, e.g. HPLC-UV. Additionally, strongly hydrophilic iridoid glycoside compounds bind strongly to the polar stationary phase and so can be difficult to separate. Triterpene saponins (also found in *Verbascum* spp.) occur in multicomponent mixtures of glycosidic forms and most triterpenes do not absorb UV or visible light.

The authors (Cieśla et al. 2011) also argue that hydrophilic interaction chromatography (HILIC) (described below) may also be a good option when dealing with strongly polar glycosidic compounds with a high affinity for aqueous mobile phases.

6.4.2 High-Performance Liquid Chromatography (HPLC)

HPLC is currently considered the most appropriate method to analyze botanicals. It has numerous advantages, including being relatively easy to operate, being fully automated with high resolution, and having selectivity and sensitivity. However, chromatographic optimization can be very difficult, expensive, and time consuming, especially when attempting to separate a variable number of compounds that have poor peak shape. There are a number of options here including column and mobile phase buffering and solvent optimization.

Chromatographic methods are coupled to detectors such as ultraviolet (UV) and diode array detectors (DAD), which are prone to extract matrix interferants from matrix compounds that absorb at the same λ_{max} as the target analytes. There can be co-elutions and silica-based columns are vulnerable to relatively basic (pH >9) and acidic (pH >2) mobile phases and high temperatures (Tistaert et al. 2011). Other disadvantages include, for example, the need for an expensive instrument and large volumes of noxious chemicals (Sudberg et al. 2010; Upton et al. 2011).

Tistaert et al. (2011) outlined some of the approaches used to optimize analytical methods for botanicals, and in particular focusing on a screening design used to optimize HPLC-UV as an analytical method for fingerprints of *Ginkgo biloba* extracts. Using the peak capacity as the measured response, the most important effects were determined as the column temperature, wavelength, and injection volume. These variables might be considered when elucidating *Verbascum* spp. using HPLC-UV.

Although there is still no standard method, validated methods are being developed. Klimek et al. (2010) reported on a RP-HPLC-UV (λ_{max} = 349 nm), method used to successfully determine simultaneously eight flavonoids and two phenylethanoids from the flowers of two species of *Verbascum: V. densiflorum* and *V. phlomoides*. High levels of diosmin and tamarixetin 7-rutinoside (2.327–2.392% of dry weight) were found in the flowers of *V. phlomoides* using a C(18) Lichrosphere 100 column (5 µm, 250 mm × 4.6 mm, i.d.). The eluate was an acetonitrile gradient using aqueous 0.5% (w/v) orthophosphoric acid solution containing 1% (v/v) tetrahydrofurane. The flowers of *V. densiflorum* were found to contain higher levels of verbascoside (0.688–0.742% dry weight) and luteolin 7-glucoside (0.204–0.279% dry weight). Validation was determined for linearity over the test ranges, high sensitivity in terms of detection limits, and repeatability (Klimek et al. 2010).

Reverse-phase liquid chromatography is also favored to separate saponins due to high column efficiency and good repeatability. However, it should be noted that separation selectivity may not always be sufficient for isomeric saponins with small differences, e.g. aldohexosyl or aldopentosyl unit (Guo et al. 2013). Reverse-phase chromatographic methods are frequently used for *Verbascum* analysis (Tatli et al. 2004a, 2007).

UHPLC uses short columns packed with small particles (sub-2 mm) working at high pressures (>400 bar). Avula et al. (2008) analyzed hoodigosides from the shrub *Hoodia* spp. and found that the method could be used for the rapid analysis of a wide range of formulations including gels, capsules, tablets, sprays, tea bags, snack bars, powders, and juices (Nguyen et al. 2006; Tistaert et al. 2011).

HILIC addresses the fact that much pharmacological processing of herbal products produces polar compounds, i.e. water extracts. Produced as an alternative to silica-based chromatography columns (Alpert 1990), this approach uses a partitioning effect between the polar stationary phase and the aqueous mobile phase.

Its advantages are reported to be shorter analysis time (15–30 minutes) compared with reverse-phase liquid chromatography (RPLC) which can require more than 60 minutes to run, in addition to better resolution and comparative separation power. However, there are also disadvantages with HILIC columns, in particular the difficulty in selecting the increasing number of stationary phases needed to separate saponins. Additionally, mobile phases with a high concentration of acetonitrile decrease saponin solubility resulting in peak fronting and low loadability, significantly affecting the volume of saponins that can be separated (Guo et al. 2013). Nevertheless, a method using hydrophilic interaction ultra-performance liquid chromatography coupled with triple-quadrupole tandem mass spectrometry (HILIC-UPLC-TQ-MS/MS) and working in multiple reaction monitoring mode was used to successfully characterize 11 nucleobases and nucleosides from *G. biloba* leaf extract simultaneously in a period of 7 minutes. The method was validated for linearity, sensitivity, and repeatability, in addition to recovery (Yao et al. 2015).

6.4.3 Gas Chromatography (GC)

GC is an effective analytical method for the characterization of volatile compounds (Tistaert et al. 2011). Typically coupled with MS, it has an excellent separation efficacy and sensitivity detection. Nevertheless, its range of use is limited to non-polar, volatile, and thermally stable compounds – for example, essential oils – and this limitation makes GC an unsuitable method for many botanicals, including *Verbascum* spp.

Armatu et al. (2011) were unique in using gas chromatography-mass spectrometry (GC-MS) to investigate butanol and ethanol extracts of *V. phlomoides* and identified 25 compounds from 2 extracts: L1 extract comprising 3 alcohols, 4 ketones, 3 aldehydes, 3 organic acids, and 7 esters; and L2 extract comprising 3 acids, 4 alcohols, 7 esters, 5 ketones, and 3 aldehydes. Esters and ketones were the major constituents in both extracts.

As an aside and not related directly to constituents of *Verbascum,* GC-triple quadrupole-MS has been used to detect quantifiable amounts of polybrominated diphenyl ethers (PCB-153) in *V. thapsus* collected from residential and rural areas of Spain (Pérez et al. 2013).

6.4.4 Ion Exchange Chromatography, Size Exclusion Chromatography, Capillary Electrophoresis

Ion exchange chromatography is a widely used form of column chromatography, whether in research, analysis, or protein purification. Proteins are ideal for this method because of their charged nature. Ion exchange chromatography also has advantages in terms of high capacity and high resolution. However, this method is not widely used for botanicals or natural products, although it was reported in the literature as having been used as a purification step for the extraction of lectin from *Pinellia ternate* (Zuo et al. 2012) and the purification of DING proteins extracted from *Hypericum perforatum* (Perera et al. 2008).

Size exclusion chromatography (gel chromatography) is widely used in the area of protein analysis, although it is also employed in lipid and starch analysis (Burgess

2018). Based on the size of the analyte, the method is commonly used to separate protein from other material or by protein shape. This method is not used with botanicals.

Capillary electrophoresis (CE), as a miniaturized technique, has the advantage of low solvent consumption and consequently decreased operational and environmental costs. Disadvantages include limited sample (injection) volume and sometimes the need for additional preconcentration (Tistaert et al. 2011). Although used for marker and fingerprint analysis (Sun and Shi 2008; Kesselring et al. 2013), additional disadvantages have been reported, including the occurrence of overlapping peaks with complex compounds and non-reproducible retention times due to high voltages causing fluctuations in the electro-osmotic flow. A study comparing CE to HPLC (radix of Scutellariae) found that the analytical time was reduced from 40 to 12 minutes but there was also a decrease in peak numbers detected, from 14 to 11 (Wang et al. 2005). Nevado et al. (2012) validated and optimized a capillary zone electrophoresis (CZE) method to analyze selected phenolic compounds (rosmarinic and caffeic acid) in olive oil. An optimized preconcentration procedure based on SPE was used.

6.4.5 Hyphenated Techniques (LC–MS, GC–MS, LC–NMR)

Chromatographic techniques such as HPLC or LC are typically connected with detectors such as Ultra Violet (UV) (herbal fingerprinting), DAD (UV absorbing compounds), evaporative light scattering detection (ELSD), and chemiluminescence detection (CL) (non-UV absorbing compounds), NMR (metabolomics profiling), and mass spectrometry (MS) (identification of separate compounds through the generation of a mass spectrum). The coupling of separation and detection methods can involve more than one separation or detection technique, e.g. LC–PDA–MS, LC–MS–MS, LC–NMR–MS, LCPDA–NMR–MS (Patel et al. 2010).

Hyphenated methods offer the advantage of assisting with structural elucidation without the need for isolating the compound, except for NMR, where compound purity remains important (Halabalaki et al. 2014). With small amounts of trace compounds, analyte enrichment is an essential step necessitating online coupling with SPE, solid-phase microextraction, or large volume injection (LVI), e.g. –SPE–LC–MS or LVI–GCMS. SPE was originally developed as a purification step for HPLC or GC analysis (Bucar et al. 2013). In addition, rutin, caffeic acid, and chlorogenic acid were identified and quantitatively determined, showing that a TLC–MS coupled system (and it is argued HPTLC) may also be an effective method of analysis.

Hyphenated methods have been reported extensively for *Verbascum* analysis including TLC/UV spectrophotometry (Bradley 2006; Alipieva et al. 2014), HPLC–MS, LC–MS, HPLC–NMR (Turker et al. 2004), GC–MS (Armatu et al. 2011), HPLC–DAD–NMR (Georgiev et al. 2011a,b), liquid chromatography–electrospray ionization mass spectrometry (HPLC–ESI–MS) (Akdemir et al. 2003, 2004a,b; Arrif et al. 2006), and Fast Atom Bombardment–MS (FAB–MS) (Abou Gazar et al. 2003a).

Finally, one of the disadvantages of bioactivity guided analysis is that it can result in repeated isolation of the same compounds. Therefore, strategies (so called dereplication strategies) have been developed to reduce this time-consuming and costly disadvantage by combining separation methods, spectroscopic detection techniques, and online database searching. For example, HPLC together with photodiode array detection (PDA), MS, and NMR, could allow crude extracts or fractions to be screened not just for biological activity but also for structural classes. In practice, multiple hyphenated coupling can be used together with bioactivity assays for effective screening of extracts including LCD–AD–UV and LC–MS/LC–MS–MS or LC–NMR and LC–UV–MS in order to obtain a large amount of analytical data on the extract constituents prior to isolation (Patel et al. 2010). Weller (2012), however, has argued over to what extent such methods can truly be considered hyphenated methods, particularly in terms of the bioactivity directed component, because of the lack of real-time analysis and the break in the time-line between the chemical analysis and biological activities.

6.4.6 TLC Bioautography

One technique that has increasingly been cited within the literature as an important screening method is TLC bioautography (Choma and Grzelak 2011). This method is considered to provide relatively quick and inexpensive separation of the constituents, together with an assessment of the antimicrobial activity of the separated constituents. It is very appropriate for plant-based compounds (Kagan and Flythe 2014). It is also been argued that it may be more reliable than some of the more traditional antimicrobial methods (Horváth et al. 2013), This method, perhaps most importantly, allows for activity-guided isolation of compounds. On the other hand, loss of activity demonstrated *in vitro* can be indicative of synergistic interaction of constituents within the plant.

The process consists of two basic parts: first, separation of plant extracts by paper or thin layer chromatography (PC or TLC); and second, exposing the chromatograms to microbial suspensions (e.g. fungi or bacteria in broth or agar) and examining for zones of microbial inhibition. The effectiveness of this screening method, known as bioautography, depends on both the quality of the chromatographic separation and the care taken with microbial culture conditions. Regarding antimicrobial activity assays, many variations of bioautography have been employed, including contact, immersion (overlay), and direct, although bioluminescent approaches (using bioluminescent bacteria) are increasingly being used (Choma and Grzelak 2011; Weller 2012). This method has not been standardized and a number of different procedures are used within the literature; for example, a contact method (the TLC plate is placed in contact with the microbial culture) or immersion/overlay method (the microbial culture is poured onto the TLC plate) or direct method (the TLC plate is dipped into or sprayed with a layer of microbial liquid culture). Redox indicators such as triphenyl tetrazolium chloride (TTC) dye are typically used to identify bacterial growth. Kagan and Flythe (2014) provide a good example of a contact method used to investigate the antimicrobial properties of separated compounds of *Trifolium pratense* cv. Kenland (phenolic compounds) against the bacterium *Clostridium sticklandii*.

Two factors that are important to the success of this method are the quality of the chromatographic separation and the care taken with microbial culture conditions. In terms of the chromatographic procedure, the number of bands was found to double in one study when the separation distance was increased (15 instead of 8.5 cm); although, regrettably, with a different sample (of the herb) from the same cultivar but grown in a separate plot on the same farm. Separation can also be in one or two directions across the plate (Kagan and Flythe 2014).

The choice of solvent (specifically, two successive developments in different solvent systems) in the same study was found to affect the number of bands derived. Problems can occur with polar compounds as they typically require a more acid or basic solvent. Microorganisms are readily killed by acid compounds, especially with a pH of less than 5.0.

The contact method has been criticized due to questions on the ability of compounds to diffuse into the growth media. Thus, at low concentrations or poor ability to diffuse, inhibition may not be detectable. Alternatively, there may be a spread from one band to a neighboring area masking the inhibitory zones. On the plus side, this method is easy to use, quick, and cheap. There is also less risk of the bands spreading than with the overlay or direct methods (Kagan and Flythe 2014).

Zampini et al. (2010) also reported on a TLC autographic assay for the rapid detection of antioxidant capacity based on the ABTS (2,2'-azino-bis (3-ethylbenzothiazoline-6-sulfonic acid)) scavenging activities. Autographic methods to detect antioxidant activity have also been developed based on xanthine oxidase inhibitors and DPPH (2,2-diphenyl-1-picrylhydrazyl). scavenging activities. The use of alternative TLC plates (C18 adsorbent or microcrystalline cellulose) has been proposed to address the previously mentioned challenges with extraction/elution of polar compounds, but this can in turn adversely affect visualization.

Akdemir et al. (2004a) used a DPPH based, TLC autography method to investigate antioxidant scavenging properties of *Verbascum salviifolium*.

6.4.7 Spectroscopic Methods

Spectroscopic techniques such as vibrational spectroscopy, mid-infrared and near-infrared (MIR and NIR), in addition to NMR are used in relation to the analysis of botanicals and are typically used in conjunction with chromatographic methods (Weller 2012).

6.4.7.1 Nuclear Magnetic Resonance (NMR) NMR offers significant advantages in research in that it has the ability to simultaneously detect numerous disparate compounds generally present at low compounds (compared to primary metabolites) and because the signal intensity is only dependent on the molar concentration in the solution, quantitation is possible (Verpoorte et al. 2007; Kim et al. 2010, 2011; Georgiev et al. 2011b). A major disadvantage is signal overlapping, although that can generally be resolved with 2D approaches (Kim et al. 2010, 2011).

NMR (1D and 2D) are used extensively across the published studies on *Verbascum* (Tatli et al. 2004a, 2006, 2007; Georgiev et al. 2011b). Although most of the papers refer to the use of NMR (1D and 2D) to elicit the structural details of the detected compounds, one paper looked at the use of ^{1}H NMR (proton nuclear magnetic resonance (proton NMR, hydrogen-1 NMR)) in combination with principle component analysis (PCA) in a metabolomics study. Five different species were found to divide into two groups based on the amount and type of metabolite detected in each species. Additionally, *Verbascum xanthophoeniceum* and *Verbascum nigrum* accumulate higher amounts of harpagoside (0.5% on dry weight basis) and verbascoside, forsythoside B, and leucosceptoside B (in total 5.6–5.8% on dry weight basis) (Georgiev et al. 2011b).

In summary, although there is no general consistency across the various separation and detection methods used to analyze *Verbascum*, HPLC (direct or reverse phase) coupled to UV-Vis and IR, MS, and NMR are the favored methods to date. The majority of the publications researched that characterized the constituents of *Verbascum* have used an IR and UV spectroscopic method (Akdemir et al. 2003, 2004a,b; Tatli et al. 2004a,b, 2006). Klimek et al. (2010) have reported a more recent (and welcome) move to validate the analytical method used (Klimek et al. 2010).

6.5 Chemical Characterization

Here, the primary concern is with secondary metabolites, i.e. those compounds produced by the plant that are not directly or primarily involved in growth, development, and reproduction but which have a defensive or ecological function. Secondary metabolites are stimulated in response to certain environmental factors such as heat, light, water, or predation to aid survival.

While primary metabolites can be produced across broad groupings, secondary metabolites can be limited to a specific species or a number of species which are linked and typically thought to give that species an evolutionary advantage, such as predator defense, resistance against disease, or reproductive advantage (Pengally 2004).

Table 6.4 presents the range of compounds typically found in the family Scrophularaceae and genus *Verbascum* plus the other families they have also been isolated from.

Table 6.4 Compounds typically found in different plant families

Compound	Families
Iridoid glycosides and non-glycosides	Wide variety of plants (and families) including Rubiaceae, Lamiaceae, Scrophulariaceae, Pedaliaceae, and Gentianaceae
Flavonoid	Universal within the plant kingdom
Phenylethanoid/phenylpropenoid glycosides	Scrophulariaceae (*Verbascum* spp., *Rhemannia glutinosa, Digitalis purpurea*), Plantaginaceae (*Plantago asiatica* and *P. lanceolate*), Asteraceae (*Echinacea pallida, E. angustifolia*), Lamiaceae (*Stachys* spp., *Teucrium* spp., *Ocimum sanctum*), and Verbenaceae (*Verbena* spp., *Lantana camara*)
Saponins	Widely distributed in approx. 500 genera of plants, mainly Liliiaceae, Dioscoreaceae, Solanaceae, Sapindaceae, and Agavaceae
Spermine alkaloids	Mainly found in Angiospermae. Approx, 9% of species (within genera) contain alkaloids but the occurrence is uneven both in terms of species number and plant organ
Polysaccharides	As a group they are universally found throughout the plant kingdom

Source: Pengally (2004); Negi et al. (2013).

Overall, the research appears to have focused principally on *V. thapsus* and *V phlomoides, V. nigrum, Verbascum lychnitis, V. thapsiforme, Verbascum undulatum,* and *Verbascum georgicum* with a larger number of compounds from these species isolated, particularly the iridoid glycosides (Tatli and Akdemir 2004; Kahraman et al. 2012; Alipieva et al. 2014).

Iridoid glycosides, flavonoids, phenylethanoid glycosides, triterpene saponins, spermine alkaloids, polysaccharides, and phenolic acids have been identified within the genus *Verbascum* across a range of parts including whole plant, aerial parts, inflorescence/flowers, leaves, seeds, roots, and capsules (Tatli and Akdemir 2004; Alipieva et al. 2014). It is not always possible to be exact as to the precise plant organs used, as the papers mainly refer to the general part as for example aerial or flowers (Alipieva et al. 2014). You will recall that the European Pharmacopeia notes that mullein flowers comprise the dried flowers, reduced to the corolla and the androecium (EMA 2008, 2018).

The iridoid glycosides are by far the most widely distributed of the compounds characterized, having been identified in 58 species/subspecies, while phenylethanoid glycosides were identified in 23 species/subspecies, flavonoids in 25, and saponins in 18. The remaining constituents have been identified in fewer species, in particular the spermine alkaloids which have only been isolated from a limited number of species, mainly the leaves of *Verbascum pseudonobile,* but also the leaves of *V. nigrum* and *Verbascum phoeniceum*. It is interesting to note that to date no saponins have been found in *V. densiflorum* although six were isolated from *V. thapsiforme*, previously used as a synonym for *V. densiflorum* in the scientific literature. Saponins, iridoid glycosides, and flavonoids have been found in *Verbascum bottae* but the specific compounds were not discussed (Mothana et al. 2008).

It should be noted that the same compounds have been isolated and characterized from different parts of the plant; for example, the flavonoid, kaempferol, has been isolated both from the flower and underground parts of *V. phlomoides*, while quercetin was found in the fruit and aboveground parts of *V. nigrum* and the aboveground, flower, and seed of *Verbascum oreophilum*. This is also seen with iridoid compounds where aucubin was isolated from the flower and root of *Verbascum lasianthum,* the leaves and inflorescence of *Verbascum saccatum* and *Verbascum sinuatum,* plus the root and whole plant of *V. thapsus* (Bianco et al. 1980; Falsone et al. 1982; Mnatsakanyan et al. 1983; Khuroo et al. 1988; Pardo et al. 1998; Akdemir et al. 2004b,c; Danchul et al. 2006; Tatli et al. 2006; Kupeli et al. 2007; Alipieva et al. 2014).

Across the range of known constituents, a number of compounds have been suggested as possible chemotaxonomic markers both for the genus (ajugol, picroside IV, and verbascoside) and/or family ((+)-genipin, α-gardiol, β-gardiol, buddlindeterpene A, buddlindeterpene B, and buddlindeterpene C) (Hussain et al. 2009). (+)-genipin, α-gardiol, β-gardiol, buddlindeterpene A, buddlindeterpene B, and buddlindeterpene C were isolated in the genus *Verbascum* and genus *Buddleja,* both of which are found within the Scrophulariaceae family. While to date no single constituent has been located in every species, ajugol has been isolated and characterized across 41 species while picroside IV was found in 2 and verbascoside in 21. Other constituents have also been isolated and characterized, e.g. catalpol across 30 species and aucubin across 42 species. Aucubin and catalpol have been isolated from a range of *Plantago* spp. (Jurisić et al. 2004) and *Veronica* spp. (Crişan et al. 2010) which was formerly included in the Scrophularaceae family before being reclassified.

Regarding activity, the saponins and polysaccharides are thought to be responsible for expectorant, demulcent, and emollient properties, while the phenolic compounds, flavonoids, and phenylethanoids are connected with anti-inflammatory, antimicrobial, and diuretic activity (Turker and Camper 2002; Tatli et al. 2004a; Armatu et al. 2011). Tatli and Akdemir (2006) found that two saponins, Ilwensisaponin A and C, isolated from the flowers of *Verbascum pterocalycinum* var. *mutense* showed antimicrobial activity against *Aspergillus fumigatus* ATCC 90906, although no activity was found against other gram-positive and gram-negative bacteria and yeasts from this study.

6.5.1 Iridoid Glycosides

In total, 144 iridoid glycosides and non-glycosidic iridoids have been isolated from nearly all 66 species/subspecies/varieties from whole plant/aerial, epigeal, flower, leaf, capsule, and root. The exceptions are the species *Verbascum ancyritanum, Verbascum austriacum, Verbascum eremobium, Verbascum fruticulosum, V. pseudonobile, Verbascum scardicolum, Verbascum schimperianum,* and subspecies *Thapsus* subsp. *thapsus* (Tatli and Akdemir 2004; Alipieva et al. 2014).

Figures for percentage content of iridoid glycosides, in the flower, have been given as 0.56% in *V. phlomoides* and 0.13% in *V. densiflorum*. The flower of *V. densiflorum* is reported to show a different concentration range with tenfold less aucubin but twofold more catalpol than the flower of *V. phlomoides* (EMA 2008, 2018).

Using the mean peak area of the characteristic signals to measure the relative quantity of constituents in the leaf of various *Verbascum* plants, the quantity of harpagide was shown to significantly vary between plants, exhibiting highest amounts in *V. phoeniceum*, followed by *V. nigrum* and *V. xanthophoeniceum*. The amount of harpagide was significantly lower in *V. phoeniceum* (7 and 33) and *V. densiflorum*. Ajugol levels were also higher in *V. xanthophoeniceum, V. nigrum,* and *V. phoeniceum*, while aucubin was present in *V. xanthophoeniceum* and *V. nigrum*, at levels several times higher compared to the other *Verbascum* species (Georgiev et al. 2011a). Harpagoside was found in similar amounts (5.8–6.4 mg/g dry weight) in both *V. xanthophoeniceum* and *V. nigrum* using an HPLC–DAD assay (Georgiev et al. 2011a).

Iridoids (structure illustrated in Figure 6.4) comprise a group of cyclopentano[c]pyran monoterpenoids, which occur naturally in most of the species of *Verbascum* studied. Structurally, they typically comprise a bicyclic H-5/H-9 β, β-*cis*-fused cyclopentanopyran ring system with a double bond between C-3 and C-4 including non-substitution at C-4 (Tatli and Akdemir 2004).

The C9-type iridoids are strongly represented in all the species investigated to date, including aucubin (41 species), catalpol (29 species), ajugol (40 species), ajugoside (24 species), harpagide (32 species), and harpagoside (36 species). C10-type iridoids have also been isolated including geniposidic acid, lychnitoside, genipin, and α-gardiol. In general, *Verbascum* spp. contain aucubin and catalpol type iridoids and acetylated derivatives modified with aliphatic and aromatic acids (acetic acid, trans-cinnanic acid, trans-*p*-coumeric acid, and ferulic acid). Glycosides also indicate the esterification position (Tatli and Akdemir 2004; Kahraman et al. 2012; Alipieva et al. 2014).

There has been more of a focus on *V. phlomoides*, *V. thapsus,* and *V. thapsiforme* in terms of the research undertaken on these constituents than there has been with other species to date: 49 compounds, both glycosidic and non-glycosidic iridoids, have been

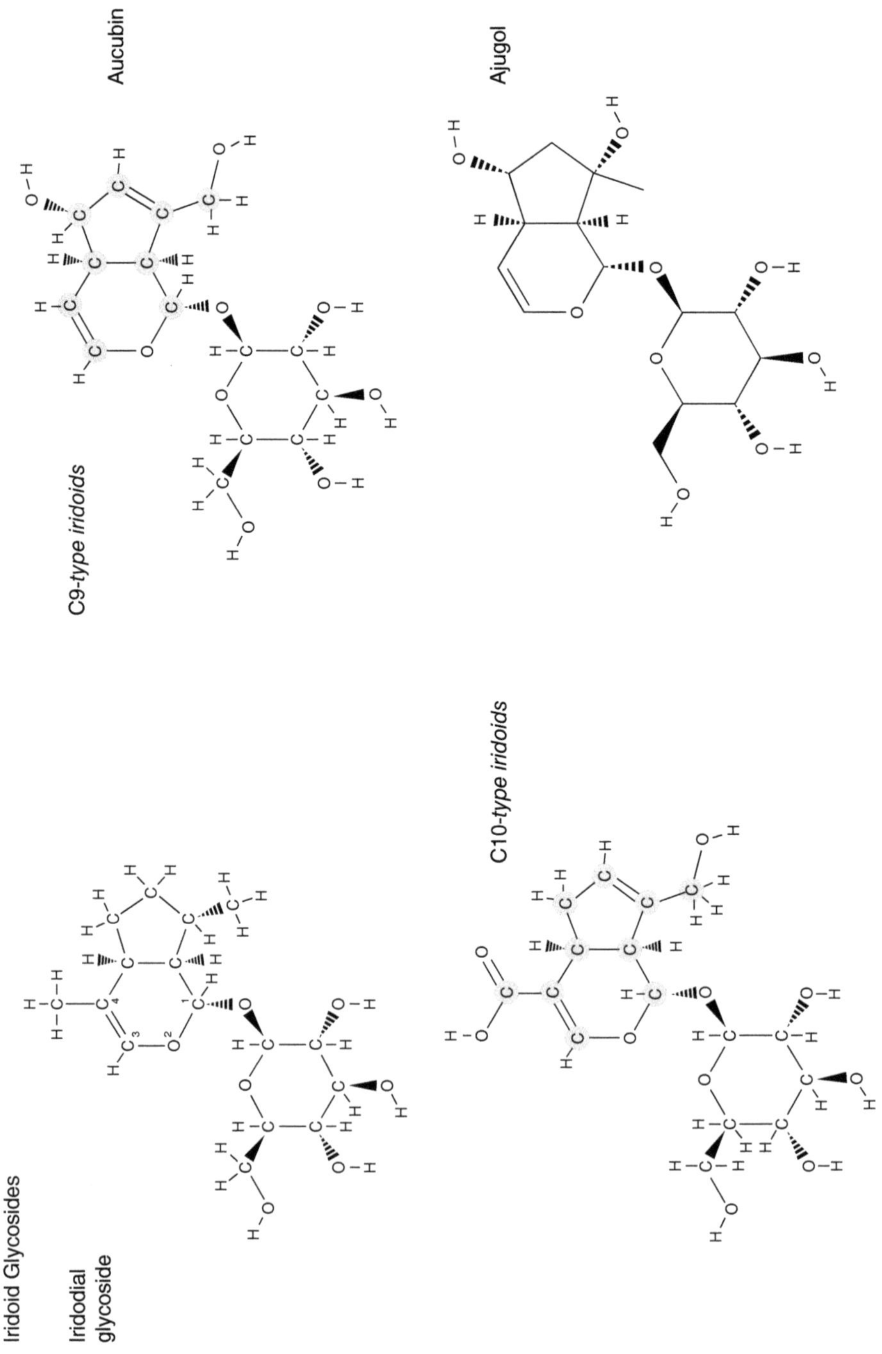

Figure 6.4 Structure of selected constituents of *Verbascum* spp.

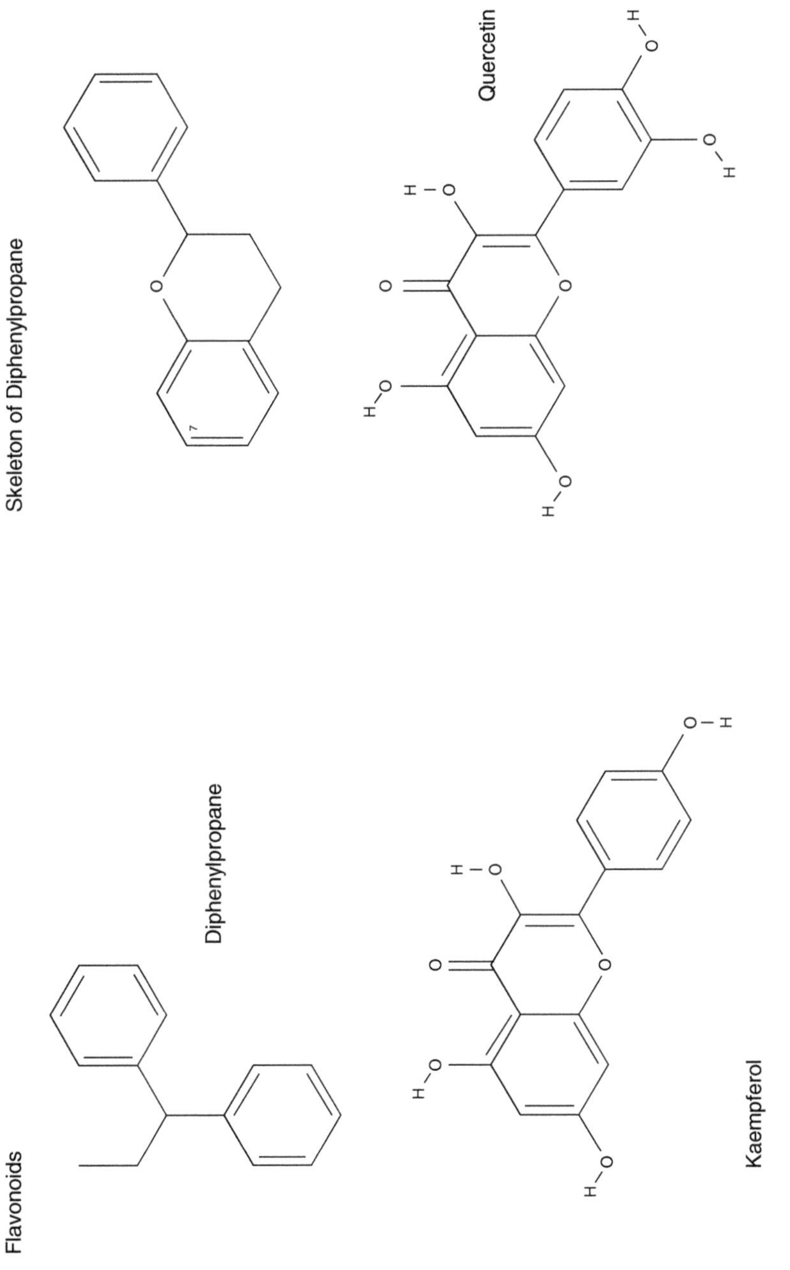

Figure 6.4 *(Continued)*

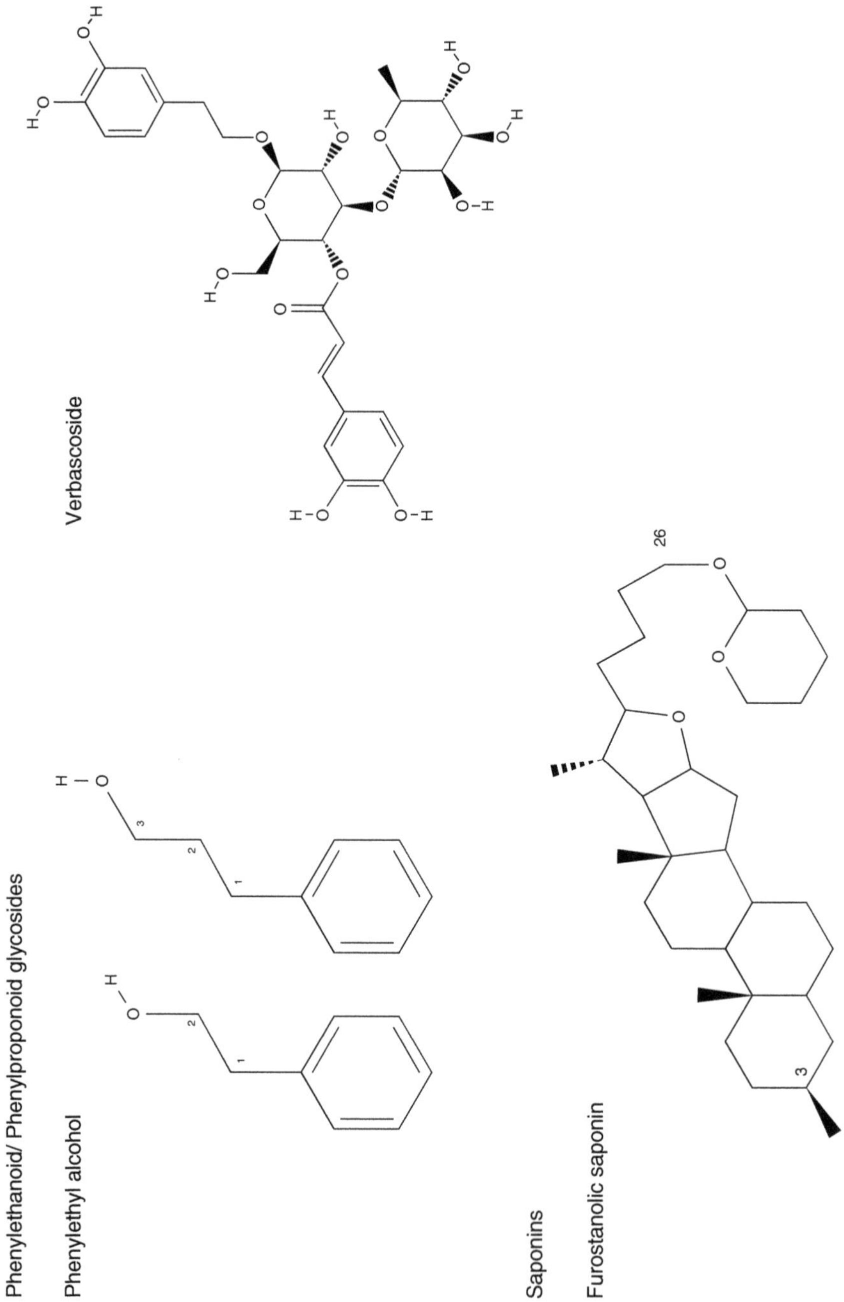

Figure 6.4 *(Continued)*

Triterpenic saponin aglycone

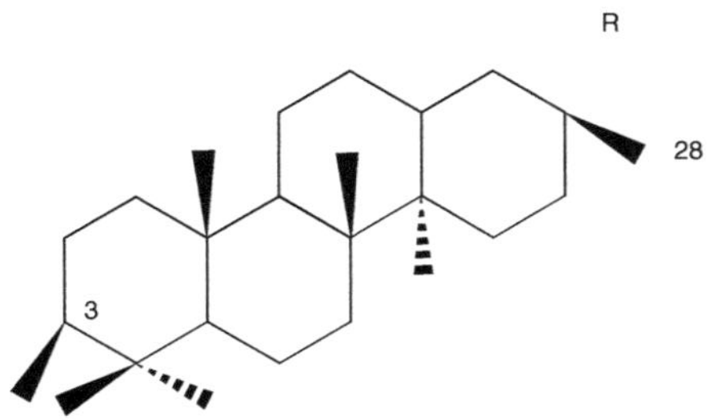

Buddlejasaponin Ia

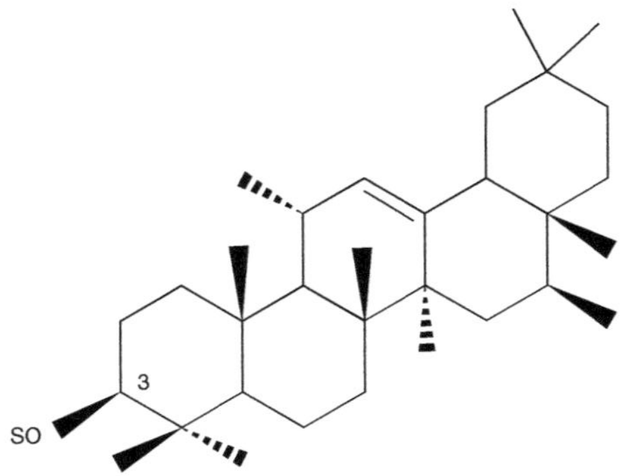

Figure 6.4 *(Continued)*

characterized from *V. thapsus*, 15 compounds from *V. phlomoides*, and 10 constituents from *V. thapsiforme* (Tatli and Akdemir 2004; Kahraman et al. 2012; Alipieva et al. 2014). Alipieva et al. (2014) commented in an extensive review of the constituents and species that constituents such as catalpol, aucubin, ajugol, harpagide, and derivatives isolated from *V. phlomoides* and *V. thapsiforme* were only characterized by means of TLC analysis, current practice employs UV, IR plus 1D, and 2D NMR spectoral analysis (Georgiev et al. 2011a,b).

Akdemir et al. (2004a) have argued that the wide range of iridoids and iridoid glycosides should be useful in terms of taxonomic evaluation of the *Verbascum* genus, noting that 6-O-β-D-glucopyranosylaucubin, 6-O-α-L- rhamnopyranosylcatalpol, verbaspinoside [6-O-(2″-O-trans-cinnamoyl)-α-L-rhamnopyranosylcatalpol], pulverulentoside I [6-O-(2″-O-trans-p-methoxycinnamoyl- 3″-O-acetyl)-α-L- rhamnopyranosylcatalpol] and buddlejoside A8 [6-O-(4″-O-trans - 3,4-dimethoxycinnamoyl) α-L-rhamnopyranosylcatalpol] were isolated across a range of species and parts. The authors noted that although rhamnopyranosyl catalpol esters and similar compounds were the predominant iridoids isolated from *V. salviifolium, Verbascum cilicicum,* and *V.l asianthum* (Tatli et al. 2003; Akdemir et al. 2004b,c) they are not unique to the Scrophularaceae family and thus have limited use as marker compounds (Helfrich and Rimpler 1999; Akdemir et al. 2005).

6.5.2 Flavonoids

Flavonoids are another group within the polyphenols and they comprise a wide range of compounds which can exist in a free form or as glycosides, including flavones, flavonals, anthocyanidins, procyanidins, calchones, and dihydroflavones, and flavans (Pengally 2004; Alipieva et al. 2014). Their chemical structure (illustrated in Figure 6.4) is based around two benzene rings (C15) connected by a three-carbon chain, which is generally closed, forming a heterocyclic C ring. Flavonoids are formed by both the shikimic acid and acetate pathways via condensation of a phenylpropanoid precursor with three malonli coenzyme A units (Pengally 2004). Flavonoids are found in a wide variety of plants, the most common, kaempferol and quercetin, being isolated from approx. 70% of plant species. Furthermore, as part of the analysis of *Verbascum* spp., flavone and flavonol as aglycones (including, apigenin, luteolin, quercetin, and kaempferol) have been characterized (Tatli and Akdemir 2004; Kahraman et al. 2012; Alipieva et al. 2014). Danchul et al. (2007) had reported the isolation of hesperidin in the stems of *Verbascum gnaphalodes*, aboveground parts and fruits of *V. nigrum*, aboveground parts and stems of *V. phlomoides,* and aboveground parts of *V. phoeniceum*. The reported presence of hesperidin has not been confirmed in subsequent investigations and it has been mooted that it was an artifact of the isolation and characterization process (EMA 2008, 2018).

Glycosylation is typically at C-7. A C-glucoside was isolated from *V. cheriathifolium* and isoflavones and flavonolignans from *V. sinaiticum* (EMA 2008, 2018).

Flavonoids as a group are not as well represented within the genus *Verbascum,* having been isolated from only 25 of the 66 species and subspecies investigated to date: 16 compounds were characterized from *V. sinaiticum*, while 10 were found in *V. lychnitis,* 14 in *V. densiflorum,* 12 in *V. thapsus,* and 22 in *V. phlomoides*. Tatli and Akdemir (2004): Kahraman et al. (2012) and Alipieva et al. (2014) list the flavonoids (flavones, flavonols, and O-glycosides) identified across species and parts in the genus

Verbascum. The constituents have been isolated from all parts of the plant. However, Danchul et al. (2007) reported that flavonoid compounds were not found in some of the species studied, including *Verbascum flavidum, Verbascum formosum* Fisch., *Verbascum hajastanicum* Bordz., *Verbascum macrocarpum* Boiss., *Verbascum pyramidatum* Bieb., *Verbascum speciosum* Shrad., *Verbascum turkestanicum* Franch., *Verbascum varians* Freyn et Sint., and *Verbascum wilhelmsianum* C. Koch.

In an analysis of total flavonoid content of *V. thapsus*, Kogje et al. (2010) found that the leaf contains 0.024, stem 0.009, and root 0.018 (mg/g dry weight).

6.5.3 Phenylethanoid/Phenylproponoid Glycosides

Phenylethanoid glycosides are another group of phenolic compounds present in *Verbascum* spp. Phenylethanoid glycosides are typically distributed widely across a number of species and families as noted in Table 6.4. As a group, phenlyethanoids are not as diverse in this genus as in other studied genera of the family, with verbascoside being reported as being the most widely distributed compound in this group and isolated from 23 species (Pengally 2004; Tatli and Akdemir 2004; Kahraman et al. 2012; Alipieva et al. 2014).

Naturally water soluble, phenylethanoid glycosides are characterized by a hydroxylphenylethyl moiety linked to a β-pyranose (apiose, galactose, rhamnose or xylose) via a glycosidic bond (Pengally 2004). The majority of phenolic compounds isolated were phenylethanoid glycosides (C6-C2) and a few phenylpropanoid glycosides (C6-C3) (structure illustrated in Figure 6.4). Most are triglycosides with the third glycosidic moiety attached to C6 of the core glucose. Figures for verbascoside content in the leaves of *V. nigrum, V. xanthophoeniceum,* and *V. phoeniceum* were found to vary greatly between 0.18% and 3.03% of the dry weight. Verbascoside was reported as being highest in *V. nigrum* (30.31 mg/g dry weight), followed by *V. xanthophoeniceum* (15.79 mg/g dry weight) and *V. phoeniceum* 7 (13.28 mg/g dry weight). Forsythoside B was highest in *V. xanthophoeniceum* (24.18 mg/g dry weight), followed by *V. nigrum* and *V. phoeniceum* (10.75 and 9.56 mg/g dry weight, respectively), while its content in *V. phoeniceum* 7 and 33, and *V. densiflorum* was below 0.3% of the dry weight. Similarly, leucosceptoside B was accumulated in higher amounts in *V. xanthophoeniceum* and *V. nigrum* (15.58–16.93 mg/g dry weight) (Georgiev et al. 2011a). The distribution of phenylethanoids across species and parts is outlined in Tatli and Akdemir 2004; Kahraman et al. 2012; Alipieva et al. 2014.

Verbascoside is the most widely distributed of the phenylethanoid glycosides and has been isolated from 21 of the 23 investigated species. Figures of 0.6% have been found in *V. densiflorum* flower, but only traces in *V. phlomoides* flower (Bradley 2006). In structure it comprises a caffeic acid and 2-(3, 4-dihydroxyphenyl) ethyl moiety (hydroxytyrosol) bound to β-(D)-glucopyranoside through ester and glycosidic links. It also has a rhamnose sugar molecule in sequence (1 → 3) to the glucose molecule. Its antioxidant activity comes from the two catechol groups and, because of its affinity for negatively charged membrane phospholipids, it tends to localize in the phospholipid bilayer of erythrocytes where it can affect its antioxidant properties. Low density lipoproteins (LDL) are similarly protected. Verbascoside has been shown to have anti-inflammatory activity (against periodontitis, the inflammation of the gums and supporting structures of the teeth) (reported in D' Imperio et al. 2014).

A proper understanding of the stability of the various compounds outlined above is still in its infancy, although verbascoside (phenylethanoid present in different plants) has been reported to be unstable at different pH conditions in a study that mimicked the pH changes that occur in the stomach (pH 3) and intestine (pH 7) (D' Imperio et al. 2014). Verbascoside was found to be stable at pH 3 with 100% recovery after 24 hours. However, Verbascoside was unstable at pH 7, with more than 62% of the original compound being transformed into isoverbascoside and other active products. The antioxidant effects of isoverbascoside (when compared to those of verbascoside) were found to have reduced.

Coniferin and syringin are two examples of phenylpropanoid glycosides isolated from a methanol extract of the fresh plant of *Verbascum letourneuxii* (Emam 2010).

6.5.4 Saponins

Saponins have an amphiphilic nature with non-polar aglycones bound to one or more sugar (polar) moieties. This combination of polar and non-polar structural elements in their molecules explains their soap/detergent-like behavior in aqueous solutions (Sparg et al. 2004; Negi et al. 2013).

Consisting of polycyclic aglycones with one or more sugars, saponins can be divided into two main groups, steroidal saponins (C27 spirostane skeleton) and triterpene saponins (C30 skeleton), depending on the number and position of the attached sugar units (illustrated in Figure 6.4). The number and length of the sugar chains can be linear or branched and can vary from 1 to 11 although 1 or 2 to 5 is most frequent. Saponins are widely distributed across the plant kingdom and tend to be present in plants in low concentrations (Vincken et al. 2007). Steroidal saponins are mainly found in monocotyledonous angiosperms (including species from the following families: Agavaceae, Alliaceae, Araliaceae, Asparagaceae, Asteraceae, Balanitaceae, Dioscoreaceae, Dracaenaceae, Leguminosae, Liliaceae, Phytolaccaceae, Solanaceae, Taccaceae, Zygophyllaceae), while triterpene saponins are found almost exclusively in dicotyledonous angiosperms (including species from the following families: Amaranthacea, Apiaceae (Umbelliferae), Aquifoliaceae, Araliaceae, Asclepiadaceae, Asteraceae, Berberidaceae, Buddlejaceae, Cactaceae, Campanulaceae, Caprifoliaceae, Caryophyllaceae, Chenopodiaceae, Combretaceae, Cucurbitaceae, Diapensiaceae, Dipsacaceae, Eupteleaceae, Hippocastanaceae, Lamiaceae, Lardizabalaceae, Lecythidaceae, Leguminosae, Lythraceae, Menispermaceae, Molluginaceae, Myrsinaceae, Passifloraceae, Phytolaccaceae, Pittosporaceae, Polygalaceae, Primulaceae, Ranunculaceae, Rhamnaceae, Rosaceae, Rubiaceae, Sapindaceae, Sapotaceae, Scrophulariaceae, Styracaceae, Ternstroemiaceae, Tiliaceae, Verbenaceae, Zygophyllaceae) (Sparg et al. 2004).

Most of the species examined have been found to contain either steroidal saponins or triterpene saponins; however, the Solanaceae (dicotyledonous) family are one exception in containing steroidal saponins in all the species examined. Other exceptions have included *Aspilia montevidensis* (Asteraceae), *Balanites aegyptiaca* (Balanitaceae), *Trigonella foenum-graecum* (Leguminosae), and *Tribulus terrestris* (Zygophyllaceae), which also contained steroidal saponins. However, saponin content has also been found to vary by plant part (Cheok et al. 2014).

All saponins (structure illustrated in Figure 6.4) have at least one sugar attached to the aglycon, typically at C3 (Monodesmosidic saponins). In bidesmosidic saponins (two sugars), the sugars are typically attached at C3 (ether linkage) and C28 (ester linkage) as in the case of triterpene saponins, and at C3 and C26 (ether linkage) as in the case of furostanol saponins. Tridesmosidic saponins with three sugars are rare and can form D and L isomers (e.g. D-glucose, D-galactose, D-glucoronic acid, D-galatronic acid, L-rhamnose, L-arabinose, and D-xylose) with interglycosidic linkages (α and β). Monosaccharides can take a pyranose or furanose form (Augustin et al. 2011). A furostene skeletal form can occur typically, in fresh plant material (where the hydroxyl group is in the 26-position and has a glycosidic linkage), the aglycone structure remains pentacyclic and open.

Steroidal saponins can be subdivided into two further groups, namely, furostanol and spiroatanol, in addition to triterpenes.

Verbascum spp. has been found to comprise 34 triterpene saponins across 18 species, the most abundant species being *V. sinaiticum* and *V. lychnitis* L, having 8 compounds isolated from each (Tatli and Akdemir 2004; Kahraman et al. 2012; Alipieva et al. 2014). The triterpene saponins located are mainly oleanane-type although ursane-type saponins (rosamutin and nigaichigoside) have been isolated, for example from *Verbascum wiedemannianum* (Abou Gazar et al. 2003b). Tatli and Akdemir (2004) have reported on the isolation of Verbascosaponin (Saponin I), (including the aglycone verbascogenin, $C_{30}H_{50}O_4$). Under acidic conditions verbascosaponin can transform into the triterpene A, $C_{30}H_{48}O_3$, converting from one to two double bonds (the difference being in the aglycone structure) (Schöderh and Haslinger 1993). Doubt has been raised that triterpene A is an artifact of this process rather than a true constituent. Additionally, De Pascual et al. (1980, 1982) noted that thapsuine B may also be an artifact due only to the extraction process.

Finally, although there is no uniformity across the saponins isolated from the various species (of *Verbascum*), the first two ursane-type saponins have been isolated from *V. wiedemannianum* (Abou Gazar et al. 2003b) which may have chemotaxonomic importance. There also appears to be some relationship between the genera *Verbascum* and *Scrophularia* in terms of chemical constituents (Klimek et al. 1992).

6.5.5 Spermine Alkaloids

The distribution of spermine alkaloids is much more restricted than the previous compounds described to date, having only been isolated from *V. nigrum, V. phoeniceum* L., *V. pseudonobile,* and *Verbascum songaricum* (Tatli and Akdemir 2004; Kahraman et al. 2012; Alipieva et al. 2014).

Drandarov and Hais (1997) reported the presence of verbacine and verballocine in the same plant material, noting that they act as precursers to the synthesis of verbascenine and verballoscenine. Verballoscenine (13-acetyl-1-(Z)-cinnamoyl-6-oxo-8-phenyl-1,5,9,13- tetraazacycloheptadecane) is a Z isomer of verbascenine (13-acetyl-10(Z)-cinnamoyl-6-oxo-8-phenyl-1,5,9,13-tetraazacycloheptadecane) (Drandarov and Hais 1997).

6.5.6 Polysaccharides

These are found mainly in the form of free monosaccharides, oligosaccharides, and polysaccharides and isolated mainly from the roots. A water-soluble acidic polysaccharide (2–3%), mainly a highly branched arabinogalactan with a β-1,6- linked galactan backbone, has been identified, plus a pair of neutral polysaccharides (arabinogalacatan and xyloglucan) from commercial mullein flower of *V. phlomoides* and *V. densiflorum* (EMA 2008, 2018).

6.5.7 Other Constituents

Interest in the fatty acid content of *V. songaricum* stemmed from its traditional use and the fact that unsaturated fatty acids have known anti-inflammatory properties (antagonistic effects against arachidonic acid, thromboxanes, and leukotrienes). The result (from a hexane extraction of the plant) showed that there were high levels of unsaturated fatty acids (principally oleic acid at 30.63%), which could have a beneficial pharmacological effect (Makhatova et al. 2015).

The seed oils (*V. thapsus*) have previously been found to contain high levels of total polyunsaturated fatty acids (PUFA), mainly linoleic acid (18:2n-6) (reported in Riaz et al. 2013). In another study, the seeds of *V. thapsus* has been found to contain 29–33% of oil comprising 11 fatty acids with up to 88–90% linoleic and oleic acid. De Pascual et al. (1978) isolated (benzene extract) a range of fatty acids including palmitic, stearic, oleic, linoleic, linolenic, arachidic, and β-sitosterol from the seed oil of *V. thapsus*. Esters of stearic acid, palmitic acid, oleic acid, and linoleic acid were obtained from a petroleum ether extract again of *V. thapsus* (reported in Riaz et al. 2013).

Neolignans consist of two phenylpropane monomers linked by a carbon-carbon or carbon-oxygen bond. Tatli and Akdemir (2004); Kahraman et al. (2012), Alipieva et al. (2014) list the compounds isolated and characterized from *V. thapsus, V. letourneuxii,* and *V. salviifolium*.

Phenolic acids, including acids of vanillin, *p*-hydroxybenzine, *p*-coumarin, ferulin, protocatechuin, and *p*-hydroxycinnanin have been identified from the flowers of *V. phlomoides* and *V. densiflorum* (Bradley 2006). *P*-coumaric acid glucoside has been isolated from the flower of *V. phlomoides* (Bradley 2006).

6.6 Discussion

A recognition of complexity is central to understanding botanical research. This complexity must be kept to the forefront in research design, in the development of regulatory guidelines, and in the design of manufacturing processes and quality control procedures. Analysis of botanicals needs to be approached from a multiperspective viewpoint rather than a purely linear one. Too often there is a search for the one regulation or the one validated method, but because botanicals are all different and have their own unique issues, one size does not fit all.

It is easy to see the complexity of botanicals in terms of their physical and chemical properties, which can vary due to a number of variables, including: (i) external factors (weather conditions during growth and/or harvesting, application of pesticides, drying processes); (ii) internal factors age of the plant, the part of the plant used (described in botanical rather than general terms); (iii) solvent extraction proposals (polarity effects leading to reduced complexity and selective enrichment of certain constituents and depletion of others); and (iv) the manufacture or research methods applied (approach to research, validation of methods, and processes).

For example, the age of the plants can affect the spatial distribution of compounds and thus the proportion and type of constituents extracted both qualitatively and quantitatively (Govindaraghavana and Sucher 2015). The polyphenol content in plants has been shown to vary (independent of the part of the plant) depending on the drying process, increasing, for example, with air drying and decreasing with oven drying. Various reasons have been proposed to explain this variability in polyphenols, including the stress response to the plant drying out and the effect of elevated oven temperatures on the polyphenols (Pferschy-Wenzig and Bauer 2015).

Authentication and identification of plants are the main starting points in any analytical and/or quality system for botanicals. This generally includes a consideration of: the (i) taxonomic features of the plant together with the macro and microscopic morphology; (ii) physio-chemical profile (physical encompassing ash content and swelling index) and chemical (encompassing constituent markers or fingerprint characteristics of the plant); and (iii) molecular markers. The need for appropriate taxonomic schemes which facilitate differentiation of species is imperative. Indeed, Govindaraghavana and Sucher (2015) mention that there is a real need to maintain the skill base in taxonomy and plant identification. The diverse morphology exhibited by the genus *Verbascum* is an illustrative example of the inherent difficulties with the taxonomic process and any further analyses thereof (Muazaz et al. 2014).

A review of the chemical constituents isolated and characterized from *Verbascum* is detailed in references Tatli and Akdemir 2004, Kahraman et al. 2012, and Alipieva et al. 2014, showing that the main groups are iridoid glycosides, flavonoids, phenylethanoid glycosides, and triterpene saponins. Of all the species investigated, *V. lychnitis, V. nigrum, V. phlomoides, V. thapsiforme, V. thapsus,* and *V. wiedemannianum* offer the greatest potential for scientific investigation as they have been shown to include all four groups. Nevertheless, if the speciation cannot be guaranteed then the chemical analysis is not built on a firm foundation. For example, observed qualitative and quantitative differences in the constituent profile of *Verbascum* spp. which has been discussed in detail in this chapter would cease to be of such significance if the speciation could not be confirmed. If there is any doubt over the species (of *Verbascum* under investigation) then the relevance of the constituent profile is in doubt. Indeed, because of the inherent variability of botanicals, when analyzing the concentration of compounds, i.e. quantitative evaluation, it is recommended to collect at least three years of data from controlled conditions. A one-off measurement is not considered sufficiently reliable (Karaveliogullari and Aytaç 2008).

Although several compounds have been proposed, there are still no definitive marker compounds for the genus *Verbascum*. No single compound has been isolated in every species, although that may be a feature of the current stage of analysis rather than a reflection of the chemistry of the plants. Nevertheless, at this stage, the science is incomplete and to date, ajugol, picroside IV, and verbascoside have been proposed as marker compounds for the genus *Verbascum* and/or (+)-genipin, α-gardiol, β-gardiol, buddlindeterpene A, buddlindeterpene B and buddlindeterpene C for the family Scrophulariaceae (Hussain et al. 2009). Ajugol and aucubin having been isolated from 41 and 42 species respectively would appear contenders, although they have also been isolated from other genera such as *Plantago* spp. (Jurisić et al. 2004) and *Veronica* spp. (Crişan et al. 2010) both of which were formerly included in the Scrophularaceae family.

Similarly, given the large number of constituents isolated and characterized across the 66 currently studied species of *Verbascum*, the lack of an indisputable marker compound impedes the discovery of new *Verbascum* species.

The specific solvent used in the extraction will determine the constituent profile of the extract (Sander et al. 2006; Sasidharan et al. 2011). For example, polar solvent will extract more polar compounds such as flavonoids, and lipophilic solvents will extract more non-polar compounds such as the essential oils and waxes. The avoidance of artifacts during the extraction process is an important consideration. The flavonoid hesperidin (*V. phlomoides*) and the saponins hydroxythapsuine B and thapsuine B isolated from *V. thapsus* were reported as artifacts. The EMA (2008) report noted that hesperidin (from *V. phlomoides*) was not confirmed in later studies.

Research (and to an extent manufacture), while offering their own particular and overlapping considerations, nevertheless both tend to push the boundaries in terms of the methods and instrumentation employed (Li and Vederas 2009; Henrich and Beutler 2013; Bilia 2014; Atanasov et al. 2015). The use of metabolic profiling to identify appropriate fingerprints has opened up quality control measures by enhancing the ability to focus chemoprofiling of, for example, specific species of botanicals across a genus, thus supporting approaches to authentication, adulteration, and stability (Pferschy-Wenzig and Bauer 2015). The development of DNA barcoding strategies for identification and adulteration has similarly assisted the commercial use of botanicals (Nybom et al. 2014; Mishra et al. 2016). The research on *Verbascum* has focused on molecular profiling (Georgiev et al. 2011a), chemotaxonomy, and phylogenetics (Srivastava and Saggoo 2014; Muazaz et al. 2014). Nevertheless, that does not mean that traditional skills, for example in taxonomy and pharmacognosy (of plants), should be discarded (Upton et al. 2011; Govindaraghavana and Sucher 2015). Sometimes analytical methods are favored for practical reasons, such as TLC as it is a relatively inexpensive method, or HPTLC where there are more samples to compare (the newly isolated compound) against, compared to HPLC which has cost implications and has a smaller library of comparative commercial samples. While HPLC is more expensive, it offers much better and more stable chromatographic separation and HPLC can be hyphenated with a wide range of detectors (UV, UV diode array, fluorescence, and MS detectors) (Chopra et al. 2006; Tian et al. 2009; Govindaraghavana and Sucher 2015).

Validated methods are a critical requirement for research and are increasingly being developed for the various analytical approaches, (Tistaert et al. 2011) including HPLC (Chopra et al. 2006), capillary-zone electrophoresis (Nevado et al. 2012), NMR, and HPLC (Klimek et al. 2010) as examples.

Interestingly, the validated HPLC method (Klimek et al. 2010) was able to differentiate between flower samples of *V. phlomoides* (high levels of diosmin and tamarixetin 7-rutinoside) and *V. densiflorum* (verbascoside and luteolin 7-glucoside). More so because mullein flower is considered to comprise the corolla and andrecium of *Verbascum* (*thapsus, phlomoides*, and *densiflorum*) and no saponins have as yet been identified in *densiflorum* while six were found in *thapsiflorme*. The species *thapsiforme* was replaced with *densiflorum* in the EMA assessment report on the three *Verbascum* species (EMA 2008, 2018).

When considering a traditional approach, it should be based on the ethnomedical use of the plant, the features in terms of taxonomy, plant chemistry, phylogenetics, and/or pharmacology (Wiesner and Knöss 2014; Atanasov et al. 2015). But it is also important to appreciate the other components of traditional use, such as growing area, cultivation, harvesting, processing, and storage. One way to look at these factors is to view them as steps in a chemical process and, if the steps are changed or modified, the end result is likely to vary.

In a global market, the process of trading between countries can be seen to force the development of regulatory harmonization. While regulation had been shown to encourage innovation, regulation that is too prescriptive can have the opposite effect. Thus, regulation based on an incomplete understanding of botanicals could have unforeseen consequences (Pelkmans and Renda 2014).

In recent years there has been some movement toward an agreed approach at a regional and global level. Regional regulatory approaches in the EU, Asia, and South America have been developed (Kroes 2014; Knöss et al. 2014; Sharma 2015; Wagner et al. 2016). The EU regulations on herbal medicines have been repeatedly noted and referenced, in respect of a common legal framework with multilateral acceptance across countries. Since the 1980s, the International Conference of Drug Regulatory Authorities has been supporting various authorities including the WHO and national and regional regulatory bodies in terms of national and international regulation of medicines and vaccines, including herbal medicine. Nevertheless, the regulatory framework for local, and even regional, levels is still extensively shaped by cultural considerations. China, Japan, and Asia maintain a strong tradition of using herbs as medicines which feeds into their broader herbal and natural product industry. The monograph could play a role in reflecting local and regional practices while fulfilling a legal and scientific quality and safety role (Bouin and Wierer 2014; Wagner et al. 2016).

Despite all this complexity, the overall aim is quite straightforward, being to show quality, safety, and efficacy, all based on sound scientific principles. (Bilia 2014; Kroess 2014; Wiesner and Knöss 2014; Pferschy-Wenzig and Bauer 2015). This requires a quality control system to ensure that these targets are met. However, scientific principles, on their own, do not provide the overarching structure on which to build a coordinated approach to any production or process. Clinical research focuses on risk benefit and evidence-based medicine. For pharmaceuticals, the ICH guidelines together with national regulations provide a framework for evaluating quality, safety, and efficacy (Govindaraghavana and Sucher 2015). The main difficulty for botanicals is that because of their complexity, the regulation and guidelines are not always directly applicable (Bilia et al. 2001) Complicated products together with complicated processes are not always helpful in this regard (Pelkmans and Renda 2014).

6.7 Conclusion

Botanicals are complex and any analysis needs to take this into account. Authentication and identification of the botanical is the starting point in a quality process which should be based primarily on taxonomic and morphological data supported by chemical marker or fingerprinting data. However, metabolic and/or molecular and DNA barcoding may provide additional information. Analytical methods are developing and improving together with regulation and research, but botanical analysis is complex and difficult. Regulation can stimulate research, but inappropriate regulation can stifle innovation, so a balance will be needed in this regard.

Following from this review, there are five main issues as highlighted:

1. Botanicals are complex and thus research should be multiperspective in approach and involve a multidisciplinary team,
2. The analytical journey starts with authentication and identification of the botanical but should take account of the full supply chain,
3. Chemical, metabolic, and molecular analysis may be required depending on the botanical.
4. Analytical methods and technology are improving with increasing development of validated methods. Nevertheless, botanical analysis is complex and challenging.
5. Regulation can stimulate research, but it needs to be appropriate to the current stage of understanding and development of the industry.

Funding and Acknowledgments

AMK was supported by Cork Institute of Technology as part of her PhD programme. The author also acknowledges the funding of a High-Resolution Sector-Field Inductively Coupled Plasma Mass Spectrometer (HR-ICP-SFMS) under the Science Foundation Ireland (SFI) Research Infrastructure Call 2012 [Proposal #12/RI/2335 (2)].

References

Abou Gazar, H., Bedir, E., Khan, I.A., and Calis, I. (2003a). Wiedemanniosides A–E: new phenylethanoid glycosides from roots of *Verbascum wiedemannianum*. *Planta Medica* **69** (9): 814–819.

Abou Gazar, H., Tasdemir, D., Ireland, C.M., and Calis, I. (2003b). Iridoids and Triterpene Saponins from *Verbascum wiedemannianum* (Scrophulariaceae). *Biochemical Systematics and Ecology* **31**: 433–436.

Akdemir, Z.S., Tatli, I.I., Bedir, E., and Khan, I.A. (2003). Two new Iridoid Glucosides from *Verbascum salviifolium* Boiss. *Zeitschrift für Naturforschung* **60b**: 113–117.

Akdemir, Z.S., Tatli, I.I., Irege, E.B., and Khan, I.A. (2004a). Neolignan and phenylethanoid glycosides from *Verbascum salviifolium* Boiss. *Turkish Journal of Chemistry* **28**: 621–628.

Akdemir, Z.S., Tatli, I.I., Bedir, E., and Khan, I.A. (2004b). Aceylated Iridoid glycosides from *Verbascum lasianthum* Boiss. *Turkish Journal of Chemistry* **28**: 101–109.

Akdemir, Z.S., Tatli, I.I., Bedir, E., and Khan, I.A. (2004c). Iridoid and phenylethanoid glycosides from *Verbascum lasianthum*. *Turkish Journal of Chemistry* **28**: 227–234.

Akdemir, Z.S., Tatli, I.I., Bedir, E., and Khan, I.A. (2005). Two new iridoid glycosides from *Verbascum salvifolium* Boiss. *Zeitschrift für Naturforschung* **60b**: 113–117.

Akdemir, Z., Kahraman, C., Tatl*ı*, I.I. et al. (2011). Bioassay-guided isolation of anti-inflammatory, antinociceptive and wound healer glycosides from the flowers of *Verbascum mucronatum* Lam. *Journal of Ethnopharmacology* **136** (3): 436–443.

Alipieva, K., Orhan, I.E., Tatli, I.I., and Georgiev, M.I. (2014). Treasure from garden: chemical profiling, pharmacology and biotechnology of mulleins. *Phytochemistry Reviews* **13**: 417–444.

Alpert, A.J. (1990). Hydrophilic-interaction chromatography for the separation of peptides, nucleic acids and other polar compounds. *Journal of Chromatography A* **499**: 177–196.

Armatu, A., Bodirlau, R., Nechita, C.B. et al. (2011). Characterization of biological active compounds from *Verbascum phlomoides* by chromatography techniques. I. Gas chromatography. *Romanian Biotechnological Letters* **16** (4): 6297–6304.

Arrif, S., Benkhaled, M., Long, C. et al. (2006). Glycosilated iridoids and a triterpene saponin from *Verbascum balii* (Batt.) M. Quaiser. *Biochemical Systematics and Ecology* **34** (3): 259–262.

Atanasov, A.G., Waltenberger, B., Pferschy-Wenzig, E.-M. et al. (2015). Discovery and resupply of pharmacologically active plant-derived natural products: a review. *Biotechnology Advances* **33**: 1582–1614.

Augustin, J.M., Kuzina, V., Andersen, S.B., and Bak, S. (2011). Molecular activities, biosynthesis and evolution of triterpenoid saponins. *Phytochemistry* **72**: 435–457.

Avula, B., Wanga, Y.H., Pawar, R.S. et al. (2008). A rapid method for chemical fingerprint analysis of *Hoodia* species, related genera, and dietary supplements using UPLC–UV–MS. *Journal of Pharmaceutical and Biomedical Analysis* **48**: 722–731.

Barbour, E.K., Al Sharif, M., Sagherian, V.K. et al. (2004). Screening of selected indigenous plants of Lebanon for antimicrobial activity. *Journal of Ethnopharmacology* **93** (1): 1–7.

Beer, A.-M. and Neff, A. (2013). Differentiated evaluation of extract-specific evidence on *Cimicifuga racemosa's* efficacy and safety for climacteric complaints. *Evidence-based Complementary and Alternative Medicine*. [Online], https://doi.org/10.1155/2013/860602.

Bennett, B.C. and Balick, M.J. (2014). Does the name really matter? The importance of botanical nomenclature and plant taxonomy in biomedical research. *Journal of Ethnopharmacology* **152**: 387–392.

Bianco, A., Guiso, M., Iavarone, C. et al. (1980). Iridoids. Part 28. 6-O-b-D-Xylopyranosylaucubin from *Verbascum sinuatum*. *Phytochemistry* **19** (4): 571–733.

Bilia, A.R. (2014). Science meets regulation. *Journal of Ethnopharmacology* **158**: 487–494.

Bilia, A.R., Bergonzi, M.C., Morgenni, F. et al. (2001). Evaluation of chemical stability of St. John's wort commercial extract and some preparations. *International Journal of Pharmaceutics* **213**: 199–208.

Bilia, A.R., Bergonzi, M.C., Mazzi, G., and Vincieri, F.F. (2002). Analysis and stability of the constituents of artichoke and St. John's wort tinctures by HPLC-DAD and HPLC-MS. *Drug Development and Industrial Pharmacy* **28** (5): 609–619.

Boğa, M., Ertaş, A., Yılmaz, M.A. et al. (2016). UHPLC-ESI-MS/MS and GC-MS analyses on phenolic, fatty acid and essential oil of *Verbascum pinetorum* with antioxidant, anticholinesterase, antimicrobial and DNA damage protection effects. *Iranian Journal of Pharmaceutical Research* **15** (3): 393–405.

Bouin, A.-S. and Wierer, M. (2014). Quality standards of the European Pharmacopoeia. *Journal of Ethnopharmacology* **158**: 454–457.

Bradley, P. (2006). Mullein. In: *British Herbal Compendium to the British Herbal Pharmacopoeia*, 296–299. Westbury on Trym: British Herbal Medicine.

British Herbal Pharmacopoeia (BHP) (1983). British Herbal Medicine Association. Bournemouth, United Kingdom.

British Herbal Pharmacopoeia (BHP) (1996). British Herbal Medicine Association. Bournemouth, United Kingdom.

Bucar, F., Wube, A., and Schmid, M. (2013). Natural product isolation – how to get from biological material to pure compounds. *Natural Product Reports* **30**: 525–545.

Burgess, R.R. (2018). A brief practical review of size exclusion chromatography: rules of thumb, limitations, and troubleshooting. *Protein Extression and Purification* **150**: 81–85.

Caixach, J., Flores, C., Spoof, L. et al. (2016). Liquid chromatography – mass spectrometry. In: *Handbook of Cyanobacterial Monitoring and Cyanotoxin Analysis* (eds. J. Meriluoto, J. Codd and L. Spoof), 218–257. Wiley.

CAMAG (2018). Instruments, tools and concepts for HPTLC – application notes [Online]. Available at: https://www.camag.com/en/tlc_hptlc/camag_laboratory/methods.cfm?kat=137 (accessed 1 March 2019).

Cheok, C.Y., Salman, H.A.K., and Sulaiman, R. (2014). Extraction and quantification of saponins: a review. *Food Research International* **59**: 16–40.

Choma, I.M. and Grzelak, E.M. (2011). Bioautography detection in thin-layer chromatography. *Journal of Chromatography A* **1218**: 2684–2691.

Chopra, S., Ahmad, F.J., Khar, R.K. et al. (2006). Validated high-performance thin-layer chromatography method for determination of Trigonelline in herbal extract and pharmaceutical dosage form. *Analytica Chimica Acta* **577** (1): 46–51.

Cieśla, L., Hajnos, M., and Waksmundzka-Hajnos, M. (2011). Application of hydrophilic interaction TLC systems for separation of highly polar glycosidic compounds from the flowers of selected *Verbascum* species. *Journal of Planar Chromatography* **24** (4): 295–300.

Crişan, G., Vlase, L., Balica, G. et al. (2010). LC/MS analysis of aucubin and catalpol of some *Veronica* species. *Forma* **58** (2): 237–242.

Cui, S., Fu, B., Sen-Chun Lee, F., and Wang, X. (2005). Application of microemulsion thin layer chromatography for the fingerprinting of licorice (*Glycyrrhiza* spp). *Journal of Chromatography B* **828**: 33–40.

D' Imperio, M., Cardinali, A., D'Antuono, I. et al. (2014). Stability–activity of verbascoside, a known antioxidant compound, at different pH conditions. *Food Research International* **66**: 373–378.

Danchul, T.Y., Khanin, V.A., and Shagova, L.I. (2006). Iridoids of the genus *Verbascum* (Scrophulariaceae). *Rastitel'Nye Resursy* **42**: 48–59.

Danchul, T.Y., Khanin, V.A., Shagova, L.I., and Shavarda, A.L. (2007). Flavonoids of some species of the genus *Verbascum* (Scrophulariaceae). *Rastitel'Nye Resursy* **43**: 92–100.

Dar, M.A., Bhat, M.F., Hassan, R. et al. (2018). Extensive phytochemistry, comprehensive traditional uses, and critical pharmacological profile of the great mullein: *Verbascum thapsus* L. *The Natural Products Journal* **8**: 1–14.

De Brabander, H.F., Noppea, H., Verheyden, K. et al. (2009). Residue analysis: future trends from a historical perspective residue analysis: future trends from a historical perspective. *Journal of Chromatography A* **1216**: 7964–7976.

De Pascual, T.J., Diaz, F., and Grande, M. (1978). Components of *Verbascum thapsus* L. I. Triterpenes. *Anales de Quimica* **74** (2): 311–314.

De Pascual, T.J., Diaz, F., and Grande, M. (1980). Components of *Verbascum thapsus* L. III. Contribution to the study of saponins. *Anales de Quimica – Serie C* **76** (2): 107–110.

De Pascual, T.J., Hernandez, J.M., Diaz, F., and Grande, M. (1982). Chemical compounds from *Verbascum lychnitis* L. *Lychnitoside. Anales de Química Serie C, Química orgánica y bioquímica* **78** (1): 108–111.

Dévier, M.-H., Mazellier, P., Ait-Aissa, S., and Budzinski, H. (2011). New challenges in environmental analytical chemistry: identification of toxic compounds in complex mixtures. *Comptes Rendus Chimie* **14** (7): 766–779.

Dhami, N. and Mishra, A.D. (2015). Phytochemical variation: how to resolve the quality controversies of herbal medicinal products? *Journal of Herbal Medicine* **5**: 118–127.

Drandarov, K. and Hais, I.M. (1997). Separation of E-Z isomeric macrocyclic spermine alkaloids of *Verbascum pseudonobile* and *Verbascum phoeniceum* and of their derivatives using thin-layer chromatography. *Journal of Chromatography* **724** (1–2): 416–423.

Dulger, B. (2006). Antimicrobial activity of some endemic Scrophulariaceae from Turkey. *Pharmaceutical Biology* **44** (9): 672–676.

Dulger, B. and Gonuz, A. (2004). Antimicrobial activity of some endemic *Verbascum, Salvia* and *Stachys* species. *Pharmaceutical Biology* **42** (4–5): 301–304.

Dulger, B. and Ugurlu, E. (2005). Evaluation of antimicrobial activity of some endemic *Scrophulariaceae* members from Turkey. *Pharmaceutical Biology* **43** (3): 275–279.
Dülger, B., Kırmızı, S., Arslan, H., and Güleryüz, G. (2002). Antimicrobial activity of three endemic *Verbascum* species. *Pharmaceutical Biology* **40** (8): 587–589.
Dulger, G., Tutenocakli, T., and Dulger, B. (2015). Antimicrobial potential of the leaves of common mullein (*Verbascum thapsus* L., Scrophulariaceae) on microorganisms isolated from urinary tract infections. *Journal of Medicinal Plants Studies* **3** (2): 86–89.
Early, R. (1995). *Total Quality Management in the Food Industry*, 1–30. Springer Science + Business Media.
EMA (2008). Assessment report on *Verbascum thapsus* L., *V. densiflorum* Bertol., *V. phlomoides* L., Flos with traditional use [Online]. Available at: https://www.ema.europa.eu/en/documents/herbal-report/superseded-assessment-report-verbascum-thapsus-l-v-densiflorum-bertol-v-phlomoides-l-flos_en.pdf (accessed 1 March 2019).
EMA (2018). Assessment report on *Verbascum thapsus* L., *V. densiflorum* Bertol. (*V. thapsiforme* Schrad) and *V. phlomoides* L., flos Final [Online]. Available at: https://www.ema.europa.eu/en/documents/herbal-report/final-assessment-report-verbascum-thapsus-l-v-densiflorum-bertol-v-thapsiforme-schrad-v-phlomoides-l_en.pdf (accessed 1 March 2019).
Emam, S.S. (2010). Glycosides of *Verbascum letourneuxii* Asch and its antioxidant activity. *Australian Journal of Basic and Applied Sciences* **4** (10): 5038–5050.
Falsone, G., Laryea, M.D., Crea, A.E.G., and Finner, E. (1982). Iridoids from *Verbascum sinuatum*. *Planta Medica* **44** (3): 150–153.
Furey, A. and Tassell, M. (2008). Towards a systematic scientific approach in the assessment of efficacy of an herbal preparation. Hawthorn (Crataegus spp.) invited editorial. *European Journal of Heart Failure* **10**: 1153–1157.
Furey, A., O'Doherty, S., O'Callaghan, K. et al. (2010). Azaspiracid poisoning (AZP) toxins in shellfish: toxicological and health considerations. Toxicon Special Issue -. *Toxins in Seafood* **56**: 173–190. (5-Year Impact Factor: 2.742).
Gabriëls, M. and Plaizier-Vercammen, J.A. (2003). Densitometric thin-layer chromatographic determination of artemisinin and its lipophilic derivatives, artemether and arteether. *Journal of Chromatographic Science* **41** (7): 359–366.
Gautam, A., Kashyap, S.J., Sharma, P.K. et al. (2010). Identification, evaluation and standardization of herbal drugs. Scholars Research Library. *Der Pharmacia Lettre* **2** (6): 302–315.
Georgiev, M.L., Ali, K., Alipieva, K. et al. (2011a). Metabolic differentiations and classification of *Verbascum* species by NMR-based metabolomics. *Phytochemistry* **72**: 2045–2051.
Georgiev, M., Alipieva, K., Orhan, K. et al. (2011b). Antioxidant and cholinesterases inhibitory activities of *Verbascum xanthophoeniceum* Griseb. and its phenylethanoid glycosides. *Food Chemistry* **128**: 100–105.
Govindaraghavana, S. and Sucher, N.J. (2015). Quality assessment of medicinal herbs and their extracts: criteria and prerequisites for consistent safety and efficacy of herbal medicines. *Epilepsy & Behavior* **52**: 363–371.
Grabias, B. and Swiatek, L. (1987). Iridoid glucosides in *Verbascum* genus. *Herba Polonica* **33** (4): 225–232.
Green, J. (2000). *Herbal Medicine Maker's Handbook*, pp. 79, 169, 177, 185. Crossing Press.
Grieve, M. (ed.) (1974). Mullein, Great. In: *A Modern Herbal*, 562. London: Jonathan Cape.
Grieve, M. (1981). Mullein, Great. In: *A Modern Herbal*, 562–566. New York: Dover Publications, Inc.

Gross, K.L. and Warner, P.A. (1978). The biology of Canadian weeds. 28. *Verbascum thapsus* L. and *V. blattaria* L. *Canadian Journal of Plant Science* **58**: 401–413.

Guo, X., Zhang, X., Feng, J. et al. (2013). Purification of saponins from leaves of *Panax notoginseng* using preparative two-dimensional reversed-phase liquid chromatography/hydrophilic interaction chromatography. *Analytical and Bioanalytical Chemistry* **405** (10): 3413–3421.

Halabalaki, M., Bertrand, S., Stefanou, A. et al. (2014). Sample preparation issues in NMR-based plant metabolomics: optimisation for Vitis wood samples. *Phytochemical Analysis* **25**: 350–356.

Heinrich, M. (2010). Ethnopharmacology in the 21st century – grand challenges. *Frontiers in Pharmacology* **1** (8): 1–3.

Helfrich, E. and Rimpler, H. (1999). Iridoid glycosides and phenolic glycosides from *Holmskioldia sanguinea*. *Phytochemistry* **50**: 619–627.

Henrich, C.J. and Beutler, J.A. (2013). Matching the power of high throughput screening to the chemical diversity of natural products. *Natural Product Reports* **30**: 1284–1298.

Hildreth, J., Hrabeta-Robinson, E., Applequist, W. et al. (2007). Standard operating procedure for the collection and preparation of voucher plant specimens for use in the nutraceutical industry. *Analytical and Bioanalytical Chemistry* **389**: 13–17.

Horváth, G., Acs, K., and Kocsis, B. (2013). TLC-direct bioautography for determination of antibacterial activity of *Artemisia adamsii* essential oil. *Journal of AOAC International* **96** (6): 1209–1213.

Hussain, H., Aziz, S., Miana, G.A. et al. (2009). Minor chemical constituents of *Verbascum thapsus*. *Biochemical Systematics and Ecology* **37** (2): 124–126.

James, K.J., Furey, A., Lehane, M. et al. (2002). First evidence of an extensive Northern European distribution of azaspiracid poisoning (AZP) toxins in shellfish. *Toxicon* **40** (7): 909–915.

James, J.K., Diaz Sierra, M., Lehane, M. et al. (2003). Detection of five new hydroxyl analogues of azaspiracids in shellfish using multiple tandem mass spectrometry. *Toxicon* **4**: 277–283.

Jurisić, R., Debeljak, Z., Vladimir-Knezević, S., and Vuković, J. (2004). Determination of aucubin and catalpol in *Plantago* species by Micellar electrokinetic chromatography. *Zeitschrift für Naturforschung C* **59**: 27–31.

Kagan, I.A. and Flythe, M.D. (2014). Thin-layer chromatographic (TLC) separations and bioassays of plant extracts to identify antimicrobial compounds. *Journal of Visualized Experiments*, [Online], Available: http://www.jove.com/video/51411 (accessed 27 March 2014).

Kahraman, C., Akdemir, Z.S., and Tatli, I.I. (2012). Promising cytotoxic activity profile, biological activities and phytochemical screening of *Verbascum* L. species. *Medicinal and Aromatic Plant Science and Biotechnology* (Special Issue 2): 63–75.

Kamil, M. (2013). Supply chain and management system based standardization of botanicals. *Planta Medica* **79**: P60.

Karaveliogullari, F.A. and Aytaç, Z. (2008). Revision of the genus *Verbascum* L. (Group A) in Turkey. *Botany Research Journal* **1** (1): 9–32.

Kesselring, H., Hamann, E., Stöcklin, J., and Armbruster, G.F. (2013). New microsatellite markers for *Anthyllis vulneraria* (Fabaceae), analyzed with spreadex gel electrophoresis. *Applications in Plant Sciences* **1** (12): 1–3.

Khan, A.M., Qureshi, R.A., Gillani, S.A., and Ullah, F. (2011). Antimicrobial activity of selected medicinal plants of Margalla Hills, Islamabad, Pakistan. *Journal of Medicinal Plants Research* **5** (18): 4665–4670.

Khuroo, M.A., Qureshi, M.A., Razdan, T.K., and Nichols, P. (1988). Sterones, iridoids and a sesquiterpene from *Verbascum Thapsus*. *Phytochemistry* **27** (11): 3541–3544.

Kim, H., Choi, Y.H., and Verpoorte, R. (2010). NMR-based metabolomic analysis of plants. *Nature Protocols* **5** (3): 536–549.

Kim, H., Choi, Y.H., and Verpoorte, R. (2011). NMR-based plant metabolomics: where do we stand, where do we go? *Trends in Biotechnology* **29** (6): 267–275.

Klimek, B., Lavaud, C., and Massiot, G. (1992). Saponins from *Verbascum nigrum*. *Phytochemistry* **31** (12): 4368–4370.

Klimek, B., Olszewska, M.A., and Tokar, M. (2010). Simultaneous determination of flavonoids and phenylethanoids in the flowers of *Verbascum densiflorum* and *V. phlomoides* by high-performance liquid chromatography. *Phytochemical Analysis* **21** (2): 150–156.

Knöss, W., Chinou, I., and Wiesner, J. (2014). Regulation of herbal and traditional medicinal products – European and global strategies (international symposium Trad Reg. 2013). *Journal of Ethnopharmacology* **158**: 447–518.

Kogje, K.K., Jagdale, V.K., Dudhe, S.S. et al. (2010). Antioxidant property and phenolic compounds of few important plants from trans-Himalayan regions of North India. *Journal of Herbal Medicine and Toxicology* **4**: 145–151.

Kroes, B.H. (2014). The legal framework governing the quality of (traditional) herbal medicinal products in the European Union. *Journal of Ethnopharmacology* **158**: 449–453.

Kumar, P.G., Kumar, R., Badere, R., and Singh, S.B. (2010). Antibacterial and antioxidant activities of ethanol extracts from trans Himalayan medicinal plants. *Pharmacognosy Journal* **2** (17): 66–69.

Kupeli, E., Tatli, I.I., Akdemir, Z.S., and Yesilada, E. (2007). Bioassay-guided isolation of anti-inflammatory and antinociceptive glycoterpenoids from the flowers of *Verbascum lasianthum* Boiss. ex Bentham. *Journal of Ethnopharmacology* **110**: 444–450.

Li, J.W.-H. and Vederas, J.C. (2009). Drug discovery and natural products: end of an era or an endless frontier? *Science* **325**: 161–165.

Makhatova, B.G., Datkhayev, U.M., Burda, N.Y., and Kyslychenko, V.S. (2015). Fatty acids from *Verbascum songaricum* herb. *Research Journal of Pharmaceutical, Biological and Chemical Sciences* **6** (6): 277–279.

Marchand, E., Atemnkeng, M.A., Vanermen, S., and Plaizier-Vercammen, J. (2007). Development and validation of a simple thin layer chromatographic method for the analysis of Artemisinin in *Artemisia annua* L. plant extracts. *Biomedical Chromatography* **22** (5): 454–459.

McCarthy, E. and O'Mahony, J.M. (2010). What's in a name? Can mullein weed beat TB where modern drugs are failing? *Evidence-based Complementary and Alternative Medicine* **2011**, 239237, 7. DOI:https://doi.org/10.1155/2011/239237.

McIntyre, E., Saliba, A.J., Wiener, K.K., and Sarris, J. (2016). Herbal medicine use behaviour in Australian adults who experience anxiety: a descriptive study. *BMC Complementary and Alternative Medicine* **16**: 60. https://doi.org/10.1186/s12906-016-1022-3
.

Mishra, P., Kumar, A., Nagiredd, A. et al. (2016). DNA barcoding: an efficient tool to overcome authentication challenges in the herbal market. *Plant Biotechnology Journal* **14**: 8–21.

Mnatsakanyan, V.A., Arutyunyan, L.S., and Eribekyan, M.I. (1983). Iridoid glycosides of *Verbascum saccatum*. *Khimiya Prirodnykh Soedinenii* (1): 38–41.

Mosihuzzaman, M. and Choudhary, M.I. (2008). Protocols on safety, efficacy, standardization, and documentation of herbal medicine (IUPAC technical report). *Pure and Applied Chemistry* **80** (10): 2195–2230.

Mothana, R.A., Abdo, S.A., Hasson, S. et al. (2008). Antimicrobial, antioxidant and cytotoxic activities and phytochemical screening of some Yemeni medicinal plants.

Evidence-based Complementary and Alternative Medicine, eCAM **7** (3): 323–330.
Muazaz, A.-H., Mohammed, M.J., Kanawapee, N. et al. (2014). Genetic diversity and relationships among *Verbascum* species in Iraq by RAPD-PCR technique. *Global Science Research Journals* **2** (2): 063–074.
Negi, J.S., Negi, P.S., Pant, G.J. et al. (2013). Naturally occurring saponins: chemistry and biology. *Journal of Poisonous and Medicinal Plant Research* **1** (1): 001–006.
Nevado, J.J., Robledo, V.R., and Callado, C.S. (2012). Monitoring the enrichment of virgin olive oil with natural antioxidants by using a new capillary electrophoresis method. *Food Chemistry* **133** (2): 497–504.
Newman, D.J. and Cragg, G.M. (2012). Natural products as sources of new drugs over the 30 years from 1981 to 2010. *Journal of Natural Products* **75**: 311–315.
Nguyen, D.T.T., Guillarme, D., Rudaz, S., and Veuthey, J.-L. (2006). Fast analysis in liquid chromatography using small particle size and high pressure. *Journal of Separation Science* **29**: 1836–1848.
NTP (National Toxicology Programme) (2016). *Report on Carcinogens*, 14e. Research Triangle Park, NC: U.S. Department of Health and Human Services, Public Health Service. [Online], Available: https://ntp.niehs.nih.gov/go/roc14 [01 Mar 2019].
Nybom, H., Weising, K., and Rotter, B. (2014). DNA fingerprinting in botany: past, present, future. *Investigative Genetics* **5** (1). [Online], Available: http://www.investigativegenetics.com/content/5/1/1 [01 Mar 2019].
Palaniappan, K. and Holley, R.A. (2010). Use of natural antimicrobials to increase antibiotic susceptibility of drug resistant bacteria. *International Journal of Food Microbiology* **140**: 164–168.
Palhares, R.M., Gonçalves Drummond, M., Dos Santos Alves Figueiredo Brasil, B. et al. (2015). Medicinal plants recommended by the world health organization: DNA barcode identification associated with chemical analyses guarantees their quality. *PLoS One* **10** (5): e0127866. https://doi.org/10.1371/journal.pone.0127866.
Pardo, F., Perich, F., Torres, R., and Delle Monache, F. (1998). Phytotoxic iridoid glucosides from the roots of *Verbascum thapsus*. *Journal of Chemical Ecology* **24** (4): 645–653.
Patel, K.N., Patel, J.K., Patel, M.P. et al. (2010). Introduction to hyphenated techniques and their applications in pharmacy. *Pharmaceutical Methods* **1** (1): 2–13.
Pelkmans, J. and Renda, A. (2014). Does EU Regulation Hinder or Stimulate Innovation? *CEPS Special Report*, No. 96 [Online]. Available at: https://www.ceps.eu/publications/does-eu-regulation-hinder-or-stimulate-innovation (accessed 1 March 2019).
Pengally, A. (2004). *Constituents of Medicinal Plants*, 2e, 46. Sydney: Allen and Unwin.
Perera, T., Berna, A., Scott, K. et al. (2008). Proteins related to St. John's Wort p27SJ, a suppressor of HIV-1 expression, are ubiquitous in plants. *Phytochemistry* **6** (4): 865–872.
Pérez, R.A., Tadeo, J.L., Albero, B. et al. (2013). Gas chromatography-triple-quadrupole mass spectrometry for analysis of selected polyhalogenated pollutants in plants. Comparison of extraction methods. *Analytical and Bioanalytical Chemistry* **405** (1): 389–400.
Pferschy-Wenzig, E.-M. and Bauer, R. (2015). The relevance of pharmacognosy in pharmacological research on herbal medicinal products. *Epilepsy & Behavior* **52**: 344–362.
Quinlan, F. (1883). A note upon the use of the mullein plant in the treatment of pulmonary consumption. *British Medical Journal* **1152**: 149.
Riaz, M., Zia-Ul-Haqb, M., and Jaafarc, H.Z.E. (2013). Common mullein, pharmacological and chemical aspects. *Revista Brasileira de Farmacognosia* **23**: 948–959.
Rivera, J.O., Loya, A.M., and Ceballos, R. (2013). Use of herbal medicines and implications for conventional drug therapy medical sciences. *Alternative & Integrative Medicine* **2**: 130. https://doi.org/10.4172/2327-5162.1000130.

Rose, F. (2006). *The Wild Flower Key: How to Identify Wild Plants, Trees and Shrubs in Britain and Ireland*. Puffin; Rev Ed edition.

Sander, L.C., Sharpless, K.E., and Wise, S.A. (2006). Dietary supplement standard reference materials. *Life Sciences* **78**: 2044–2048.

Sarris, J. (2018). Herbal medicines in the treatment of psychiatric disorders: 10-year updated review. *Phytotherapy Research* **32** (7): 1147–1162.

Sasidharan, S., Chen, Y., Saravanan, D. et al. (2011). Extraction, isolation and characterization of bioactive compounds from plants' extracts. *African Journal of Traditional, Complementary and Alternative Medicines* **8** (1): 1–10.

Schöderh, H. and Haslinger, E. (1993). The structure of verbascosaponin. *Liebigs Annalen der Chemie* **4**: 413–418.

Searo.who.int. (2019). Sixty-Seventh World Health Assembly, WHA 67.18, Agenda item 15.1 (24 May 2014).

Sharma, S. (2015). Current status of herbal product: regulatory overview. *Journal of Pharmacy and Bioallied Sciences* **7** (4): 293–296.

Sparg, S.G., Light, M.E., and van Staden, D. (2004). Biological activity & distribution of saponins. *Journal of Ethnopharmacology* **94** (2–3): 219–243.

Srivastava, D.K. and Saggoo, M.I.S. (2014). Molecular identification of *Verbascum thapsus* L. (Ban Tambaaku) and its ITS sequence comparison with other *Verbascum* L. species medicinal plants. *International Journal of Phytomedicines and Related Industries* https://doi.org/10.5958/j.0975-6892.6.1.0.

Sudberg, S., Sudberg, E.M., Terrazas, J. et al. (2010). Fingerprint analysis and the application of HPTLC to the determination of identity and quality of botanicals, from an industry perspective. *Journal of AOAC International* **93** (5): 1367–1375.

Sun, G. and Shi, C. (2008). The overall quality control of radix Scutellariae by capillary electrophoresis fingerprint. *Journal of Chromatographic Science* **46** (5): 454–460.

Świątek, L., Salama, O., and Sticher, O. (1982). 6-O-β-D-xylopyranosylcatalpol, a new iridoid glycoside from *Verbascum thapsiforme*. *Planta Medica* **45** (7): 153.

Tachjian, A., Maria, V., and Jahangir, A. (2010). Use of herbal products and potential interactions in patients with cardiovascular diseases. *Journal of the American College of Cardiology* **55** (6): 515–525.

Talib, W.H. and Mahasneh, A.M. (2010). Antimicrobial, cytotoxicity and phytochemical screening of Jordanian plants used in traditional medicine. *Molecules* **15**: 1811–1824.

Tassell, M.C., Kingston, R., Gilroy, D. et al. (2010). Hawthorn (Crataegus spp.) in the treatment of cardiovascular disease: a review. *Pharmacognosy Reviews* **4** (7): 32–41.

Tatli, I.I. and Akdemir, Z.S. (2004). Chemical constituents of *Verbascum* L. species. *FABAD Journal of Pharmaceutical Sciences* **29**: 93–107.

Tatli, I.I. and Akdemir, Z.S. (2006). Traditional uses and biological activities of *Verbascum* species. *FABAD Journal of Pharmaceutical Sciences* **31**: 85–96.

Tatli, I.I., Akdemir, Z.S., Bedir, E., and Khan, I.A. (2003). 6-O-α-L-Rhamnopyranosylcatalpol derivative iridoids from *Verbascum cilicicum*. *Turkish Journal of Chemistry* **27**: 765–772.

Tatli, I.I., Akdemir, Z.S., Bedir, E., and Khan, I.A. (2004a). Saponin, iridoid, phenylethanoid and monoterpene glycosides from *Verbascum pterocalycinum* var. *mutense* Hub.- Mor. *Turkish Journal of Chemistry* **28**: 111–122.

Tatli, I.I., Akdemir, Z.S., Bedir, E., and Khan, I.A. (2004b). Phenylethanoid glycosides from *Verbascum siniaticum*. *Turkish Journal of Chemistry* **28**: 111–115.

Tatli, I.I., Khan, I.A., and Akdemir, Z.S. (2006). Acylated iridoid glycosides from the flowers of *Verbascum lasianthum* Boiss. ex Bentham. *Zeitschrift für Naturforschung* **61b**: 1183–1187.

Tatli, I.I., Akdemir, Z.S., and Schuhly, W. (2007). Secondary metabolites from bioactive methanolic extract of *Verbascum pycnostachyum* Boiss. and Helder flowers. *Hacettepe University Journal of the Faculty of Pharmacy* **27**: 23–32.

Tian, R.-T., Xieb, P.-S., and Liua, H.-P. (2009). Evaluation of traditional Chinese herbal medicine: *Chaihu* (*Bupleuri* radix) by both high-performance liquid chromatographic and high-performance thin-layer chromatographic fingerprint and chemometric analysis. *Journal of Chromatography A* **216** (11): 2150–2155.

Tistaert, C., Dejaegher, B., and Vander Heyden, Y. (2011). Chromatographic separation techniques and data handling methods for herbal fingerprints: a review. *Analytica Chimica Acta* **690**: 148–161.

Turker, A.U. and Camper, N.D. (2002). Biological activity of common mullein, a medicinal plant. *Journal of Ethnopharmacology* **82**: 117–125.

Turker, A.U., Camper, N.D., and Gürel, E. (2004). High-performance liquid chromatographic determination of a saponin from *Verbascum thapsus* L. *Biotechnology & Biotechnological Equipment* **18** (1): 54–59.

Upton, R., Graff, A., Jolliffe, G. et al. (2011). *American Herbal Pharmacopoeia, Botanical Pharmacognosy microscopic Characterization of Botanical Medicines*. Boca Raton: CRC Press.

Verpoorte, R., Choi, Y.H., and Kim, H.K. (2007). NMR-based metabolomics at work in phytochemistry. *Phytochemistry Reviews* **6**: 3–14.

Vincken, J.-P., Heng, L., de Groot, A., and Gruppen, H. (2007). Saponins, classification and occurrence in the plant kingdom. *Phytochemistry* **68**: 275–297.

Wagner, H. and Bladt, S. (1996). *Plant Drug Analysis: A Thin Layer Chromatography Atlas*, 2e, 88. Berlin: Springer-Verlag.

Wagner, H. and Ulrich-Merzenich, G. (2009). Synergy research: approaching a new generation of phytopharmaceuticals. *Phytomedicine* **16**: 97–110.

Wagner, H. and Ulrich-Merzenich, G. (eds.) (2013). *Evidence and Rational Based Research on Chinese Drugs*. Springer.

Wagner, H., Bauer, R., and Melchart, D. (2016). New analytical monographs on TCM herbal drugs for quality proof. *Forschende Komplementärmedizin* **23** (Suppl 2): 16–20.

Wang, L.C., Cao, Y.H., Xing, X.P., and Ye, J.N. (2005). Fingerprint studies of *Radix Scutellariae* by capillary electrophoresis and high-performance liquid chromatography. *Chromatographia* **62** (5): 283–288.

Weller, M.G. (2012). A unifying review of bioassay-guided fractionation, effect-directed analysis and related techniques. *Sensors* **12**: 9181–9209.

Welz, A.N., Emberger-Klein, A., and Menrad, K. (2018). Why people use herbal medicine: insights from a focus-group study in Germany. *BMC Complementary and Alternative Medicine* **18** (1): 92. https://doi.org/10.1186/s12906-018-2160-6.

WHO (2003). *Guidelines on Good Agricultural and Collection Practices (GACP) for Medicinal Plants*. Geneva, Switzerland: WHO, [Online], Available: http://apps.who.int/medicinedocs/en/d/Js4928e [01 Mar 2019].

WHO (2005). National Policies on Traditional Medicine and Regulation of Herbal Medicines. Report of a WHO Global Survey [Online]. Available at: http://apps.who.int/medicinedocs/en/d/Js7916e (accessed 1 March 2019).

WHO (2011). Quality Control Methods for Herbal Materials [Online]. Available at: http://apps.who.int/medicinedocs/en/d/Jh1791e (accessed 1 March 2019)

WHO (2013). WHO Traditional Medicine Strategy: 2014–2023 [Online]. Available at: http://www.who.int/medicines/publications/traditional/trm_strategy14_23/en (accessed 1 March 2019).

Wiesner, J. and Knöss, W. (2014). Future visions for traditional and herbal medicinal products – a global practice for evaluation and regulation? *Journal of Ethnopharmacology*

158 (Pt B): 516–518.
Xia, J., Gao, J., Kokudo, N. et al. (2013). Methicillin-resistant *Staphylococcus aureus* antibiotic resistance and virulence. *Bioscience Trends* **7** (3): 113–121.
Yadav, P., Mahour, K., and Kumar, A. (2011). Standardization and evaluation of herbal drug formulations. *Journal of Advanced Laboratory Research in Biology* **2** (4): 161–166.
Yao, X., Zhou, G., Tang, Y. et al. (2015). HILIC-UPLC-MS/MS combined with hierarchical clustering analysis to rapidly analyze and evaluate nucleobases and nucleosides in *Ginkgo biloba* leaves. *Drug Testing and Analysis* **7** (2): 150–157.
Yin, S.-Y., Wei, W.-C., Jian, F.-Y., and Yang, N.-S. (2013). Therapeutic applications of herbal medicines for cancer patients. *Evidence-based Complementary and Alternative Medicine* 302426, 15 [Online], http://dx.doi.org/10.1155/2013/302426.
Zampini, I.C., Ordoñez, R.M., and Isla, M.I. (2010). Autography assay for the rapid detection of antioxidant capacity of liquid, semi-solid pharamceutical formulations using ABTS immobilized in a gel entrapment. *AAPS PharmSciTech* **11** (3): 1159–1163.
Zhao, Y.L., Wang, S.F., Li, Y. et al. (2011). Isolation of chemical constituents from the aerial parts of *Verbascum thapsus* and their antiangiogenic and antiproliferative activities. *Archives of Pharmacal Research* **34** (5): 703–707.
Zuo, Z., Fan, H., Wang, X. et al. (2012). Purification and characterization of a novel plant Lectin from *Pinellia ternata* with antineoplastic activity. *Springerplus* **1**: 13. https://doi.org/10.1186/2193-1801-1-13.

7
Purification and Isolation Techniques for Enrichment of Bioactive Phytochemicals from Herbs and Spices

Ramón Aznar and Dilip K. Rai
Food Bioscience, Teagasc Food Research Centre, Ashtown, Dublin D15KN3K, Ireland

7.1 Introduction

Herbs and spices are rich in bioactive phytochemicals, most notably antioxidant polyphenols (Aksel 2010). Polyphenols are secondary plant metabolites eliciting pharmacological or toxicological effects in human and animals (Aksel 2010), such as antimicrobial (Hemalatha et al. 2016), antiviral (Aboubakr et al. 2016), and anti-inflammatory (Thanekar et al. 2016), as well as possessing high antioxidant capacity (Jassbi et al. 2016). Studies on polyphenols are challenging because of the complexity of their chemical nature (simple phenols, phenolic acids, coumarins, flavonoids, and stilbenes), the numerous steps needed to achieve a good purification and isolation, and their extended occurrence in herbs and spices material.

To obtain the desired bioactive phytochemical(s), first they need to be extracted from the matrix as described previously in this book (see Chapters 4 & 5), using the appropriate choice of solvent(s) and techniques. Some of the extraction techniques can be used for purification purposes too. For instance, supercritical fluid extraction (SFE) can serve both as an extraction and purification method (Ivanovic et al. 2013). However, because of the fact that the extraction step is usually a non-selective procedure, several undesirable components are also co-extracted. These undesired components may interfere with the targeted chemicals and affect the biological characterization of bioactive phytochemicals. Therefore, the use of extra selective techniques is needed to achieve more precise and reliable results.

Herbs, Spices and Medicinal Plants: Processing, Health Benefits and Safety, First Edition.
Edited by Mohammad B. Hossain, Nigel P. Brunton, and Dilip K. Rai.

Most of the characterization studies related to bioactive compounds are carried out by non-chromatographic spectrophotometric methods (Politeo et al. 2010; Misharina et al. 2015; Jin et al. 2016) or chromatographic methods coupled with detectors such us ultraviolet (UV) or diode ray (Costa et al. 2015), where very often a fractionation of the extract may be mandatory to avoid false quantification or interferences with other compounds (Robards 2003). Moreover, due to the continuous discovery of novel compounds in plants, including herbs and spices, absolute characterization is necessary. When mass spectrometry is not enough to establish a definitive structure, due to structural complexity, isolation and purification of the novel compound is required to perform nuclear magnetic resonance (NMR) spectroscopy in order to establish the structural information. Besides structural identification, the purified compounds can be assessed for various biological activities, as many natural compounds are known to possess a wide range of properties that can be useful (Costa et al. 2015). For example, new compounds are replacing existing ones in the food industry due to the customer demand for natural and no toxic colorants and preservatives (Xie et al. 2015).

This chapter aims to provide a comprehensive review of different purification techniques used to clean-up and isolate bioactive phytochemicals in well-known and widely used herbs and spices as well as to evaluate the current state of the art and reflect future trends.

7.2 How to Approach Purification and Isolation

Traditionally, compounds have been purified and isolated mainly by knowing the matrix and then fractioning the extract several times before identifying the compounds without following any biological screen (Figure 7.1). This process is called pure-compound screening. However, better approaches have been followed recently. Bioassay-guided fractionation has been the state-of-the art method for identifying bioactive natural products (Figure 7.1). This approach involves preparative-scale fractioning and assessment of the biological activity desired up to the isolation and purification of the compounds that present higher activity (Brusotti et al. 2014).

Until now, bioactivity-guided fractionation has been successfully applied in only a few studies in regards to the matrices of interest for this book. For example, from mace and nutmeg, a novel compound 3′-methyl-5′-pentyl-furylarylic acid along with 16 known compounds were isolated using column chromatography (CC) (Kimura et al. 2010). Three compounds from nutmeg and turmeric were isolated using flash CC (Radwan et al. 2014). Antimicrobial compounds were isolated from thyme (*Thymus vulgaris*) essential oil using layer chromatography (Moricz et al. 2012). From celery (*Apium graveolens* L.), three phthalides, two furanocoumarins, and one phenylpropanoid were isolated using thin-layer chromatography (TLC) and CC guided fractionation (Sbai et al. 2017) and the isolation of the major polyphenol compounds in marjoram (*Origanum majorana* L.) was achieved using flash CC (Hossain et al. 2014).

Although this approach guides you through isolation of the fraction that has the higher biological activity, it still presents some drawbacks:

- it requires a huge amount of initial sample;
- it presents a risk of losing activity due to the wide range of preparative techniques involved in the process of isolation;
- it is expensive, due to solvents and material;
- and although it targets much better the desired compounds, it is still labor-intensive and time-consuming.

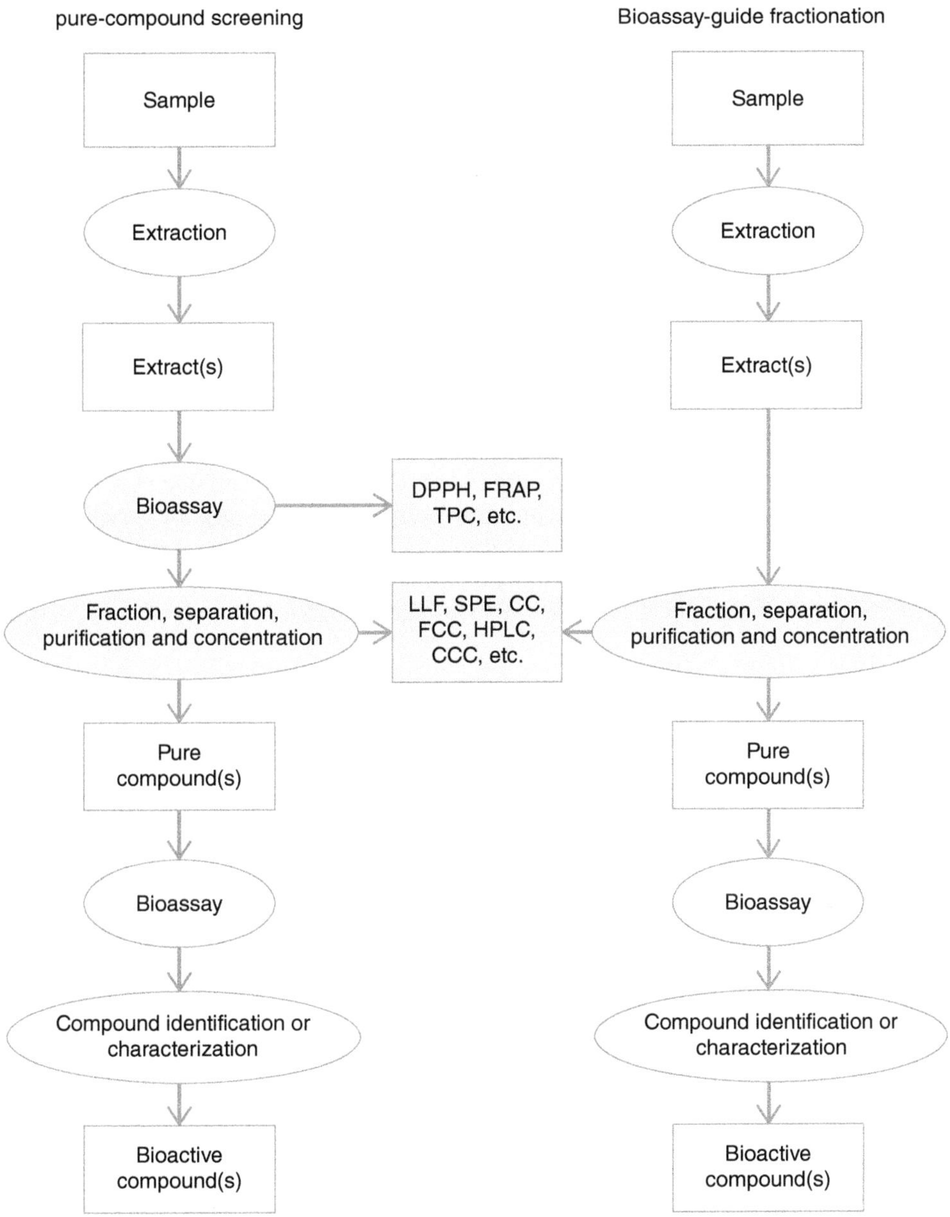

Figure 7.1 Diagram showing steps involved in pure-compound screening and bioassay-guided fractionation. *Source:* Adapted from (Li et al. 2016). LLP, liquid–liquid partitioning; SPE, solid-phase extraction; CC, column chromatography; FCC, flash column chromatography; HPLC, high-pressure liquid chromatography; CCC, counter-current chromatography.

Recently, the micro-fractionation bioactivity-integrated fingerprint has taken over as the best approach to purify and isolate bioactive compounds. It is mainly a miniaturization of the previously described approach of bioassay-guided fractionation, but uses fewer solvents and less starting material. It uses high-pressure liquid chromatography (HPLC) micro-fractionation to divide the crude extract, which is placed onto a microplate for direct biological screening. The microplate can be connected to a detector to recognize the compounds that produce the biological activity tested, making the identification of the compounds of interest easier and faster. So far this approach has been performed successfully in plants (Hou et al. 2012; Grosso et al. 2013), but no studies have been carried out yet on spices and herbs.

7.3 Purification Techniques

The selection of the most suitable purification or isolation technique is not an easy task. Sometimes, the automated techniques available are expensive and/or difficult to use, while the manual ones are time-consuming. Below we review some of the most commonly used techniques to accomplish purification of a wide range of bioactive compounds in herbs and spices, which can be used as a guide.

7.3.1 Liquid–Liquid Fractionation

Liquid–liquid fractionation (LLF) or liquid–liquid partitioning (LLP) is widely used to purify and isolate compounds since it is straightforward to perform. It is based on the distribution of the target analytes in two liquid phases (partition coefficient). These liquids with different partition coefficients can be separated into two different fractions. Decantation is used to separate liquids that are immiscible and form a well-defined layer. However, if they are miscible, a rotavapor can be used to separate solvents because they may present different boiling points. There are various factors involved during the process of LLP, where the affinity of the analytes to the solvent is the most important. Table 7.1 summarizes the most used solvents in the LLP technique to target the most well-known bioactive compounds in herbs and spices. Other critical decisions

Table 7.1 Bioactive compounds in order of polarity from more polar to less polar

Water	Methanol	Ethanol	Acetone	Dichloromethanol	Chloroform	Ether
Anthocyanins Tannins Saponins Terpenoids	Anthocyanin Terpenoids Saponins Tannins Flavones Polyphenols	Tannins Polyphenols Flavonol Terpeniods Alkaloids	Flavonoids	Terpenoids	Terpenoids Flavonoids	Alkaloids Terpenoids

Source: Adapted from (Cowan 1999; Reichardt and Welton 2010).

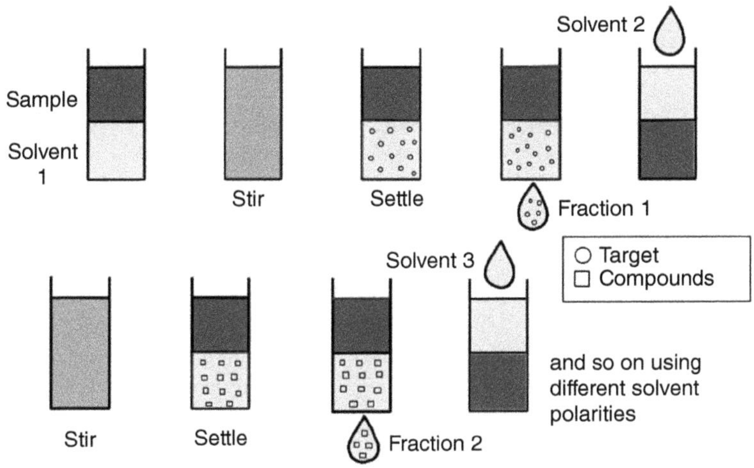

Figure 7.2 Liquid–liquid fractionation involving immiscible solvents are used to separate compounds in the extracted sample into different fractions.

to make are the volume of solvent(s) used and time. Sometimes an exhaustive fractionation is carried out, which involves large amounts of solvent and a long period of time. This process can be accelerated by shaking or be ultrasound assisted, among other techniques.

As can be seen in Figure 7.2, LLF or the partition technique can be used to collect different fractions, i.e. one for each solvent used. Normally LLP is used in a sequential way (Table 7.2) using more than two solvents with different polarities to achieve several fractions containing different groups of compounds as outlined in Table 7.1.

LLP is an easy and cheap technique to implement in any laboratory; no expensive material (mainly glassware) or experienced employees are required. For these reasons, it is widely used and quite often used before other purification techniques to separate compounds creating different fractions. In Table 7.2 some examples of LLP are described, such as the work of Ryu and co-authors that used LLP with butanol, hexane, and ethyl acetate in clove (*Syzygium aromaticum*) extract to create different fractions (Ryu et al. 2016a); or in bay leaves (*Laurus nobilis*), when LLP was used after methanolic extraction to isolate sesquiterpenes (Barla et al. 2007). However, LLP presents some drawbacks, the most important being that it is time-consuming and the high use of organic solvent(s) (some of them toxic) goes against the trend of using more eco-friendly methods.

7.3.2 Solid-Phase Extraction

Solid-phase extraction (SPE) is a powerful technique for universal, rapid, and selective sample preparation (extraction or purification). The versatility of SPE allows its use for a wide number of purposes during sample clean-up such as purification and enrichment of target analytes (Thurman and Mills 1998).

Purification takes place when an aqueous extract passes through a cartridge (sorbent), and the analytes are retained on the stationary phase. An elution with a solvent

Table 7.2 Applications of liquid–liquid partitioning in herbs and spices

Sample	Solvents	Compound	Reference
Clove (*S. aromaticum*)	Sequential purification BuOH, *n*-hexane, and EtAC. And then, CH_2Cl_2 (soluble and insoluble fractions)	Fluvanol glucoronides and flovoniods were isolated after extra purification	Ryu et al. (2016a)
Clove (*S. aromaticum*)	Sequential purification BuOH, *n*-hexane, water, and EtAC. And then, CH_2Cl_2 (soluble and insoluble fractions)	Acetophenone, chromone glycosides, phenylpropanoid, sesquiterpenoid and triterpenoid, sterol, and tannin were isolated after extra purification	Ryu et al. (2016b)
Bay (*Laurus nobilis*)	After methanol extraction, LLP was done with hexane and dichloromethane	A new sesquiterpene, lauroxepine, and six known sesquiterpene lactones	Barla et al. (2007)
Thyme (*T. vulgaris* L.)	After extraction with water, different fractions were collected using different concentrations of ethanol	Acidic polysaccharide	Chun et al. (2001)
Bay (*L. nobilis*)	After methanol extraction, LLP was done with hexane, ethyl acetate, and *n*-butanol	Six sesquiterpene lactones	Fang et al. (2005)
Mace (*Myristica fragrans*)	After methanol extraction, LLP was done with *n*-hexane, EtAC, n-BuOH, and water	A novel furan derivative and 16 known compounds	Kimura et al. (2010)

BuOH, Butanol; EtAC, ethyl acetate; CH_2Cl_2, dichloromethane.

that presents affinity to the biomolecules targeted is required to extract them from the cartridge. The schematic diagram in Figure 7.3 summarizes the four basic steps needed in SPE: (i) conditioning of the cartridge; (ii) loading of the sample; (iii) washing of the interferences; and (iv) finally elution and collection of the desired compounds.

SPE is becoming more popular due to the possibility of purifying and enriching the crude extract in one step. Moreover, there is a wide variety of cartridges and discs

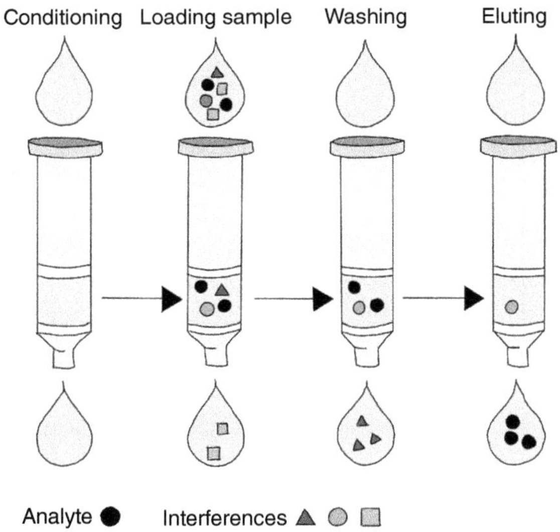

Figure 7.3 Solid-phase extraction workflow, starting with conditioning the column, loading the sample, washing interferences, and finally elution to isolate a compound.

with different sorbents (alumina, activated charcoal, Florisil, C18, C8, PSA, Chlorofiltr, among others) and sizes, which combined with different polarity solvents and pH variation makes SPE a really versatile technique. From nutmeg (*Maristica fragrans*), different SPE sorbents (silica amino, C8, C18) were used to purify several biocompounds (Radwan et al. 2014). Fecka and Turek used a C18 sorbent to purify 26 polyphenolic compounds from sage (*Salvia officinalis folium*) (Fecka and Turek 2007). SPE is a fast and cheap technique used to purify compounds that can even be automated or online with analytical techniques (Exarchou et al. 2003). Another advantage that SPE presents is the possibility of miniaturization thereby reducing the amount of sample and solvents used. Table 7.3 present examples of the use of the SPE technique to purify biocompounds.

7.3.2.1 Molecular Imprinted Polymers Molecular imprinted polymers (MIPs) are synthetic materials obtained by co-polymerizing a monomer with a cross-linker in the presence of a template molecule (Figure 7.4), which can be tailored to target and purify the desired compounds. This method is fast and more selective than SPE and it uses less solvent, which makes it an environmentally friendly technique. MIPs offer other advantages such as higher loading capacities of target analytes (than conventional sorbents C18, silica, etc.), higher efficiency for the retention of analytes, and improved selectivity during the retention process (Ashley et al. 2017), and can even be reused reducing costs.

MIPs are routinely used in the separation of environmental contaminants (Diaz-Alvarez et al. 2014). Recently, MIP has been used for the extraction of caffeic acid from fruits (Fan et al. 2016), glycosides from soybeans (Peng et al. 2016), a mixture of polyphenols from peanut meal (Schwarz et al. 2016), saponins from ginseng (*Panax notoginseng*) (Hou et al. 2015), and hypericin from herbal extract of *Hypericum perforatum* L. (Li et al. 2014). However, only few papers have been

Table 7.3 Solid-phase extraction for clean-up of a specific class of phytochemicals

Sample	SPE	Compound	Reference
Sage (*Salvia officinalis folium*)	SPE C18	26 polyphenolic compounds	Fecka and Turek (2007)
Oregano (*Origanum vulgare* subsp. *hirtum*)	Online SPE for peak storage. Hysphere GP cartridges	Flavonoids taxifolin, aromadendrin, eriodictyol, naringenin, and apigenin, the phenolic acid rosmarinic acid, and the monoterpene carvacrol were identified.	Exarchou et al. (2003)
Sage (*Salvia officinalis*)	Chromabond SB	Oleanolic acid and ursolic acid	Janicsak et al. (2003)
Nutmeg (*Maristica fragrams*)	Silica, Amino, C8, and C18 SPE	Erythro-(7R,8R)-Δ8′-4,7-dihydroxy-3,3′,5′-trimethoxy-8-0-4′-neolignan, erythro-(7R,8R)-Δ8′-7-acetoxy-3,4,3′,5′-tetra-methoxy-8-0-4′-neolignan, and 5-hydroxy-eugenol	Radwan et al. (2014)
Sage (*Salvia officinalis folium*)	Sepra C18-E	Low-molecular components containing oxygen atoms; ketones (α- and β-thujone, camphor, borneol), alcohols (linalool, isoborneol, terpinen-4-ol, α-terpienol, iso-3-thujanol), and cyclic ether (eucalyptol).	Dawidowicz and Dybowski (2010)
Thyme (*T. vulgaris* L.)	Polymeric RP-105 SPE	Phenolic acids (gallic, protocatechuic, *p*-hydroxybenzoic, chlorogenic, vanilic, caffeic, syringic, *p*-coumaric, ferulic, sinapic, benzoic, *m*-coumaric, *o*-coumaric, osmarinic, cinnamic acids) and 3,4-dihydroxybenzaldehyde, syringaldehyde, *p*-hydroxybenzaldehyde, and vanillin	Sterbova et al. (2004)
Mixed spice	Bond-Elut C18 SPE	Coumarin	Scotter et al. (2011)

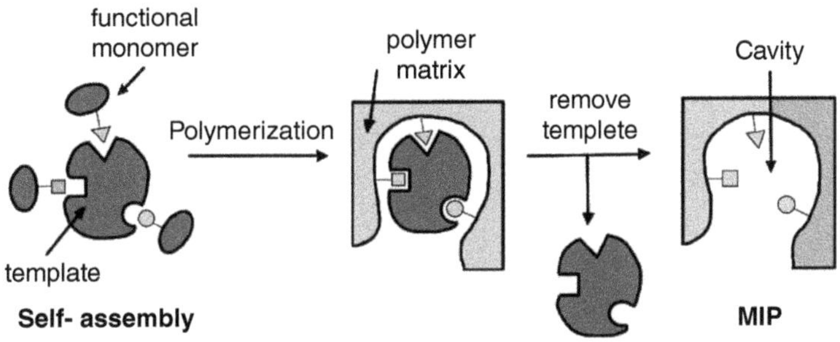

Figure 7.4 Diagram showing highly selective molecular imprinted polymer design. *Source:* Adapted from (Sarafraz-Yazdi and Razavi 2015).

published on their applications to herbs and spices, in particular in the isolation of curcumin and its derivatives (demethoxycurcumin and bisdemethoxycurcumin) from turmeric (*Curcuma longa* L.) (Kitabatake et al. 2013; Wulandari et al. 2015).

The lesser application of MIPs in the isolation of compounds could be because MIPs target low molecular weight compounds, while most of the compounds are relatively high molecular weight for this technique. Consequently, an improvement in the synthesis is needed to increase the applicability of MIPs. Moreover, although MIP technology appears to be a promising technique, it is notable that its main strength (selectivity) is also its main drawback. MIPs cannot be used yet to target multicompounds as different specific tailored MIPs will be needed for each compound or family of compounds.

7.3.3 Preparative Liquid Chromatography

Chromatography is the most common technique used to separate and purify compounds. In particular, liquid chromatography is based on a sample transported by a solvent (mobile phase) through a structure held by a matrix (stationary phase). The sample travels at different speeds through the stationary phase causing the separation of the compounds and eluting at different times (retention time) based on the polarity of the mobile phase. This separation is based on differential partitioning of the analytes between the mobile and stationary phases (affinity). Liquid chromatography techniques can be used with preparative or analytical purpose (coupled with a detector). A variety of preparative chromatographic techniques exist, and Figure 7.5 and Table 7.4 summarize the most frequently used.

This section will detail the most relevant uses of preparative chromatographic techniques to purify and isolate bioactive compounds from herbs and spices. In the literature, this is the most frequently used technique to date, which could be due to the wide range of sub-techniques and the advances developed over the last two decades mostly driven by environmental awareness to develop novel techniques that reduce the use of toxic solvents (Azmir et al. 2013).

7.3.3.1 Thin-Layer Chromatography TLC is a chromatographic technique where a liquid sample migrates by capillarity through a solid adsorbent medium (such as

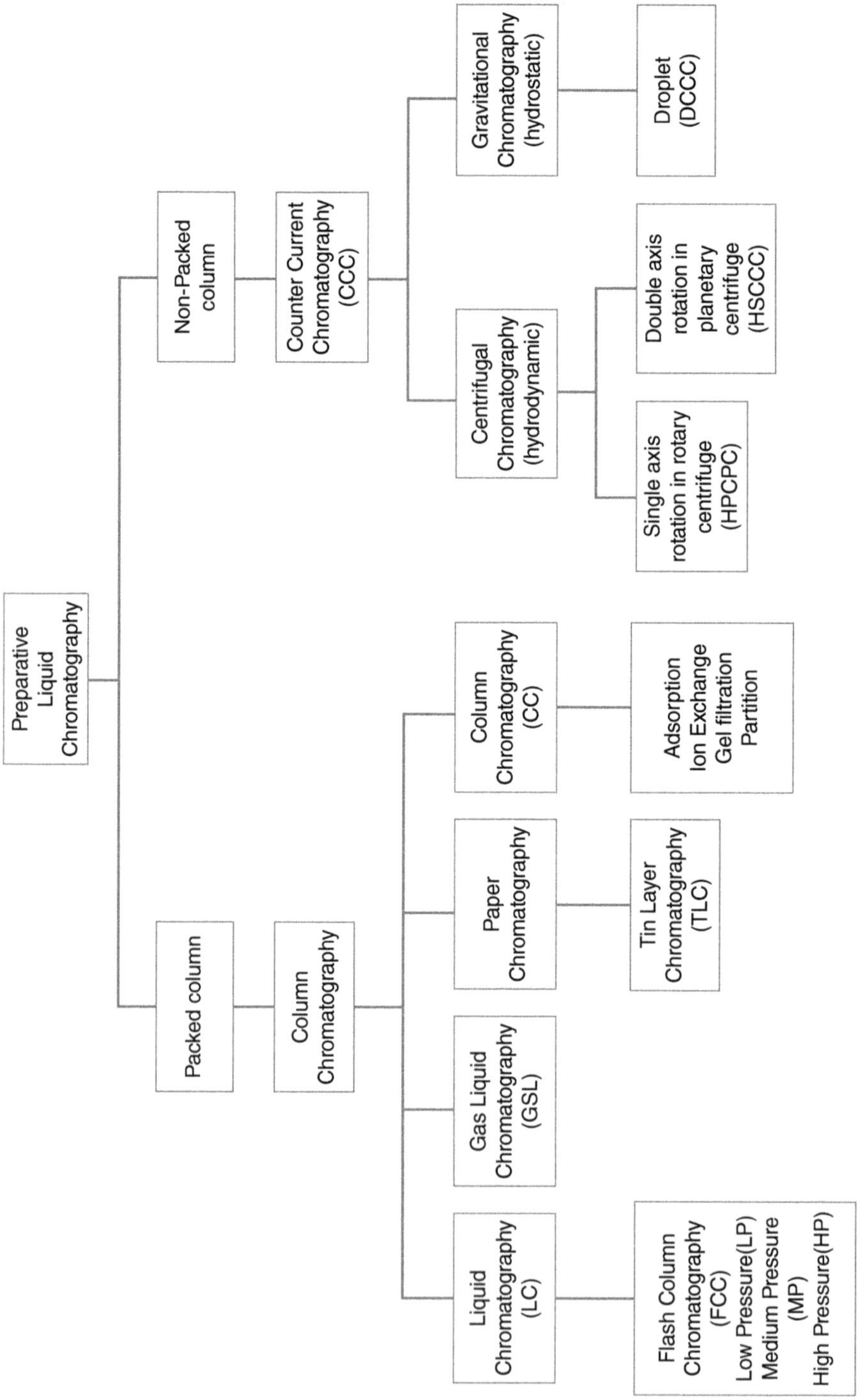

Figure 7.5 Diagram presenting the most common preparative liquid chromatographic techniques used for isolation and purification.

Table 7.4 Liquid chromatographic techniques for purification and isolation based on pressure

Technique	Pressure	Amount of sample	Type of sample
Flash Chromatography column (FCC)	1–2 bar	1–200 g	Crude, semipurified
Low Pressure (LP)	<5 bar	1–50 g	semipurified
Medium Pressure (MP)	5–20 bar	1–50 g	semipurified
High Pressure or high performance (HP)	>20 bar	0.5–1 g or less	semipurified

Source: Adaptation of (Claeson et al. 1993).

alumina or silica gel), which is arranged as a thin layer on a rigid support (such as a glass or plastic plate).

Nowadays, the main use of TLC is to optimize other chromatographic techniques such as column or flash CC, which involves multiple preliminary steps (solvent selection, column conditioning, retention volume, band volume, resolution, and corresponding analyte fraction numbers) (Fair and Kormos 2008). The use of TLC is easy, fast, and reduces costs during method development (Ignat et al. 2011). After optimization at a small scale, TLC can be used at a larger scale using other preparative chromatographic techniques (described below) that can hold a higher volume of sample. TLC has been successfully applied to cinnamon (*Cinnamomum zeylanicum*) and celery (*A. graveolens*) to target cinnamaldehyde and sedanolide, respectively (Babu et al. 2007; Momin and Nair 2001).

7.3.3.2 Column Chromatography (CC) CC is a labor-intensive and solvent-consuming technique, and it provides large volumes of fractions that need subsequent concentration for isolation and identification of pure substances. The typical sorbent materials used in this column as the stationary phase are silica gel, resins, RP-C18, Toyopearl, and LH-20 combined with solvents of different polarities to achieve a good separation.

CC is a technique widely used in research and industry laboratories, and the common stages taken during separation are shown in Figure 7.6. First, the correct column

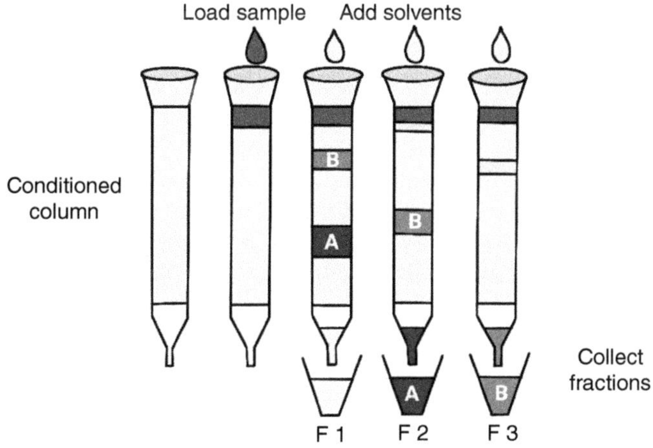

Figure 7.6 Description of sample purification by column chromatography using different solvents to collect several fractions.

size and sorbent have to be selected according to the amount of sample that needs to be loaded, as well as the physico-chemical characteristics of the target compounds. Second, the column has to be conditioned, and then the sample loaded. Solvent or solvents will be added to wash the sample and achieve separation through the column (the flow goes with the gravity). Different fractions can be collected F1 (solvent), F2 (compound A), and F3 (compound B) as exemplified in Figure 7.6

The same principle of CC shown in Figure 7.6 can be applied to other preparative column techniques, but with the assistance of pressure pumps to achieve a more effective separation of the compounds in a shorter time plus the use of fewer solvents and sorbents. The CC has been widely applied as Table 7.5 shows. For example, CC using a sephadex LH-20 column to purify rosmarinic acid was successfully applied to basil (*Ocimum basilicum*) matrix (Jayasinghe et al. 2003), and sephadex G75 to achieve pigments on cinnamon (*C. zeylanicum*) (Tan et al. 2011).

7.3.3.3 Flash Column Chromatography Flash column chromatography (FCC) has become a routine technique to purify organic chemicals in laboratories (Fair and Kormos 2008). It can be automatized and different fractions can be obtained by using different solvents; it is relatively fast and robust, easy to use, with a wide range of columns and different sizes to adapt to any purification process, and with a reasonable price considering the good results obtained. However, although it is an efficient technique, due to the excessive use of solvents it will be replaced by preparative liquid chromatography techniques which are more effective and environmentally friendly.

As shown in Table 7.4, the pressure working range is about 1–2 bar and the columns used are mainly silica gel with different mesh and C-18 column. FCC can be coupled to a detector, such as UV, to improve detection and fraction collection. Some examples of purification are displayed in Table 7.5, including its application on oregano (*Origanum vulgare*) by a silica gel column to achieve isolated glycosides (Milos et al. 2000) and sesquiterpenes from bay leaves (*L. nobilis*) (Julianti et al. 2012).

7.3.3.4 High-Pressure Liquid Chromatography HPLC is a separation technique that finds its application mostly as an analytical technique. HPLC involves the injection of a small volume of liquid sample into a packed column with tiny particles (stationary phase) where components of the sample are moved through the column with a liquid (mobile phase) forced through it by high pressure delivered by a pump. The compounds present in the sample are separated by various chemical and/or physical interactions between their molecules and the packing particles. Once the compounds are separated, they can be detected and/or collected in fractions.

The principles of all LC techniques work the same way as HPLC. But HPLC excels in speed, efficiency, and sensitivity. HPLC has been successfully applied on herbs and spices to purify gingerols in ginger (*Zingiber officinale*) (Wang et al. 2011) and lauropenes in bay (*L. nobilis*) (Chen et al. 2014) among other specific applications (see Table 7.5). Moreover, HPLC can be coupled to a wide range of detectors such as FIA, UV, RI, ELSD, MS, etc. However, HPLC equipment is expensive and requires more qualified personnel than most of the techniques previously described. The main drawback is the low applicability of this technique in a preparative scale due to the small amount of crude sample that one is able to load in comparison to the other techniques.

Table 7.5 Preparative chromatographic techniques used to purify and isolate compounds in herbs and spices

Sample	Technique	Separation	Compound	Reference
Clove (*S. aromaticum*)	FCC, CC, MPLC, and HPLC	Redi Sep-C18, Silica gel 230-400 mesh, Sephadex LH-20, LiChroprep RP-18 and reverse phase YMC Pack ODS-A column	Nineteen flavonoids, of which four were novel compounds	Ryu et al. (2016a)
Clove (*S. aromaticum)*	FCC and CC	Redi Sep-C18, Sephadex LH-20 and Reverse phase YMC gel, Silica gel 230-400 mesh, LiChroprep RP-18 column	A novel acetophenone along with 21 known compounds	Ryu et al. (2016b)
Oregano (*Origanum vulgare* subsp. *hirtum*)	HPLC	Hysphere GP	Flavonoids (taxifolin, aromadendrin, eriodictyol, naringenin, apigenin)	Exarchou et al. (2003)
Turmeric (*C. xanthorrhiza* Roxb)	MPLC	Silica gel	Germacrone and curzerenone	Claeson et al. (1993)
Clove (*S. aromaticum)*	Sequential chromatography AEC, HICC, SEC	DEAE-Toyopearl 650 (Cl^-), Butyl-Toyoperl 650 M, Sephadex G-75 gel, Sepharose CL^-6B column	Two antithrombotic polysaccharides	Lee et al. (2001)
Clove (*S. aromaticum)*	TLC and CC	Silica gel F_{254} (TLC) and for CC Toyopearl HW-40C, Sep-pack C18, YMC-gel ODS-AQ, and Sephadex LH-20 column	Phenolic compounds and 6′-O-acetylisobiflorin	Yoshimura et al. (2011)
Basil (*Ocimum basilicum* L.)	CC	Sephadex LH-20 column	Rosmarinic acid along with 22 polyphenols	Jayasinghe et al. (2003)

(continued)

Table 7.5 *(continued)*

Sample	Technique	Separation	Compound	Reference
Oregano (*O. vulgare* L. subsp. *hirtum*)	FCC	Silica gel column	Glycosides	Milos et al. (2000)
Pimento (*Pimenta. dioica*)	CC	Toyopearl HW-40C, Sep-pack C18, YMC-gel ODS-AQ and Sephadex LH-20 column	Phenolic compounds and (2S)-3-(4-hydroxy-3-methoxyphenyl)-propane-1,2-diol 1-O-(6′-O-galloyl)-β-D-glucoside for the first time after further hydrolysis	Yoshimura et al. (2011)
Bay leave (*L. nobilis*)	CC and HPLC	Silica gel column and Zorbax Rx-sil	From CC (reynosin and santamarine) and from HPLC fraction (10-epigazaniolide, gazaniolid, spirafolide, and costunolid)	Fang et al. (2005)
Cinnamon (*Cinnamomum burmannii*)	CC	Sephadex G75	Pigments	Tan et al. (2011)
Coriander seeds (*Coriandrum sativum* L.)	VLC and MPLC	Silica gel and CombiFlash silica gel column, respectively	Tripetroselinin, petroselinic acid, 1,3-dipetroselinin, 2-C-methyl-D-erythritol, 2-C-methyl-D-erythritol 4-O-beta-D-glucopyranoside and linalool	Zhang et al. (2015)
Thyme (*T. vulgaris* L.)	CC and HPLC	DEAE-Toyopearl 650C (Cl^-), Butyl- Toyopearl 650 M and Sepharose Cl-6B for CC anf for HPLC Shodex OHpak KB*05 column	Acidic polysaccharide	Chun et al. (2001)

Ginger (*Z. officinale*)	HSCCC, CC, and HPLC	Solvents, silica gel, and VP-ODS column, respectively	Three gingerols	Wang et al. (2011)
Cumin (*Cuminum cyminum* L.)	HSCCC	Solvent n-hexane, methanol, and water	Cuminaldehyde and *p*-Menta-1,4-dien-7-al	Chen et al. (2011)
Cinnamon (*Cinnamomum zeylanicum* Blume.)	CC and TLC	Silica gel column and silica gel and a F_{254} 0.25 mm TLC plate was used to optimize the isolation	Cinnamaldehyde	Babu et al. (2007)
Bay (*L. nobilis*)	CC, MPLC, and HPLC	Silica gel column, ODS, and YMC-pack ODS-AM, respectively	Two new compounds (Laurupene) and six known sesquiterpenes	Chen et al. (2014)
Cinnamon (*Cinnamomum burnanni*) among other varieties	CC and HPLC	LH-20 and L, SymmetryPrep C18, respectively	Doubly linked procyanidin type-A polymers	Anderson et al. (2004)
Bay (*L. nobilis*)	CC	Silica gel	A new sesquiterpene, lauroxepine, and six known sesquiterpene lactones	Barla et al. (2007)
Cinnamon (*Cinnamomum tamala*)	CC and HPLC	C18, Toyopearl HW-40F gel and ODS C18 gel for CC and for HPLC C18 column	*O*-methylated epimers of cinnamtannin	Chen et al. (2016)
Bay (*L. nobilis*)	CC and HPLC	Silica gel and a Zorbax Rx-sil normal phase column, respectively	Detected for the first time in bay 10-epigazaniolid, gazaniolid and the known compounds spirafolide, costunolid, reynosinand santamarine	Fang et al. (2005)

(continued)

Table 7.5 *(continued)*

Sample	Technique	Separation	Compound	Reference
Cinnamon (*C. zeylanicum*)	CC	Diaion HP-20SS resin, Diaion HP-20 column, and Sephadex LH-20 columns	Five phenolic compounds, protocatechuic acid, cinnamtannin B-1, urolignoside, rutin, and quercetin-3-*O*-R-L-rhamnopyranoside	Jayaprakasha et al. (2006)
Bay (*L. nobilis*)	FCC and HPLC	Normal-phase silica and YMC ODS-A column normal and reversed phase	22 sesquiterpenes including 10 previously unreported compounds, eudesmane lactones and their corresponding methyl esters	Julianti et al. (2012)
Bay (*L. nobilis*)	CC and HPLC	Silica gel and Sephadex LH-20 and semi-preparative HPLC analysis on μ-Bondapak C18 reverse phase	Major flavonol (L-EA-IIa-3-H2)	Kang et al. (2002)
Cinnamon (*Cinnamomum cassia* Blum.)	CC, MPLC, and HPLC	Slica gel column, RP-18, and open column chromatography, respectively	Six phenylpropanoids: syringaresinol, medioresinol, coumarin, 2-hydroxycinnamaldehyde, cryptamygin A, and 3′,5,7-trimethoxy epicatechin	Kang et al. (2016)
Paprika (*Capsicum annuum* L. var. *grossum* BAILEY)	CC	Diaion HP-20, ODS, and silica gel	Three new acyclic diterpene glycosides: capsianoside XVII, capsianoside V methyl ester, and capsianoside XIV	Lee et al. (2008)

Turmeric (*C. longa*)	FCC and CC	Silica gel and LH-20, respectively	Three pure curcumenoids: curcumin, demethoxyated curcumin, and bisdemethoxy curcumin	Radwan et al. (2014)
Bay (*L. nobilis*)	CC	Silica gel	Three trypanocidal compounds: lactone, zaluzanin-D and 1-hydroperoxy-*p*-menthan-2-en-8-ol acetate	Uchiyama et al. (2002)
Rosemary (*Rosmarinus officinalis*)	CPC	Hexane/ethyl acetate/methanol/water (3 : 2 : 3 : 2, v/v/v)	Carnosic acid and carnosol	Grace et al. (2017)
Garlic (*Allium sativum*)	SEC	Bio-Gel P-2 Column (1800 Da exclusion limit)	Fructans	Chandrashekar et al. (2011)
Sea fennel (*Crithmum maritimum* L.)	CC	Silica gel 60 and Sephadex LH-20	Falcarindiol	Meot-Duros et al. (2010)
Celery (*A. graveolens* L.)	CC assisted by TLC	Silica gel 60 and Sephadex LH-20	Three phthalides (senkyunolide A, (3S)-butylphthalide, and sedanolide), two furanocoumarins (bergapten and scopoletin), and one phenylpropanoid (*p*-hydroxyphenethyltransferulate).	Sbai et al. (2017)
Celery seeds (*A. graveolens* L.)	CC, MPLC, and preparative TLC	Silica gel	Sedanolide, senkyunolide-N, and senkyunolide-J	Momin and Nair (2001)

AEC, anion exchange chromatography; CC, column chromatography; CPC, centrifugal partition chromatography; FCC, flash column chromatography; HICC, hydromorphic interaction column chromatography; HPLC, high-pressure liquid extraction; HSCCC, high-speed counter-current chromatography; MPLC, medium-pressure liquid extraction; SEC, size exclusion chromatography; VLC, vacuum liquid chromatography.

7.3.3.5 Counter-Current Chromatography Counter-current chromatography (CCC) uses a biphasic liquid system to separate compounds. The phases' density difference and a centrifugal field are the parameters allowing the equilibrium between the two liquid phases (Ignat et al. 2011). CCC eliminates the possible irreversible adsorption of the analytes to the stationary phase (sorbents) and eliminates the carry-over, resulting in improved recovery (Wang et al. 2011). Sometimes, it is a challenge to obtain pure compounds by conventional chromatography separation methods due to the structural similarities of the target compound. In such situations CCC comes as a method of choice but as it is a quite novel technique compared with other more conventional methods, it is not widely used and implemented in laboratories.

Centrifugal partition chromatography (CPC) is an advanced form of CCC. The separation is accomplished by pressure and the centrifugal force of the rotational motion of coiled columns. High-speed counter-current chromatography (HSCCC) is another improved CCC technology (Figure 7.7), which is a promising technique to isolate compounds from crude extracts, where their concentration is quite small. HSCCC has been used successfully applied to isolate two structurally similar bio-compounds (culminaldehyde and *p*-menta-1,4-dien-7-al as shown in Figure 7.8) from cumin oil (Chen et al. 2011).

7.3.4 Hydrolysis

Most of the time, hydrolysis is used to target bioactive phytochemicals from cell walls or other complexes and to break polymers into monomers to achieve a more reliable quantification, due to the lack of standard for high molecular weight polyphenols. Hydrolysis can be performed via enzymatic or chemical (acidic or alkaline) routes. The most common factors that need to be optimized are concentration, temperature,

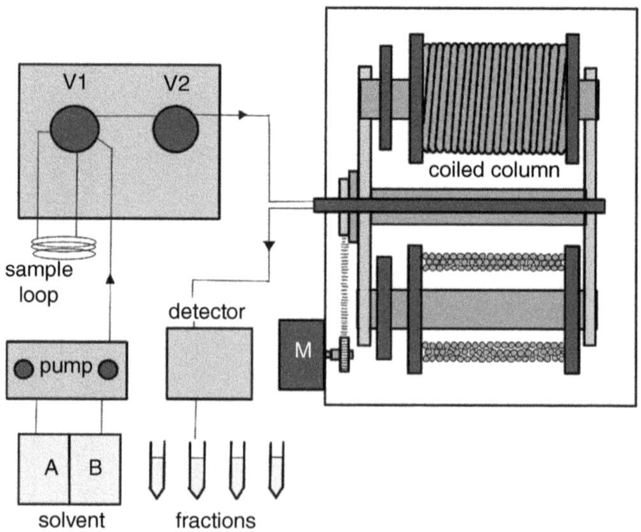

Figure 7.7 High-speed counter-current chromatography with the most important parts of the equipment to collect fractions.

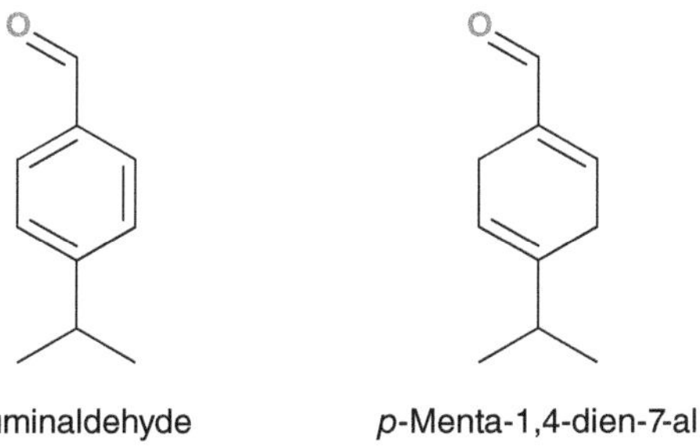

Figure 7.8 Chemical structure of two similar biocompounds (culminaldehyde and *p*-menta-1,4-dien-7-al) separated and isolated using HSCCC. *Source:* Adapted from (Chen et al. 2011).

pH, and time to achieve a successful recovery yield. Regarding phenolic compounds in spices and herbs, one of the major challenges is to break the glycosidic complex (polyphenols bound to cellulose wall components), where hydrolysis is needed, without reducing the activity of the biocompounds. Table 7.6 highlights the use of hydrolysis to purify biocompounds from herbs and spices such as acid hydrolysis (HCl) to purify pigments from cinnamon (*Cinnamomum burmannii*) (Tan et al. 2011) or basic Potassium hydroxide (KOH) to isolate piperic acid from black pepper (*Piper nigrum*) (Zarai et al. 2013).

7.3.5 Membrane Filtration

A membrane is a thin layer of semi-permeable material that separates substances; when a driving force is applied across the membrane, separation of substances based on molecular mass is achieved. This technique is easy to use and efficient but time-consuming.

Membrane processes can be classified as microfiltration, nanofiltration, reverse osmosis, and ultrafiltration (UF), where UF is the most commonly used. As an example, antithrombotic polysaccharides were isolated from clove (*S. aromaticum*) using UF 100 and 10 kDa (Lee et al. 2001). The acidic polysaccharide was isolated from ginger (*Z. officinale*) using UF 100 and 300 kDa (Chun et al. 2001) and from garlic (*Allium sativum*) matrix, fructans were isolated using ultrafiltration with a 3 kDa membrane and 3.5 kDa cut-off (Chandrashekar et al. 2011).

7.3.6 Recrystallization

Recrystallization or fractional crystallization is a procedure used to purify an impure compound in a solution. This method of purification is based on the principle that the solubility of most solids increases with increased temperature. This means that as temperature increases, the amount of solute that can be dissolved in a solvent also increases. The main disadvantage of recrystallization is that it takes a long time to isolate a compound.

Recrystallization has been applied in a few works related to herbs and spices. In clove (*S. aromaticum*) using methanol as a solvent, a flavonoid compound was isolated

Table 7.6 Summary of different hydrolysis techniques to isolate bioactive compounds from herbs and spices

Sample	Hydrolysis	Compound	Reference
Pimento (*P. dioica*)	Enzymatic (tannase)	(2S)-3-(4-hydroxy-3-methoxyphenyl)-propane-1,2-diol 1-O-(6′-O-galloyl)-β-D-glucoside for the first time	Yoshimura et al. (2011)
Clove (*S. aromaticum*)	Acid HCl	Two novel compounds Rhamnazin-3-O-β-D-glucuronide-6″-methyl ester and Rhamnocitrin-3-O-β-D-glucuronide-6″-methyl ester	Ryu et al. (2016a)
Cinnamon (*C. burmannii*)	Acid HCl	Pigments	Tan et al. (2011)
Oregano (*O. vulgare* L. subsp. *hirtum*)	Enzymatic (β-glucosidase)	Aglycones	Milos et al. (2000)
Paprika (*Capsicum annuum*)	Basic KOH	Tocopherols and carotenoids	Daood et al. (2008)
Ginger (*Z. officinale* Rosc.)	Enzymatic (cellulolytic and pectinolytic)	4-, 6-, 8-, and 10-gingerol and 6- and 8-shogaol	Schweiggert et al. (2008)
Ginger (*Z. officinale* Z.)	Acid and basic	Diosmin, thymol, and carvacrol	Alu'datt et al. (2016)
Black pepper (*Piper nigrum* L.)	Basic KOH	Piperic acid	Zarai et al. (2013)
Sweet, hot, and chili peppers	Acid HCl	Flavanone, naringenin, and hesperetin	Baranowska et al. (2016)

(Ryu et al. 2016a), a triterpenoid, and a tannin compound using the same solvent (Ryu et al. 2016b). From turmeric (*Curcuma xanthorrhiza* Roxb), a diarylheptanoid was isolated using methanol as a solvent (Claeson et al. 1993).

7.3.7 Other Techniques

7.3.7.1 Supercritical Fluid Extraction SFE is an environmentally friendly technique. It uses critical fluid with densities similar to liquids but with a lower viscosity, which makes the extraction faster than with traditional organic solvents (Ahmed 2001). Carbon dioxide (CO_2) is the fluid most often used (low toxicity and compatible with food processes) (Ignat et al. 2011). The main advantages of SFE are speed, use of eco-friendly solvents, and it is automatable. Moreover, the absence of air and light during the selective extraction reduces the degradation of compounds. (Figure 7.9).

SFE carries out extraction, purification, and fraction collection all at once. It is mostly used to extract oils from aromatic herbs and spices with medical purpose (Dima et al. 2014), but lately it has also found application in the food industry to extract natural preservatives and colorants. The main drawbacks of this technique are the price, equipment cost, and the fact that CO_2 as a supercritical fluid is not suitable for highly polar or ionic compounds. For more information, refer to recent review carried out regarding SFE in herbs (Fornari et al. 2012).

7.3.7.2 Capillary Electrophoresis Capillary electrophoresis (CE) is a method used to separate medium molecular weight, polar, and charged compounds. The CE is based on a differential movement or migration of solutes caused by the attraction or repulsion forces in an electric field. The main advantages of CE are high separation and resolution efficiency, shorter time analysis, and less consumption of reagents and sample. However, it is not as robust and reproducible technique as HPLC.

As an example, this method was successfully applied to isolate daidzein, rutin, and quercetin from *Cinnamomum camphora* (L.) Presl. (Chen et al. 2000).

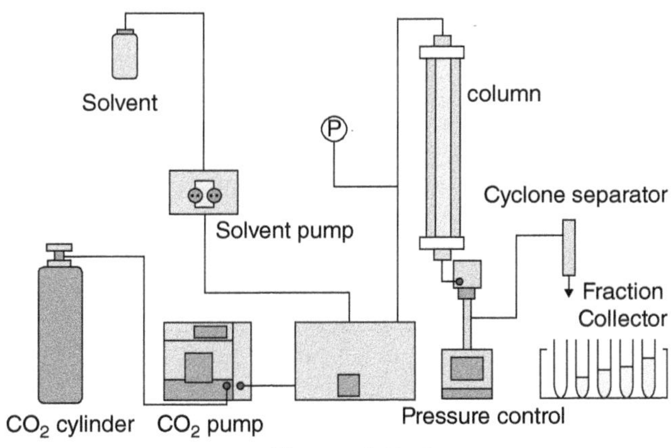

Figure 7.9 Supercritical fluid extraction equipment with CO_2 as the supercritical fluid used to collect fractions of a sample.

Hurtado-Fernandez et al. have comprehensively reviewed the application of CE separation to purify polyphenols in herbs and spices among other plant matrices (Hurtado-Fernandez et al. 2010).

7.3.7.3 QuEChERS Quick, Easy, Cheap, Effective, Rugged, and Safe (QuEChERS) methodology consists of two steps: first, extraction of the analytes from the matrix (solid–liquid extraction) followed by a dispersive solid-phase extraction (dSPE) clean-up. The advantages of the QuEChERS method include rapidity, simplicity and robustness, low solvent consumption, practically no glassware requirements, and low cost (Albero et al. 2014). These characteristics and advantages make QuEChERS an interesting procedure to implement in laboratories. The QuEChERS method was initially developed for the multiresidue determination of pesticides in fruits and vegetables (Anastassiades et al. 2003). As an example of versatility, this technique has been miniaturized and adapted to extract and purify other compounds such as (polycyclic aromatic hydrocarbons (PAHs), polybrominated diphenyl ethers (PBDEs), polychlorinated biphenyls (PCBs), and organophosphate and pyrethroid pesticides) in a complex matrix (Aznar et al. 2014).

Since then, this technique has been applied to many matrices and diverse target compounds, and was recently used to detect 160 pesticides in herbs (Taha and Gadalla 2017) and 154 pesticides in cardamom (*Elettaria cardamomurn*) (Jadhav et al. 2017). Despite several advantages, QuEChERS has the drawback of not being powerful enough to be used for isolation of biocompounds. Thus, further modification needs to be done in the future to the initially described QuEChERS method to achieve purification of biocompounds. Despite these facts, the versatility of QuEChERS makes it a promising technique to be improved and adapted in the near future to extract biocompounds from plants.

7.3.7.4 Cell Membrane Chromatography Cell membrane chromatography (CMC) is a biological affinity chromatographic technique useful for screening bioactive compounds in complex matrices. It uses silica coated with appropriate active cell membranes as a stationary phase. It is a favorable technique to target biocompounds as CMC can directly seek out active compounds based on target receptors from complex samples (such as herbs and spices). However, it presents two major limitations. First, the separation ability of CMC is lower than conventional HPLC and hence compounds can easily co-elute as a single peak; and, second, this method cannot be directly coupled with MS due to restriction of the mobile phase used (Li et al. 2016).

Human embryonic kidney 293 cells with a steadily high expression of epidermal growth factor receptors (EGFRs) were used to prepare the cell membrane stationary phase in a CMC model for screening active compounds in turmeric (*C. longa*), and separation of bioactive compounds ar-turmerone, curcumin, demethoxycurcumin, and bisdemethoxycurcumin was achieved (Sun et al. 2013).

7.4 Example of Purification and Isolation

In this chapter, the most common techniques for purification and isolation of bioactive compounds applied to herb and spice matrices have been reviewed. The present work can be useful to understand the complexity of the process of isolation and how difficult it is to achieve good yields of isolation of natural products. A few researchers have presented a flowchart of the steps carried out (Fang et al. 2005; Chandrashekar et al. 2011; Tan et al. 2011; Zeng et al. 2015), which is highly recommended to gain a better understanding of the work involved. Recently, Ryu and co-authors isolated bioactive phytochemicals in clove (*S. aromaticum*) (Ryu et al. 2016a) using a complex separation protocol, which is illustrated in Figure 7.10.

Bioactive compounds from dried clove (2 kg of initial sample) were exhaustively extracted using methanol, which yielded crude extract of 625 g. Then, the crude extract was fractionated into four fractions using LLP with *n*-hexane, ethyl acetate (EtOAc), *n*-butanol (BuOH), and water (H_2O). Each fraction was divided into dichloromethane (CH_2Cl_2) soluble and insoluble fractions. Moreover, different preparative liquid chromatographic techniques were applied, such as CC, medium-pressure liquid chromatography (MPLC), HPLC, and flash column (FC) with a wide range of column chemistries and solvents. Recrystallization was also performed to isolate and purify bioactive compounds. As many as 19 compounds were isolated, including four novel flavonol glucuronides, namely rhamnetin-3-*O*-beta-D-glucuronide, rhamnazin-3-*O*-beta-D-glucuronide, rhamnazin-3-*O*-beta-D-glucuronide-6″-methyl ester, and rhamnocitrin-3-*O*-beta-D-glucuronide-6″-methyl ester, where identification was achieved by 1D- and 2D-NMR spectroscopy.

7.5 Challenges and Future Trends

In crude extracts, generally extracted in methanol, the content of lipids, sugars, and other co-extracted compounds are higher than the amount of bioactive phytochemicals (secondary metabolites such as alkaloids, terpenes, and phenolic compounds) (Azmir et al. 2013). Moreover, several phytochemicals are bound to plant cell wall components, such as carbohydrates and proteins, making the separation difficult. This would require application of chemical or enzymatic hydrolysis. However, while removing the undesired hydrolyzed products, there may be a loss of the compounds of interests. Thus, one of the main challenges is to develop simple methods of extraction and purification to minimize the loss of target compounds and improve recoveries. The purification may depend on the choice of separation technique, type of solvents (varying polarities and pH), temperature and time, ratio of sample to solvent, as well as the chemical characteristics of the target analytes and the matrix. Hence, regarding future applications, MIPs technology maybe one of the most promising techniques, due to the high level of recovery of target compounds, and its selectivity, enrichment, and purification from complex samples such as spices and herbs. MIPs are efficient, rapid, and inexpensive (for the low amount of consumed solvents and instrumentation used) and even reusable, which makes it an eco-friendly technique. These characteristics make MIPs a promising candidate for scale-up, clean-up, and isolation experiments, and therefore potentially suitable for industrial (food and pharmacological) applications (Li et al. 2014). Recently, work has developed MIPs with nanoparticles (increasing the surface solvent ratio) or magnetic MIPs, increasing the applicability of this technique (Wackerlig and Lieberzeit 2015).

The other challenge that needs to be overcome is the risk of loss of bioactivity during the purification and isolation process. Often the bioactive compound can be easily oxidized or degraded when exposed to harsh chemicals and temperature during the long purification process (Dai and Mumper 2010). Thus, techniques that minimize dead

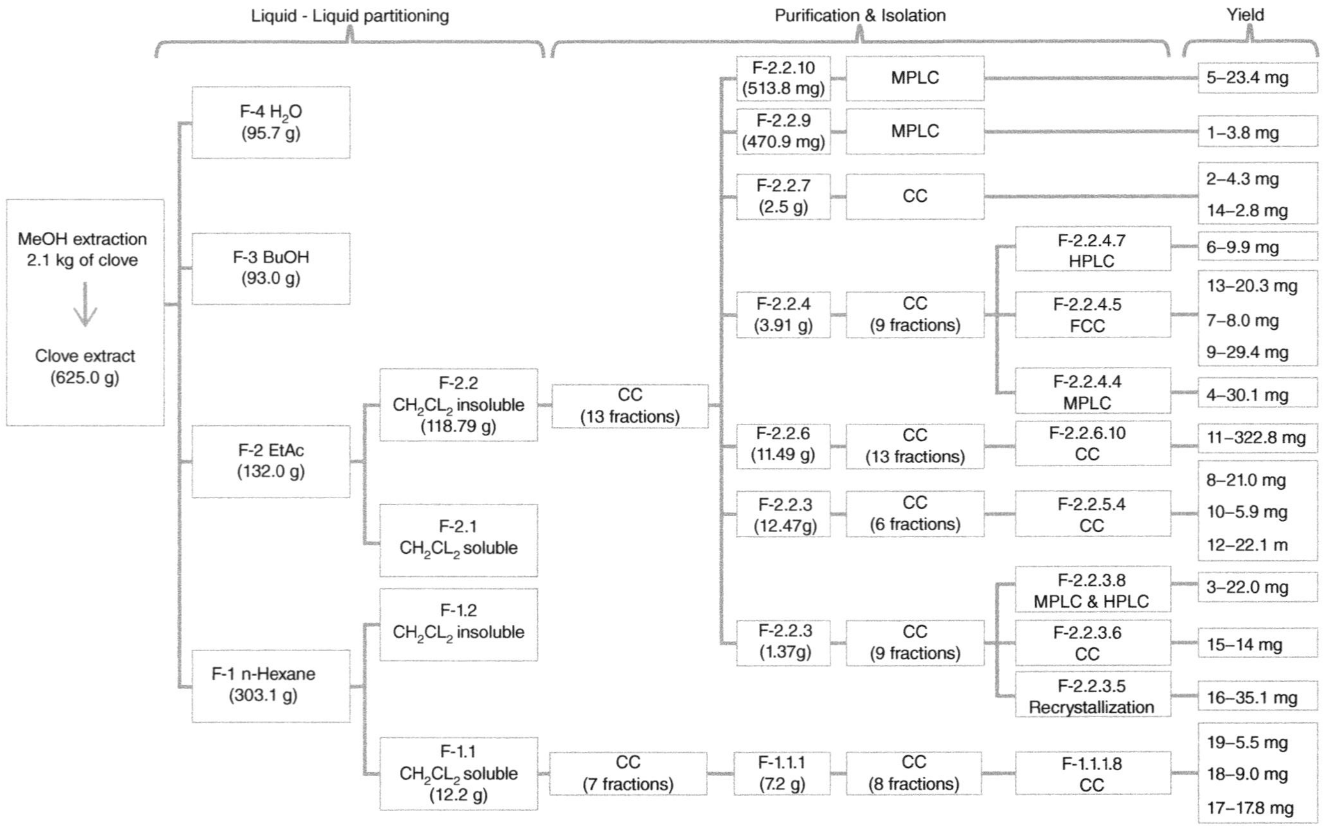

Figure 7.10 Flow chart describing the isolation of biocompounds from clove extract. *Source:* Adapted (Ryu et al. 2016a). (CC, column chromatography; FCC, flash column chromatography; HPLC, high-pressure liquid extraction; MPLC, medium-pressure liquid extraction).

time or reduce oxygen exposure are necessary. This is where SFE plays an important role, as it has been identified as the best method for isolating polyphenol compounds from spices (Palenzuela et al. 2004). More applications of this technique are expected in the near future with most of them related to extracting biocompounds from herbs and spice oils.

The time-consuming process to purify a single compound with good yield for structural identification by NMR spectroscopy is another bottle-neck in the purification process (Molnar-Perl and Fuzfai 2005), which will be solved in the future through the use of hyphenated techniques such as HPLC coupled to NMR spectroscope.

Finally, it is necessary to highlight the low yield of isolated compounds. As presented in Figure 7.10, 2 kg of starting material of clove could yield 625 g of powdered methanolic extract, which further results in the isolation of 19 bioactive compounds in the range of 2.8 to 322.8 mg. The isolated compounds in percentage represent only between 1.3×10^{-4} to 0.015% of the initial sample. Micro-fractionation bioactivity-integrated fingerprinting will be the best way to approach the discovery and isolation of new compounds. Although it has not yet been applied to herb and spice matrices, it has performed well in other plants solving some of the major issues, such as the use of a high mass of the initial sample, the amount of solvent used, the long time period and tedious process with consequent loss of activity of bioactive compounds.

References

Aboubakr, H.A., Nauertz, A., Luong, N.T. et al. (2016). In vitro antiviral activity of clove and ginger aqueous extracts against feline calicivirus, a surrogate for human norovirus. *Journal of Food Protection* **79**: 1001–1012.

Ahmed, F.E. (2001). Analyses of pesticides and their metabolites in foods and drinks. *TrAC Trends in Analytical Chemistry* **20**: 649–661.

Aksel, B. (2010). A brief review on bioactive compounds in plants. *The Norwegian Academy of Science and Letters*, Oslo, Norway: 11–17.

Albero, B., Sanchez-Brunete, C., Miguel, E. et al. (2014). Rapid determination of natural and synthetic hormones in biosolids and poultry manure by isotope dilution GC-MS/MS. *Journal of Separation Science* **37**: 811–819.

Alu'datt, M.H., Rababah, T., Alhamad, M.N. et al. (2016). Optimization of phenolic content, antioxidant, and inhibitory activities of alpha-glucosidase and angiotensin converting (AC) enzymes from *Zingiber officinale* Z. *International Journal of Food Properties* **19**: 1303–1316.

Anastassiades, M., Lehotay, S.J., Stajnbaher, D., and Schenck, F.J. (2003). Fast and easy multiresidue method employing acetonitrile extraction/partitioning and "dispersive solid-phase extraction" for the determination of pesticide residues in produce. *Journal of AOAC International* **86**: 412–431.

Anderson, R.A., Broadhurst, C.L., Polansky, M.M. et al. (2004). Isolation and characterization of polyphenol type-a polymers from cinnamon with insulin-like biological activity. *Journal of Agricultural and Food Chemistry* **52**: 65–70.

Ashley, J., Shahbazi, M.A., Kant, K. et al. (2017). Molecularly imprinted polymers for sample preparation and biosensing in food analysis: progress and perspectives. *Biosensors & Bioelectronics* **91**: 606–615.

Azmir, J., Zaidul, I.S.M., Rahman, M.M. et al. (2013). Techniques for extraction of bioactive compounds from plant materials: a review. *Journal of Food Engineering* **117**: 426–436.

Aznar, R., Albero, B., Sanchez-Brunete, C. et al. (2014). Multiresidue analysis of insecticides and other selected environmental contaminants in poultry manure by gas chromatography/mass spectrometry. *Journal of AOAC International* **97**: 978–986.

Babu, P.S., Prabuseenivasan, S., and Ignacimuthu, S. (2007). Cinnamaldehyde – a potential antidiabetic agent. *Phytomedicine* **14**: 15–22.

Baranowska, I., Hejniak, J., and Magiera, S. (2016). Development and validation of a RP-UHPLC-ESI-MS/MS method for the chiral separation and determination of flavanone, naringenin and hesperetin enantiomers. *Talanta* **159**: 181–188.

Barla, A., Topcu, G., Oksuz, S. et al. (2007). Identification of cytotoxic sesquiterpenes from *Laurus nobilis* L. *Food Chemistry* **104**: 1478–1484.

Brusotti, G., Cesari, I., Dentamaro, A. et al. (2014). Isolation and characterization of bioactive compounds from plant resources: the role of analysis in the ethnopharmacological approach. *Journal of Pharmaceutical and Biomedical Analysis* **87**: 218–228.

Chandrashekar, P.M., Prashanth, K.V.H., and Venkatesh, Y.P. (2011). Isolation, structural elucidation and immunomodulatory activity of fructans from aged garlic extract. *Phytochemistry* **72**: 255–264.

Chen, G., Zhang, H.W., and Ye, J.N. (2000). Determination of rutin and quercetin in plants by capillary electrophoresis with electrochemical detection. *Analytica Chimica Acta* **423**: 69–76.

Chen, Q.Q., Hu, X.F., Li, J.M. et al. (2011). Preparative isolation and purification of cuminaldehyde and p-menta-1,4-dien-7-al from the essential oil of *Cuminum cyminum* L. by high-speed counter-current chromatography. *Analytica Chimica Acta* **689**: 149–154.

Chen, H.Q., Xie, C.F., Wang, H. et al. (2014). Sesquiterpenes inhibiting the microglial activation from *Laurus nobilis*. *Journal of Agricultural and Food Chemistry* **62**: 4784–4788.

Chen, L., Wang, T., Yuan, P.L. et al. (2016). Preparation of methylated products of A-type procyanidin trimers in cinnamon bark and their protective effects on pancreatic beta-cell. *Journal of Food Science* **81**: 1062–1069.

Chun, H., Shin, D.H., Hong, B.S. et al. (2001). Purification and biological activity of acidic polysaccharide from leaves of *Thymus vulgaris* L. *Biological & Pharmaceutical Bulletin* **24**: 941–946.

Claeson, P., Tuchinda, P., and Reutrakul, V. (1993). Some empirical aspects on the practical use of flash chromatography and medium pressure liquid-chromatography for the isolation of biologically-active compounds from plants. *Journal of the Science Society of Thailand* **19**: 73–86.

Costa, D.C., Costa, H.S., Albuquerque, T.G. et al. (2015). Advances in phenolic compounds analysis of aromatic plants and their potential applications. *Trends in Food Science & Technology* **45**: 336–354.

Cowan, M.M. (1999). Plant products as antimicrobial agents. *Clinical Microbiology Reviews* **12**: 564–579.

Dai, J. and Mumper, R.J. (2010). Plant phenolics: extraction, analysis and their antioxidant and anticancer properties. *Molecules* **15**: 7313–7352.

Daood, H.G., Korbasz, M., Hamdan, S., and Beczner, J. (2008). Simultaneous LC determination of ergosterol, tocopherols and carotenoids in foods. *Chromatographia* **68**: 137–140.

Dawidowicz, A.L. and Dybowski, M.P. (2010). SPE isolation of low-molecular oxygen compounds from essential oils. *Journal of Separation Science* **33**: 3213–3220.

Diaz-Alvarez, M., Barahona, F., Turiel, E., and Martin-Esteban, A. (2014). Supported liquid membrane-protected molecularly imprinted beads for micro-solid phase extraction of sulfonamides in environmental waters. *Journal of Chromatography A* **1357**: 158–164.

Dima, C., Cotarlet, M., Alexe, P., and Dima, S. (2014). Microencapsulation of essential oil of pimento *Pimenta dioica* (L) Merr. by chitosan/k-carrageenan complex coacervation method. *Innovative Food Science & Emerging Technologies* **22**: 203–211.

Exarchou, V., Godejohann, M., Van Beek, T.A. et al. (2003). LC-UV-solid-phase extraction-NMR-MS combined with a cryogenic flow probe and its application to the identification of compounds present in Greek oregano. *Analytical Chemistry* **75**: 6288–6294.

Fair, J.D. and Kormos, C.M. (2008). Flash column chromatograms estimated from thin-layer chromatography data. *Journal of Chromatography A* **1211**: 49–54.

Fan, D.X., Li, H., Shi, S.Y., and Chen, X.Q. (2016). Hollow molecular imprinted polymers towards rapid, effective and selective extraction of caffeic acid from fruits. *Journal of Chromatography A* **1470**: 27–32.

Fang, F., Sang, S.M., Chen, K.Y. et al. (2005). Isolation and identification of cytotoxic compounds from bay leaf (*Laurus nobilis*). *Food Chemistry* **93**: 497–501.

Fecka, I. and Turek, S. (2007). Determination of water-soluble polyphenolic compounds in commercial herbal teas from *Lamiaceae*: peppermint, melissa, and sage. *Journal of Agricultural and Food Chemistry* **55**: 10908–10917.

Fornari, T., Vicente, G., Vazquez, E. et al. (2012). Isolation of essential oil from different plants and herbs by supercritical fluid extraction. *Journal of Chromatography A* **1250**: 34–48.

Grace, M.H., Qiang, Y., Sang, S.M., and Lila, M.A. (2017). One-step isolation of carnosic acid and carnosol from rosemary by centrifugal partition chromatography. *Journal of Separation Science* **40**: 1057–1062.

Grosso, C., Jager, A.K., and Staerk, D. (2013). Coupling of a high-resolution monoamine oxidase-a inhibitor assay and HPLC-SPE-NMR for advanced bioactivity profiling of plant extracts. *Phytochemical Analysis* **24**: 141–147.

Hemalatha, R., Nivetha, P., Mohanapriya, C. et al. (2016). Phytochemical composition, GC-MS analysis, in vitro antioxidant and antibacterial potential of clove flower bud (*Eugenia caryophyllus*) methanolic extract. *Journal of Food Science and Technology* **53**: 1189–1198.

Hossain, M.B., Camphuis, G., Aguilo-Aguayo, I. et al. (2014). Antioxidant activity guided separation of major polyphenols of marjoram (*Origanum majorana* L.) using flash chromatography and their identification by liquid chromatography coupled with electrospray ionization tandem mass spectrometry. *Journal of Separation Science* **37**: 3205–3213.

Hou, Y.Y., Cao, X.L., Wang, L.Q. et al. (2012). Microfractionation bioactivity-based ultra performance liquid chromatography/quadrupole time-of-flight mass spectrometry for the identification of nuclear factor-kappa B inhibitors and beta(2) adrenergic receptor agonists in an alkaloidal extract of the folk herb *Alstonia scholaris*. *Journal of Chromatography. B, Analytical Technologies in the Biomedical and Life Sciences* **908**: 98–104.

Hou, S.Y., Yang, S.L., He, H.L. et al. (2015). Multi-templates molecularly imprinted polymer for the specific solid-phase extraction of saponins from *Panax notoginseng* herbal extract. *Current Pharmaceutical Analysis* **11**: 292–299.

Hurtado-Fernandez, E., Gomez-Romero, M., Carrasco-Pancorbo, A., and Fernandez-Gutierrez, A. (2010). Application and potential of capillary electroseparation methods to determine antioxidant phenolic compounds from plant food material. *Journal of Pharmaceutical and Biomedical Analysis* **53**: 1130–1160.

Ignat, I., Volf, I., and Popa, V.I. (2011). A critical review of methods for characterisation of polyphenolic compounds in fruits and vegetables. *Food Chemistry* **126**: 1821–1835.

Ivanovic, J., Dimitrijevic-Brankovic, S., Misic, D. et al. (2013). Evaluation and improvement of antioxidant and antibacterial activities of supercritical extracts from clove buds. *Journal of Functional Foods* **5**: 416–423.

Jadhav, M., Thekkumpurath, A.S., Nakade, M. et al. (2017). Multiresidue method for targeted screening of pesticide residues in spice cardamom (*Elettaria cardamomurn*) by liquid chromatography with tandem mass spectrometry. *Journal of AOAC International* **100**: 603–609.

Janicsak, G., Veres, K., Kallai, M., and Mathe, I. (2003). Gas chromatographic method for routine determination of oleanolic and ursolic acids in medicinal plants. *Chromatographia* **58**: 295–299.

Jassbi, A.R., Zare, S., Firuzi, O., and Xiao, J.B. (2016). Bioactive phytochemicals from shoots and roots of salvia species. *Phytochemistry Reviews* **15**: 829–867.

Jayaprakasha, G.K., Ohnishi-Kameyama, M., Ono, H. et al. (2006). Phenolic constituents in the fruits of *Cinnamomum zeylanicum* and their antioxidant activity. *Journal of Agricultural and Food Chemistry* **54**: 1672–1679.

Jayasinghe, C., Gotoh, N., Aoki, T., and Wada, S. (2003). Phenolics composition and antioxidant activity of sweet basil (*Ocimum basilicum* L.). *Journal of Agricultural and Food Chemistry* **51**: 4442–4449.

Jin, S.K., Choi, J.S., Jeong, J.Y., and Kim, G.D. (2016). The effect of clove bud powder at a spice level on antioxidant and quality properties of emulsified pork sausage during cold storage. *Journal of the Science of Food and Agriculture* **96**: 4089–4097.

Julianti, E., Jang, K.H., Lee, S. et al. (2012). Sesquiterpenes from the leaves of *Laurus nobilis* L. *Phytochemistry* **80**: 70–76.

Kang, H.W., Yu, K.W., Jun, W.J. et al. (2002). Isolation and characterization of alkyl peroxy radical scavenging compound from leaves of *Laurus nobilis*. *Biological & Pharmaceutical Bulletin* **25**: 102–108.

Kang, Y.J., Seo, D.G., and Park, S.Y. (2016). Phenylpropanoids from cinnamon bark reduced beta-amyloid production by the inhibition of beta-secretase in Chinese hamster ovarian cells stably expressing amyloid precursor protein. *Nutrition Research* **36**: 1277–1284.

Kimura, Y., Ito, H., and Hatano, T. (2010). Effects of mace and nutmeg on human cytochrome P450 3A4 and 2C9 activity. *Biological & Pharmaceutical Bulletin* **33**: 1977–1982.

Kitabatake, T., Tabo, H., Matsunaga, H., and Haginaka, J. (2013). Preparation of monodisperse curcumin-imprinted polymer by precipitation polymerization and its application for the extraction of curcuminoids from *Curcuma longa* L. *Analytical and Bioanalytical Chemistry* **405**: 6555–6561.

Lee, J.I., Lee, H.S., Jun, W.J. et al. (2001). Purification and characterization of antithrombotics from *Syzygium aromaticum* (L.) Merr. & Perry. *Biological & Pharmaceutical Bulletin* **24**: 181–187.

Lee, J.H., Kiyota, N., Ikeda, T., and Nohara, T. (2008). Three new acyclic diterpene glycosides from the aerial parts of paprika and pimiento. *Chemical & Pharmaceutical Bulletin* **56**: 582–584.

Li, Z.Z., Qin, C.L., Li, D.M. et al. (2014). Molecularly imprinted polymer for specific extraction of hypericin from *Hypericum perforatum* L. herbal extract. *Journal of Pharmaceutical and Biomedical Analysis* **98**: 210–220.

Li, D.Q., Zhao, J., Wu, D., and Li, S.P. (2016). Discovery of active components in herbs using chromatographic separation coupled with online bioassay. *Journal of Chromatography. B, Analytical Technologies in the Biomedical and Life Sciences* **1021**: 81–90.

Meot-Duros, L., Cerantola, S., Talarmin, H. et al. (2010). New antibacterial and cytotoxic activities of falcarindiol isolated in *Crithmum maritimum* L. leaf extract. *Food and Chemical Toxicology* **48**: 553–557.

Milos, M., Mastelic, J., and Jerkovic, I. (2000). Chemical composition and antioxidant effect of glycosidically bound volatile compounds from oregano (*Origanum vulgare* L. ssp hirtum). *Food Chemistry* **71**: 79–83.

Misharina, T.A., Alinkina, E.S., and Medvedeva, I.B. (2015). Antiradical properties of essential oils and extracts from clove bud and pimento. *Applied Biochemistry and Microbiology* **51**: 119–124.

Molnar-Perl, I. and Fuzfai, Z. (2005). Chromatographic, capillary electrophoretic and capillary electrochromatographic techniques in the analysis of flavonoids. *Journal of Chromatography A* **1073**: 201–227.

Momin, R.A. and Nair, M.G. (2001). Mosquitocidal, nematicidal, and antifungal compounds from *Apium graveolens* L. seeds. *Journal of Agricultural and Food Chemistry* **49**: 142–145.

Moricz, A.M., Ott, P.G., Boszormenyi, A. et al. (2012). Bioassay-guided isolation and identification of antimicrobial compounds from thyme essential oil by means of overpressured layer chromatography, bioautography and GC-MS. *Chromatographia* **75**: 991–999.

Palenzuela, B., Arce, L., Macho, A. et al. (2004). Bioguided extraction of polyphenols from grape marc by using an alternative supercritical-fluid extraction method based on a liquid solvent trap. *Analytical and Bioanalytical Chemistry* **378**: 2021–2027.

Peng, M.J., Xiang, H.Y., Hu, X. et al. (2016). Boronate affinity-based surface molecularly imprinted polymers using glucose as fragment template for excellent recognition of glucosides. *Journal of Chromatography A* **1474**: 8–13.

Politeo, O., Jukic, M., and Milos, M. (2010). Comparison of chemical composition and antioxidant activity of glycosidically bound and free volatiles from clove (*Eugenia caryophyllata Thunb.*). *Journal of Food Biochemistry* **34**: 129–141.

Radwan, M.M., Tabanca, N., Wedge, D.E. et al. (2014). Antifungal compounds from turmeric and nutmeg with activity against plant pathogens. *Fitoterapia* **99**: 341–346.

Reichardt, C. and Welton, T. (2010). *Solvents and Solvent Effects in Organic Chemistry*. Weinheim: Wiley-VCH Verlag GmbH & Co. KGaA.

Robards, K. (2003). Strategies for the determination of bioactive phenols in plants, fruit and vegetables. *Journal of Chromatography A* **1000**: 657–691.

Ryu, B., Kim, H.M., Lee, J.S. et al. (2016a). New flavonol glucuronides from the flower buds of *Syzygium aromaticum* (clove). *Journal of Agricultural and Food Chemistry* **64**: 3048–3053.

Ryu, B., Kim, H.M., Woo, J.H. et al. (2016b). A new acetophenone glycoside from the flower buds of *Syzygium aromaticum* (cloves). *Fitoterapia* **115**: 46–51.

Sarafraz-Yazdi, A. and Razavi, N. (2015). Application of molecularly-imprinted polymers in solid-phase microextraction techniques. *TrAC Trends in Analytical Chemistry* **73**: 81–90.

Sbai, H., Zribi, I., Dellagreca, M., and Haouala, R. (2017). Bioguided fractionation and isolation of phytotoxic compounds from *Apium graveolens* L. aerial parts (Apiaceae). *South African Journal of Botany* **108**: 423–430.

Schwarz, L.J., Danylec, B., Harris, S.J. et al. (2016). Sequential molecularly imprinted solid-phase extraction methods for the analysis of resveratrol and other polyphenols. *Journal of Chromatography A* **1438**: 22–30.

Schweiggert, U., Hofmann, S., Reichel, M. et al. (2008). Enzyme-assisted liquefaction of ginger rhizomes (*Zingiber officinale* Rosc.) for the production of spray-dried and paste-like ginger condiments. *Journal of Food Engineering* **84**: 28–38.

Scotter, M.J., Roberts, D.P.T., and Rees, G.O. (2011). Development and single-laboratory validation of an HPLC method for the determination of coumarin in foodstuffs using internal standardization and solid-phase extraction cleanup. *Analytical Methods* **3**: 414–419.

Sterbova, D., Matejicek, D., Vlcek, J., and Kuban, V. (2004). Combined microwave-assisted isolation and solid-phase purification procedures prior to the chromatographic determination of phenolic compounds in plant materials. *Analytica Chimica Acta* **513**: 435–444.

Sun, M., Ma, W.N., Guo, Y. et al. (2013). Simultaneous screening of four epidermal growth factor receptor antagonists from *Curcuma longa* via cell membrane chromatography online coupled with HPLC-MS. *Journal of Separation Science* **36**: 2096–2103.

Taha, S.M. and Gadalla, S.A. (2017). Development of an efficient method for multi residue analysis of 160 pesticides in herbal plant by ethyl acetate hexane mixture with direct injection to GC-MS/MS. *Talanta* **174**: 767–779.

Tan, M.X., Gan, D.H., Wei, L.X. et al. (2011). Isolation and characterization of pigment from *Cinnamomum burmannii* peel. *Food Research International* **44**: 2289–2294.

Thanekar, D., Dhodi, J., Gawali, N. et al. (2016). Evaluation of antitumor and anti-angiogenic activity of bioactive compounds from *Cinnamomum tamala*: in vitro, in vivo and in silico approach. *South African Journal of Botany* **104**: 6–14.

Thurman, E.M. and Mills, M.S. (1998). *Solid-Phase Extraction*. New York: Wiley.

Uchiyama, N., Matsunaga, K., Kiuchi, F. et al. (2002). Trypanocidal terpenoids from *Laurus nobilis L. Chemical & Pharmaceutical Bulletin* **50**: 1514–1516.

Wackerlig, J. and Lieberzeit, P.A. (2015). Molecularly imprinted polymer nanoparticles in chemical sensing – synthesis, characterisation and application. *Sensors and Actuators B: Chemical* **207**: 144–157.

Wang, X., Zheng, Z.J., Guo, X.F. et al. (2011). Preparative separation of gingerols from *Zingiber officinale* by high-speed counter-current chromatography using stepwise elution. *Food Chemistry* **125**: 1476–1480.

Wulandari, M., Urraca, J.L., Descalzo, A.B. et al. (2015). Molecularly imprinted polymers for cleanup and selective extraction of curcuminoids in medicinal herbal extracts. *Analytical and Bioanalytical Chemistry* **407**: 803–812.

Xie, Y.J., Yang, Z.L., Cao, D.Y. et al. (2015). Antitermitic and antifungal activities of eugenol and its congeners from the flower buds of *Syzygium aromaticum* (clove). *Industrial Crops and Products* **77**: 780–786.

Yoshimura, M., Amakura, Y., and Yoshida, T. (2011). Polyphenolic compounds in clove and pimento and their antioxidative activities. *Bioscience Biotechnology and Biochemistry* **75**: 2207–2212.

Zarai, Z., Boujelbene, E., Ben Salem, N. et al. (2013). Antioxidant and antimicrobial activities of various solvent extracts, piperine and piperic acid from *Piper nigrum*. *LWT Food Science and Technology* **50**: 634–641.

Zeng, Q.H., Lu, C.L., Zhang, X.W., and Jiang, J.G. (2015). Isolation and identification of ingredients inducing cancer cell death from the seeds of *Alpinia galanga*, a Chinese spice. *Food & Function* **6**: 431–443.

Zhang, C.R., Dissanayake, A.A., Kevseroglu, K., and Nair, M.G. (2015). Evaluation of coriander spice as a functional food by using in vitro bioassays. *Food Chemistry* **167**: 24–29.

8

Medicinal Properties of Herbs and Spices: Past, Present, and Future

Celia Rodríguez-Pérez[1,2] and Ramón Aznar[3]

[1]*Department of Nutrition and Food Science, University of Granada Campus of Cartuja, Granada, 18071, Spain*

[2]*Institute of Nutrition and Food Technology (INYTA), José Mataix, Biomedical Research Centre, University of Granada, Avenida del Conocimiento s/n, Granada, E-18071, Spain*

[3]*Food Bioscience, Teagasc Food Research Centre, Ashtown, Dublin D15KN3K, Ireland*

8.1 Introduction

The latest report from the World Health Organization (WHO) estimated that USD 7.3 trillion was spent on health worldwide in 2015, close to 10% of global Gross Domestic Product (WHO 2017). This fact, together with the coexistence of huge advances in human wellbeing and extreme deprivation in many parts of the world (WHO 2005), has positioned traditional medicine (TM) as one of the leading research topics in the area of public health. Nowadays, interest in natural products as a source of potential chemotherapeutic agents in developed countries is coming back, and is reflected in the clinical use of them and their derivatives. Natural products represent more than 50% of all the drugs in clinical use in the world. In this context, plants contribute over 25% of the total (Gurib-Fakim 2006). In fact, the WHO estimated that more than 60% of the population relies on TM for their primary health care (Gragg et al. 2012). So much so that the same organization developed and launched the WHO Traditional Medicine Strategy 2014–2023, with the objective of keeping the population healthy through the prioritization of traditional and complementary medicine products (WHO 2013).

According to the WHO, traditional medicine is defined as a comprehensive term that includes various forms of indigenous medicine and also TM systems, i.e. traditional Chinese medicine, Indian Ayurveda, and Arabic Unani medicine (WHO 2002). Traditional medicine is based on skills and practices derived from theories, beliefs, and experiences indigenous to different cultures to maintain health but also to prevent or treat physical and mental illnesses (WHO 2013). Specifically, the employment of

Herbs, Spices and Medicinal Plants: Processing, Health Benefits and Safety, First Edition.
Edited by Mohammad B. Hossain, Nigel P. Brunton, and Dilip K. Rai.

herbs and spices is known as medication therapy, which is also included within TM practices. The terms "herbs" and "spices" have more than one definition but, roughly speaking, herbs are defined as any plant with leaves, seeds, or flowers mainly used for flavoring, food, or medicine, e.g. rosemary, oregano, garlic, onion, or cumin, among others. Spices are defined as a part of a plant or a powder made from that part which is commonly added to foods to increase or enhance its flavor. Spices differ from other plants used in food because they are used in small amounts to impart flavor rather than nutrients (Martínez-Graciá et al. 2015). In many cultures, they are employed as colorants and preservatives. For example, basil, oregano, thyme, and rosemary are employed for fresh food preservation (Martínez-Graciá et al. 2015). The main advantage that their uses present is that they are considered as generally recognized as safe (GRAS) and consequently are potential alternatives to synthetic chemical additives. The most recent example is the approval of the use of rosemary extract as a food additive by the European Union (EU) (EFSA 2015). Herbs and spices are widely available on the EU market in the form of food supplements. However, currently there is no EU legislation specifically for botanicals (which include herbs and spices) and, for that reason, the European Food Safety Authority (EFSA) is working on the harmonization of that market (EFSA 2016).

Scientific knowledge about herbs and spices commonly employed in TM has determined that they may contain one or many bioactive constituents that could be therapeutic (Rodríguez-Pérez et al. 2016). These bioactive compounds are known as components with health benefits that typically occur in small quantities in certain plant-based foods (Singh et al. 2016) and are attracting research attention. In this regard, *in vitro* assays, *in vivo* assays, and clinical studies are demonstrating the dynamic relationship between bioactive compounds and health. Thus, this chapter encompasses the most recent research about the effect of the most frequently used herbs and spices in the treatment and prevention of the most common diseases and pathologies, i.e. cardiovascular (CV), hepatic and inflammatory diseases, cancer, obesity, diabetes, digestive stimulation, hypertension, and Alzheimer's disease (AD).

8.2 Historical Uses of Herbs and Spices

Herbs and spices have been employed for thousands of years as ornaments, condiments, preservatives, fragrances, dyes, and even medicines. In this last regard, written documents prove their employment to treat different ailments from ancient times.

The first written evidence appeared during the thirtieth century BCE in Mesopotamia, where prescription medicines were recorded on cuneiform tablets (Borchardt 2002). For example, garlic (*Allium sativum*) was used as early as 3000 BCE for the treatment of intestinal disorders and is now known for its fibrinolytic activity and its possible role in lowering blood cholesterol (Al-Qattan 2009). As shown in the timeline in Figure 8.1, in ancient Egypt the first recorded use of herbs to treat illnesses was found in sixteenth century BCE in the Ebers and Edwin Smith papyrus.

Around the thirteenth century BCE, Shennong established the fundamentals of China's agriculture and herbal medicine (Bagley 1999). In India, it was not until the sixth century BCE that Sushruta wrote *The Compendium of Suśruta* and established the fundamentals of Ayurvedic medicine with a compilation of medicinal substances. In Ancient Greece, around the fourth century BCE, Hippocrates – the "father of

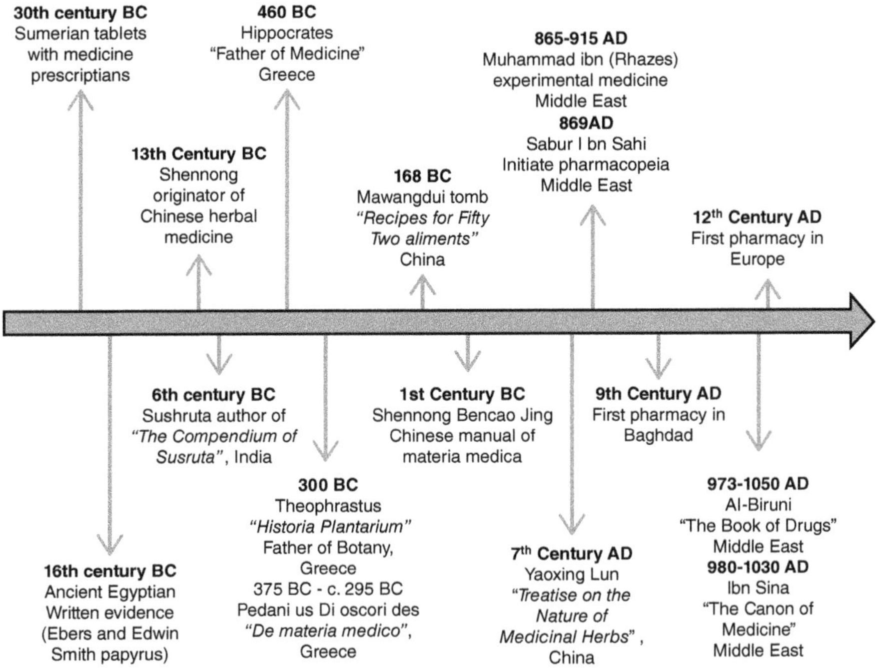

Figure 8.1 Timeline of the history of pharmacology.

medicine" – was already saying "Let food be thy medicine and medicine be thy food." Between 371 and 287 BCE, Theophrastus wrote *Historia Plantarum* and gained the title the "father of botany." And in 375–295 BCE, Pedanius Dioscorides wrote *De materia medica,* a five-volume book of pharmacopeia about herbal medicine and related medicinal substances that was used for many centuries.

Around 168 BCE, inside the Mawangdui tomb in China, the book *Recipes for Fifty-Two Ailments* was written. And also around the first century BCE, Shennong Bencao Jing wrote the *Chinese Manual of Materia Medica,* influenced by the *De Materia Medica* book of Pedanius. Thus, the use of herbs and spices to treat and prevent illnesses started to develop in the Middle East. Around 865–915 AD, Muhammad Ibn (known as Rhazes) was an early proponent of experimental medicine. In 869, Sabur Ibn Sahi set the bases of pharmacopeia and during the ninth century AD the first pharmacy opened in Baghdad. Between 973 and 1050, Al-Biruni wrote *The Book of Drugs* and Ibn Sina in 980–1030 wrote *The Canon of Medicine.*

Medical and pharmaceutical manuscripts of Persian medicine from the tenth century AD reveal concepts of insomnia treatment using herbal remedies (Petramfar et al. 2014). Likewise, several traditional Persian medicine textbooks relate the treatment of Alzheimer's disease using herbal remedies (Shirbeigi et al. 2018). Finally, it was around the twelfth century that the first pharmacy opened in Europe.

The components of these herbs and spices and their mechanisms of action against disease and illness remained obscure, despite being used traditionally to treat various ailments (Table 8.1). Herbs and spices have been indispensable for daily human health, and over the last few years, several bioactive compounds have been isolated

Table 8.1 Traditional uses of some spices and herbs, based on (Nadkarni and Nadkarni 1999; Kunnumakkara et al. 2009) for various ailment treatments

Spices and herbs	Traditional uses
Pepper (*Piper nigrum*)	Improve appetite, cure cold, cough dyspnea, diseases of the throat, fever, colic, worms and piles, anti-inflammatory
Cardamom (*Elettaria cardamomum*)	Diuretic, digestive, urinary disorders, gastrointestinal protective, anti-inflammatory and antibacterial, constipation, dysentery
Cinnamon (*Cinnamomum zeylanicum*)	Antipyretic, antiseptic, astringent, balsamic, carminative, fungicidal, stimulant, stomachic
Cloves (*Syzygium aromaticum*)	Painkiller, analgesic, anesthetic, antibacterial, antiparasitic, digestive, antiperspirant
Garlic (*Allium sativum*)	Antidyspeptic, antifungal, ear infection, duodenal ulcer, skin diseases
Ginger (*Zingiber officinale*)	Sialagogue, heart and blood diseases, antinausea, abdominal spasm, respiratory and rheumatic disorders, anti-inflammatory
Cumin (*Cuminum cyminum*)	Antispasmodic, carminative, digestive stimulant
Rosemary (*Rosmarinus officinalis*)	Stimulant, carminative, diuretic, hepatoprotective, antirheumatic, expectorant, analgesic
Turmeric (*Curcuma longa*)	Anti-inflammatory, diuretic, laxative, antirheumatism, body ache, diarrhea, hepatic diseases, stress and depression
Onion (*Allium cepa*)	Diuretic, expectorant, useful for bleeding piles

from the spices described in Table 8.1, providing a scientific basis for their use in our diet (Kunnumakkara et al. 2009); although more work needs to be done to assess their mechanism of action.

8.3 Herbs and Spices in the Prevention and Treatment of Chronic Diseases

Many herbs and spices have been tested to treat and prevent the most common illnesses *in vitro* (Figure 8.2). Thus, a considerable amount of literature concerning the *in vitro* health properties of herbs and spices can be found. However, since *in vivo* studies and clinical trials on humans are the most reliable assays, this chapter focuses on updating the state-of-the-art of the effect of the most used herbs and spices against cancer, inflammation, obesity, diabetes, hypertension, digestive disorders, Alzheimer, and liver damage, which are discussed below (Tables 8.2 and 8.3, respectively).

8.3.1 Anticancer Properties

Scientists have discovered an inverse association of spice consumption with oncological incidences. In this regard, curcumin (diferuloylmethane), a naturally occurring phenolic compound of turmeric (*Curcuma longa*), has been probably the most

Spice	Active biochemical	Properties	Reference
Turmeric *Curcuma longa)* 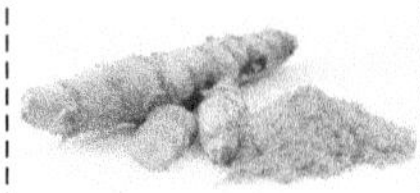	Curcumin 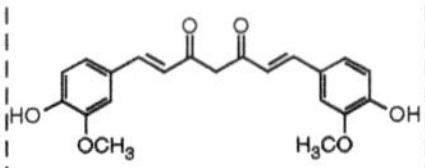	Anticancer Anti-inflammatory Antimicrobial Cardiac diseases Neuropsychiatric disorders Alzheimers disease	Zhang et al. (2018) Shehzad et al. (2017) Kunnumakkara et al. (2017b) Jaing et al. (2017) Lopresti et al. (2017) Hamaguchi et al. (2010)
Cinnamon *Cinnamomum cassia)* 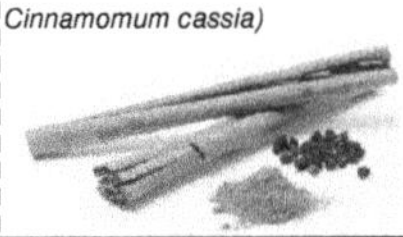	Cinnamaldehy de 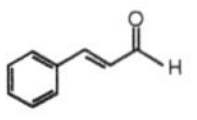	Antifungal Anticancer Antiallergic Neuro protective Antimicrobial	Taguchi et al. (2010) Ng Wu (2011) Kageyama-Yahara et al. (2011) Lv et al. (2017) Shreaz et al. (2017)
Ginger *Zingiber officinale)* 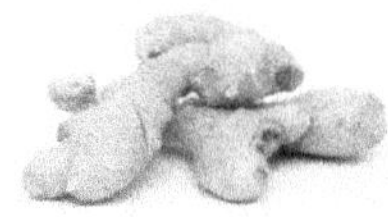	Gingerol 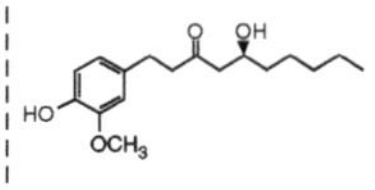	Anticancer Anti-inflammatory Antiausea Antiallergic Colonic motility Antiobesity	Zhang et al. (2017) Choi et al. (2017) Marx et al. (2017) Murata et al. (2017) Cai et al. (2015) Misawa et al. (2015)
Clove *Syzygium aromaticum)* 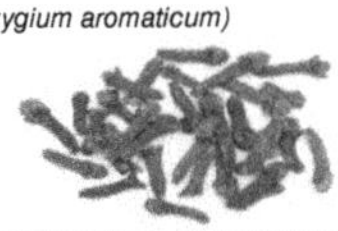	Eugenol 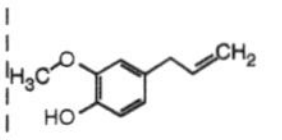	Antifungal Antimicrobial Anti-inflammatory Antidiabetic Enhance immune responses	Sharma et al. (2017) Marchese et al. (2017) Tsai et al. (2017) Tahir et al. (2016) Dibazar et al. (2014)
Nutmeg and Mace *Myristica fragrans)* 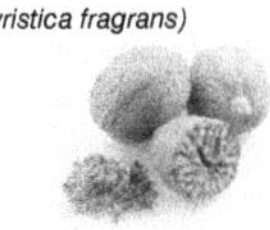	Licarin 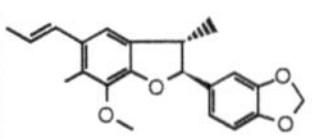	Insulin resistance Anticancer Inhibit NO Antiphotoaging agent Anti-allergic	Shyni et al. (2016) Acuna et al. (2016) Cao et al. (2013) Kwon et al. (2011) Matsui et al. (2015)
Rosemary *Rosmarinus Officinalis)* 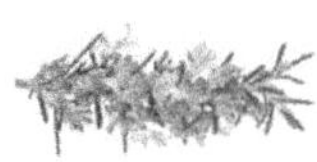	Rosmarinic acid 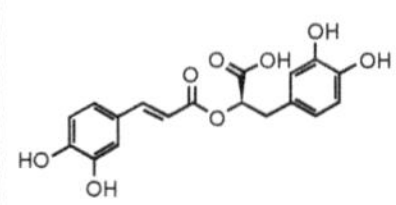	Antidiabetic Anticancer Anticancer Antibacterial Neuro protective	Naimi et al. (2017) Lou et al. (2016) Moore et al. (2016) Sacco et al. (2015) Ghaffari et al. (2014)

Figure 8.2 Bioactive compounds from herbs and spices that present medicinal effect *in vitro*.

studied bioactive compound against cancer. In addition to *in vitro* studies, a wide range of literature evidences the role of curcumin in diverse transcription factors, inflammatory cytokines, enzymes, kinases, growth factors, and receptor modulation in clinical and preclinical studies (Kunnumakkara et al. 2017a). The most recognized mechanism of action of curcumin is the inhibition of cyclooxygenase 2 (COX-2) at the transcriptional level (Sharma et al. 2005). In this context, an early dose-escalation pilot study was carried out on 15 patients with colorectal cancer. In that study, a 220 mg capsule containing 18 mg of curcumin and 2 mg of desmethoxycurcumin suspended in 200 mg of turmeric essential oils was administered daily for 29 days. The researchers measured the cyclooxygenase 2 COX-2 activity and gene expression in whole blood indirectly using plasma prostaglandin E_2 (PGE_2) concentration and Western blotting. The results showed a dose-dependent inhibition of basal

Table 8.2 Bioactivity of herbs and spices evaluated in animal models

Matrix	Bioactive compound	Properties	Study design	n	Mechanism of action	Ref.
Black pepper (*Piper nigrum*)	Piperine	Antihypertensive	Wistar rats were administered for 6 wk clear water or L-NAME (40 mg/kg/d) dissolved in water, piperine (20 mg/kg/d), curcumin (100 mg/kg/d) or their combination in corn oil by oral gavage	48	↓ (p <0.01) BP compared to L-NAME group but BP remained above the control until the end of the experiment	Hlavačková et al. (2011)
Celery (*Apium graveolens*)	Not defined	Antihypertensive	Male Wistar rats were randomly divided into nine groups: all groups except group 9 (normotensive rats), received DOCA for 7 wk (20 mg/kg, twice weekly, s.c.) 300 mg/kg of exanic, methanolic, and aqueous-ethanolic (20/80, v/v) seed celery extracts	54	↓ BP and increased the ↑ HR in hypertensive rats with no effect on normotensive rats	Moghadam et al. (2013)
Cinnamon (*Cinnamomum zeylanicum*)	Not defined	Hepatoprotective	(CCl_4)-induced liver damage male Wistar rats consumed cinnamon extracts (0.01, 0.05, and 0.1 g/kg) for 28 d	63	↓ (p <0.05) ALT, ALP, AST in 3 cinnamon groups compared to CDR treatment group	Eidi et al. (2012)

Cinnamon (*Cinnamomum zeylanicum*)	water soluble phenols	Antidiabetic	36 animals were divided into six groups (Group 1 to 6) such that each group contains three animals per sex with similar weight, and treated with various cinnamon polyphenol extracts at 200 mg/kg BW and Glibenclamide at 5 mg/kg BW. was administered as the positive control (Group 4)	36	Improvement in blood sugar, serum insulin, lipid profile, and liver enzymes were observed among STZ-induced diabetic rats when supplemented with *Cinnamomum zeylanicum* extracts containing 45% polyphenol (procynZ-45) and 75% polyphenol content (procynZ-75), as compared to the standard aqueous extract containing 15% polyphenol	Krishnakumar et al. (2014)
Cumin (*Cuminum cyminum*)	Not defined	Antihypertensive	Hypertensive rats received 200 mg/kg BW of a cumin standardized aqueous extract for 9 wk	—	Improved plasma NO and ↓SBP in hypertensive rats	Kalaivani et al. (2013)
Fennel (*Foeniculum vulgare*)	Not defined	Antidiabetic	Albino Wistar rats were divided into 4 groups: Group 1: Control ($n = 4$); Group 2: Normal rats treated with the extract ($n = 4$); Group 3: Diabetic animals ($n = 4$); Group 4: diabetic rats ($n = 4$) treated with 100 mg/kg of *F. vulgare* extract for 14 d	16	*F. vulgare* partially restored levels of glucose in diabetic rats; ↓ BW; ↑ water intake	Mhaidat et al. (2015)

(continued)

Table 8.2 *(continued)*

Matrix	Bioactive compound	Properties	Study design	n	Mechanism of action	Ref.
Fennel (*Foeniculum vulgare*)	Not defined	Hepatoprotective	Albino Wistar rats were divided into 4 groups: Group 1: Control ($n = 4$); Group 2: Normal rats treated with the extract ($n = 4$); Group 3: Diabetic animals ($n = 4$); Group 4: diabetic rats ($n = 4$) treated with 100 mg/kg of *F. vulgare* extract for 14 d	16	Attenuation of the elevation of ALT and AST in diabetic rats	Mhaidat et al. (2015)
Ginger (*Zingiber officinale*)	Not defined	Anti-inflammatory	Arthritis induced rats were randomized and received orally water (control), indomethacin (1.0 mg/kg BW) or 200 mg/kg BW ginger rhizomes powder suspended in 1 ml of water for 28 d	54	↓ Blood total leucocyte, granulocyte and agranulocyte counts after treatment compared to healthy control group ($p < 0.05$); Modulation of the changes in IL-6 ($p < 0.001$) and anti-inflammatory cytokines ($p > 0.05$) of arthritic rats compared to healthy rats	Ramadan et al. (2011)
Mixes of different spices	Not defined	Digestive stimulation	Wistar rats weighing were maintained on three experimental diets along with a parallel basal control diet for 8 wk Mix I: coriander, turmeric, red chili, black pepper and cumin; Mix II: Mix I + ginger; Mix III: Mix I + onion	32	All the 3 spices mixes↑ activities of pancreatic lipase, chymotrypsin and amylase; stimulation of bile flow and of bile acid secretion. Mix III had the highest stimulatory influence particularly on bile secretion, bile acid output, and the activities of pancreatic enzymes.	Platel et al. (2002)

Mixes of different spices	Not defined	Digestive stimulation	Adult female Wistar rats were fed on diets containing (g %): curcumin (0.5), capsaicin (0.015), piperine (0.02), ginger (0.05), cumin (1.25), fenugreek (2.0), mustard (0.25), asafoetida (0.25), ajowan (0.2), fennel (0.5), coriander (2.0), mint (1.0), garlic (0.5), and onion (2.0) for 6 wk	—	All the test spices except fenugreek and mustard produced a significant (p <0.05) shortening of the food transit time.	Platel and Srinivasan (2001)
Mixes of different spices	Not defined	Digestive stimulation	Adults female Wistar rats ($n = 8$ per group) were provided by (i) a single intragastic dose mg/kg BW of cumin, 600; coriander, 400; ajowan, 80; fennel, 200; mint, 400; and garlic oil, 0.02 dose and (ii) a continued dietary intake: Groups of animals were maintained for 8 wk on the following spice diets: cumin (1.25%), coriander (2.0%), ajowan (0.2%), fennel (0.5%), mint (1.0%), and garlic (0.5%)	112	Dietary spices: Cumin, coriander, ajowan, fennel, and mint ↑ (p <0.05) the percentage of bile solids compared to control. Cumin, ajowan, and garlic ↑ (p <0.05) the bile flow rate compared to control. Oral administration: ajowan ↑ (p <0.05) the percentage of bile solids and cumin ↑ (p <0.05) the bile flow rate compared to control	Platel and Srinivasan (2000)
Rosemary (*Rosmarinus officinalis*)	Rosmarinic acid	Anti-inflammatory	Rosmarinic acid was administered at 10, 25, and 50 mg/kg, and the extract was administered at 10 and 25 mg/kg (equivalent doses to rosmarinic acid groups) to male Wistar rats (carrageenan-induced paw oedema model in the rat)	64	↓ Paw edema by 60% at the dose of 25 mg/kg of extract and rosmarinic acid compared with the control group exhibiting a dose–response effect.	Rocha et al. (2015)

(continued)

Table 8.2 (*continued*)

Matrix	Bioactive compound	Properties	Study design	n	Mechanism of action	Ref.
Rosemary (*Rosmarinus officinalis*)	Not defined	Antidiabetic	Male Sprague-Dawley rats that consumed Rosemary 70% ethanol extract as drinking water at 250 and 500 mg/kg BW	60	No difference in serum glucose	Nusier et al. (2007)
Rosemary (*Rosmarinus officinalis*)	Essential oils	Antidiabetic	Adult male Wistar rats were divided in 4 groups: group 1: Control treated with distilled water; Group 2: diabetic rats treated with distilled water; Group 3: non-diabetic rats treated with essential oils (30 mg/kg); Group 4: diabetic rats treated with essential oils (30 mg/kg.) for 15 d	48	↓ Blood glucose concentration ($p < 0.05$) in group of diabetic rats treated with essential oils from rosemary compared to diabetic control	Selmi et al. (2017)
Rosemary (*Rosmarinus officinalis*)	Not defined	Antiobesity	Male Sprague-Dawley rats that consumed Rosemary 70% ethanol extract as drinking water at 250 and 500 mg/kg BW	60	No difference in body weight	Nusier et al. (2007)
Rosemary (*Rosmarinus officinalis*)	Carnosic acid	Antiobesity	C57BL/6 J- ob/ob leptin-deficient mice ($n = 30$) were divided into 3 groups: 1 control group and 2 groups with diets containing 0.01 and 0.02% (w/w) of carnosic acid for 4 wk	30	↓BW and food intake ($p < 0.05$) in group fed with 0.02% of CA compared to control group	Park and Sung (2015)

Saffron (*Crocus sativus*)	Not defined	Hepatoprotective	Male Wistar rats were made diabetic with a single injection of streptozotocm. Rats were randomly separated into four groups: Group 1, healthy control rats; Group 2 non-diabetic rats were treated with 40 mg/kg BW/d mtrapentoneal (i.p.) injection of Saffron extract; Group 3, diabetic rats; Group 4, diabetic rats were treated with saffron extract (40 mg/kg BW/d, i.p.) for 8 wk	40	↓ ($p < 0.05$) MDA contents of the liver tissue and serum levels of ALT, AST, and bilirubin in Group 4 compared to Group 3	Rahbani et al. (2012)
Saffron (*Crocus sativus*)	Crocin	Hepatoprotective	Male Wistar rats consumed corn oil (control), DZN (15 mg/kg/d, orally) and crocin (12.5, 25, and 50 mg/kg/d, intraperitoneally in combination with DZN) for 4 wk	6	↓ ($p < 0.001$) MDA level in the group that received DZN plus 25 mg crocin	Lari et al. (2015)
Saffron (*Crocus sativus*)	Crocin	Hepatoprotective	Male Wistar rats were divided in 4 groups: control, acrylamide (25 mg/kg), crocin (50 mg/kg), acrylamide + crocin (25 mg/kg acrylamide and 50 mg/kg crocin) groups	40	↓ ($p < 0.05$) ALT, ALP, SOD, and CAT activities and MDA levels after crocin treatment	Gedik et al. (2017)

(continued)

Table 8.2 *(continued)*

Matrix	Bioactive compound	Properties	Study design	n	Mechanism of action	Ref.
Saffron (*Crocus sativus*)	Crocin	Hypolipidemic	Albino Wistar rats of either sex were used. The animals fed either with NFD or HFD were administered orally saffron (25, 50, and 100 mg/kg) or crocin (4.84, 9.69, and 19.38 mg/kg) in their respective groups for five consecutive days	112	NFD + 25 mg/kg saffron: ↓ TG, TC, LDL ($p < 0.05$); NFD + 50 and 100 mg/kg saffron: ↓ TG, TC, LDL ($p < 0.001$), ↑ HDL ($p < 0.05$ and $p < 0.001$, respectively) NFT + 4.84 mg/kg crocin: ↓ LDL ($p < 0.05$); NFD + 19.38 mg/kg crocin ↓ TG, TC, LDL, ↑ HDL ($p < 0.001$) 25, 50, and 100 mg/kg saffron: ↓ TG, TC, LDL ($p < 0.001$), ↑ HDL ($p < 0.01$ and $p < 0.001$, respectively) HFD + all concentration crocin: ↓ TG, TC, LDL ($p < 0.001$) HFD + 6.69 and 19.38 mg/kg crocin: ↑ HDL ($p < 0.05$ and $p < 0.05$, respectively)	Asdaq and Inamdar (2010)
Saffron (*Crocus sativus*)	Not defined	Digestive stimulation	Wistar rats were divided into 3 groups, N-L-Nitro-L- arginine methyl ester (LNAME) + saffron and control groups. In saffron group 100 mg/kg aqueous saffron extract was administered orally for 5 d	8	↑Basal and stimulated acid ($p = 0.006$) and peptin secretions ($p = 0.008$)	Nabavizadeh et al. (2009)

Turmeric (*Curcuma longa*)	Curcuminoids	Influence on Alzheimer's disease	Male, Sprague–Dawley rats were employed and different doses of the test compounds (mixture of curcuminoids: curcumin, bisdemethoxycurcumin, and demethoxycurcumin) were administered intra-peritoneally. Morris water maze test was carried out.	—	Curcuminoids and the individual components had inhibitory effect ($p < 0.05$) in the ex vivo AChE assay and exhibited memory enhancing effect in Morris water maze test	Ahmed and Gilani (2009)
Turmeric (*Curcuma longa*)	Curcumin	Antihypertensive	Wistar rats were administered for 6 wk clear water or L-NAME (40 mg/kg/d) dissolved in water, piperine (20 mg/kg/d), curcumin (100 mg/kg/d) or their combination in corn oil by oral gavage	48	↓ ($p < 0.01$) SBP by 28.9 mm Hg at the end of the experiment compared to control	Hlavačková et al. (2011)
Turmeric (*Curcuma longa*)	Curcumin	Anti-inflammatory	Male and female Wistar rats with induced colitis were randomly divided and 25–100 mg/kg of curcumin was administered by gavage 48, 24, and 1 h prior to the induction of colitis and 24 h later	—	↓ degree of colonic injury, the index of neutrophil infiltration, Th1 cytokine secretion, colonic levels of nitrites, and reduced COX-2 and iNOS overexpression; ↑ IL-10 production.	Sánchez-Calvo et al. (2009)

(continued)

Table 8.2 *(continued)*

Matrix	Bioactive compound	Properties	Study design	n	Mechanism of action	Ref.
Turmeric (*Curcuma longa*)	Not defined	Anti-inflammatory	Arthritis induced rats were randomized and received orally water (control), indomethacin (1.0 mg/kg BW) or 200 mg/kg BW turmeric powder suspended in 1 ml of water for 28 d	54	↓blood total leucocyte, granulocyte and agranulocyte counts after treatment compared to healthy control group ($p < 0.05$); Completely modulation in pro-inflammatory and anti-inflammatory cytokines of arthritic rats compared to healthy rats	Ramadan et al. (2011)
Turmeric (*Curcuma longa*)	Curcumin	Antiobesity	Rats were divided into four groups (*n* = 6 per group). A normal diet group comprised rats fed the AIN76A rodent diet; a high-fat diet-induced obese group comprised rats fed a 60% high-fat diet; a *Garcinia cambogia* treated group (positive control) comprised rats fed a 60% high-fat diet with *G. cambogia* 500 g/kg BW/d; and a fermented *C. longa* treated group comprised rats fed a 60% high-fat diet with FCE50 500 g/kg BW/d.	24	16% reduction in body weight gain; 31% reduction in organ WAT weight	Kim et al. (2016)

ALP, alkaline phosphate; ALT, alanine aminotransferase; AST, aminotransferase; BP, Blood pressure; BW, Body weight; CAT, Catalase; CC14, Carbon tetrachloride; CDR, Clinical Dementia Rating; COX-2, cyclo-oxygenase 2; DOCA, Deoxycorticosterone acetate; DZN, Diazinon; HDL, High density lipoprotein; HFD, high fat diet; HR, Heart rate; IL, Interleukin; iNOS, Inducible nitric oxide synthase; LDL, Low density lipoprotein; MDA, Malondialdehyde; NFD, Normal fat diet; NO, Nitric oxide; SBP, Systolic blood pressure; SOD, Superoxido dismutase; TG, Triglycerides; WAT, White adipose tissue.

Table 8.3 Clinical studies based on herb and spice consumption

Matrix	Bioactive compound	Properties	Study design	n	Mechanism of action	Ref.
Bay (*Laurus nobilis*)	Not defined	Antidiabetic	People with T2DM were divided in 4 groups: groups with given capsules containing 1, 2, or 3 g of bay leaves and placebo and placebo for 30 d.	40	Significant (p 0.05)↓ serum glucose, TC and LDL in volunteers who consumed 1, 2, or 3 g of bay; ↑HDL and ↓ TG in volunteers who consumed 1 and 2 g of bay	Khan et al. (2009)
Bay (*Laurus nobilis*)	Not defined	Antidiabetic	Randomized crossover study in which 20 volunteers consumed cookies supplemented with 3 or 6% of bay leaf extract	20	↓ Blood glucose concentration at 30 ($p = 0.014$) and 45 ($p = 0.010$) min in group who consumed cookies with 6% of bay leaf extract compared to control	Khan et al. (2017)
Black cumin (*Nigella sativa*)	Not defined	Anticancer	40 children with acute lymphoblastic leukemia were divided into 2 groups: Group I: 20 patients under methotrexate therapy and Black seeds 80 mg/kg/d for 1 wk; Group 2: 20 patients under methotrexate therapy and placebo. Control group: 20 healthy children of matched age and sex as a control group	60	Significant differences in prognosis regarding remission, relapse, death, and disease-free survival	Hagag et al. (2013)

(continued)

Table 8.3 *(continued)*

Matrix	Bioactive compound	Properties	Study design	n	Mechanism of action	Ref.
Chili (*Capsicum annuum* L.)	Capsinoids	Antiobesity	12-wk, placebo-controlled, double-blind, randomized study. Forty overweight or obese women and 40 men were randomly assigned to a capsinoid (6 mg/d) or placebo group	80	Abdominal adiposity decreased more ($p = 0.049$) in the capsinoid group ($-1.11 \pm 1.83\%$) than in the placebo group ($-0.18 \pm 1.94\%$); ↓BW ($p < 0.0001$) in capsinoid group; fat oxidation was higher at the end of the study in the capsinoid group	Snitker et al. (2008)
Cinnamon (Cinnamomum zeylanicum)	Not defined	Antiobesity	A double blind, randomized, placebo controlled clinical trial was conducted on patients with T2DM. Participants were randomly assigned to take either 3 g/d cinnamon supplement ($n = 22$) or a placebo ($n = 22$) for 8 wk.	44	↓ BW, BMI, fat body mass ($p < 0.05$) after intervention in cinnamon group.	Vafa et al. (2012)
Cinnamon (*Cinnamomum zeylanicum*)	Not defined	Antidiabetic	Randomized placebo-controlled trial with 60 volunteers who were divided into 6 groups: Groups 1, 2, and 3 consumed 1, 3, or 6 g of cinnamon daily, respectively, and groups 4, 5, and 6 were given placebo capsules for 5 wk	60	Significant ($p < 0.05$)↓ in FPG, serum glucose, TG, LDL, TC	Khan et al. (2003)

Cinnamon (*Cinnamomum zeylanicum*)	Polyphenol type-A polymers	Antidiabetic	Pre-diabetic and metabolic syndrome volunteers were randomly assigned to supplement their diet with 500 mg of Cinnulin PF® (2 capsules/d) for 12 wk ($n = 12$). Placebo group ($n = 10$).	22	↓ FBG ($p < 0.01$), SBP ($p < 0.001$) and body fat ($p < 0.02$). ↑lean mass ($p < 0.02$) in Cinnulin PF® group compared to control	Ziegenfuss et al. (2006)
Cloves (*Eugenia aromaticum*)	Not defined	Antidiabetic	Thirty-six people, with T2DM were divided into 4 groups and given capsules containing 0, 1, 2, or 3 g of cloves/d for 30 d followed by a 10 d washout period. Since the responses to the three levels of cloves were not significantly different, the three groups were combined	36	↓ Serum glucose in control group, no significant changes in the placebo group	Khan et al. (2006)
Cloves (*Eugenia aromaticum*)	Cinnamaldehyde, eugenol, allicin and curcumin	Hypolipidemic	Mild to moderate hyperlipidemics volunteers were divided into 3 groups ($n = 15$ each): 2 supplementation groups, one with cloves (500 mg/d) and one with turmeric (500 mg/d) and control group for 3 mo	45	↓ ($p < 0.01$) TC, TG, LDL and VLDL and ↑ ($p < 0.01$) HDL	Balasasirekha and Lakshmi (2012)

Table 8.3 (*continued*)

Matrix	Bioactive compound	Properties	Study design	n	Mechanism of action	Ref.
Cloves (*Eugenia aromaticum*)	Not defined	Hypolipidemic	Thirty-six people, with type 2 DM were divided into 4 groups and given capsules containing 0, 1, 2, or 3 g of cloves/d for 30 d followed by a 10 d washout period. Since the responses to the three levels of cloves were not significantly different, the three groups were combined	36	↓ TG, TC, LDL, ~HDL in treatment group, no significant changes in the placebo group	Khan et al. (2006)
Garlic (*Allium sativum*)	Allicin	Hypolipidemic	Single-blind, placebo controlled study carried out in hyperlipidemic patients. They were divided in 3 groups ($n = 50$ each): enteric-coated garlic powder tablet (equal to 400 mg garlic, 1 mg allicin) twice daily, anethum tablet (650 mg) twice daily, and placebo tablet for 6-wk	150	↓ TC, LDL and ↑ HDL $p = 0.000$. No significant changes in TG ($p = 0.222$)	Kojuri et al. (2007)
Garlic (*Allium sativum*)	Allicin	Hypolipidemic	Randomized double-blinded crossover design in which volunteers (serum cholesterol>250 gm/dc) were divided into two groups: 45 were in the trial group (take garlic tablets) and the remaining 55 in the control group in the first 3 mo, placebo in the second 3 mo and discontinue all tablets in the last 3 mo (total = 9 mo)	100	No significant differences in the TC levels between the two groups at the end of the study	Tanamai et al. (2004)

Garlic (*Allium sativum*)	Not defined	Hypolipidemic	Adults with LDL-C concentrations of 130 to 190 mg/dl were randomly assigned to 1 of the following 4 treatment arms: raw garlic, powdered garlic supplement, aged garlic extract supplement, or placebo for 6 mo	192	No statistically significant effects of the 3 forms of garlic on LDL-C, HDL, TG or TC plasma concentrations	Gardner et al. (2007)
Garlic (*Allium sativum*)	Allicin	Antihypertensive	Double-blind parallel randomized placebo-controlled trial in patients with uncontrolled hypertension who consumed 4 capsules of aged garlic extract (960 mg containing 2.4 mg S-allylcysteine) daily for 12 wk	50	↓ Blood pressure by 10.2 ± 4.3 mm Hg ($p = 0.03$) in garlic group compared to control	Ried (2011)
Ginger (*Zingiber officinale*)	Not defined	Hypolipidemic	Double blind controlled multicenter clinical trial study carried out in patients with hyperlipidemia treatment group (receiving ginger capsules 3 g/d in 3 divided doses) and placebo group for 45 d	85	↓ ($p < 0.05$) TG, TC, LDL, and VLDL in treatment group	Alizadeh-Navaei et al. (2008)
Ginger (*Zingiber officinale*)	Not defined	Anticancer	Obese woman with breast cancer were randomly assigned into four groups; placebo, water-based exercise, ginger supplement and water-based exercise + ginger supplement groups. Inger supplementation consisted on 4 capsules (750 mg each)/7 d a week for 6 wk	40	Ginger supplementation: significant increase of GPx ($p < 0.05$); Water-based exercise + ginger: significant increase of adiponectin, GPx, NO, MDA	Karimi and Roshan (2013)

(continued)

Table 8.3 *(continued)*

Matrix	Bioactive compound	Properties	Study design	n	Mechanism of action	Ref.
Ginger (*Zingiber officinale*)	Not defined	Antidiabetic	Randomized, double-blind, placebo-controlled trial in which 88 participants affected by diabetes were randomly assigned into ginger (GG) and placebo (PG) groups. The GG received 3 one-gram capsules containing ginger powder whereas the PG received 3 one-gram microcrystalline-containing capsules daily for 8 wk.	88	↓ The mean of FBG by 10.5% ($p = 0.003$); ↑ the mean of FBG by 21% in the PG ($p = 0.01$). Variation in HbA1c mean was in line with that of FBS. Statistical difference was found in the two groups before and after the intervention in terms of median of fasting insulin level, S%, and HOMA-IR ($p < 0.005$).	Mozaffari-Khosravi et al. (2014)
Onion (*Allium cepa*)	Not defined	Anticancer	Daily intake of 20 g of fresh garlic	—	Reduction of nitrite formation by the inhibition of nitrate-reducing bacteria	Xing et al. (1982)
Onion (*Allium cepa*)	Not defined	Anticancer	Three periods were designed. Period 1: basal diet; Period 2: basal diet +300 mg of sodium nitrate in water and 500 mg of L-proline; Period 3: 5 g of garlic pieces in capsules + basal diet + sodium nitrate and proline	9	Significantly reduction ($p < 0.01$) of amount of N-nitrosoprolien when garlic is consumed	Xing et al. (1989)

Onion (*Allium cepa*)	Not defined	Antidiabetic	T1DM and T2DM diabetic patients consumed 100 g of the crude fresh slices of *Allium cepa*	42	Ingestion of *Allium cepa* reduces FBG levels by 40 mg/dl, compared to glibenclamide (81 mg/dl)	Taj Eldin et al. (2010)
Rosemary (*Rosmarinus officinalis*)	Not defined	Hypolipidemic	Healthy adults were randomly selected and given 2, 5, or 10 g/d of rosemary leaves powder for a period of 8 wk	48	↓ TC and TG in the three treated groups ($p < 0.01$). ↓ LDLc ($p < 0.01$) and ↑HDLc ($p = 0.023$) in the group given 10 g of the herb powder, ↓ fasting serum glucose the group given 5 and 10 g ($p < 0.01$).	Labban et al. (2014)
Rosemary (*Rosmarinus officinalis*)	Essential oil	Antihypertensive	Prospective study in which patients with primary hypotension received in the first stage 1 ml placebo (olive oil) every 8 h; 2nd stage 1 ml rosemary essential oil every 8 h and 3th stage 1 ml placebo every 8 h.	32	↑ SBP values is observed during the first stage which is maintained during treatment with Rosemary essential oil and which ↓ after this period.	Fernández et al. (2014)
Rosemary (*Rosmarinus officinalis*)	Not defined	Influence on Alzheimer's disease	Double-blinded randomized controlled trial where 68 participating students randomly received 500 mg rosemary and placebo twice daily for 1 mo	68	Enhancement of prospective and retrospective memory	(Nematolahi et al. 2018)

(continued)

Table 8.3 *(continued)*

Matrix	Bioactive compound	Properties	Study design	n	Mechanism of action	Ref.
Sage (*Salvia officinalis*)	Not defined	Influence on Alzheimer's disease	Four-month, parallel group, placebo-controlled trial were participants with mild-AD were randomly assigned to receive either *Salvia officinalis* extract using a fixed dose (60 drops/d) or no treatment during each 10-d period	111	Better outcome on cognitive functions than placebo (ADAS-cog $p = 0.03$ and CDR-SB $p < 0.003$)	Akhondzadeh et al. (2003)
Turmeric (*Curcuma longa*)	Curcumin	Anticancer	A dose-escalation pilot study of a standardized formulation of turmeric extract (220-mg capsule of P54FP contained 18 mg of curcumin and 2 mg of desmethoxycurcumin suspended in 200 mg of turmeric essential oils) in patients with advanced colorectal cancer	15	Dose-dependent inhibition of basal and LPS-induced PGE_2	Plummer et al. (2001)
Turmeric (*Curcuma longa*)	Curcumin	Anticancer	Phase II trial in which patients with pancreatic cancer took 8 g curcumin by mouth daily until disease progression	25	Downregulation of the expression of NF-κB, cyclooxygenase-2, and phosphorylated signal transducer and activator of transcription 3 in peripheral blood mononuclear cells	Dhillon et al. (2008)

Turmeric (*Curcuma longa*)	Curcumin	Anticancer	Patients under treatment for solid tumors were enrolled in a controlled study to assess its efficacy in alleviating the side effects of cancer chemo- and radiotherapy using a semi-quantitative evaluation (visual analogue scale) of the side effects, assessing also the plasma free radical status in all patients	160	Lecithinized curcumin might alleviate the burden of side effects associated to chemo- and radiotherapy	Belcaro et al. (2014)
Turmeric (*Curcuma longa*)	Malondialdehyde	Antidiabetic	Standard metformin treatment with turmeric supplementation (2 g)	60	Turmeric has a beneficial effect on blood glucose, oxidative stress, and inflammation	Selvi et al. (2015)
Turmeric (*Curcuma longa*)	Curcumin	Influence on Alzheimer's disease	Patients with AD consumed curcumin 1 g daily or 3 g daily or placebo for 6 mo	34	No differences on MMSE scores or β-amyloid plasma levels among groups	Baum et al. (2008)
Turmeric (*Curcuma longa*)	Curcumin	Influence on Alzheimer's disease	22 patients with AD and 11 controls consumed curcumin 2 g daily or 4 g daily or placebo for 6 mo	33	No differences on cognitive performance and plasma CSF biomarkers	Ringman et al. (2012)

AD, Alzehimer's disease; ADAS-cog, Alzheimer's Disease Assessment Scale; BMI, Body mass index; BW, Body weight; CDR-SB, Clinical Dementia Rating Sum of Boxes; CSF, Cerebrospinal fluid; FPG, Fasting plasma glucose; GPx, Glutation peroxidase; HDL, High density lipoprotein; LDL, Low density lipoprotein; LPS, Lipopolysaccharide; MDA, Malondialdehyde; MMSE, Mini-Mental State Examination; NO, Nitric oxide; PGE_2, Prostaglandin E2; SBP, Systolic blood pressure; T2DM, Type 2 diabetes mellitus; TG, Triglycerides; VLDL, Very low density lipoprotein.

and lipopolysaccharide (LPS)-induced PGE_2 values, highlighting the importance of developing a useful biomarker of drug efficacy based on COX-2 assessment (Plummer et al. 2001). Additionally, in a more recent phase II trial, 25 patients with pancreatic cancer experienced a downregulation of the expression of COX-2. Likewise, they were shown to downregulate the nuclear factor (NF)-κB, phosphorylated signal transducer and activator of transcription 3 in peripheral blood mononuclear cells (Dhillon et al. 2008). Despite the fact that curcumin presents limited absorption due to its low water solubility, it has proven to be well-tolerated, safe, and biologically active in some types of cancer (Adiwidjaja et al. 2017; Kunnumakkara et al. 2017a).

In itself, garlic is popularly recognized as health promoter. In the case of its anticancer properties, Xing et al. (1982) had already observed that the mortality from gastric cancer in one area of China, where the consumption of garlic was 20 g/d, was significantly lower than in areas where garlic was not commonly included in the diet. This may be explained by the reduction of nitrite formation due to the inhibition of nitrate-reducing bacteria. Nitrates, nitrites, and nitrosamines have been potentially related to the risk of suffering several cancers and especially linked to gastric cancer (Song et al. 2015). The blocking effect of N-nitroso compounds in the human body was later supported by Xing et al., who demonstrated this effect when 5 g of fresh garlic was consumed per day (Xing et al. 1982). One of the main bioactive compounds in garlic is allicin, an organosulfur compound that has been demonstrated to be a promising candidate to treat several diseases (Borlinghaus et al. 2014). Other works carried out with allicin have revealed it induces the expression of pro-apoptotic protein *in vitro* in colon, breast, and gastric cancer cells (Bat-Chen et al. 2010; Zhang et al. 2010; Shao et al. 2012; Rahimi-Moghaddam et al. 2015). However, clinical and preclinical trials are still needed to confirm its role in cancer prevention or treatment.

Black cumin (*Nigella sativa*) gave an improved prognosis for leukemia remission and disease-free survival in children, in comparison to the control group (Hagag et al. 2013). The etiology of cancer has been also associated with continued oxidative stress, which can lead to chronic inflammation (Reuter et al. 2010). Some spices, e.g. ginger (*Zingiber officinale*), have verified their clinical relevance in improving adiponectin and biomarkers related to oxidative stress, e.g. adiponectin or glutation peroxidase in obese women with breast cancer when they took 3 g/d for six weeks (Karimi and Roshan 2013). However, despite the fact that ginger has been traditionally employed for treating nausea (Palatty et al. 2013), recent clinical studies have failed to demonstrate the reduction of nausea severity in patients with breast and ovarian cancers (Shokri et al. 2017; Thamlikitkul et al. 2017).

8.3.2 Anti-inflammatory Properties

Inflammation plays an important role in various diseases with high prevalence within populations, such as atherosclerosis or asthma. It is well-known that during inflammation, different mediators, e.g. pro-inflammatory cytokines such as interleukin (IL)-1, tumor necrosis factor (TNF), interferon (INF)-γ, IL-6, IL-12, IL-18, and the granulocyte–macrophage colony-stimulating factor, are released (Mueller et al. 2010). In this regard, Ghasemian et al. (2016) reviewed the anti-inflammatory effects of a few herbs highlighting the potential role of herbs in activation or inhibition of pro-inflammatory cytokines. Among herbs and spices, one of the most studied so far has been turmeric. It has been shown to increase the anti-inflammatory cytokine IL-10 and to decrease the degree of colonic injury in Wistar rats with induced ulcerative colitis (Sánchez-Calvo et al. 2009). Turmeric also showed a significant anti-arthritic activity by alleviating hind paw erythema or oedema, cellular toxicity, loss in body weight or bone marrow, and spleen hypertrophy, among other effects, in animal models (Ramadan et al. 2011). Specifically, 200 mg/kg body weight (BW) of turmeric powder modulated the changes in pro- and anti-inflammatory cytokines of arthritic rats. Similar effects but to a lesser extent were found in the same study when 200 mg/kg BW of ginger rhizome powder was administered to the arthritis-induced rats. Additionally, 25 mg/kg of rosemary (*Rosmarinus officinalis*) extract and its isolated bioactive compound rosmarinic acid showed a reduction by 60% of paw edema in carrageenan-induced paw edema Wistar rats compared to control, exhibiting a dose-response effect (Rocha et al. 2015). Among the reviewed herbs and spices, turmeric is the most promising spice as regards the treatment of inflammatory disorders. Despite several clinical trials registered on the clinicaltrials .gov webpage regarding inflammation and turmeric, there is a lack of relevant results that have already been published.

8.3.3 Antidiabetic Properties

According to the latest global report on diabetes from the WHO, it is a fact that diabetes is on the rise: 422 million adults were living with diabetes in 2014, compared to 108 million in 1980 (WHO 2016). Before the introduction of insulin as a therapeutic treatment for diabetes, diet was the only way to treat this disease. According to Yeh and Dham, 400 herbs and plant preparations are reported to have beneficial effects in dealing with diabetes mellitus illness (Yeh et al. 2003; Dham et al. 2006). Among them, cinnamon *(Cinnamomum cassia)* showed significant improvement ($p < 0.05$) in Streptozotocin (STZ)-induced diabetic rats in blood sugar, serum insulin, lipid profile, and liver enzymes, when a cinnamon extract containing 45% and 75% of phenolic compounds was consumed compared to the control (aqueous extract containing 15% of phenolic compounds) (Krishnakumar et al. 2014). Similar results were found by Khan et al. in a double-blind randomized controlled trial conducted in 60 volunteers with type 2 diabetes mellitus (T2DM) who consumed 1, 3, or 6 g of cinnamon daily for five weeks, showing that all three levels of cinnamon consumption significantly reduced fasting plasma glucose, triglycerides (TG), total cholesterol (TC), and low-density lipoprotein (LDL) (Khan et al. 2003). Moreover, there are nutraceuticals made up with cinnamon already on the market, which have been also clinically tested, i.e. Cinnulin PF®, a water-soluble cinnamon extract. Twenty-two prediabetic and metabolic syndrome volunteers received 500 mg of Cinnulin PF® daily, which is equivalent to approximately 10 g of whole cinnamon powder, for 12 weeks. The results demonstrated that fasting blood glucose (FBG), systolic blood pressure (SBP), and body fat were significantly reduced ($p < 0.01$; $p < 0.001$; $p < 0.02$, respectively) compared to control (Ziegenfuss et al. 2006). The intake of 1, 2, or 3 g of cloves (*Syzygium aromaticum*) per day for 30 days has also shown a positive response in decreasing serum glucose in a clinical trial of 36 volunteers with T2DM (Khan et al. 2006). The results obtained by Mozaffari-Khosravi et al. (2014) were in line with this. They conducted a clinical trial including 88 T2DM volunteers who consumed a 1 g capsule of ginger powder daily for 8 weeks, concluding that the intake of the 1 g capsule of ginger ameliorated the glycemic status of the participants via improving insulin resistance indices and decreasing FBG and glycated hemoglobin (HbA1c). Additionally, fresh red onion (*Allium cepa*) has been considered as a potential dietary supplement in the management of type 1 diabetes (T1DM) and DMT2 due to its capacity to reduce FBG levels by about 89 mg/dl in relation to insulin (145 mg/dl), and by 40 mg/dl, compared to glibenclamide (81 mg/dl) in type 1 diabetic patients and type 2 diabetic patients, respectively (Taj Eldin et al. 2010). Treatment with supplementation of turmeric on T2DM metformin patients ($n = 60$) was also effective for FBG and HbA1c reduction, together with a significant improvement in the lipid profile of participants (Selvi et al. 2015).

Additionally, studies demonstrating the insulin-enhancing activity of bay (*Laurus nobilis*) leaves are emerging. In this regard, low levels (1–3 g/d) of bay leaves, consumed in capsules, significantly ($p < 0.05$) reduced serum glucose and improved the lipid profile in 40 volunteers with T2DM (Khan et al. 2009). In a recent study, the same authors tested the effect of supplemented cookies containing 3% (w/w) bay leaf powder, and cookies containing 6% (w/w) bay leaf powder in postprandial glycemia in 20 volunteers (Khan et al. 2017). Results showed a significant reduction in blood glucose concentration at 30 and 45 minutes in the group who took the cookies which contained 6% of bay leaf powder compared to the control group. Conversely, the role of rosemary as an antidiabetic may remain controversial. Despite some authors concluding that this plant has antidiabetic effect, mainly attributable to its composition in phenolic diterpenes and phenolic acids, e.g. carnosol and rosmarinic acid (Sedighi et al. 2015), other *in vivo* studies carried out in male Sprague-Dawley rats that consumed rosemary 70% ethanol extract as drinking water at 250 and 500 mg/kg BW failed to find differences in serum glucose (Nusier et al. 2007). Nevertheless, a latest *in vivo* study showed the effectiveness of an intake of 30 mg/kg of essential oils from rosemary in induced-diabetic adult male Wistar rats in blood sugar reduction ($p < 0.05$) (Selmi et al. 2017). Thus, it is crucial to determine the composition of rosemary and choose the correct bioactive compounds before carrying out additional clinical trials that help to determine the mechanism underpinning the observed physiological effects in animal models.

Fennel (*Foeniculum vulgare*) is a well-known Mediterranean aromatic plant which has been employed as a spice in TM as a diuretic or analgesic (Choi and Hwang 2004). However, recent *in vivo* studies have demonstrated that fennel could also have positive effects in treating diabetes via restored levels of glucose and enhancing some of the CV complications associated with diabetes. The positive effects could be attributable to its composition in triterpenes, steroids, phenolic compounds, and saponins (Mhaidat et al. 2015). However, despite these promising results, further preclinical and clinical studies are necessary to confirm the real effect of fennel in treating diabetes.

Not only have the abovementioned herbs and spices demonstrated antidiabetic properties, but also in a pilot, double-blind, placebo-controlled, randomized clinical trial, the combination of *Lagerstroemia speciosa, Berberis aristata,* and turmeric with alpha-lipoic acid and folic acid showed a significant improvement in TG, high-density lipoprotein (HDL), fasting plasma insulin (FPI), and homeostatic model assessment (HOMA)-Index in 40 adult subjects with impaired fasting glucose (Cicero et al. 2017). Thus, the potential synergic effect of one or more herbs and spices should not be forgotten.

8.3.4 Antiobesity Properties

Traditionally, obesity has not been considered a disease to be treated. However, currently it is considered a global epidemic of the developed world (Rodríguez-Pérez et al. 2017). Despite the increasing interest in finding bioactive compounds from plants capable of helping obesity management, only a few *in vivo* studies have demonstrated the antiobesity effect of herbs and spices. In the case of rosemary, Park et al. evaluated the effect on the thymus and spleen of genetically obese (C57BL/6 J- ob/ob) leptin-deficient mice ($n = 30$) fed carnosic acid, one of the main bioactive compounds from rosemary. They found that mice fed with 0.02% (w/w) of carnosic acid, decreased BW and food intake in a significant way ($p < 0.05$) (Park and Sung 2015). Conversely, Nusier et al. (2007) failed to find a decrease in BW in male Sprague-Dawley rats that consumed rosemary 70% ethanol extract as drinking water at 250 and 500 mg/kg. Despite the different results described, it should not be forgotten that the mechanism of action will depend not only on the studied extract but also on the animal model that is employed for the study (Rodríguez-Pérez et al. 2017). The potential role of rosemary in obesity has been recently reviewed by Hassani et al. (Hassani et al. 2016). In spite of the high *in vitro* and *in vivo* antiobesity evidence of rosemary, once again the authors concluded with the necessity of performing clinical studies that confirm the effectiveness and safety of rosemary in humans. In another *in vivo* study, the administration of 500 g/kg BW/day of a 50% ethanolic fermented turmeric extract in high-fat diet-induced obese rats showed a significant 16% reduction ($p < 0.05$) in BW gain and reduction (by 31%; $p < 0.05$) in organ white adipose tissue (Kim et al. 2016). However, information that supports the clinical abovementioned effects is scarce. On the other hand, a double-blind, randomized, placebo-controlled clinical trial showed that the intake of 3 g/day of cinnamon significantly reduced ($p < 0.05$) BW, body mass index (BMI), and fat body mass in patients with T2DM (Vafa et al. 2012).

Currently, brown adipose tissue is emerging as a promising target to treat obesity (Rodríguez-Pérez et al. 2017). In spite of the controversy regarding the existence of this tissue in human adults, different bioactive compounds – e.g. capsainoids from red pepper (*Capsicum annuum*) – are being investigated due to their capability of activating thermogenesis, increasing energy expenditure (Kang et al. 2010; Ono et al. 2011). Results from a double-blind, randomized, placebo-controlled trial carried out in 80 overweight or obese volunteers, who were randomized to take 6 g/d of capsinoids from red pepper for 12 weeks, revealed the suitability of these compounds for decreasing abdominal fat and BW, and increasing fat oxidation (Snitker et al. 2008). However, not enough sets of well-designed trials supporting the antiobesity effect of phenolic compound-based products are available. Hence, more effort and longer intervention trials are necessary to confirm or complete the results already published.

8.3.5 Hypolipidemic Properties

Hyperlipidaemia is defined as an abnormally elevated level of any or all lipids or lipoproteins in the blood. According to the data provided by the Global Health Observatory (GHO) and from the WHO, a third of ischemic heart disease is attributable to high cholesterol, and raised cholesterol is estimated to cause 2.6 million deaths. Together with obesity, hyperlipidemia is considered a CV risk factor

(Wilson et al. 2002) and, on its own, it is considered the major risk factor for suffering atherosclerosis (Kojuri et al. 2007).

Among herbs and spices, garlic is probably one of the most promoted cholesterol-lowering agents. However, conflicting results can be found in the literature. A randomized double-blind crossover study failed to find any significant difference in TC concentrations after the intake of garlic tablets containing 500 mg of allicin for nine months (Tanamai et al. 2004). It is remarkable that even though Tanamai and co-authors employed more concentrated tablets, the results were not significant in terms of total cholesterol concentrations compared to those showed by Kojuri et al. (Kojuri et al. 2007). These negative findings were supported by another trial that was conducted employing raw garlic and two different commercial tablets in 192 patients with high levels of serum LDL cholesterol (Gardner et al. 2007). In this study, no significant changes in LDL, HDL, TG, and TC were found with any of the three garlic treatments. However, a clinical trial carried out in 150 hyperlipidemic patients showed a significant reduction in TC, LDL, and a significant increase of HDL after the intake of enteric-coated garlic powder tablets, equal to 400 mg of garlic, which contained 1 mg of allicin (Kojuri et al. 2007). In spite of the non-conclusive results, a more recent meta-analysis which included 26 studies, conducted in 2012, concluded that garlic powder and aged garlic extract could reduce TC, while garlic oil could be more effective for TG level reduction (Zeng et al. 2012).

Fewer studies, but with positive results regarding the clinical effect of ginger and cloves on lipid plasma composition, are available. In this regard, 3 g/day of ginger significantly improved the TG, TC, LDL, and very low-density lipoprotein (VLDL) plasma composition ($p < 0.05$) in hyperlipidemic patients after treatment, but not compared to placebo group except for TC and TG (Alizadeh-Navaei et al. 2008). This effect could be attributed to the capacity of ginger to inhibit cholesterol biosynthesis, which is related to plasma LDL reduction (Fuhrman et al. 2000). Additionally, cloves have also demonstrated their hypolipidemic effect in 45 mild to moderate hyperlipidemic volunteers: 500 mg of cloves in the form of four capsules a day for a period of three months reduced TC, TG, LDL, and VLDL and increased HDL (Balasasirekha and Lakshmi 2012). This could be explained by its high composition in bioactive compounds, i.e. cinnamaldehyde (19.6 mg), eugenol (0.04 mg), allicin (1.39 mg), and curcumin (0.09 mg). Moreover, in agreement with the previous work, similar results were displayed in a study that involved 36 patients with T2DM given capsules containing 0, 1, 2, or 3 g of cloves/d for 30 days, except for HDL which did not change its concentration in a significant way after the treatment (Khan et al. 2006).

Again, as has been proven in other herbs and spices, the synergistic behavior of bioactive compounds from plant matrices was manifested in an *in vivo* study with saffron (*Crocus sativus*) and its isolated carotenoid crocin (Asdaq and Inamdar 2010). In this study, the intake of a normal fat diet supplemented with 25 mg/kg saffron showed decreasing TG ($p < 0.05$), TC ($p < 0.05$), and LDL ($p < 0.01$) compared to a control group. More promising results were shown when animals with a normal fat diet were supplemented with 50 and 100 mg/kg saffron in terms of TG, TC, and LDL decrease ($p < 00.001$) and HDL increase (50 mg/kg, $p < 0.05$; 100 mg/kg, $p < 0.001$). Similar results were found in animals fed a high-fat diet, despite being supplemented with crocin, that also showed good hypolipidemic results. Thus, the use of entire saffron was more effective, and this may be explained by the synergistic behavior of the bioactive compounds present in it.

8.3.6 Influence on Digestive Stimulation

Several spices, including anise (*Pimpinella anisum*) seeds, black pepper (*Piper nigrum*), cardamom (*Elettaria cardamomum*), clove, cinnamon, coriander (*Coriandrum sativum*), cumin, fennel, turmeric, garlic, ginger, and mint (*Mentha spicata*), have been traditionally employed against digestive disorders (Platel and Srinivasan 2004). However, it has not been until recent years that the effects of these compounds have started to be investigated *in vitro* and *in vivo*. One of the most accepted theories regarding digestive stimulation resides in the capacity of some spices to stimulate the activity of enzymes responsible for digestion, i.e. amylase, lipase, and chymotrypsin. In this context, an early study of Ramakrishna et al. (2003) investigated the effect of different spices on digestive enzyme activities and demonstrated the effect of several spices – garlic, onion, ginger, mint, fennel, or cumin – on pancreatic digestive enzymes (lipase, amylase, and chymotrypsin) stimulation. They showed that a lower concentration (0.1 mg) of garlic, onion, ginger, fennel, or mint appeared to exert a beneficial influence on digestion, increasing the lipase activity, while the same concentration of coriander, mustard (*Brassica juncea*), and cumin increased (p <0.05) the amylase activity. Moreover, 1 mg of garlic, onion, ginger, coriander, mustard, or mint increased the amylase activity and 1 mg of fennel and showed a significant increase in lipase activity. The majority of these herbs and spices did not show an effect on chymotrypsin activity, except for the addition of 1 mg of garlic, ginger, or mint that significantly decreased its activity (Ramakrishna et al. 2003). Nabavizadeh et al. (2009) also found a significant increase in basal and stimulated acid and peptin secretions ($p = 0.006$ and $p = 0.008$, respectively) in Wistar rats that consumed 100 mg/kg of aqueous saffron extract.

Animal studies have revealed that a good number of spices can enhance the secretion of bile with higher bile acid content (Srinivasan 2005). Bile secretion is important in the digestion process for fat emulsification and absorption. Platel and co-authors performed a study aimed to determine the effect of several spices, i.e. cumin, coriander, ajowan (*Trachyspermum ammi*), fennel, mint, and garlic on bile acid secretion through a dietary study and a single dose study (Platel and Srinivasan 2000). For this, they employed eight adult female Wistar rats per group and tested a single intragastic dose five times the concentration normally employed in traditional pharmacological preparations or dietary treatment for eight weeks. They found that a single dosage of ajowan and cumin had a significant positive influence on bile flow rate and in the percentage of bile solids, respectively (Platel and Srinivasan 2000).

The synergistic effect of different mixes of spices – i.e. coriander, turmeric, red chili (*Capsicum annuum*), black pepper, cumin, ginger, and onion – also demonstrated their positive effect on amylase, lipase, and chymotrypsin enhancement in Wistar rats compared to control (Platel et al. 2002). The abovementioned mixes of spices stimulated the secretion of bile acid and bile flow, thus allowing better fat digestion and absorption (Platel et al. 2002).

The beneficial influence of some spices on digestive enzyme stimulation or bile secretion has been directly correlated with the reduction of food transit time (Platel and Srinivasan 2001). In this regard, Platel and co-authors demonstrated an acceleration of food transit effect when consuming spices such as ginger, cumin, ajowan, fennel, coriander, mint, garlic, and onion and bioactive compounds (i.e. curcumin, capsaicin, piperine) which could play an additional role in the prevention of colon cancer through combating constipation (Platel and Srinivasan 2001).

Despite the traditional uses and the *in vivo* favorable results, the lack of preclinical and clinical trials with standardized concentrations of spices or their main bioactive compounds makes it hard to claim a digestive stimulation effect of spices.

8.3.7 Antihypertensive Properties

Hypertension, also known as high blood pressure (BP), is a chronic medical condition where the BP in the arteries is more elevated than it should be. According to data from the WHO, globally, the overall prevalence of raised blood pressure in adults aged 25 and over was around 40% in 2008. Among the mechanisms of action involved in hypertension reduction, Al Disi et al. reported several pathways which converge in the reduction of oxidative stress which could later enhance vasodilatation and decrease vasoconstriction, thus ameliorating hypertension (Al Disi et al. 2016). In this context, garlic has been traditionally employed to manage high BP. The beneficial effect of garlic has been attributed to the increment of nitric oxide production, which allows muscle relaxation and vasodilatation. A meta-analysis carried out by Reinhart et al. (2008) where randomized double-blind placebo-controlled trials were included, concluded that garlic reduces BP in patients with an elevated systolic blood pressure. Later studies have shown that the intake of 4 capsules of aged garlic extract daily, containing 2.4 mg of S-allylcysteine for 12 weeks, significantly ($p = 0.03$) reduced the systolic BP in patients with uncontrolled hypertension (Ried 2011). Likewise, celery (*Apium graveolens*) has been reported as an antihypertensive plant. In this case, 300 mg/kg of hexanic, methanolic, and aqueous-ethanolic (20/80, v/v) extracts from seed celery showed a 38, 24, and 23 mmHg significant decrease in BP, respectively accompanied by an increase in the heart rate in hypertensive Wistar rats (Moghadam et al. 2013). Similar effects were found in hypertensive rats that have consumed 200 mg/kg BW of a cumin standardized aqueous extract for nine weeks. After the ingestion of cumin extract, the plasma nitrogen oxide (NO) concentration was improved and the systolic BP decreased (Kalaivani et al. 2013). Additionally, a study performed to assess the effectiveness of curcumin and piperine in rats with NO-deficient hypertension to increase blood pressure demonstrated that these compounds isolated from curcuma and black pepper, respectively, prevented the increase of blood pressure caused by chronic N(ω)-nitro-L-arginine methyl ester (L-NAME) administration. However, contrary to expectations, their combination did not show any significant synergic effect (Hlavačková et al. 2011). On the other hand, rosemary essential oil has been shown to be effective on the treatment of primary hypotension through protecting against low diastolic blood pressure (Fernández et al. 2014).

8.3.8 Protection Against Alzheimer's Disease

The prevalence of Alzheimer's disease (AD) nowadays is alarming. According to the 2015 World Alzheimer report, it is expected that by 2050 its occurrence among the population will be near 106 million. This means that 1 in 85 persons worldwide will live with this disease, which may have health costs of US $818 billion (Brookmeyer et al. 2007). Among the pharmacologic effect from plants which have been studied for cognitive-enhanced effects, those that involve antioxidant, anti-inflammatory or anticholinesterase (AChE) effects are the most representative for AD prevention (Howes et al. 2003). The anti-AChE effect is getting most attention from researchers due to naturally-occurring compounds with anti-AChE activity from plants (Murray et al. 2013). An *in vitro* study showed the inhibitory effect of ursolic acid isolated from oregano (*Origanum vulgare*) (Chung et al. 2001). Recent *in vivo* studies concluded that ursolic acid significantly reversed the amyloid beta protein in induced learning and memory deficits in mice (25–35, respectively), attenuating the accumulation of malondialdehyde and depletion of glutathione in the hippocampus (Liang et al. 2016).

Ahmed and Gilani investigated the *ex vivo* effect of turmeric on memory in rats by measuring the anti-AChE activity (Ahmed and Gilani 2009). A mixture of curcuminoids, curcumin, bisdemethoxycurcumin, and demethoxycurcumin and each individual compound had an inhibitory effect ($p < 0.05$) in the *ex vivo* AChE assay and exhibited a memory enhancing effect for the Morris water maze test in scopolamine-induced amnesia in rats. However, a clinical trial carried out with 34 patients with AD who consumed 1 or 3 g of curcumin or placebo daily for six months failed to find significant differences in mini-mental state examination scores or β-amyloid plasma levels (Baum et al. 2008). In addition, no differences in cognitive performance and plasma cerebrospinal biomarkers were found among groups of patients with AD who consumed 2 or 4 g of curcumin daily for six months or placebo (Ringman et al. 2012). Most of the studies hypothesized that the low effectivity of these compounds could be explained due to the poor absorption of curcumin when it is administered orally, which tends to be better when it is consumed with food (Mishra and Palanivelu 2008). It has been also pointed out that curcumin has limited penetration into the brain (Pan et al. 1999), which may explain, at least in part, the low activity at different concentrations on AD patients.

On the other hand, peroxynitrite ($ONO^{-}{}_2$) seems to be responsible for the cognitive dysfunction induced by amyloid beta protein. In this regard, 0.25 mg/kg of rosmarinic acid, which is the most abundant compound from rosemary, demonstrated that it has protective effects against memory impairments observed in AD due to its scavenging of peroxynitrite (Alkam et al. 2007). Other work reported that memory improvement with rosemary may be explained by its inhibitory effect on AChE in the brain (Miraj 2016).

The absence of a cure for AD and the difficulties in diagnosis in the preclinical phase make herbs and spices a good source for extracting bioactive compounds that may play an important role in future research to prevent, slow, or even cure Alzheimer's disease.

8.3.9 Hepatoprotective Properties

The liver is one of the most important organs in the body. In the liver, essential functions, e.g. those related to digestion, metabolism, detoxification, immunity, or the storage of nutrients within the body, are performed. Several herbs and spices have been shown to act as liver protectives. A study carried out in diabetic-induced albino Wistar rats showed that the intake of 100 mg/kg of fennel extract attenuates the increase of the transaminases alanine aminotransferase (ALT) and aminotransferase (AST), which are an indicator of liver injury, protecting the liver from complications associated with diabetes (Mhaidat et al. 2015). Similar results were found by Rahbani et al. who employed an ethanolic extract of saffron to evaluate its hepatoprotective properties as a complication of diabetes mellitus in STZ-induced diabetes in rats. The administration of 40 mg/kg of BW/day for eight weeks significantly decreased the serum level concentrations of ALT, AST, and bilirubin (Rahbani et al. 2012), where the levels of ALT, AST, alkaline phosphate (ALP), and plasma malondialdehyde are considered an indicator of liver injury. In this regard, another study conducted in rats exposed to diazonin to induce hepatic problems, using 25 mg/kg/day for four weeks of crocin – one of the most bioactive compounds from saffron – decreased ($p < 0.001$) the malondialdehyde (MAD) (Lari et al. 2015). The hepatoprotective effect of crocin has been closely related to its high antioxidant properties (Vahdati Hassani et al. 2017). In order to verify this hypothesis, Gedik et al. (2017) induced oxidative stress using acrylamide in Wistar rats. The biochemical and histological results showed that after crocin treatment, the levels of ALT, AST, ALP, catalase, and superoxide dismutase activities significantly decreased. The same happened with MAD plasma levels (Gedik et al. 2017). Additionally, 0.01, 0.05, and 0.1 g/kg of cinnamon bark ethanolic extract consumed over 28 days also demonstrated a positive effect against carbon tetrachloride (CCl4)-induced liver damage in Wistar rats by reducing levels of ALT, ALP, and AST (Eidi et al. 2012). Thus, fennel, cinnamon, and especially saffron appear to be interesting matrices for further clinical study development.

8.4 Interaction and Potential Side Effects

Herbal–drug interaction can be divided in pharmacokinetic interaction (quantitative), such as drug absorption, distribution, elimination, etc., and pharmacodynamics (qualitative), including antagonist, additive, and synergistic effects (Gupta et al. 2017).

Some compounds present in herbs and spices have proven their benefits in human health but some of them have also been shown to possess a synergistic influence, increasing the efficiency of the pharmaceutical drugs (Zhou et al. 2016). Thus, this fact could explain the existence of an increasing tendency of patients to seek assistance from complementary and alternative medicines, which includes the use of herbs and spices in combination with prescribed medication (Ting et al. 2017). For example, Seo and co-workers, using a mixture of curcumin extracted from turmeric and NVP-BEZ 235 drug (a potent dual inhibitor of phosphatidylinositide 3-kinases [PI3K] and mechanistic target of rapamycin [mTOR]), proved synergistically-induced apoptosis in human renal carcinoma Caki-1 cells (Seo et al. 2014). Another study performed on rats with STZ- induced diabetes found a significant reduction of 7.9% of non-FBG using glibenclamide (5 mg/kg). However, when combined with ginger extract, the reduction was increased up to 25% (Al-Omaria et al. 2012). Also, garlic can affect the pharmacokinetics of the drug metformin, reducing blood glucose levels in rat plasma (Chourey et al. 2011).

There is a general belief that spices and herbs as natural products are inherently safe for human consumption. However, some active compounds present in them may have side effects too. In this regard, as has been discussed in the text, curcumin compound has been shown to be one of the most promising spices to treat and prevent several diseases. However, assays performed in rats have demonstrated that the chronic use of curcumin could cause liver toxicity (Mishra and Palanivelu 2008; Balaji and Chempakam 2010). Cinnamon supplement can cause acute hepatitis, with abdominal pain, diarrhea, and vomiting (Brancheau et al. 2015). Regarding garlic intake, high consumption of garlic-containing supplements may enhance the effects of anticoagulant drugs, resulting in a higher risk of bleeding (Pandey and Awasthi 2015). The same effect has been found in ginger extract when combined with the anticoagulant warfarin in a study of 171 adults (Shalansky et al. 2007). Moreover, the ingestion of high doses of clove essential oil (10 ml) has caused intravascular coagulation and renal failure (Janes et al. 2005).

Although the number of studies aiming to understand herb–drug interaction has increased overall since 2000 (Choi et al. 2017), and the consumption of herbs and spices rich in bioactive components for seasoning of foods at low-dosage is recommended (Bi et al. 2017), more rigorous scientific research is urgently needed to guide clinical practice as well as to safeguard the wellbeing of patients (Gupta et al. 2017).

8.5 Future Trends

The reviewed diseases in this chapter not only lead to complications in many parts of the body, which can increase the risk of dying prematurely, but can also pose a high economic impact on families and health systems. In this context, the use of several herbs and spices, which have been commonly employed in traditional practices, may cushion the economic impact due to their low price. For this reason, the efforts that researchers are making to identify bioactive compounds from herbs and spices and to understand their role in health promotion, individually and in the context of a dietary cuisine, are not suprising. It should not be forgotten that despite the fact that the reviewed diseases have multifactorial etiology, they have a common associated nexus: nutrition. However, methodological shortcomings and clinical heterogeneity limit the trustworthiness and clinical applicability of existing TM (Chung et al. 2015). Other important factors to take into consideration are the following. On the one hand, each herb or spice can contain thousands of compounds and only some of them have therapeutic effects. Also, the bioactive compound profiles and concentrations of the plants may be affected by the part of the plant harvested, seasons, cultivars, and growing area, among other things. On the other hand, the time-consuming job of isolating, identifying, and testing biocompounds is a necessary work that needs to be done in order to be able to assess properly the possible effects on human health.

In spite of the growing evidence regarding the potential efficacy of some herbs and spices, further well-controlled standardized studies that include greater numbers are necessary in order to achieve a stronger evidence-based medicine approach. These approaches will allow the establishment of recommendations on the uses of herbs and spices in dietary guidelines. Moreover, additional studies are necessary in order to establish the optimum dosage and the mechanism of action underlying the above-mentioned health effects.

Abbreviations

AChE	Anticholinesterase
AD	Alzheimer's disease
ALP	Alkaline phosphate
ALT	Alanine aminotransferase
AST	Aminotransferase
BMI	Body mass index

BP	Blood pressure
BW	Body weight
CC14	Carbon tetrachloride
COX-2	Cyclooxygenase
CV	Cardiovascular disease
EFSA	European Food Safety Authority
EU	European Union
FBG	Fasting blood glucose
FPI	Fasting plasma insulin
GHO	Global health observatory
GRAS	Generally recognized as safe
HbA1c	Glycated haemoglobin
HDL	High-density lipoprotein
HOMA	Homeostatic model assessment
IL	Interleukin
INF	Interferon
LDL	Low-density lipoprotein
L-NAME	N(ω)-nitro-L-arginine methyl ester
LPS	Lipopolysaccharide
MAD	Malondialdehyde
mTOR	Mechanistic target of rapamycin
NF	Nuclear factor
NO	Nitrogen oxide
ONO_2^-	Peroxinitrite
PGE_2	Prostaglandin E_2
PI3K	Phosphatidylinositide 3-kinases
SBP	Systolic blood pressure
STZ	Streptoxotocin
T1DM	Type 1 diabetes
T2DM	Type 2 diabetes
TC	Total cholesterol
TG	Triglycerides
TM	Traditional medicine
TNF	Tumor necrosis factor
VLDL	Very low-density lipoprotein
WHO	World Health Organization

References

Acuna, U.M., Carcache, P.J.B., Matthew, S., and de Blanco, E.J.C. (2016). New acyclic bis phenylpropanoid and neolignans, from *Myristica fragrans* Houtt., exhibiting PARP-1 and NF-kappa B inhibitory effects. *Food Chemistry* **202**: 269–275.

Adiwidjaja, J., McLachlan, A.J., and Boddy, A.V. (2017). Curcumin as a clinically-promising anti-cancer agent: pharmacokinetics and drug interactions. *Expert Opinion on Drug Metabolism & Toxicology* **13**: 953–972.

Ahmed, T. and Gilani, A.H. (2009). Inhibitory effect of curcuminoids on acetylcholinesterase activity and attenuation of scopolamine-induced amnesia may explain

medicinal use of turmeric in Alzheimer's disease. *Pharmacology Biochemistry and Behavior* **91** (4): 554–559.
Akhondzadeh, S., Noroozian, M., Mohammadi, M. et al. (2003). Salvia officinalis extract in the treatment of patients with mild to moderate Alzheimer's disease: a double blind, randomized and placebo-controlled trial. *Journal of Clinical Pharmacy and Therapeutics* **28** (1): 53–59.
Al Disi, S.S., Anwar, M.A., and Eid, A.H. (2016). Anti-hypertensive herbs and their mechanisms of action: part I. *Frontiers in Pharmacology* **6**: 323–329.
Alizadeh-Navaei, R., Roozbeh, F., Saravi, M. et al. (2008). Investigation of the effect of ginger on the lipid levels. A double blind controlled clinical trial. *Saudi Medical Journal* **29**: 1280–1284.
Alkam, T., Nitta, A., Mizoguchi, H. et al. (2007). A natural scavenger of peroxynitrites, rosmarinic acid, protects against impairment of memory induced by Aβ25–35. *Behavioural Brain Research* **180**: 139–145.
Al-Omaria, I.L., Afifib, F.U., and Salhaba, A.S. (2012). Therapeutic effect and possible herb drug interactions of ginger (Zingiber officinale Roscoe, Zingiberaceae) crude extract with glibenclamide and insulin. *World* **9**: 11.
Al-Qattan, M.M. (2009). Garlic burns: case reports with an emphasis on associated and underlying pathology. *Burns* **35**: 300–302.
Asdaq, S.M.B. and Inamdar, M.N. (2010). Potential of *Crocus sativus* (saffron) and its constituent, crocin, as hypolipidemic and antioxidant in rats. *Applied Biochemistry and Biotechnology* **162**: 358–372.
Bagley, R. (1999). *The Cambridge History of Ancient China. Shang Archaeology*. Cambridge, UK: Cambridge University Press.
Balaji, S. and Chempakam, B. (2010). Toxicity prediction of compounds from turmeric (*Curcuma longa* L.). *Food and Chemical Toxicology* **48** (10): 2951–2959.
Balasasirekha, R. and Lakshmi, U. (2012). Effect of cloves and turmeric on hyperlipidemics. *Journal of Human Ecology* **37**: 125–132.
Bat-Chen, W., Golan, T., Peri, I. et al. (2010). Allicin purified from fresh garlic cloves induces apoptosis in colon cancer cells via Nrf2. *Nutrition and Cancer* **62**: 947–957.
Baum, L., Lam, C.W., Cheung, S.K. et al. (2008). Six-month randomised, placebo-controlled, double-blind, pilot clinical trial of curcumin in patients with alzheimer disease. *Journal of Clinical Psychopharmacology* **28**: 110–113.
Belcaro, G., Hosoi, M., Pellegrini, L. et al. (2014). A controlled study of a lecithinized delivery system of curcumin (Meriva®) to alleviate the adverse effects of cancer treatment. *Phytotherapy Research* **28** (3): 444–450.
Bi, X.Y., Lim, J., and Henry, C.J. (2017). Spices in the management of diabetes mellitus. *Food Chemistry* **217**: 281–293.
Borchardt, J.K. (2002). The beginnings of, drug therapy: ancient Mesopotamian medicine. *Drug News & Perspectives* **15**: 187–192.
Borlinghaus, J., Albrecht, F., Gruhlke, M.C.H. et al. (2014). Allicin: chemistry and biological properties. *Molecules* **19**: 12591–12618.
Brancheau, D., Patel, B., and Zughaib, M. (2015). Do cinnamon supplements cause acute hepatitis? *The American Journal of Case Reports* **16**: 250–254.
Brookmeyer, R., Johnson, E., Ziegler-Graham, K., and Arrighi, H.M. (2007). Forecasting the global burden of Alzheimer's disease. *Alzheimer's & Dementia: The Journal of the Alzheimer's Association* **3**: 186–191.
Cai, Z.X., Tang, X., Wang, F.Y. et al. (2015). Effect of gingerol on colonic motility via inhibition of calcium channel currents in rats. *World Journal of Gastroenterology* **21**: 13466–13472.

Cao, G.Y., Yang, X.W., Xu, W., and Li, F. (2013). New inhibitors of nitric oxide production from the seeds of *Myristica fragrans*. *Food and Chemical Toxicology* **62**: 167–171.

Choi, E. and Hwang, J. (2004). Antiinflammatory, analgesic and antioxidant activities of the fruit of *Foeniculum vulgare*. *Fitoterapia* **75**: 557–565.

Choi, J., Kim, K.J., Kim, B.H. et al. (2017). 6-Gingerol suppresses adipocyte-derived mediators of inflammation in vitro and in high-fat diet-induced obese zebra fish. *Planta Medica* **83**: 245–253.

Chourey, S., Narsinghani, T., and Soni, L.K. (2011). Effect of Allium Sativum on the pharmacokinetic of Metformin in rat plasma: A herb-drug interaction study. *Der Pharma Chemica* **3**: 287–291.

Chung, Y., Heo, H., Kim, E. et al. (2001). Inhibitory effect of ursolic acid purified from *Origanum majorana L.* on the acetylcholinesterase. *Molecules and Cells* **11**: 137–143.

Chung, V.C., Ho, R.S., Wu, X. et al. (2015). Are meta-analyses of chinese herbal medicine trials trustworthy and clinically applicable? A cross-sectional study. *Journal of Ethnopharmacology* **162**: 47–54.

Cicero, A.F.G., Fogacci, F., Morbini, M. et al. (2017). Nutraceutical effects on glucose and lipid metabolism in patients with impaired fasting glucose: a pilot, double-blind, placebo-controlled, randomised clinical trial on a combined product. *High Blood Pressure and Cardiovascular Prevention* **24**: 283–288.

Dham, S., Shah, V., Hirsch, S., and Banerji, M.A. (2006). The role of complementary and alternative medicine in diabetes. *Current Diabetes Reports* **6**: 251–258.

Dhillon, N., Aggarwal, B.B., Newman, R.A. et al. (2008). Phase II trial of curcumin in patients with advanced pancreatic cancer. *Clinical Cancer Research: An Official Journal of the American Association for Cancer Research* **14**: 4491–4499.

Dibazar, S.P., Fateh, S., and Daneshynandi, S. (2014). Clove (*Syzygium aromaticum*) ingredients affect lymphocyte subtypes expansion and cytokine profile responses: an in vitro evaluation. *Journal of Food and Drug Analysis* **22**: 448–454.

EFSA (2016). Botanicals added to EFSA Data Warehouse. [Online]. Available at: https://www.efsa.europa.eu/en/press/news/160705 (accessed 18 February 2018).

EFSA Panel on Food Additives and Nutrient Sources added to Food (ANS) (2015). Extension of use of extracts of rosemary (E 392) in fat-based spreads. *EFSA Journal* **13** (5): 4090.

Eidi, A., Mortazavi, P., Bazargan, M., and Zaringhalam, J. (2012). Hepatoprotective activity of cinnamon ethanolic extract against CCI4-induced liver injury in rats. *EXCLI Journal* **11**: 495–507.

Fernández, L.F., Palomino, O.M., and Frutos, G. (2014). Effectiveness of *Rosmarinus officinalis* essential oil as antihypotensive agent in primary hypotensive patients and its influence on health-related quality of life. *Journal of Ethnopharmacology* **151**: 509–516.

Fuhrman, B., Rosenblat, M., Hayek, T. et al. (2000). Ginger extract consumption reduces plasma cholesterol, inhibits LDL oxidation and attenuates development of atherosclerosis in atherosclerotic, apolipoprotein E-deficient mice. *The Journal of Nutrition* **130**: 1124–1131.

Gardner, C.D., Lawson, L.D., Block, E. et al. (2007). Effect of raw garlic vs commercial garlic supplements on plasma lipid concentrations in adults with moderate hypercholesterolemia: a randomised clinical trial. *Archives of Internal Medicine* **167**: 346–353.

Gedik, S., Erdemli, M.E., Gul, M. et al. (2017). Hepatoprotective effects of crocin on biochemical and histopathological alterations following acrylamide-induced liver injury in wistar rat. *Biomedicine & Pharmacotherapy* **95**: 764–770.

Ghaffari, H., Venkataramana, M., Jalali Ghassam, B. et al. (2014). Rosmarinic acid mediated neuroprotective effects against H_2O_2-induced neuronal cell damage in N_2A cells. *Life Sciences* **113**: 7–13.

Ghasemian, M., Owlia, S., and Owlia, M.B. (2016). Review of anti-inflammatory herbal medicines. *Advances in Pharmacological Sciences* **2016**: 9130979: 1–11.

Gragg, G.M., Grothaus, P.G., and Newman, D.J. (2012). *Plant Bioactives and Drug Discovery: Principles, Practice and Perspectives*. Wiley.

Gupta, R.C., Chang, D., Nammi, S. et al. (2017). Interactions between antidiabetic drugs and herbs: an overview of mechanisms of action and clinical implications. *Diabetology & Metabolic Syndrome* **9** (1): 59.

Gurib-Fakim, A. (2006). Medicinal plants: traditions of yesterday and drugs of tomorrow. *Molecular Aspects of Medicine* **27**: 1–93.

Hagag, A.A., Elaal, A.M.A., Elsheik, A., and Elzamarany, E.A. (2013). Protective effect of *Nigella sativa* oil against methotrexate induced hepatotoxicity in children with acute lymphoblastic leukemia. *Journal of Leukemia*: 1–8.

Hamaguchi, T., Ono, K., and Yamada, M. (2010). Curcumin and Alzheimer's disease. *CNS Neuroscience & Therapeutics* **16**: 285–297.

Hassani, F.V., Shirani, K., and Hosseinzadeh, H. (2016). Rosemary (*Rosmarinus officinalis*) as a potential therapeutic plant in metabolic syndrome: a review. *Naunyn-Schmiedeberg's Archives of Pharmacology* **389**: 931–949.

Hlavačková, L., Janegová, A., Uličná, O. et al. (2011). Spice up the hypertension diet-curcumin and piperine prevent remodeling of aorta in experimental L-NAME induced hypertension. *Nutrition and Metabolism* **8**: 72.

Howes, M.R., Perry, N.S., and Houghton, P.J. (2003). Plants with traditional uses and activities, relevant to the management of Alzheimer's disease and other cognitive disorders. *Phytotherapy Research* **17**: 1–18.

Janes, S.E.J., Price, C.S.G. et al. (2005). Essential oil poisoning: N-acetylcysteine for eugenol-induced hepatic failure and analysis of a national database. *European Journal of Pediatrics* **164** (8): 520–522.

Jiang, S., Han, J., Li, T. et al. (2017). Curcumin as a potential protective compound against cardiac diseases. *Pharmacological Research* **119**: 373–383.

Kageyama-Yahara, N., Wang, X.Y., Katagiri, T. et al. (2011). Suppression of phospholipase C gamma 1 phosphorylation by cinnamaldehyde inhibits antigen-induced extracellular calcium influx and degranulation in mucosal mast cells. *Biochemical and Biophysical Research Communications* **416**: 283–288.

Kalaivani, P., Saranya, R.B., Ramakrishnan, G. et al. (2013). *Cuminum cyminum*, a dietary spice, attenuates hypertension via endothelial nitric oxide synthase and NO pathway in renovascular hypertensive rats. *Clinical and Experimental Hypertension* **35**: 534–542.

Kang, J., Tsuyoshi, G., Han, I. et al. (2010). Dietary capsaicin reduces obesity-induced insulin resistance and hepatic steatosis in obese mice fed a high-fat diet. *Obesity* **18**: 780–787.

Karimi, N. & Roshan, V.D. (2013). Change in adiponectin and oxidative stress after modifiable lifestyle interventions iChange in adiponectin and oxidative stress after modifiable lifestyle interventions in breast cancer cases. *Asian Pacific Journal of Cancer Prevention* **14**: 2845–2850.

Khan, A., Safdar, M., Ali Khan, M.M. et al. (2003). Cinnamon improves glucose and lipids of people with type 2 diabetes. *Diabetes Care* **26**: 3215–3218.

Khan, A., Qadir, S.S., Khattak, K.N., and Anderson, R.A. (2006). Cloves improve glucose, cholesterol and triglycerides of people with type 2 diabetes mellitus. *The FASEB Journal* **20**: A990–A990.

Khan, A., Zaman, G., and Anderson, R.A. (2009). Bay leaves improve glucose and lipid profile of people with type 2 diabetes. *Journal of Clinical Biochemistry and Nutrition* **44**: 52–56.

Khan, I., Shah, S., Ahmad, J. et al. (2017). Effect of incorporating bay leaves in cookies on postprandial glycemia, appetite, palatability, and gastrointestinal well-being. *Journal of the American College of Nutrition* **36**: 514–519.

Kim, J.H., Kim, O., Yoon, H. et al. (2016). Anti-obesity effect of extract from fermented *Curcuma longa* L. through regulation of adipogenesis and lipolysis pathway in high-fat diet-induced obese rats. *Food & Nutrition Research* **60**: 30428.

Kojuri, J., Vosoughi, A.R., and Akrami, M. (2007). Effects of anethum graveolens and garlic on lipid profile in hyperlipidemic patients. *Lipids in Health and Disease* **6** (1): 5.

Krishnakumar, I., Issac, A., Johannah, N. et al. (2014). Effects of the polyphenol content on the anti-diabetic activity of *Cinnamomum zeylanicum* extracts. *Food & Function* **5**: 2208–2220.

Kunnumakkara, A.B., Koca, C., Dey, S. et al. (2009). Traditional uses of spices: an overview. In: *Molecular Targets and Therapeutic Uses of Spices* (eds. B. Aggarwal and A. Kunnumakkara), 1–24. World Scientific.

Kunnumakkara, A.B., Bordoloi, D., Harsha, C. et al. (2017a). Curcumin mediates anticancer effects by modulating multiple cell signaling pathways. *Clinical Science* **131**: 1781–1799.

Kunnumakkara, A.B., Bordoloi, D., Padmavathi, G. et al. (2017b). Curcumin, the golden nutraceutical: multitargeting for multiple chronic diseases. *British Journal of Pharmacology* **174**: 1325–1348.

Kwon, Y.Y., Kim, D., Kim, J., and Hwang, J.K. (2011). Effects of Licarin E on expression of matrix metalloproteinase-1 and Type-1 procollagen in UVB-irradiated human skin fibroblasts. *Phytotherapy Research* **25**: 1891–1894.

Labban, L., Mustafa, U.E.S., and Ibrahim, Y.M. (2014). The effects of rosemary (Rosmarinus officinalis) leaves powder on glucose level, lipid profile and lipid perodoxation. *International Journal of Clinical Medicine* **5** (06): 297–304.

Lari, P., Abnous, K., Imenshahidi, M. et al. (2015). Evaluation of diazinon-induced hepatotoxicity and protective effects of crocin. *Toxicology and Industrial Health* **31**: 367–376.

Liang, W., Zhao, X., Feng, J. et al. (2016). Ursolic acid attenuates beta-amyloid-induced memory impairment in mice. *Arquivos de Neuro-Psiquiatria* **74**: 482–488.

Lopresti, A.L. (2017). Curcumin for neuropsychiatric disorders: a review of in vitro, animal and human studies. *Journal of Psychopharmacology* **31**: 287–302.

Lou, K.H., Yang, M., Duan, E.D. et al. (2016). Rosmarinic acid stimulates liver regeneration through the mTOR pathway. *Phytomedicine* **23**: 1574–1582.

Lv, C., Yuan, X., Zeng, H.W. et al. (2017). Protective effect of cinnamaldehyde against glutamate-induced oxidative stress and apoptosis in PC12 cells. *European Journal of Pharmacology* **815**: 487–494.

Marchese, A., Barbieri, R., Coppo, E. et al. (2017). Antimicrobial activity of eugenol and essential oils containing eugenol: a mechanistic viewpoint. *Critical Reviews in Microbiology* **43**: 668–689.

Martínez-Graciá, C., González-Bermúdez, C.A., Cabellero-Valcárcel, A.M. et al. (2015). Use of herbs and spices for food preservation: advantages and limitations. *Current Opinion in Food Science* **6**: 38–43.

Marx, W., Ried, K., McCarthy, A.L. et al. (2017). Ginger mechanism of action in chemotherapy-induced nausea and vomiting: a review. *Critical Reviews in Food Science and Nutrition* **57**: 141–146.

Matsui, T., Ito, C., Masubuchi, S., and Itoigawa, M. (2015). Licarin A is a candidate compound for the treatment of immediate hypersensitivity via inhibition of rat mast cell line RBL-2H3 cells. *Journal of Pharmacy and Pharmacology* **67**: 1723–1732.

Mhaidat, N.M., Abu-Zaiton, A.S., Alzoubi, K.H. et al. (2015). Antihyperglycemic properties of *Foeniculum vulgare* extract in streptozocin-induced diabetes in rats. *International Journal of Pharmacolog Y* **11**: 72–75.

Miraj, S. (2016). An evidence-based review on herbal remedies of *Rosmarinus officinalis*. *Der Pharmacia Letter* **8**: 426–436.

Misawa, K., Hashizume, K., Yamamoto, M. et al. (2015). Ginger extract prevents high-fat diet-induced obesity in mice via activation of the peroxisome proliferator-activated receptor delta pathway. *Journal of Nutritional Biochemistry* **26**: 1058–1067.

Mishra, S. and Palanivelu, K. (2008). The effect of curcumin (turmeric) on alzheimer's disease: an overview. *Annals of Indian Academy of Neurology* **11**: 13–19.

Moghadam, M.H., Imenshahidi, M., and Mohajeri, S.A. (2013). Antihypertensive effect of celery seed on rat blood pressure in chronic administration. *Journal of Medicinal Food* **16**: 558–563.

Moore, J., Yousef, M., and Tsiani, E. (2016). Anticancer effects of rosemary (*Rosmarinus officinalis* L.) extract and rosemary extract polyphenols. *Nutrients* **8**: 32–38.

Mozaffari-Khosravi, H., Talaei, B., Jalali, B. et al. (2014). The effect of ginger powder supplementation on insulin resistance and glycemic indices in patients with type 2 diabetes: a randomised, double-blind, placebo-controlled trial. *Complementary Therapies in Medicine* **22**: 9–16.

Mueller, M., Hobiger, S., and Jungbauer, A. (2010). Anti-inflammatory activity of extracts from fruits, herbs and spices. *Food Chemistry* **122**: 987–996.

Murata, K., Ishida, Y., Nishio, A. et al. (2017). Screening of spice extracts possessing anti-acetylcholinesterase activity and active principle of bitter ginger, rhizome of *Zingiber zerumbet*. *Natural Product Communications* **12**: 1053–1056.

Murray, A.P., Faraoni, M.B., Castro, M.J. et al. (2013). Natural AChE inhibitors from plants and their contribution to Alzheimer's disease therapy. *Current Neuropharmacology* **11**: 388–413.

Nabavizadeh, F., Salimi, E., Sadroleslami, Z. et al. (2009). Saffron (*Crocus sativus*) increases gastric acid and pepsin secretions in rats: role of nitric oxide (NO). *African Journal of Pharmacy and Pharmacology* **3**: 181–184.

Nadkarni, K.M. and Nadkarni, A.K. (1999). *Indian Materia Medica with Ayurvedic, Unani-Tibbi, Siddha, Allopathic, Homeopathic*. Naturopathic and Home Remedies. Popular Prakashan Privated Limited.

Naimi, M., Vlavcheski, F., Shamshoum, H., and Tsiani, E. (2017). Rosemary extract as a potential anti-hyperglycemic agent: current evidence and future perspectives. *Nutrients* **9**: 1–9.

Nematolahi, P., Mehrabani, M., Karami-Mohajeri, S., and Dabaghzadeh, F. (2018). Effects of Rosmarinus officinalis L. on memory performance, anxiety, depression, and sleep quality in university students: a randomized clinical trial. *Complementary Therapies in Clinical Practice* **30**: 24–28.

Ng, T. and Wu, S.J. (2011). Antiproliferative activity of *Cinnamomum cassia* constituents and effects of Pifithrin-alpha on their apoptotic signaling pathways in hep G2 cells. *Evidence-based Complementary and Alternative Medicine*: 1–6.

Nusier, M.K., Bataineh, H.N., and Daradkah, H.M. (2007). Adverse effects of rosemary (*Rosmarinus officinalis* L.) on reproductive function in adult male rats. *Experimental Biology and Medicine (Maywood, N.J.)* **232**: 809–813.

Ono, K., Tsukamoto-Yasui, M., Hara-Kimura, Y. et al. (2011). Intragastric administration of capsiate, a transient receptor potential channel agonist, triggers thermogenic sympathetic responses. *Journal of Applied Physiology* **110**: 789–798.

Palatty, P.L., Haniadka, R., Valder, B. et al. (2013). Ginger in the prevention of nausea and vomiting: a review. *Critical Reviews in Food Science and Nutrition* **53**: 659–669.

Pan, M.H., Huang, T.M., and Lin, J.K. (1999). Biotransformation of curcumin through reduction and glucuronidation in mice. *Drug Metabolism and Disposition: The Biological Fate of Chemicals* **27**: 486–494.

Pandey, H. and Awasthi, P. (2015). Effect of processing techniques on nutritional composition and antioxidant activity of fenugreek (Trigonella foenum-graecum) seed flour. *Journal of Food Science and Technology – Mysore* **52** (2): 1054–1060.

Park, M. and Sung, M. (2015). Carnosic acid attenuates obesity-induced glucose intolerance and hepatic fat accumulation by modulating genes of lipid metabolism in C57BL/6J-Ob/Ob mice. *Journal of the Science of Food and Agriculture* **95**: 828–835.

Petramfar, P., Zarshenas, M.M., Moein, M., and Mohagheghzadeh, A. (2014). Management of insomnia in traditional persian medicine. *Forschende Komplementärmedizin* **21**: 119–125.

Platel, K. and Srinivasan, K. (2000). Influence of dietary spices and their active principles on pancreatic digestive enzymes in albino rats. *Nahrung – Food* **44**: 42–46.

Platel, K. and Srinivasan, K. (2001). Studies on the influence of dietary spices on food transit time in experimental rats. *Nutrition Research* **21**: 1309–1314.

Platel, K. and Srinivasan, K. (2004). Digestive stimulant action of spices: a myth or reality? *Indian Journal of Medical Research* **119**: 167–179.

Platel, K., Rao, A., Saraswathi, G., and Srinivasan, K. (2002). Digestive stimulant action of three indian spice mixes in experimental rats. *Nahrung – Food* **46**: 394–398.

Plummer, S.M., Hill, K.A., Festing, M.F. et al. (2001). Clinical development of leukocyte cyclooxygenase 2 activity as a systemic biomarker for cancer chemopreventive agents. *Cancer Epidemiology, Biomarkers & Prevention: A Publication of the American Association for Cancer Research, cosponsored by the American Society of Preventive Oncology* **10**: 1295–1299.

Rahbani, M., Mohajeri, D., Rezaie, A., and Nazeri, M. (2012). Protective effect of ethanolic extract of saffron (dried stigmas of *Crocus sativus* L.) on hepatic tissue injury in streptozotocin-induced diabetic rats. *Journal of Animal and Veterinary Advances* **11**: 1985–1994.

Rahimi-Moghaddam, P., Hashemi-Setobadi, H., and Ghazinejhadian-Shooshtari, F. (2015). Effect of allicin on tamoxifen-sensitive MCF-7 breast cancer cells. *Journal of Medicinal Plants* **14**: 101–110.

Ramadan, G., Al-Kahtani, M.A., and El-Sayed, W.M. (2011). Anti-inflammatory and anti-oxidant properties of *Curcuma longa* (turmeric) versus *Zingiber officinale* (ginger) rhizomes in rat adjuvant-induced arthritis. *Inflammation* **34**: 291–301.

Ramakrishna Rao, R., Platel, K., and Srinivasan, K. (2003). In vitro influence of spices and spice-active principles on digestive enzymes of rat pancreas and small intestine. *Nahrung – Food* **47**: 408–412.

Reinhart, K.M., Coleman, C.I., Teevan, C. et al. (2008). Effects of garlic on blood pressure in patients with and without systolic hypertension: a meta-analysis. *Annals of Pharmacotherapy* **42**: 1766–1771.

Reuter, S., Gupta, S.C., Chaturvedi, M.M., and Aggarwal, B.B. (2010). Oxidative stress, inflammation, and cancer: how are they linked? *Free Radical Biology and Medicine* **49**: 1603–1616.

Ried, K. (2011). Garlic, chocolate, or tomatoes for (pre-) hypertension? *Journal Fur Hypertonie* **15**: 7–10.

Ringman, J.M., Frautschy, S.A., Teng, E. et al. (2012). Oral curcumin for alzheimer's disease: tolerability and efficacy in a 24-week randomised, double blind, placebo-controlled study. *Alzheimer's Research & Therapy* **4**: 43–51.

Rocha, J., Eduardo-Figueira, M., Barateiro, A. et al. (2015). Anti-inflammatory effect of rosmarinic acid and an extract of *Rosmarinus officinalis* in rat models of local and systemic inflammation. *Basic & Clinical Pharmacology & Toxicology* **116**: 398–413.

Rodríguez-Pérez, C., Jiménez Sánchez, C., Lozano-Sánchez, J. et al. (2016). Emerging green technologies for the extraction of phenolic compounds from medicinal plants. In:

Recent Progress in Medicinal Plants. Volume 41 Analytical and Processing Techniques, 81–104 (ed. M.P.J.N. Govil). Houston, USA: Studium Press LLC.

Rodríguez-Pérez, C., Segura-Carretero, A., and del Mar Contreras, M. (2017). Phenolic compounds as natural and multifunctional anti-obesity agents: a review. *Critical Reviews in Food Science and Nutrition* **20**: 1–18.

Sacco, C., Bellumori, M., Santomauro, F. et al. (2015). An in vitro evaluation of the antibacterial activity of the non-volatile phenolic fraction from rosemary leaves. *Natural Product Research* **29** (16): 1537–1544.

Sánchez-Calvo, J.M., Villegas, I., Sánchez-Fidalgo, S., Camacho-Barquero, L., Talero, E., Motilva, V. & Alarcón De La Lastra, C. (2009). Protective effect of curcumin, a Curcuma longa constituent, in early colonic inflammation in rats. *Drug Development Research* **70**: 425–437.

Sedighi, R., Zhao, Y., Yerke, A., and Sang, S. (2015). Preventive and protective properties of rosemary (*Rosmarinus officinalis* L.) in obesity and diabetes mellitus of metabolic disorders: a brief review. *Current Opinion in Food Science* **2**: 57–80.

Selmi, S., Rtibi, K., Grami, D. et al. (2017). Rosemary (*Rosmarinus officinalis*) essential oil components exhibit anti-hyperglycemic, anti-hyperlipidemic and antioxidant effects in experimental diabetes. *Pathophysiologu* **24**: 297–303.

Selvi, N.M.K., Sridhar, M., Swaminathan, R., and Sripradha, R. (2015). Efficacy of turmeric as adjuvant therapy in type 2 diabetic patients. *Indian Journal of Clinical Biochemistry* **30**: 180–186.

Seo, B.R., Min, K.J., Cho, I.J. et al. (2014). Curcumin significantly enhances dual PI3K/Akt and mTOR inhibitor NVP-BEZ235-induced apoptosis in human renal carcinoma Caki cells through down-regulation of p53-dependent Bcl-2 expression and inhibition of Mcl-1 protein stability. *PloS one* **9** (4): e95588.

Shalansky, S., Lynd, L., Richardson, K. et al. (2007). Risk of warfarin-related bleeding events and supratherapeutic international normalized ratios associated with complementary and alternative medicine: A longitudinal analysis. *Pharmacotherapy* **27** (9): 1237–1247.

Shao, S., Zhang, W., and Li, F. (2012). Apoptosis of human gastric cancer cell line SGC-7901 induced by allicin. *Advanced Materials Research* **343**: 1285–1289.

Sharma, R., Gescher, A., and Steward, W. (2005). Curcumin: the story so far. *European Journal of Cancer* **41**: 1955–1968.

Sharma, A., Rajendran, S., Srivastava, A. et al. (2017). Antifungal activities of selected essential oils against *Fusarium oxysporum* f. sp lycopersici 1322, with emphasis on *Syzygium aromaticum* essential oil. *Journal of Bioscience and Bioengineering* **123**: 308–313.

Shehzad, A., Qureshi, M., Anwar, M.N., and Lee, Y.S. (2017). Multifunctional Curcumin mediate multitherapeutic effects. *Journal of Food Science* **82**: 2006–2015.

Shirbeigi, L., Dalfardi, B., Abolhassanzadeh, Z., and Nejatbakhsh, F. (2018). Dementia etiologies and remedies in traditional persian medicine; a review of medicinal plants and phytochemistry. *Current Drug Metabolism* **19** (5): 414–423.

Shokri, F., Gharebaghi, P.M., Esfahani, A. et al. (2017). Comparison of the complications of platinum-based adjuvant chemotherapy with and without ginger in a pilot study on ovarian cancer patients. *International Journal of Women's Health and Reproduction Sciences* **5**: 324–331.

Shreaz, S., Sheikh, R.A., Rimple, B. et al. (2010). Anticandidal activity of cinnamaldehyde, its ligand and Ni(II) complex: effect of increase in ring and side chain. *Microbial Pathogenesis* **49**: 75–82.

Shyni, G.L., Sasidharan, K., Francis, S.K. et al. (2016). Licarin B from *Myristica fragrans* improves insulin sensitivity via PPAR gamma and activation of GLUT4 in the IRS-1/PI3K/AKT pathway in 3T3-L1 adipocytes. *RSC Advances* **6**: 79859–79870.

Singh, A., Gupta, R., Saikia, S.K. et al. (2016). Diseases of medicinal and aromatic plants, their biological impact and management. *Plant Genetic Resources: Characterisation and Utilisation* **14**: 370–383.

Snitker, S., Fujishima, Y., Shen, H. et al. (2008). Effects of novel capsinoid treatment on fatness and energy metabolism in humans: possible pharmacogenetic implications. *The American Journal of Clinical Nutrition* **89**: 45–50.

Song, P., Wu, L., and Guan, W. (2015). Dietary nitrates, nitrites, and nitrosamines intake and the risk of gastric cancer: a meta-analysis. *Nutrients* **7**: 9872–9895.

Srinivasan, K. (2005). Role of spices beyond food flavoring: nutraceuticals with multiple health effects. *Food Reviews International* **21**: 167–188.

Taguchi, Y., Takizawa, T., Ishibashi, H. et al. (2010). Therapeutic effects on murine oral candidiasis by oral administration of cassia (*Cinnamomum cassia*) preparation. *Japanese Journal Medicine Mycology* **51**: 13–21.

Tahir, H.U., Sarfraz, R.A., Ashraf, A., and Adil, S. (2016). Chemical composition and antidiabetic activity of essential oils obtained from two spices (*Syzygium aromaticum* and *Cuminum cyminum*). *International Journal of Food Properties* **19**: 2156–2164.

Taj Eldin, I.M., Ahmed, E.M., and Elwahab, H.M.A. (2010). Preliminary study of the clinical hypoglycemic effects of *Allium cepa* (red onion) in type 1 and type 2 diabetic patients. *Environmental Health Insights* **4**: 71–77.

Tanamai, J., Veeramanomai, S., and Indrakosas, N. (2004). The efficacy of cholesterol-lowering action and side effects of garlic enteric coated tablets in man. *Journal of the Medical Association of Thailand* **87**: 1156–1161.

Thamlikitkul, L., Srimuninnimit, V., Akewanlop, C. et al. (2017). Efficacy of ginger for prophylaxis of chemotherapy-induced nausea and vomiting in breast cancer patients receiving adriamycin–cyclophosphamide regimen: a randomised, double-blind, placebo-controlled, crossover study. *Supportive Care in Cancer* **25**: 459–464.

Ting, C.T., Kuo, C.J., Hu, H.Y. et al. (2017). Prescription frequency and patterns of Chinese herbal medicine for liver cancer patients in Taiwan: a cross-sectional analysis of the National Health Insurance Research Database. *BMC Complementary and Alternative Medicine* **17** (1): 118.

Tsai, T.H., Huang, W.C., Lien, T.J. et al. (2017). Clove extract and eugenol suppress inflammatory responses elicited by Propionibacterium acnes in vitro and in vivo. *Food and Agricultural Immunology* **28**: 916–931.

Vafa, M., Mohammadi, F., Shidfar, F. et al. (2012). Effects of cinnamon consumption on glycemic status, lipid profile and body composition in type 2 diabetic patients. *International Journal of Preventive Medicine* **3**: 531–536.

Vahdati Hassani, F., Mehri, S., Abnous, K. et al. (2017). Protective effect of crocin on BPA-induced liver toxicity in rats through inhibition of oxidative stress and downregulation of MAPK and MAPKAP signaling pathway and miRNA-122 expression. *Food and Chemical Toxicology* **107**: 395–405.

Wilson, P.W., D'agostino, R.B., Sullivan, L. et al. (2002). Overweight and obesity as determinants of cardiovascular risk: the Framingham experience. *Archives of Internal Medicine* **162**: 1867–1872.

World Health Organization. (2002). WHO Traditional Medicine Strategy 2002–2005. Available at: http://www.wpro.who.int/health_technology/book_who_traditional_medicine_strategy_2002_2005.pdf (accessed 18 December 2019).

World Health Organization. (2005). WHO Global Atlas of Traditional, Complementary and Alternative Medicine. Available at: https://apps.who.int/iris/bitstream/handle/10665/43108/9241562862_map.pdf?sequence=1&isAllowed=y (accessed 18 December 2019).

World Health Organization (2013). WHO Traditional Medicine Strategy 2014–2023. Available at: https://www.who.int/medicines/publications/traditional/trm_strategy14_23/en/ (accessed 18 December 2019).

World Health Organization. (2016). Global Report on Diabetes. Available at: https://www.who.int/diabetes/global-report/en/ (accessed 18 December 2019).

World Health Organization (2017), WHO estimates cost of reaching global health targets by 2030. [Online]. Available at: http://www.who.int/mediacentre/news/releases/2017/cost-health-targets/en/ (accessed 18 February 2018).

Xing, M., Wang, M., Xu, H. et al. (1982). Garlic and gastric cancer–the effect of garlic on nitrite and nitrate in gastric juice. *Acta Nutrimenta Sinica Journal* **4**: 53–56.

Xing, M., Xinying, L., Jinzhou, L. et al. (1989). The blocking effect of garlic on the formation of n-nitrosoproline in the human body. *Acta Nutrimenta Sinica* **11**: 141–145.

Yeh, G.Y., Eisenberg, D.M., Kaptchuk, T.J., and Phillips, R.S. (2003). Systematic review of herbs and dietary supplements for glycemic control in diabetes. *Diabetes Care* **26**: 1277–1294.

Zeng, T., Guo, F., Zhang, C. et al. (2012). A meta-analysis of randomised, double-blind, placebo-controlled trials for the effects of garlic on serum lipid profiles. *Journal of the Science of Food and Agriculture* **92**: 1892–1902.

Zhang, W., Ha, M., Gong, Y. et al. (2010). Allicin induces apoptosis in gastric cancer cells through activation of both extrinsic and intrinsic pathways. *Oncology Reports* **24**: 1585–1592.

Zhang, F., Zhang, J.G., Qu, J. et al. (2017). Assessment of anti-cancerous potential of 6-gingerol (Tongling White ginger) and its synergy with drugs on human cervical adenocarcinoma cells. *Food and Chemical Toxicology* **109**: 910–922.

Zhang, H.H., Zhang, Y., Cheng, Y.N. et al. (2018). Metformin incombination with curcumin inhibits the growth, metastasis, and angiogenesis of hepatocellular carcinoma in vitro and in vivo. *Molecular Carcinogenesis* **57**: 44–56.

Zhou, X., Seto, S.W., Chang, D. et al. (2016). Synergistic effects of Chinese herbal medicine: a comprehensive review of methodology and current research. *Frontiers in Pharmacology* **7**: 201.

Ziegenfuss, T.N., Hofheins, J.E., Mendel, R.W. et al. (2006). Effects of a water-soluble cinnamon extract on body composition and features of the metabolic syndrome in pre-diabetic men and women. *Journal of the International Society of Sports Nutrition* **3**: 45.

9
Synergy in Whole Plant Medicine: *Crataegus* spp.: An Example

Mary C. Tassell[1], Anne-Maria Keaveney[2,3], Rosari Kingston[4], Deirdre Gilroy[3], Mary Lehane[1], Brigid Lucey[3], and Ambrose Furey[1,2]

[1]*Mass Spectrometry Research Group, Department of Physical Science, Cork Institute of Technology, Bishopstown, Cork, Co. Cork, T12 P928, Ireland*
[2]*CREATE (Centre for Research in Advanced Therapeutic Engineering) and BioExplore, Cork Institute of Technology, Rossa Avenue, Bishopstown, T12 P928, Ireland*
[3]*Department of Biological Sciences, Cork Institute of Technology, Bishopstown, Cork, Co. Cork, T12 P928, Ireland*
[4]*West Cork Herb Farm, Knockeens, Churchcross, Co. Cork, P81 FE82, Ireland*

9.1 Introduction

Traditionally, phytomedicines have been considered to work via synergistic interactions between the constituents in the whole plant (Williamson 2001). Indeed, this has been one of the arguments for the effectiveness of phytomedicines at low or subtherapeutic doses (Ma et al. 2009). However, from a pharmacological viewpoint it has not always been clear whether this was the case, and where it was considered as a possibility, it was difficult to establish whether synergistic or additive effects were in fact being observed. In recent years, several papers have been published which have specifically focused upon the phenomenon of synergistic interactions in phytomedicines (Williamson 2001; Gilbert and Ferreira Alves 2003; Li and Zhang 2008; van Vuuren and Viljoen 2008; Li and Meng 2009; Wagner and Ulrich-Merzenich 2009). This body of research has contributed considerably to our understanding of the pharmacological actions demonstrated by the traditional use of phytomedicines.[1]

An important point that is not always appreciated is that the concept of synergy in combination effects is not restricted to phytomedicines but is discussed and debated

[1] In relation to these papers, synergistic effects are also referred to as supra-additive or more than additive effects.

Herbs, Spices and Medicinal Plants: Processing, Health Benefits and Safety, First Edition.
Edited by Mohammad B. Hossain, Nigel P. Brunton, and Dilip K. Rai.

across a variety of medical and scientific fields including toxicology, endocrinology, and clinical microbiology (Geary 2013).

9.2 Cardiovascular Diseases

Cardiovascular diseases (CVD) comprise a range of conditions including rheumatic heart disease, hypertensive heart disease, ischemic heart disease/coronary artery disease, cerebrovascular disease, inflammatory heart disease, congenital heart disease, and heart failure. It is reported to be the primary cause of death globally with an estimated 17.5 million people dying from CVD in 2012, amounting to 31% of all global deaths. Of these, 7.4 million were due to coronary heart disease and 6.7 million were due to stroke (WHO 2015).

CVD and the pathophysiology of heart failure is a complex area with numerous causes, risk factors, as well as the signs and symptoms listed in Table 9.1 . This necessitates a system-wide approach to prevention and aftercare.

Most patients confirmed to have heart failure are on a variety of medications including hypotensive, hypolipidemic, plus antiarrhythmic drugs (Guo et al. 2008). The medications aim to address the variety of symptoms associated with CVD.

9.3 *Crataegus* spp.

Crataegus, also known as whitethorn, mayflower, and maybush, is a member of the *Rosaceae* family. It is characterized by being a deciduous tree and shrub with thorny branches, bearing clusters of white to pink flowers in the spring and bright red berries in autumn. Native to the northern temperate zones (North America, East and Central Asia, Europe) estimates of 150–200 and up to 300 different species of *Crataegus* worldwide have been made (Edwards et al. 2012; Jurikova et al. 2012). *Crataegus laevigata* (Poir.) DC., *Crataegus oxyacanthoides,* Thuill., synonym of *C. laevigata* (Poir.) DC. and *Crataegus monogyna* Jacq. are common throughout the British Isles and Northern Europe (Brown et al. 1997; Jurikova et al. 2012). *Crataegus pentagyna* Waldst. & Kit. ex Willd.; *Crataegus nigra* Waldst. & Kit., and *Crataegus azarolus* L. are native in Southern and South Eastern Europe while hawthorn species *Crataegus pinnatifida* Bunge and *Crataegus scabrifolia* (Franch.) Rehder are native to Asia (China) and *Crataegus*

Table 9.1 Cardiovascular diseases: causes and symptoms

	Causes and risk factors	
Hypertension	**Atherosclerosis**	**Previous heart attack**
Heart valve defects	Heart muscle disease	Severe lung disease
Smoking	Diabetes	Obesity
	Symptoms and effects	
Dyspnoea	**Orthopnoea**	**Fatigue**
Heart muscle damage/hypertrophy	Coughing and wheezing	Hypertension
Nausea	Raised heart rate/palpitations	Oedema

Source: Adapted from Stern et al. (2003).

aronia (L.) Bosc ex DC., synonym of *C. azarolus var. aronia* L. is native within the Middle East (Edwards et al. 2012; Jurikova et al. 2012; Wang et al. 2013).

All species are used medicinally within their own traditions for a variety of conditions, including CVD plus its associated effects (hyperlipidaemia or hypertension, for example) plus gastrointestinal and respiratory disorders (Ljubuncic et al. 2005; Cui et al. 2006a; Furey and Tassell 2008; Tassell et al. 2010; Wang et al. 2013). The flowers, leaves, berries, bark, and seeds are all used, although the flowers, leaves, and berries have been the focus of most research to date. Similarly, most research reflects European and Asian species and ethnobotany, although, increasingly, North and South American species have been the focus of research analysis (Dewick 2002; Wang et al. 2013; Hernández-Pérez et al. 2014).

There have been a number of recent and extensive reviews (Edwards et al. 2012; Jurikova et al. 2012; Wang et al. 2013; Wu et al. 2014) on the phytochemistry of *Crataegus*. These reviews have focused on the botany (species), isolated compounds, method of extraction, ethnobotanical, pharmacology, and evidence of activity. They have examined the range and details of constituents (mainly from the leaves, flowers, and fruit) currently identified in up to 27 different species of *Crataegus* (Edwards et al. 2012). These constituents include sugars and sugar alcohols, organic and phenolic acids, terpenes, essential oils, and phenylpropanoids (flavonoid compounds, hydroxycinnamic acids, and lignins). Edwards et al. (2012) reviewed the genus *Crataegus;* Wang et al. (2013) focused on *Crataegus oxyacantha* while Jurikova et al. 2012 and Wu et al. 2014 evaluated *C. pinnatifida.*

Edwards et al. (2012) reported considerable variability among the results with regard to the constituents, which has made generalization difficult. The author reported that no consistent or specific concentration (of flavonoids and proanthocyanidins) and no specific constituents (flavonoids) could be determined from the reported literature. Flavonoid content was found to vary as much within species as between species. The authors also pointed out that where similarities and differences were observed (for example in volatile alkene, terpene, and phenylpropanoid content) it was unclear whether they were species-specific or were due to inter-individual variation. The reported research on the phytochemistry did not address the extent to which the results was dependent on factors such as environmental conditions, time of collection, species and genetics, time of year, and tissue type. In terms of activity, they noted that only six constituents have been specifically purified and examined in terms of their biological effect, namely, vitexin, hyperoside, rutin, vitexcin-2″-O-rhamnoside, acetylvitexin-2″-O-rhamnoside, and luteolin-7-O-glucoside. It appears that further research is needed to identify all of the pharmacologically active compounds present in *Crataegus* (Edwards et al. 2012).

Regarding constituent distribution in different plant parts, the flowers have been found to contain concentrations of flavonol glycosides, while the leaves contain mostly flavone derivatives and polymers of (−)-epicatechin and/or (+)-catechin. In general, the fruits are reported as chemically similar to the other parts of the plant, although they have been found to contain more hyperoside than the flowers, and less vitexin than the leaves (Edwards et al. 2012). Wu et al. (2014) detail an extensive list of constituents from the seeds and stem in addition to the fruit, leaves, and flowers. Wen et al. (2015) noted that procyanidins and triterpenoids dominated in the fruits (*C. pinnatifida*), while flavonoids were abundant in the leaves.

Earlier research by Cui et al. (2006a) on the constituents of *C. pinnatifida* provides a good example of some of the variability that can be seen between species and between plant parts (fruit and leaf). The results of this study showed that organic acid was a major constituent of the fruit (seed removed) of this species (up to 5%) but also suggested that procyanidin may lack catechin units, thereby reflecting a composition more similar in bioactive compounds to grapes, apples, and cocoa than typical European varieties of *Crataegus*. Additionally, the average degree of polymerization (of condensed tannins) in the fruit of *C. pinnatifida* was found to be lower than has been typically reported for European varieties (Svedström et al. 2002). One explanation that has been proposed to explain this variation is that the high content of organic acids (*C. pinnatifida*) may enhance procyanidin decomposition or inhibit polymerization (Cui et al. 2006a). However, in the leaf (Chinese variety) the main polyphenol components are glycosylflavones, and vitexin-2-rhamnoside, similar to that found in European varieties.

The European Scientific Co-operative on Phytotherapy (ESCOP) monograph (ESCOP 2003) lists the major constituents of *Crataegus* spp. (*C. monogyna, C. laevigata, C. oxyacanthoides* [or their hydrids] plus *C. pentagyna* and *C. azarolus*) as;

- Flavonoids (up to 2%) including vitexin-2″-rhamnoside, acetylvitexin-2″-rhamnoside, herperoside, vitexin, and rutin.
- Procyanidins, in particular oligomeric procyanidins (OPC) (approx. 3%) with 2–8 monomeric units. The procyanidins are based on condensation of catechin and/or epicatechin with varying degrees of polymerization.
- Triterpenes (ursolic acid, oleanolic acid, and crataegolic acid).
- Phenolic acids (chlorogenic acid, caffeic acid).
- Amines (Choline, Xanthines).
- Minerals (potassium salts).

The flavonoids and proanthocyanidins are considered the main components responsible for the pharmacological activity of *Crataegus* spp.

WS 1442 (45% ethanol extract) and LI 132 (70% methanol extract) are two commercial products that are used predominantly in clinical trials. They are standardized to contain 18.75% OPC and 2.25% flavonoids respectively. Dosages used within clinical trials report daily intakes between 160 and 1800 mg (Dahmer and Scott 2010). Table 9.2 outlines a number of pharmacopeias detailing the requirements in terms of species, constituents, and amounts.

9.4 Synergy

One of the central issues that needs to be addressed when considering synergy or synergistic reactions is, in fact, its definition. A number of published papers have sought to define and measure synergistic interactions accurately (Bliss 1939; Loewe 1957; Berenbaum 1989; Tallarida 2006; Chou 2010; Tallarida 2011 2012). This has led to many different definitions and confusion regarding the true meaning of synergy.

As a starting point, synergy can be defined where the combined effect of two or more agents is greater than expected from their individual effects (Williamson 2001). Therefore, synergy defined as more than the expected effect raises the possibility that there could be a less than expected effect or no interactive effect. Non-interactive effects are in most cases taken as the baseline against which greater than and less than expected effects are defined and measured.

Table 9.2 Levels of *Crataegus* constituents for medicinal use

	Species	Constituents
Pharmacopeia Commission of the People's Republic of China 2005	*C. pinnatifida* and *C. pinnatifida* var. *major*	Fruits – 0.05% Hyperoside
European pharmacopeia	*C. monogyna* Jacq. (Lindm.) and *C. laevigata* (Poiret) D.C. (*C. oxyacanthoides* Thuill.), their hybrids, and a number of less common species in the preparation of phytomedicines	Berries – minimum 1.0% procyanidins Leaf and flower – minimum of 1.5% flavonoids, expressed as hyperoside
American Herbal Pharmacopeia	*C. monogyna* Jacq. (Lindm.) or *C. laevigata* (Poiret) D.C. (*C. oxyacanthoides* Thuill.) Plus hybrids and any other *Crataegus* species	Berries – 1.0% procyanidins expressed as cyanidin chloride Leaf and flower – 1.5% flavonoids, expressed as hyperoside
United States Pharmacopeia (USP)	*C. monogyna* Jacq. (Lindm.) or *C. laevigata* (Poiret) D.C. (*C. oxyacanthoides* Thuill.)	Berries – 1.0% procyanidins expressed as cyanidin chloride Leaf and flower – 1.5% flavonoids, expressed as hyperoside

Source: Adapted from Edwards et al. (2012).

Combination effects can result from each of the following three scenarios;

1. each agent has its own individual effect;
2. only one agent has an individual effect;
3. neither of the agents has an individual effect.

Where a greater than expected effect is found then scenarios 1 and 2 are termed synergistic interactions; however, the term coalism is used in the case of scenario 3. In the case of non-interaction, only scenario 1 is considered a true additive effect (in some cases this is referred to as Bliss independence, which will be discussed later). Scenarios 2 and 3 use the term inertism. Finally, where the effect is less than expected, this is known as antagonism (scenarios 1 and 2), or alternatively, inhibition (Greco et al. 1995; Williamson 2001). Chou (2010) has also argued that synergy and antagonism require both agents to have some effect (scenario 1). Where one or neither agent has an effect (scenarios 2 and 3), this has been variously termed enhancement, potentiation, or augmentation and does not constitute a true synergistic effect. The inconsistency in terminology and lack of precision adds to the difficulty; nevertheless, the terms synergy, additive, antagonism are typically used and are accepted nomenclature.

Further problems occur when contemplating an appropriate method of analysis. In fact, despite many years and a considerable amount of discussion there is still no single standard method to measure combination effects (Berenbaum 1977, 1989; Greco et al. 1995; Chou 2010; Foucquier and Guedj 2015).

A 1995 review article (Greco et al.), reported by Chou (2010) listed 13 different approaches to synergy. Chou (2010) explained that he worked on this topic over a

Table 9.3 Different methods employed to measure synergistic interactions

Different methods used to measure synergy	
Dose-response approaches (Loewe additivity)	
Isobologram	Iso-effect graphed representation where individual dosage effects are plotted against each other in a fixed ratio combination.
Interaction index calculation of Berenbaum (1977)	Algebraic analog of the basic isobologram method.
Median-effect method of Chou and Talalay (1984)	General framework for enzyme kinetic mechanisms, based on median-effect equation derived from the mass-action law principle, encompassing the Michaelis–Menten, Hill, Henderson–Hasselbalch, and Scatchard equations.
Method of Berenbaum (1985) (Loewe additivity surface method)	Graphed method applicable for all non-parametric and parametric response surface approaches.
Non-parametric response surface approaches (3D spline fitting, contours – Suhnel (1990))	Response surface approach where the data from combination experiments with bivariate splines (non-parametric structural and random models) is analyzed without and with smoothing. The resulting simulated 3D surface and contours is analyzed against a predicted surface with no interaction.
Parametric response surface approaches (Greco et al. 1990)	Response surface approach to a quantitative assessment of drug interaction. A model was fitted using non-linear regression to the data from each separate experiment, and parameters were estimated.
Parametric response surface approaches (Weinstein et al. 1990)	Based on enzyme kinetics models.
Effect-based approaches (Bliss independence)	
Fractional product method (Webb) (1963)	Based on independent action (of the enzymes) and assumes classic Michaelis–Menten kinetics. Involves summation of the effects of two or more drugs. Observed and predicted responses are compared.
Method of Valeriote and Lin (1975)	Webb's fractional product method (1963) is followed, plus there is a further subdivision of the less-than-additive region into sub-additive, interference, and antagonism sub-regions.
Method of Drewinko et al. (1976)	Webb's fractional product method (1963) is followed, plus the predicted effect (calculated from the Bliss independence model) is subtracted from the observed effect for the combination points.
Method of Steel and Peckham (1979)	Graphed iso-effect plot with envelope of additivity developed in relation to combined radiotherapy–chemotherapy treatments. Concept of spatial cooperation used to indicate non-interaction between agents (radiotherapy and chemotherapy).
Bliss (1939) Independence response surface approach	Graphed version of the fractional product method of Webb (1963).
Method of Prichard and Shipman (1990)	Graphical, 3D version of the fractional product method of Webb (1963).

Source: Adaptsed from Greco *et al.* 1995

40-year period, of which 10 years were directed to defining additive effects (and from this synergy and antagonism). Nevertheless, within the numerous methods that have been used, two main divisions – namely a dose–response approach and an effect-based approach – can be identified (Foucquier and Guedj 2015). These approaches are outlined in Table 9.3. This chapter does not include a full discussion on all the approaches employed, but has focused on the main approaches and different models used to report synergy in *Crataegus* spp.

9.4.1 Dose–Effect Approaches

Dose–effect methods are generally considered more rigorous in terms of their ability to accurately assess agents given in combination (Williamson 2001; Chou 2010; Foucquier and Guedj 2015). The methods involve comparing dose–response curves for each agent (in a combination) at a concentration that can produce the same therapeutic effect, i.e. typically half maximal effective dose (ED-50), half maximal lethal dose (LD-50), or half maximal inhibitory concentration (IC-50). They are also independent of the mechanism of interaction.

9.4.1.1 Loewe Additivity From a mathematical perspective (Loewe 1957; Berenbaum 1989; Tallarida 2001, 2006, 2011, 2012), synergy can be defined in terms of Loewe additivity (Loewe 1957) based on the premise that two identical compounds will exhibit a combined effect that is additive in terms of their individual dose–response curves. Two principles underpin this premise: dose equivalence (which assumes that an equally effective dose of one can substitute for the other when the two are simultaneously present) and the sham combination principle (a compound cannot have a synergistic effect with itself).

Loewe additivity assumes a constant potency ratio between agents and by extension equal individual maximum effects (Tallarida 2012). Effects greater than additive are considered synergistic effects, while effects less than additive are antagonistic.

While statistically robust (Williamson 2001; Goldoni and Johansson 2007; Chou 2010), the Loewe additivity model requires a large number of data points for a full dose–response curve and is thus considered more suited to simple and well understood systems. Therefore, issues such as cost, complexity, and as yet unknown factors have been raised as reasons why there has been limited usage of the model in assessing biological systems and, in particular, complex herbal solutions. It has also been argued that the Loewe additivity model could tend to overestimate antagonism in situations where there was some form of partial independence between the combined agents (Foucquier and Guedj 2015).

9.4.1.2 Combination Index (CI) Based on Loewe additivity, the combination of two or more agents to produce an effect can be described by the combination index (CI) (Berenbaum 1977; Chou and Talalay 1983, 1984). The CI can be calculated using the following equation;

$$\frac{\text{dose of A}}{A_e} + \frac{\text{dose of B}}{B_e} = 1$$

A_e and B_e are the equi-effective dose for agent A and agent B.

Synergistic effects are by definition less than expected and so are indicated where the CI < 1. Antagonistic effects are more than expected and are indicated by CI > 1.

9.4.1.3 Isobole Method The isobole method is generally considered one of the most appropriate tools for measuring synergistic interactions between compounds. Isobolic curves are considered capable of detecting synergy (more than additive), zero effects (additive), and antagonism (reduction) within compound mixtures and have been used for this purpose since 1870 (Berenbaum 1989; Greco et al. 1995).

The isobologram (Figure 9.1a) offers a graphical representation of combination interactions and is a quantitative method where individual dosage effects are plotted against each other in a fixed ratio combination. Figure 9.1a illustrates this graphically showing the combined effect of dose–response curves at a constant potency ratio. Where the combination (of agents) is based on constant relative potency, linear additive isoboles or lines of constant effect indicate additive interactions. Again, as illustrated in Figure 9.1b, the combined effect (illustrated as E) of doses of drug A and drug B form a line of additivity or additive effects. A combined effect less than expected is considered synergistic while a combined effect more than expected is considered antagonistic.

Measurement of synergy based on the isobole assumes a number of concepts:

- that the system involves a combination of drugs (as full agonist) that produce similar effects;
- it is based around the concept of dose equivalence and constant potency ratio;
- that individual drug dose–effect relations can be graphed;
- that measurement is independent of the mechanism (Loewe 1957; Tallarida 2006, 2011, 2012).

However, although the isobole method offers a more rigorous and verifiable determination of synergy, as it is based on Loewe additivity, it suffers from the same issues as discussed above (Foucquier and Guedj 2015). That is, it is laborious, requires the establishment of dose–response curves, and can be expensive to complete. This may be difficult enough to define accurately within combinations of known constituents, but it also adds another layer (or two) of complexity to plant-based multiconstituent mixtures with unknown constituents. It is also restrictive in terms of the number of combinations that can be analyzed at any given time.

There has also been some debate in the literature over whether this method is applicable in situations such as where the potency (of the constituents) varies (e.g. partial agonist effects) resulting in non-linear additive isobolograms (Grabovsky & Tallarida 2004), with Tallarida (2012) strongly arguing that, although difficult, it is technically feasible.

9.4.1.4 Median Effect Chou and Talalay (1983, 1984) outlined a median effect approach based on the principles of mass action as a means of measuring combination effects (Chou 1976; Chou and Talalay 1977; Chou and Talalay 1981; Chou 2006, 2010). The authors maintain that the method is relatively simple (median-effect plot analyzed using logarithmic conversion and linear regression to obtain the dose–effect relationship). In addition, they also maintain that it is not limited by: (i) the shape of the dose–effect relationships; (ii) whether the agents act independently or competitively; (iii) the effect of the agents, i.e. agonist or antagonist; nor (iv) the number of drugs involved. Nevertheless, these mathematical assumptions have been challenged by Greco et al. (1995).

9.4.1.5 Response Surface Analysis Response surfaces analysis is a computerized graphical approach involving a contour plot of drug interactions. Drug concentrations

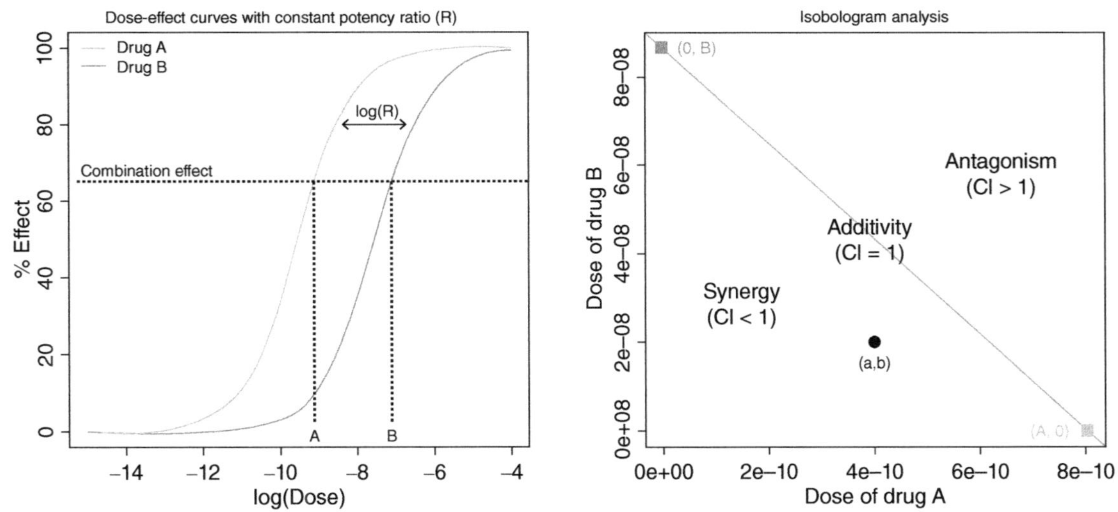

Figure 9.1 (a) Dose–response curves for two drugs A and B (here with constant potency ratio R) allow estimation of the single doses AE and BE reaching the combination effect E produced by the combination of doses a of drug A and b of drug B. (b) Isobologram analysis at the combination effect E. The single doses AE and BE are used to draw the line of additivity. The localization of the experimental point (a, b) corresponding to the doses actually needed for a combination effect E with respect to the line of additivity can be translated in term of synergy, additivity, and antagonism (Foucquier and Guedj 2015). Copyright © 2015 The Authors. *Pharmacology Research & Perspectives* published by John Wiley & Sons Ltd., British Pharmacological Society and American Society for Pharmacology and Experimental Therapeutics. This is an open access article under the terms of the Creative Commons Attribution License, which permits use, distribution and reproduction in any medium, provided the original work is properly cited.

of each drug alone are plotted as a horizontal x–y plane (dependent variables), and the effect is plotted on the z axis (independent variables). The individual dose–response points can be graphed forming a smooth response surface which serves as a reference surface for the effects (zero interaction model [additive] or interaction model [synergistic]) of the drug combination. Actual drug combination data can then be examined for deviation from the reference surface as an indication of synergism (significantly over the response surface) or antagonism (significantly under the response surface) (Berenbaum 1989; Greco et al. 1995; Tallarida 2001). Figure 9.2 illustrates an example of a surface topography for a pair of agonists in terms of their additive effects. Synergistic pairs will plot above the surface while antagonistic pairs will plot below the surface.

9.4.2 Effect-Based Approaches

Effect-based approaches directly compare the effect of combinations of agents with the effect of the individual agents and do not address dose effects. Figure 9.2 illustrates the main effect-based methods employed in measuring synergy, namely combination sub-thresholding, highest single agent, response additivity, and Bliss independence.

9.4.2.1 Combination Sub-threshold The combination sub-threshold method involves showing that a combination of drugs at a non-effective dose can give a significant effect. Synergy is declared in terms of a statistically significant p-value compared to an untreated control group at or below the 0.05 level (Foucquier and Guedj 2015).

9.4.2.2 Highest Single Agent Originally suggested by Gaddum (1957), the highest single agent (also referred to as the Gaddum's non-interaction (Berenbaum 1989) or cooperative effect (Geary 2013)) requires the combined effect (of two or more constituents) to be greater than that of each of the individual constituents, (i.e. effect of da,db > effect of da; and effect da,db > effect of db). A positive result is similarly indicated by statistically significant p-values comparing the combination to the highest single agent. This method only considers the effect of one constituent added to another although it has the advantage that it is independent of the mechanism of action (Lehár et al. 2007; Foucquier and Guedj 2015).

Although, this method does provide evidence of the superiority of combinations compared to single agents, it has been widely criticized (Berenbaum 1989; Williamson 2001; Chou 2010) as providing very limited or no evidence of synergy. The typical illustration (Berenbaum 1989; Williamson 2001) used to show why this method does not actually show synergy describes the scenario where 2 men can individually cut down 10 trees but together cut down 15 trees. Thus, finding that the combined effect is greater than the individual constituents (even at the same concentration) does not show the presence of synergy. Greco et al. (1996) also came to the same conclusion when differentiating between therapeutic synergism (where the combined effect is better than each individual effect) and *in vitro* synergy (true synergy).

9.4.2.3 Response Additivity The response additivity method (also referred to as linear interaction effect or arithmetic summation) provides a positive response when the combined effect denoted as the CI is greater than the expected effect given by the sum (E_{AB}) of the individual effects E_A and E_B.

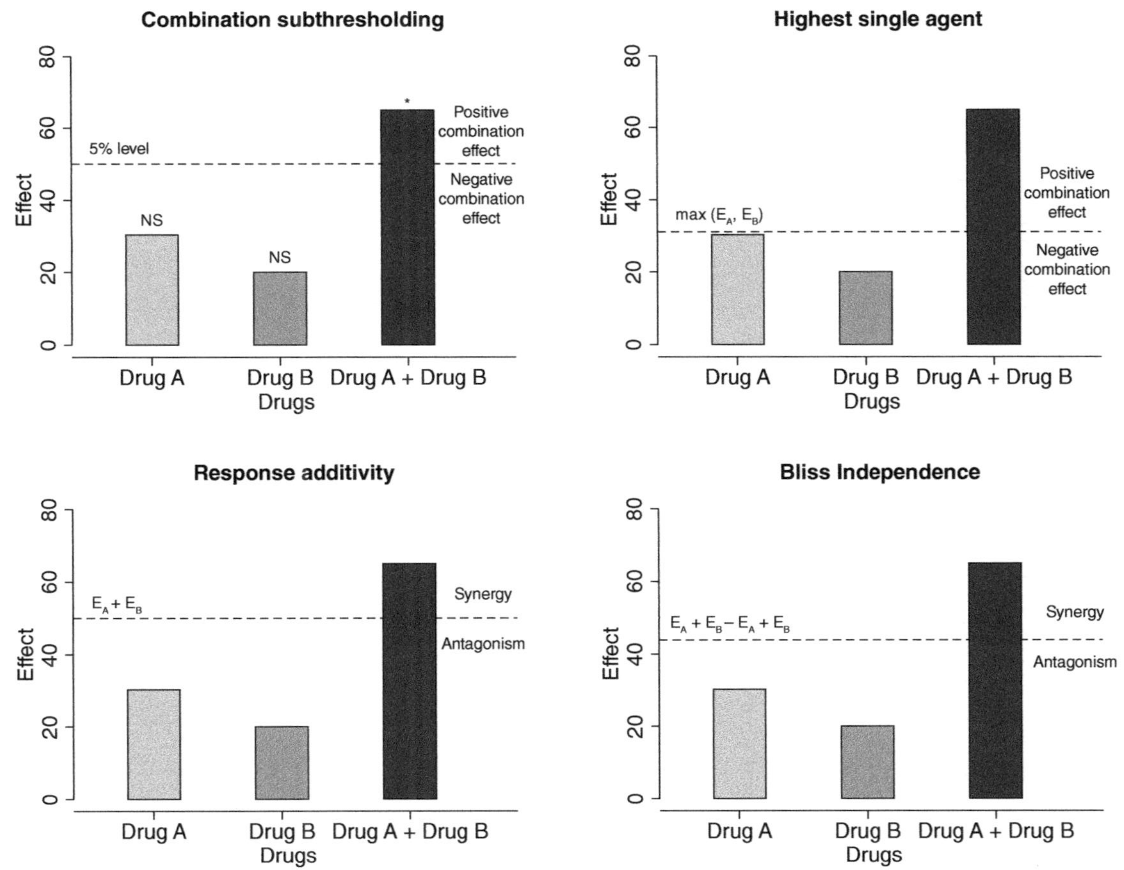

Figure 9.2 Illustration of the four effect-based approaches. (a) Combination sub-threshold, (b) highest single agent, (c) response additivity, (d) Bliss independence. (Based on EA = 20, EB = 30 and EAB = 65) NS, Non-significant; *, Significant at the 5% level (Foucquier and Guedj 2015.)

The Combination Index can be calculated as CI = $\frac{E_A+E_B}{E_{AB}}$. The p-value should be calculated using a two-way analysis of variance ANOVA of the individual and combination effects (Berenbaum 1989).

Although this approach is considered an improvement (over the highest single agent method) in that it compares the combined effects to the individual effects (Foucquier and Guedj 2015), it requires a linear response in terms of the drug/receptor interaction and dose–response curves. This is not typically common in biological systems, which tend to have logistic or curvilinear shapes (Berenbaum 1977, 1989; Caudle and Williams 1993; Geary 2013; Foucquier and Guedj 2015).

Geary (2013) commented on 44 published studies in the field of anesthesia which used this method, noting its ad hoc nature and intuitive appeal. He noted that it violated the principle of sham combinations, i.e. that a compound cannot have a synergistic effect with itself. He also mentioned that the principle of sham combinations is not universally accepted, thereby validating the use of the response additivity method (Boucher and Tam 2006).

9.4.2.4 Bliss Independence The Bliss independence model assumes that the agents are acting on independent, mutually exclusive, sites of action. The effect of the combination of agents needs only to be based on the individual drug effects without regard to the underlying dose–effect relations (Bliss 1939; Berenbaum 1989; Greco et al. 1995; Tallarida 2012) and is expressed as a fractional effect or a probability value between 0 and 1.

Although used widely in a number of settings, it is considered deficient due to a number of issues. For example, non-independent and partial overlapping combinations can give false synergistic results (Goldoni and Johansson 2007), while the underlying assumption of exponential dose–response curves does not always hold leading to anomalies in interpretation (Berenbaum 1989). Additionally, Chou (2010) has argued that synergy is not an issue of statistics but of the CI, while Chou and Talalay (1984) noted that dose–response curves from cellular and animal systems tend to be sigmoidal rather than exponential. They argue that the shape of the dose–response curve, and not only potency, needs to be considered.

9.5 Mechanisms of Action

The concept of pharmacokinetic or pharmacodynamic synergistic interactions was discussed in a publication by Spinella (2002). Pharmacokinetic synergy refers to the processes of herb absorption, distribution, biotransformation, and elimination. Pharmacodynamic synergy occurs where two or more differing constituents are directed at a similar receptor target or physiological system (Figure 9.3).

Spinella (2002) provides a number of examples of both pharmacodynamic and pharmacokinetic synergistic effects using *Hypericum perforatum, Kava kava,* and *Valeriana officinalis* by way of illustration.

In the case of *H. perforatum,* Spinella (2002) links the antidepressant action of phloroglucinol hyperforin synergistically with the sub-therapeutic monoamine oxidase (MAO) and catechol-omethyltransferase (COMT) effects of naphtodianthrone hypericin, flavonols, and xanthones. In terms of pharmacokinetic synergy, the author

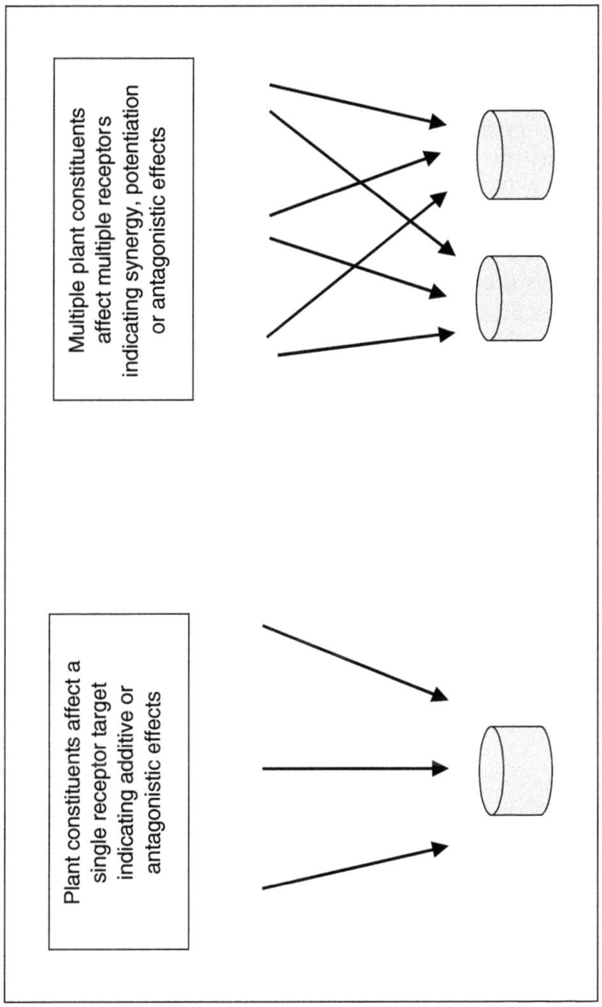

Figure 9.3 Single and multireceptor target effects from complex plant constituents. *Source:* Adapted from Wagner and Ulrich-Merzenich (2009).

uses the example of enhanced bioavailability (increased activity and solubility in water) of naphtodianthrones in the presence of procyanidins.

Wagner and Ulrich-Merzenich (2009), further distinguish between additive and synergistic interactions in this discussion of four different mechanisms.

9.5.1 Multitarget Effects

The single constituents of either a mono-extract or a multi-extract combination affect several targets rather than one. In this scenario an individual constituent may interact with a multiplicity of differing targets, thus eliciting a broad array of physiological effects. This effect is illustrated in Figure 9.3. The left-hand side of the diagram describes the proposed mechanism of non-interactive additive effects where each of a number of plant constituents is shown to have an effect on the same target, e.g. receptor, while the right-hand side of the diagram shows the proposed mechanism for synergistic effect where each of the plant constituents affects multiple targets or receptors within the body.

This approach echoes the pharmacodynamic model proposed by Spinella (2002) but offers the additional advantage that additive and synergistic effects can be distinguished from each other. Within the multitarget model, synergistic interactions require each relevant constituent to affect multiple targets, whereas with additive interactions, each constituent would only interact with a single target.

9.5.2 Pharmacokinetic or Physicochemical Effects (Enhanced Bioavailability, Improved Solubility, or Improved Resorption Rate)

Again, this approach corresponds to the model proposed by Spinella (2002) showing increased absorption and bioavailability and decreased elimination, among other effects. Indeed, Wagner and Ulrich-Merzenich (2009) offer the same increased bioavailability of hypericin example (shown above) in their discussion.

9.5.3 Interactions with the Antibiotic Resistance Mechanisms of Bacteria

This model employs the use of a combination of some agent (for example, natural products), often with little or no antimicrobial effect, together with an antibiotic in order to overcome antibiotic resistance mechanisms. The bacterial antibiotic resistance mechanisms are directly targeted, for example: the agent works directly or indirectly with the antibiotic to inhibit bacterial enzymes or to affect the bacterial cell wall; the agent blocks the efflux pump (so that the antibiotic is not eliminated from the microbe); the agent enhances antibiotic penetration (of the bacteria) by enhancing outer membrane permeability. Thymol and carvacrol have been shown to destabilize the bacterial membrane enhancing the antibiotic penetration of gram-negative bacteria. Reserpin or carnosic acid (*Rosmarinus officinalis*) can reduce the effectiveness or block bacterial efflux pumps (Hemaiswarya et al. 2008; Wagner & Ulrich-Merzenich 2009) (Figure 9.4).

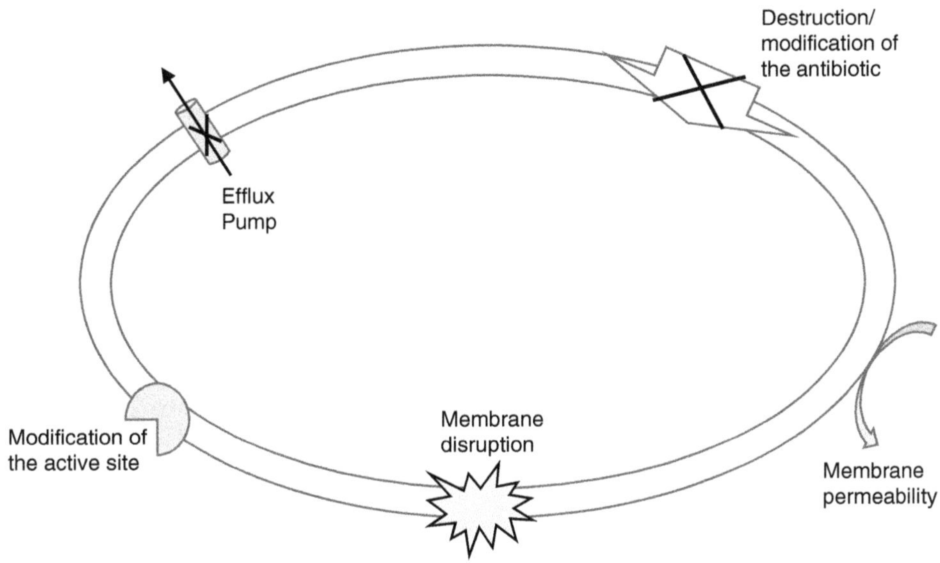

Figure 9.4 Bacterial antibiotic resistance mechanisms and natural products which can overcome these resistance mechanisms. *Source:* Adapted from Hemaiswarya et al. (2008), Wagner and Ulrich-Merzenich (2009), and Langeveld et al. (2014). indicates bacterial resistance mechanisms involving modification of the active site of the target resulting in reduction in the efficiency of binding of the drug, e.g. PBP 2a receptor (penicillin-binding proteins). Corilagin from *Arctostaphylos uva-ursi* and tellimagrandin Id (*Rosa canina*) have been shown to inhibit PBP 2a receptors. indicates direct destruction or modification of the antibiotic by enzymes produced by the organism. Natural products such as EGCg (Epigallocatechin gallate) from green tea inhibit the β-lactamase. Thymol and carvacrol are two of the main compounds in the essential oil of *Thymus vulgaris* (thyme) consisting of approximately 40% of the extracted essential oil. Their mechanism of action is to increase the permeability of bacterial membranes. In this way they facilitate the penetration of antibiotics into gram-negative bacteria. Reserpine or carnosic acid (*Rosmarinus officinalis*) use different mechanisms to either inhibit or reduce the effectiveness of the efflux pump in bacteria, thereby preventing the removal of antibiotics from the bacteria and increasing their effectiveness. Thymol and cinnamic acid can cause membrane disruption which could inhibit the efflux pump.

9.5.4 Improved Effectiveness by, for Example, Elimination or Neutralization of Adverse or Toxic Effects

This can be achieved either by constituents already contained in the extract, added to it, or formed in the extract (by heating or other processes).

This model is not considered a true synergistic effect but points to traditional processes or combinations which are known to reduce toxic effects. The authors (Wagner and Ulrich-Merzenich 2009) give the example of "pretreated drugs" and the fact that there are at least four methods used to reduce aconitine concentration (the toxic component of *Aconiti* root) so that it can be used therapeutically.

9.6 *Crataegus* spp. – a Review

This review seeks to explore whether there is evidence of a synergistic effect in a selected herbal product and discusses the considerations that arise in this process. *Crataegus* offers a good prospect for analyzing synergistic effects as there are known multiple clinical effects, which have been linked with specific constituents, and there are published reports of synergistic effects.

- There is a considerable body of research, *in vitro, in vivo,* and *ex vivo,* supporting its[2] cardiovascular effects (positive inotropic activity, ability to increase the integrity of the blood vessel wall and improve coronary blood flow, and positive effects on oxygen utilization) resulting in improved cardiac function, reduction in blood pressure, reduction in lipid levels, plus antioxidant effects (Tankanow et al. 2003; Daniele et al. 2006, Furey and Tassell 2008; Guo et al. 2008; Tassell et al. 2010).
- Flavonoids and procyanidins are considered the main pharmacologically active constituent fractions, including (to date) a wide range of individual active compounds such as hyperoside, vitexin, rutin, quercitrin, chlorogenic acid, ursolic acid, epicatechin, catechin, and procyanidins (B2, B5, C1) (Edwards et al. 2012; Jurikova et al. 2012; Wang et al. 2013; Wu et al. 2014).
- A recent Cochrane review by Guo et al. (2008)[2] supports a significant benefit in symptom control and physiologic outcomes from *Crategus* as an adjunctive treatment for chronic heart failure. A meta-analysis of 14 randomized, double-blind, placebo-controlled trials found that *Crataegus* was superior to placebo in its effects in the following areas: maximal workload, pressure–heart rate product, exercise tolerance, dyspnea, and fatigue.
- *Crataegus* (hydroalcoholic extracts of leaf and flower discussed in Table 9.2) is indicated in the ESCOP monograph for the treatment of declining cardiac performance corresponding to Functional Capacity Class II, as defined by the New York Heart Association (NYHA) (ESCOP 2003).
- Researchers[3] of *Crataegus* and its isolated constituents and fractions have reported that synergistic or enhanced effects may occur (Rajendran et al. 1996; Cirico and Omaye 2006; Sokół-Łętowska et al. 2007; Bernatonienė et al. 2008; Liu et al. 2010; Ye et al. 2010; Hernández-Pérez et al. 2014).

9.6.1 Published Papers

Hernández-Pérez et al. (2014) showed that a methanol extract (macerated dried leaves of *C. gracilor*) relaxed smooth muscle (isolated rat aortic rings) in a concentration-dependent manner, having an EC50 of 8.69 ± 4.34 μg/ml, comparable to the positive control acetylcholine (8.7 ± 0.8 μg/ml) but with a higher E_{max} or maximal effect ($94.6 \pm 11.3\%$ compared to $69.5 \pm 5.7\%$). Two fractions (F8 and F9) from the methanol extract were found to have relaxant effects but at a reduced

[2] These results come mainly from research on standardized extracts WS 1442 and LI 132 which have been discussed previously in this chapter and in Tassell et al. 2010.
[3] This review has focused on English language publications and single herbs (or constituents) as active agents. It does not include combination formulations.

potency. The major components of F8 and F9 were found to be ursolic acid and corosolic acid, respectively. The authors argued that the higher effect with the methanol extract (compared to F8 and F9) was due to synergy.

There does not appear to have been a direct investigation of synergistic affects in this study, but their analysis mirrors the highest single agent model with a % vaso-relaxation value of 94.60 ± 11.30 (methanol extract) against 54.07 ± 2.51(F8) and 89.19 ± 12.76 (F9). The values were +/– standard error of the mean, and significant at $p < 0.05$.

F8 and F9 contain multiple constituents, so this research is incomplete. The increased effect may have been due to additive effects rather than synergy, and these results do not appear to differentiate between the two as it has been argued that single dose points are not sufficient to measure synergy (Greco et al. 1995; Chou 2010). Alternatively (and mentioned by the authors), it is possible that F8 and F9 may have contained antagonistic compounds which might decrease the vaso-relaxant effects. Table 9.4 details the inhibition rates for the various constituents and combinations.

Liu et al. 2010 also refers to an enhanced antioxidant effect for crude extracts of the fruit of *C. pinnatifida* Bge. var. *major* (70% water: ethanol) compared to more purified fractions. However, although the authors consider that this enhanced effect is due to synergy, they also mention that the crude extracts contain a more complex series of procyanidins with higher mean degree of polymerization, including tetramers, pentamers, and hexamers (citing earlier studies by Sokół-Łętowska et al. 2007). Since monomers have lower antioxidant activity than dimers, etc. the enhanced effects could be due to the enhanced degree of polymerization rather than a synergistic effect.

Ye et al. (2010) investigated *in vitro* (3-hydroxy-3-methylglutaryl coenzyme A reductase (HMGR inhibitors)) and *in vivo* antihyperlipidemic effects of a crude ethanol extract (dried and powdered) and various fractions of *C. pinnatifida* fruit, employing an activity-led approach. Their investigations showed that increased purification of the crude ethanol extract reduced the inhibitory activity against HMGR, raising the prospect of a synergistic effect. Additional investigations by Ye et al. (2010) showed that the combined effect of four monomers (quercetin, hyperoside, rutin, and chlorogenic acid) in the same concentration as in the crude extract had a greater effect than the sum of the four individual monomers (mixture).

Here, the authors appear to have used the response additivity model (assuming that the mixture is greater than the sum of its constituent parts) to assess combination effects. As has already been argued, additive effects are not merely the arithmetic sum of the effects (Williamson 2001; Chou 2006, 2010). Additionally, there were

Table 9.4 Inhibition rate (IR) of *C. pinnatifida* fruit to HMG Co-A reductase (Ye et al. 2010)

Inhibition rate (IR) of *C. pinnatifida* fruit to HMG Co-A reductase matched according to their ratio in the fruit extract (*C. pinnatifida*).

Quercetin	Hyperoside	Rutin	Chlorogenic acid	Total[a]	Mixture[b]
0.16	0.32	1.42	0.95	2.85	2.85
6.28	9.64	23.53	10.56	50.01	79.5

[a] Total indicates the sum of compounds.
[b] Mixture indicates compounds.

insufficient dose points available to determine synergy from the method employed (Chou 2010).

Although only the abstract is in English (full article in Chinese), Huang et al. (2010) appears to refer to the same basic research as discussed by Ye et al. (2010) above. It would appear that they also employed the same assumptions in terms of synergy and its determination.

Jurikova et al. (2012) reference Bernatonienė et al. (2008) as evidence of synergy, although Bernatonienė et al. (2008) do not appear to consider that these results show synergy and only refer to an increased effect (free-radical scavenging) for the extracts and combined flavonoids compared to individual constituents.

The possibility of a synergistic or more than additive effect is also raised by Sokol-Letowska et al. (2007) and Cirico and Omaye (2006) in relation to the antioxidant effect.

Sokol-Letowska et al. (2007) investigated the antioxidant activity of a procyanidin preparation (extracted from *C. oxyacantha* bark) and five fractions isolated from the procyanidin preparation (monomer (−) epicatechin; dimers of (−) epicatechin; procyanidins Bs, B4, B5, and a trimer procyanidin C1). Comparisons between the procyanidin preparation and the five fractions were made as all contained the same concentrations.

It should be pointed out that Sokol-Letowska et al. (2007) do not specifically mention synergy, but the authors comment that the average activity of the procyanidin preparations were greater than those of the individual fractions. Specifically, the procyanidin preparation inhibited linoleic acid oxidation by an average of 90%, while epicatecin isolated from the same procyanidin preparation (and at the same concentration) only exhibited approximately 84% activity (inhibition of linoleic acid oxidation) and procyanidin B2 had approximately 70% activity (inhibition of linoleic acid oxidation). The authors therefore appear to be arguing for synergy, in terms of the highest single agent model discussed above.

Cirico and Omaye (2006) examined a wide range of constituents individually (catechin, hisperidin, ferulic acid, and quercetin) reporting none, pro-, and anti-oxidant effects in each case and reporting a lack of pro-oxidant effect with mixtures. Indeed, in this analysis, the possibility of an additive effect was specifically discounted as the predicted pro-oxidant effect for mixtures was not observed. These results appear to have been based on the observed effects rather than a specific model used to measure synergy.

Rajendran et al. (1996) raised the possibility of a synergistic effect due to the multiple effects observed with a tincture of *C. oxyacantha* fed to rats on an atherogenic high-fat diet (upregulation of hepatic low-density lipoproteins (LDL)-receptors, increased bile acid excretion, and depression of hepatic cholesterol synthesis). This will be discussed in more detail in the following section, which investigates multitarget effects. Rajendran et al. (1996) did not employ any specific method to measure synergy but based their observation on multiple effects.

All investigations effectively used different approaches and models, although all employed effect-based approaches. None of the studies employed the use of dose–effect approaches, including the use of the isobolegram. It is important to also add that research on combination effects should be considered at the outset, in the planning stages, and not become an observation from the results (Chou 2010). The method to be used should be clearly outlined and discussed. It is unclear to what extent any of the published studies can be said to have addressed this issue.

Additionally, a number of other authors (Zhang et al. 2001; Quettier-Deleu et al. 2003; Ljubuncic et al. 2005; Cui et al. 2006a; Yoo et al. 2007) found a dose-dependent concentration or dependent activity, or a strong relationship, between polyphenol concentrations and activity with no reference to synergistic effects.

Quettier-Deleu et al. (2003) reported that antioxidant capacity was positively linked to the content of the total polyphenols, proanthocyanidins (both global and oligomeric forms, and including the dimeric flavanol procyanidin B2) and hyperoside (a flavonol glycoside). Flavanol-type phenolics showed a higher activity than most of the flavonoid fractions tested (resulting from inhibition of cuprate-induced LDL peroxidation).

Zhang et al. (2001) also reported a dose-dependent oxidant activity (direct and indirect) for a range of pure phenol compounds. Interestingly, this is one example of both pro- and antioxidant activity which appears to be concentration dependent.

Cui (2006a) also appears to have shown concentration-dependent effects for extracts of *C. pinnatifida*. The polyphenol fraction (Hawthorn polyphenol (HP)) is an ethyl acetate extract from a crude ethanol extract (Hawthorn ethanol (HE)) of the fruit of *C. pinnatifida*. HP showed an 8.5-fold increase in polyphenols (related to concentration), and a 9.2-fold increase in antioxidant activity over the ethanol extract (HE). However, HP also showed enhanced antioxidant activity compared to test compounds of epicatechin, chlorogenic acid, and rutin, raising suggestions that the combination of polyphenols may have enhanced activity over the individual compounds. Additionally, both the HP (polyphenol fraction) and Hawthorn flavonoid (HF) (commercial extract) extracts showed equivalent effects on peroxidase inhibition. Nevertheless, the information available on the concentrations used in these experiments is incomplete, and there is no information regarding dosage concentration, which prevents confirmation of synergy in this case. *Crataegus* leaf extract (HF) was found to contain C-glycosylflanones, predominantly vitexin-2-Rhamnoside (20.5%), exhibiting a flavonoid profile similar to the leaf of European varieties. The preparation lacked procyanidines and other phenols (no peaks were shown for catechin or procyanidin dimers [B1, B3, and B4] using high-performance liquid chromatography (HPLC) analysis).

Ljubuncic et al. (2005) also found a significant dose-dependent response for *C. aronia* over a number of antioxidant assays including: induced inhibition of B-carotene oxidation, AAPH-induced plasma oxidation (AAPH - 2,2′-azobis(2-amidinopropane) dihydrochloride), Fe^{+2}-induced lipid peroxidation, and at the higher levels superanion scavenging ability.

Finally, Yoo et al. (2007) noted that high levels of total phenolics and total flavonoids in *Crataegus* (and chamomile, rosehip, lemon verbena, and green tea) correlated with (though not directly) high levels of 2,2-diphenyl-1-picrylhydrazyl (DPPH) radical scavenging activity, increased cell viability (dose-dependent), inhibition of H_2O_2-induced oxidative stress, protection of gap–junction intercellular communication (GJIC), and enhanced superoxide dismutase (SOD) and catalase (CAT) activities. The authors also mentioned (data not reported) that they found a higher correlation between total phenols ($r^2 = 0.822$) and flavonoids ($r^2 = 0.717$) and total antioxidant capacity.

However, it was also mentioned that quantitative analysis may not fully explain the relationships between particular antioxidants and antioxidant activity, and that the level of antioxidants plus interactions between them and other constituents might have an influence on the antioxidant activity.

Although both Sokol-Letowska[4] et al. (2007) and Cui[5] et al. (2006a) found that procyanidins exhibited antioxidant properties, only Sokol-Letowska et al. (2007) reported a synergistic effect. It is not clear whether this discrepancy is due to the use of different species of *Crataegus* (for example, the difference in polymerization, catechin, and epicatechin content as discussed in Cui et al. (2006a)), or to the different methodologies employed in the respective studies.

Long et al. (2006) also comment that the observed activity (decreased frequency of contraction, prolonged refractory period, and increased action potential duration) is not attributable to a single compound. Quettier-Deleu et al. (2003) mentions, however, that lipoprotein lipase expression is positively linked to total polyphenol content, but again, does not mention synergistic effect. Similarly, Schüssler et al. (1995); Kim et al. (2000); Zhang et al. (2001); Zhang (2002a); Long et al. (2006) all report dose-dependent effects.

Finally, a dose-dependent response does not of itself exclude the possibility of synergy. In a series of experiments on analgesic effects, Shafer et al. (2008) examined the relationship between synergy, additivity, and fractional receptor occupancy. The authors determined that the primary determinant, as a means of confirming the presence of receptors at multiple sites, is the relationship between the concentration of drug associated with the effect of interest and the concentration associated with 50% receptor occupancy, or kd. These interactions can be additive or synergistic. The authors report that at low concentrations they are more likely to be additive, while at concentrations at or above 50% receptor occupancy synergistic interactions are more likely.

9.6.2 Multitarget Effects

The four mechanisms suggested by Wagner and Ulrich-Merzenich (2009) may offer a way forward to understanding the molecular mechanisms involved in synergistic interactions and distinguishing them from additive effects.

The multitargeted model would appear to offer the best prospect in terms of the current discussion on *Crataegus* as studies have already confirmed the multiconstituent and multitarget effects of this herb (Wang et al. 2013).

Some studies have shown that flavonoid components (fractionated from *Crataegus*) affect a number of organs, including the heart (through inhibition of 3′5′ cyclic adenosine mono-phosphodiesterase), direct and indirect antioxidant effects, vaso-dilation via nitric oxide endothelial dependent reactions, and reduction of LDL and triglycerides (Edwards et al. 2012; Wu et al. 2014). OPC are strongly associated with maintaining heart function in cardiovascular disease and this is in part due to their remarkable effect on endothelium-dependent vaso-relaxation, even at low dosages. *Crataegus* extract WS 1442 used in the majority of clinical trials is standardized to OPCs (Tassell et al. 2010; Wang et al. 2013; Wu et al. 2014).

Rajendran et al. (1996) described the lipid lowering effect of an alcoholic extract of the fruit of *C. oxyacantha* including increased binding (increased receptor numbers) and enhancement of LDL-receptor activity, increased bile acid excretion, and

[4] *C. oxyacantha* used.
[5] *C. pinnatifida* used.

reduction of hepatic cholesterol synthesis. These affects were, unfortunately, not associated with any specific constituents or combination of constituents.

Antioxidant activity can occur by direct inhibition of reactive oxidative species generation, or indirectly, by scavenging free radicals already formed, or both. Research to date (on *Crataegus*) has included both direct and indirect antioxidant effects, focusing on three different antioxidant approaches, namely: (i) quenching free radicals to terminate the radical chain reaction (Reactive Oxidative Stress (ROS))(Cheng et al. 2013); (ii) stimulating the antioxidative enzyme reactions (ACE and SOD enzyme activity and chelating transition metals [such as copper]) (Ganie et al. 2014); and (iii) acting as reducing agents (Elango et al. 2009). Certain studies have indicated that *Crataegus* may be equally effective in inhibiting oxidative processes as scavenging free radicals (Cui et al. 2006a; Sokol-Letowska et al. 2007). There is also evidence to indicate that *Crataegus* may increase retention of alpha-tocopherol levels in the cell (Zhang et al. 2001).

While several phenolic compounds are strongly associated with antioxidant effects, including flavonoids such as vitexin, hyperoside, rutin, quercetin, epicatechin, and catechin; and phenolic acids such as chlorogenic acid, procyanidins have specifically been reported as exhibiting the strongest antioxidant effects (Skegert 2005; Cui et al. 2006a, 2006b; Yoo et al. 2007).

In terms of individual constituents (extracted from various species of *Crataegus*), the following offers an example of the available information (Edwards et al. 2012; Jurikova et al. 2012; Wang et al. 2013; Wu et al. 2014);

- Hyperoside, vitexin, and quercetin exhibit a diverse range of effects including increased coronary flow, contractile force/relaxation, and contraction velocities (Jurikova et al. 2012).
- Hyperoside, vitexin, rutin (with other flavonoids and glycosylated derivatives), plus proanthocyanins, catechin, and epicatechins have pharmacological effects such as vaso-relaxant, hypertensive, hyperlipidaemic, and myocardial effects to varying degrees (Jurikova et al. 2012; Wang et al. 2013) as listed below:
  - O-glycosides luteolin-7-glucoside, hyperoside, and rutin showed an increase in coronary flow;
  - luteolin-7-glucoside, hyperoside, and rutin resulted in an increase in the relaxation velocity of coronary flow;
  - C-glycosides of vitexin, vitexin rhamnoside, and monoacetylvitex rhamnoside have increased coronary flow and relaxation velocity but less intensively than the previous examples.
- Epicatechin, hyperoside, and chlorogenic acid have been shown to exhibit free radical scavenging activity, thereby inhibiting oxidation of LDLs both in cell and cell free systems (Cui et al. 2006b; Bernatonienė et al. 2008; Jurikova et al. 2012).
- Ursolic acid, hyperoside, isoquercetin, epicatechin, chlorogenic acid, quercetin, rutin, and protocatechuic acid have antioxidant properties (Bernatonienė et al. 2008; Jurikova et al. 2012).
- Quercetin and catechin exhibit biphasic oxidant effects, acting as pro-oxidants at low concentration and antioxidants at higher concentrations; and ferulic acid exhibits pro-oxidant effects at all concentrations (Jurikova et al. 2012; Wu et al. 2014).
- Myricetin was found to inhibit oxidation of sunflower oils, while free flavones (apigenin and luteolin) and flavonols (kaempferol, myricetin, and quercetin) showed

pro-oxidant effects. On the other hand, only apigenin showed pro-oxidant effects in an aqueous emulsion system of β-carotene and linoleal.

- Quercetin, hyperoside, rutin, and chlorogenic acid are associated with a decrease in lipoprotein levels via inhibition of isolated 3-hydroxyl-3-methylglutaryl coenzyme A reductase.
- Hyperoside, rutin, quercetin, chlorogenic acid, and ursolic acid have exhibited hypolipidemic activity in animal models (Jurikova et al. 2012).

Thus, the evidence points to multiple pathways and multiple target tissues for *Crataegus* spp. Within this multitarget model, *Crataegus* appears to demonstrate the ability to provide therapeutic benefits for many of the associated pathologies pertaining to cardiovascular disease, and thereby affects multiple targets within this system. However, it is not clear whether individual constituents affect multiple targets at the constituent level. The absence of comparable concentration-related information, together with a dearth of receptor occupancy data, makes it impossible to give a definitive differentiation of synergistic and additive interactions. Indeed, Edwards et al. (2012) point to a lack of consistency in analytical methodology even with regard to the compounds studied in each species.

9.7 General Considerations

Finally, this last section examines some of the issues that arose when reviewing the papers in this study. These are important considerations as they make definitive conclusions difficult, if not impossible. These are the types of issue that need to be addressed in all studies of this kind.

9.7.1 Lack of a Precise Definition for Combination Effects

There is no single defined method for measuring combination effects, and thus distinguishing synergy, additive, or antagonistic effects. This makes it extremely difficult to come to any definitive decision, whether from the point of view of the researcher determining the method of analysis, or the reader trying to come to a conclusion on the significance of the published results presented after research.

The debate has raged for many years (Greco et al. 1995; Goldoni and Johansson 2007; Geary 2013; Foucquier and Guedj 2015), and, while each method comes with its own advantages and disadvantages, there is no general agreement or consensus on the best and most appropriate method to be used. Advice on the best way forward differs and has included rejecting previous models (Boucher and Tam 2006; Geary 2013), integrating Loewe additivity and Bliss independence (Koizumi and Iwami 2014), case-by-case determination (Goldoni and Johansson 2007), and applying a screening approach (Foucquier and Guedj 2015), to strong advocates of the Loewe additivity (Berenbaum 1989; Greco et al. 1995; Chou 2006, 2010; Tallarida 2012) and Bliss independence models (Calzetta et al. 2015).

Nevertheless, there does appear to be some consensus that the Loewe additivity and Bliss independence methods are the two main models in contention as possible reference methods (Greco et al. 1995; Goldoni and Johansson 2007; Geary 2013; Foucquier and Guedj 2015). Of these two, Loewe additivity is considered slightly ahead ("still standing after the dust settles" [Greco et al. 1995]) and holding high biological plausibility (Goldoni and Johansson 2007). However, there is still strong support for the Bliss independent method, especially in terms of determining the combination effects of two or more antimicrobials used together (Calzetta et al. 2015).

9.7.2 Heterogeneity of Studies

One of the major difficulties when comparing information is the fact that different species are often used (*C. monogyna, C. oxyacanthoides, C. pinnatifida*, and *C. aronia*), different parts of the plant are used (leaf, fruit, bark, or combination thereof), *in vitro* and *ex vivo* techniques are both represented, and considerable heterogeneity is evident within the test methodologies. The effect of this is that the results may not be equivalent, particularly when extrapolating *in vitro* results to an *in vivo* system. (Edwards et al. 2012; Zumdick et al. 2012).

Additionally, conflicting results have also been noted in some studies. For example, Zhang published two papers in 2002. In one, (Zhang 2002a) lipid lowering activity was found to be related in part to raised excretion of bile acids via upregulation of activity of cholesterol 7 ά hydroxylase (study in hamsters). However, in the other paper (Zhang et al. 2002b), no significant increase in activity of cholesterol 7 ά hydroxylase was observed (study in rabbits).

Possible potential differences in terms of methodologies would appear to be: (i) treatment of the plant material (dried berries and ethanolic extracts); and (ii) the species of animal used for testing (rabbits and hamsters). The authors did not state why they chose an ethanolic extract for one piece of research and dried powdered plant material for another. The difference this would make in terms of outcome is uncertain, but it should be noted that alcoholic extracts were used extensively in practice and research. Another possible reason for the difference in outcomes may lie with the use of different animal species, thus highlighting the need for *ex vivo* or *in vivo* data on human subjects in order to avoid confounding results. It should be remembered that not all animals respond in the same way. For example, rabbits and hamsters, when subjected to cholesterol loading, respond by reducing hepatic LDL-receptor activity, whereas rats, with a higher cholesterol synthetic rate, initially suppress *de novo* cholesterol synthesis and bring in other compensatory mechanisms as needed (Rajendran et al. 1996).

9.7.3 Preparations Used

Most of the research has been conducted on whole herb extracts (water, hydro alcoholic) or fractions, rather than individual constituents. Ethanolic extracts (70% ethanol via percolation of *C. monogyna* fruit) have been found to have higher free-radical scavenging activity than water extracts (20 g in 100 ml) (Bernatonienė et al. 2008). Most of the clinical research has been conducted using standardized extracts WS 1442 and LI 132 (Tassell et al. 2010; Edwards et al. 2012; Wang et al. 2013). While this is generally considered a benefit in terms of whole herb research, in terms of synergy there is a need to identify the exact constituent receptor interaction for each activity in order to ascertain the mechanisms involved and possible combination effects.

It has also been emphasized that molecules in polyphenol mixtures (as in the *Crataegus* extractions under investigation) can undergo rearrangement, even during the experiment, which can affect the resulting activity (Sokol-Letowska, et al. 2007). Although the data were not supplied, Sokol-Letowska et al. (2007) reported both a reduction (3–40%) and an increase (figure not stated) in effectiveness over the course of their experiments.

Previous studies by Frankel et al. (1996) and Salah et al. (1995) found that stability (in terms of its antioxidant effect) depended on the composition of the compound. Additionally, trimers of phenolic compounds have been shown to have greater antioxidant activity than dimers which have greater antioxidant activity than monomers. Differences in activity among and within various polyphenols result from the chemical structure, individual ability to transfer a hydrogen atom as a radical (OH substitution and solubility in water), and the experimental system (Sokol-Letowska et al. 2007). Specifically, procyanidin and catechin (*Crataegus*) antioxidant activity have been shown to be dependent on both the type of molecules in the mixture and on different mechanisms of free radical formation (Sokol-Letowska et al. 2007). Cirico and Omaye (2006) reported that the more hydroxyl substitutions that occur, the stronger the antioxidant effects. Therefore, the cases of enhanced effects discussed above could be due to the chemical structure rather than combination effects.

9.7.4 Absorption and Bioavailability

These studies, additionally, fail to address the *in vivo* effect of *Crataegus* and whether these results are likely to occur in the human subject. Constituents including chlorogenic acid, hyperoside, isoquercitic acid, and vitexin rhamnoside have been shown to have reduced absorption or no absorption via the gut. It is therefore unclear to what extent the constituents contained in the extracts are in fact absorbed via the gut and thus to what extent they are available for pharmacological processes in the body (Chang et al. 2005; Liang et al. 2007).

It may be interesting to note, however, that studies conducted on the pharmacokinetics of *H. perforatum* (St. John's Wort) have indicated that the presence of proanthocyanidin B2 and hyperoside enhanced the bioavailability of the purported active constituent hypericin (Butterweck et al. 2003). As these phytochemicals are also present in *Crataegus,* they may serve similar functions, in addition to having possible therapeutic benefits in their own right. The lipophilicity of terpenoids, (also present in *Crataegus*), allows transport of substances across cell membranes, therefore facilitating interaction with intercellular targets (Wagner and Ulrich-Merzenich 2009). The need for further bioavailability studies, for individual phytochemicals which may influence (enhance or suppress) this effect in *Crataegus,* suggests an attractive area for further research. It should be pointed out that Chang et al. (2005) also observed that there was no difference in the pharmacokinetic profile between phenolic extract and individual constituents, i.e. epicatechin, chlorogenic acid, hyperoside, and isoquercitin. This still leaves the possibility that a non-phenolic compound may be involved in the process of enhancing bioavailability.

9.8 Conclusion

This chapter serves to highlight specific areas of further research needed in relation to *Crataegus* spp. in order to fully understand the effect of this herb.

From a physiological perspective, the information to date is strongly supportive of a multiconstituent and multitarget effect on the cardiovascular system, (involving various constituents, and specifically, polyphenols [procyanidines] and flavonoids affecting various receptors [liver, heart], tissues [vascular endothelial], and molecules [LDL] [Wagner and Ulrich-Merzenich 2009]). Although this evidence is gaining ground, it continues to be piecemeal and uncoordinated, resulting in research that has gaps, is overlapping, mismatched, and not fit for purpose.

In this respect, it should be remembered that synergy has a mathematical basis and not a physiological one. The call for more clinical enhancement-based approaches (Boucher and Tam 2006; Geary 2013), while intuitively attractive for many reasons, fails to take account of mathematical and biological reality.

Nevertheless, effect approaches could have a role to play. Foucquier and Guedj (2015) recommend using such approaches for initial screening followed by more detailed dose–effect analysis. While not perfect, preliminary screening approaches are widely used in many different research areas, such as cancer (Mazzio and Soliman 2009) or infection (Bag and Chattopadhyay 2015), before utilizing more detailed approaches. For now, the search for new approaches to this old problem continues (Greco et al. 1995; Yan et al. 2010; Novick 2013).

Therefore, the fact that only effect-based approaches have been conducted to date does not allow for a precise determination of the combination effects.

There needs to be a move toward a more coordinated and collaborative interdisciplinary model for testing herbal preparations, including testing the synergistic versus individual effects. There is a need to follow standard practice (adapted and validated to take account of complex active compounds) within the pharmaceutical industry, including Design of Experiments (DoE) so that data can be collected and collated in a systematic fashion. This could therefore take account of confounding factors and enable proper, informative statistical testing methods to be applied. Research strategies for complex compounds such as phytomedicines need to reflect their multiconstituent profile, while being robust and flexible enough to accommodate the interactions that can occur between constituents. To address this issue, a number of models are being increasingly used, including activity-guided, "omic" research, systems biology, and reverse analysis approaches.

Any approach to research on herbs needs to be based on a detailed understanding of the phytochemistry and constituent profile of the herbs in order to ensure that the specific chemical profile is associated with the specific bioactivity. In this chapter, *Crataegus* has been studied, but whichever plant that is being researched, basic information compliant with good agricultural and collecting practice, ethnobotanical and medical information, and appropriate and consistent research methods needs to be the norm, not just for the registration of products, but in all aspects including research. This is difficult, expensive, and time-consuming but it could in the long run save money, time, and energy, as it might allow information to be built upon rather than, as now, merely noted (Efferth and Greten 2012).

It is also important to remember the pharmacokinetic effect on *Crataegus* and the fact that many of its constituents (e.g. OPCs) have a low bioavailability. It is important to confirm that certain constituents are not metabolized to other compounds (possibly more active ones) rather than automatically assuming loss of function.

Activity-led approaches (Ye et al. 2010) offer a way through the unknown, concentrating on the constituents that give a positive result using the relevant bioassay. This might be expected to also point to combination effects, including synergy, where activity is lost on fractionation. "Omic" technologies (e.g. genomic, proteomic, and metabolomics) are still considered part of the way forward (Sheridan et al. 2012). These technologies potentially provide the level of sophistication necessary to assess the interactions of multiple constituents on a number of levels with the complex matrix that is the human body. Ethnobotany and ethnomedicine can be used as a starting point for reverse analysis using a complete product with verified effectiveness and going backwards to identify the activity and mechanisms. Reverse analysis is often associated with systems biology approaches in practice (Sheridan et al. 2012).

These approaches can help to move the study of health and illness away from purely reductionist methods and closer to that of more traditional approaches to medicine in terms of testing constituent interaction and underlying paradigms. This will hopefully lead to a more realistic and integrated approach to medicine in which a combination of knowledge bases may be acknowledged and utilized, including that of the traditional practitioner of herbal medicine.

Funding and Acknowledgments

MT was supported under the Council of Directors, Technological Sector Research – Strand III 2006 Scheme [Project #: 06/CR05]. AMK was supported by Cork Institute of Technology as part of her PhD programme. The author also acknowledges the funding of a High-Resolution Sector-Field Inductively Coupled Plasma Mass Spectrometer (HR-ICP-SFMS) under the Science Foundation Ireland (SFI) Research Infrastructure Call 2012 [Proposal #12/RI/2335 (2)].

References

Bag, A. and Chattopadhyay, R.R. (2015). Evaluation of synergistic antibacterial and antioxidant efficacy of essential oils of spices and herbs in combination. *PLoS One* **10** (7): e0131321. https://doi.org/10.1371/journal.pone.0131321.

Berenbaum, M.C. (1977). Synergy, additivism and antagonism in immunosuppression – a critical review. *Clinical and Experimental Immunology* **28**: 1–18.

Berenbaum, M.C. (1985). The expected effect of a combination of agents: the general solution. *Journal of Theoretical Biology* **114**: 413–431.

Berenbaum, M.C. (1989). What is synergy? *Pharmacological Reviews* **41** (2): 93–141.

Bernatonienė, J., Masteikova, R., Majienė, D. et al. (2008). Free radical-scavenging activities of *Crataegus monogyna* extracts. *Medicina-Lithuania* **44**: 706–712.

Bliss, C.I. (1939). The toxicity of poisons applied jointly. *Annals of Applied Biology* **26** (3): 585–615.

Boucher, A.N. and Tam, V.H. (2006). Mathematical formulation of additivity for antimicrobial agents. *Diagnostic Microbiology and Infectious Disease* **55**: 319–325.

Brown, D., Austin, S., and Reichert, R. (1997). *Early-Stage Congestive Heart Failure*. Seattle: Natural Products Research Consultants.

Butterweck, V., Liefländer-Wulf, U., Winterhoff, H., and Nahrstedt, A. (2003). Plasma levels of hypericin in presence of procyanidin B2 and hyperoside: a pharmacokinetic study in rats. *Planta Medina* **69** (3): 189–192.

Calzetta, L., Matera, M.G., and Cazzola, M. (2015). Pharmacological interaction between LABAs and LAMAs in the airways: optimizing synergy. *European Journal of Pharmacology* **761**: 168–173.

Caudle, R.M. and Williams, G.M. (1993). The misuse of analysis of variance to detect synergy in combination drug studies. *Pain* **55** (3): 313–317.

Chang, Q., Zuo, Z., Ho, W.K., and Chow, M.S. (2005). Comparison of the pharmacokinetics of hawthorn phenolics in extract versus individual pure compound. *The Journal of Clinical Pharmacology* **45** (1): 106–112.

Cheng, N., Wang, Y., Gao, H. et al. (2013). Protective effect of extract of *Crataegus pinnatifida* pollen on DNA damage response to oxidative stress. *Food and Chemical Toxicology* **59**: 709–714.

Chou, T.C. (1976). Derivation and properties of Michaelis-Menten type and hill type equations for reference ligands. *Journal of Theoretical Biology* **59**: 253–276.

Chou, T.C. (2006). Theoretical basis, experimental design, and computerized simulation of synergism and antagonism in drug combination studies. *Pharmacological Reviews* **68**: 621–681.

Chou, T.C. (2010). Drug combination studies and their synergy quantification-using the Chou-Talalay method. *Cancer Research* **70**: 440–446. https://doi.org/10.1158/0008-5472.CAN-09-1947.

Chou, T.C. and Talalay, P. (1977). A simple generalized equation for the analysis of multiple inhibitions of Michaelis-Menten kinetic systems. *Journal of Biological Chemistry* **252**: 6438–6442.

Chou, T.C. and Talalay, P. (1981). Generalized equations for the analysis of inhibitions of Michaelis-Menten and higher-order kinetic systems with two or more mutually exclusive and nonexclusive inhibitors. *European Journal of Biochemistry* **115** (1): 207–216.

Chou, T.C. and Talalay, P. (1983). Analysis of combined drug effects: a new look at a very old problem. *Trends in Pharmacological Sciences* **4**: 450–454.

Chou, T.C. and Talalay, P. (1984). Quantitative analysis of dose-effect relationships: the combined effects of multiple drugs or enzyme inhibitors. *Advances in Enzyme Regulation* **22**: 27–55.

Cirico, T.L. and Omaye, S.T. (2006). Additive or synergetic effects of phenolic compounds on human low density lipoprotein oxidation. *Food and Chemical Toxicology* **44**: 510–516.

Cui, T., Nakamura, K., Tian, S. et al. (2006a). Polyphenolic content and physiological activities of Chinese hawthorn extracts. *Bioscience, Biotechnology, and Biochemistry* **70** (12): 2948–2956.

Cui, T., Li, J.Z., Kayahara, H. et al. (2006b). Quantification of the polyphenols and triterpene acids in Chinese hawthorn fruit by high-performance liquid chromatography. *Journal of Agricultural and Food Chemistry* **54**: 4574–4581.

Dahmer, S. and Scott, E. (2010). Health effects of hawthorn. *American Family Physician* **81** (4): 465–468. 469.

Daniele, C., Mazzanti, G., Pittlemr, M.H., and Ernst, E. (2006). Adverse-event profile of *Crataegus* spp.: a systematic review. *Drug Safety* **29** (6): 523–535.

Dewick, P.M. (2002). *Medicinal Natural Products, a Biosynthetic Approach*, 2e. Wiley.

Drewinko, B., Loo, T.L., Brown, B. et al. (1976). Combination chemotherapy *in vitro* with adriamycin. observations of additive, antagonistic, and synergistic effects when used in two-drug combinations on cultured human lymphoma cells. *Cancer Biochemistry Biophysics* **1**: 187–195.

Edwards, J.E., Brown, P.N., Talent, N. et al. (2012). A review of the chemistry of the genus *Crataegus*. *Phytochemistry* **79**: 5–26.

Efferth, T. and Greten, H.J. (2012). Quality control for medicinal plants. *Medicinal & Aromatic Plants* **1**: e131. https://doi.org/10.4172/2167-0412.1000e131.

Elango, C., Jayachandaran, K.S., and Niranjali Devaraj, S. (2009). Hawthorn extract reduces infarct volume and improves neurological score by reducing oxidative stress in rat brain following middle cerebral artery occlusion. *International Journal of Developmental Neuroscience* **27** (8): 799–803.

ESCOP (European Scientific Co-operative On Phytotherapy) (2003). Crataegi folium cum flore (Hawthorn leaf and flower). In: *ESCOP Monographs: The Scientific Foundation for Herbal Medicinal Products*, 2e, 98–106. Exeter/Stuttgart: ESCOP/Thieme Medical Publishers.

Foucquier, J. and Guedj, M. (2015). Analysis of drug combinations: current methodological landscape. *Pharmaceutical Research* **3** (3) https://doi.org/10.1002/prp2.149.

Frankel, E.N., Huang, S.-W., Aeschbach, R., and Prior, E. (1996). Antioxidant activity of a rosemary extract and its constituents, carnosic acid, carnosol, and rosmarinic acid in bulk oil and oil-inwater emulsions. *Agricultural and Food Chemistry* **44**: 131–135.

Furey, A. and Tassell, M. (2008). Towards a systematic scientific approach in the assessment of efficacy of an herbal preparation: hawthorn (*Crataegus* spp.). *European Journal of Heart Failure* **10** (12): 1153–1157.

Gaddum, J.H. (1957). Theories of drug antagonism. *Pharmacological Reviews* **9**: 211–218.

Ganie, S.A., Dar, T.A., Zargar, B. et al. (2014). Antioxidant and hepatoprotective effects of *Crataegus songarica* methanol extract. *Journal of Environmental Pathology, Toxicology and Oncology* **33** (2): 131–143.

Geary, N. (2013). Understanding synergy. *American Journal of Physiology- Endocrinology and Metabolism* **304**: E237–E253. 0929-8673/03.

Gilbert, B. and Ferreira Alves, L. (2003). Synergy in plant medicines. *Current Medicinal Chemistry* **10**: 13–20.

Goldoni, M. and Johansson, C. (2007). A mathematical approach to study combined effects of toxicants *in vitro*: evaluation of the bliss independence criterion and the Loewe additivity model. *Toxicology In Vitro* **21**: 759–769.

Grabovsky, Y. and Tallarida, R.J. (2004). Isobolographic analysis for combinations of a full and partial agonist: curved Isoboles. *Journal of Pharmacology and Experimental Therapeutics* **310** (3): 981–986.

Greco, W.R., Park, H.S., and Rustum, Y.M. (1990). An application of a new approach for the quantitation of drug synergism to the combination of cis-diamminedichloroplatinum and 1-ɩ3-D-arabinofuranosylcytosine. *Cancer Research* **50**: 5318–5327.

Greco, W.R., Bravo, G., and Parsons, J.C. (1995). The search for synergy: a critical review from a response surface perspective. *Pharmacological Reviews* **47**: 331–385.

Greco, W.R., Faessel, H., and Levasseur, L. (1996). The search for cytotoxic synergy between anticancer agents: a case of Dorothy and the ruby slippers? *Journal of the National Cancer Institute* **88** (11): 699–700.

Guo, R., Pittler, M.H., and Ernst, E. (2008). Hawthorn extract for treating chronic heart failure. *Cochrane Database Systematic Reviews* (1) (Art. No.: CD005312): https://doi.org/10.1002/14651858.CD005312.pub2.

Hemaiswarya, S., Kruthiventi, A.K., and Doble, M. (2008). Synergism between natural products and antibiotics against infectious diseases. *Phytomedicine* **15** (8): 639–652. https://doi.org/10.1016/j.phymed.2008.06.008.

Hernández-Pérez, A., Bah, M., Ibarra-Alvarado, C. et al. (2014). Aortic relaxant activity of *Crataegus gracilior* Phipps and identification of some of its chemical constituents. *Molecules* **19** (12): 20962–20974.

Huang, W., Ye, X., Li, X. et al. (2010). The inhibition activity of chemical constituents in hawthorn fruit and their synergistic action to HMG-CoA Reductase [Article in Chinese] *Zhongguo Zhong Yao Za Zhi* [Translated as. *China Journal of Chinese Materia Medica* **18**: 2428–2431.

Jurikova, T., Sochor, J., Rop, O. et al. (2012). Polyphenolic profile and biological activity of Chinese hawthorn (*Crataegus pinnatifida* BUNGE) fruits. *Molecules* **17** (12): 14490–14509.

Kim, S.H., Kang, K.W., Kim, K.W., and Kim, N.D. (2000). Procyanidins in *Crataegus* extract evoke endothelium-dependent vasorelaxation in rat aorta. *Life Sciences* **67**: 121–131.

Koizumi, Y. and Iwami, S. (2014). Mathematical modelling of multi-drugs therapy: a challenge for determining the optimal combinations of antiviral drugs. *Theoretical Biology and Medical Modelling* **11**: 41–50.

Langeveld, W.T., Veldhuizen, E.J.A., and Burt, S.A. (2014). Synergy between essential oil components and antibiotics: a review. *Critical Reviews in Microbiology* **40** (1): 76–94.

Lehár, J., Zimmermann, G.R., Krueger, A.S. et al. (2007). Chemical combination effects predict connectivity in biological systems. *Molecular Systems Biology* **3**: 80–94.

Li, J. and Meng, Z. (2009). The role of sulfur dioxide as an endogenous gaseous vasoactive factor in synergy with nitric oxide. *Nitric Oxide* **20** (3): 166–174.

Li, J. and Zhang, H.-Y. (2008). Synergy in natural medicines: implications for drug discovery. *Trends in Pharmacological Sciences* **7**: 331–332.

Liang, M., Xu, W., Zhang, W. et al. (2007). Quantitative LC/MS/MS method and *in vivo* pharmacokinetic studies of vitexin rhamnoside, a bioactive constituent on cardiovascular system from hawthorn. *Biomedical Chromatography* **21** (4): 422–429.

Liu, T., Cao, Y., and Zhao, M. (2010). Extraction optimization, purification and antioxidant activity of procyanidins from hawthorn (*C. pinnatifida Bge.* var. *major*) fruits. *Food Chemistry* **119**: 1656–1662.

Ljubuncic, P., Portnaya, I., Cogan, U. et al. (2005). Antioxidant activity of *Crataegus aronia* aqueous extract used in traditional Arab medicine in Israel. *Journal of Ethnopharmacology* **101** (1–3): 153–161.

Loewe, S. (1957). Antagonism and antagonists. *Pharmacological Reviews* **9**: 237–242.

Long, S.R., Carey, R.A., Crofoot, K.M. et al. (2006). Effect of hawthorn (*Crataegus oxyacantha*) crude extract and chromatographic fractions on multiple activities in a cultured cardiomyocyte assay. *Phytomedicine* **13**: 643–650.

Ma, X.H., Zheng, C.J., Han, L.Y. et al. (2009). Synergistic therapeutic actions of herbal ingredients and their mechanisms from molecular interaction and network perspectives. *Drug Discovery Today* **14** (11–12): 579–588.

Mazzio, E.A. and Soliman, K.F. (2009). *In vitro* screening for the tumoricidal properties of international medicinal herbs. *Phytotherapy Research* **23** (3): 385–398.

Novick, S.J. (2013). A simple test for synergy for a small number of combinations. *Statistics in Medicine* **32** (29): 5145–5155.

Prichard, M.N. and Shipman, C. (1990). A three-dimensional model to analyse drug-drug interactions. *Antiviral Research* **14**: 181–205.

Quettier-Deleu, C., Voiselle, G., Fruchart, J.C. et al. (2003). Hawthorn extracts inhibit LDL oxidation. *Die Pharmazie* **58** (8): 577–581.

Rajendran, S., Deepalakshmi, P.D., Parasakthy, K. et al. (1996). Effect of tincture of *Crataegus* on the LDL-receptor activity of hepatic plasma membrane of rats fed an atherogenic diet. *Atherosclerosis* **123**: 235–241.

Salah, N., Miller, N.J., Paganga, G. et al. (1995). Polyphenolic flavanols as scavengers of aqueous phase radicals and as chain breaking antioxidants. *Archives of Biochemistry and Biophysics* **322**: 339–346.

Schüssler, M., Hölzl, J., and Fricke, U. (1995). Myocardial effects of flavonoids from *Crataegus* species. *Drug Research* **45**: 842–845.

Shafer, S.L., Hendrick, J.F., Flood, P. et al. (2008). Additivity versus synergy: a theoretical analysis of implications for anaesthetic mechanisms. *Anesthesia & Analgesia* **107** (2): 507–524.

Sheridan, H., Krenn, L., Jiang, R. et al. (2012). The potential of metabolic fingerprinting as a tool for the modernisation of TCM preparations. *Journal of Ethnopharmacology* **140**: 482–491.

Skegert, M. (2005). Phenols, procyanidins, flavones and flavonols in some plant materials and their antioxidant activities. *Food Chemistry* **89**: 191–198.

Sokół-Łętowska, A., Oszmiański, J., and Wojdyło, A. (2007). Antioxidant activity of the phenolic compounds of hawthorn, pine and skullcap. *Food Chemistry* **103** (3): 853–859.

Spinella, M. (2002). The importance of pharmacological synergy in psychoactive herbal medicines. *Alternative Medicine Review* **7** (2): 130–137.

Steel, G.G. and Peckham, M.J. (1979). Exploitable mechanisms in combined radiotherapy-chemotherapy: the concept of additivity. *International Journal of Radiation Oncology, Biology, Physics* **5**: 85–91.

Stern, S., Behar, S., and Gottlieb, S. (2003). Cardiology patient page. Aging and diseases of the heart. *Circulation* **108** (14): e99–e101. https://doi.org/10.1161/01.CIR.0000086898.96021.B9.

Suhnel, J. (1990). Evaluation of synergism and antagonism for the combined action of antiviral agents. *Antiviral Research* **13**: 23–40.

Svedström, U., Vuorela, H., Kostiainen, R. et al. (2002). Isolation and identification of oligomeric procyanidins from *Crataegus* leaves and flowers. *Phytochemistry* **60** (8): 821–825.

Tallarida, R.J. (2001). Drug synergism: its detection and applications. *The Journal of Pharmacology and Experimental Therapeutics* **298** (3): 865–872.

Tallarida, R.J. (2006). An overview of drug combination analysis with isobolograms. *The Journal of Pharmacology and Experimental Therapeutics* **319**: 1–7.

Tallarida, R.J. (2011). Quantitative methods for assessing drug synergism. *Genes & Cancer* **2** (11): 1003–1008.

Tallarida, R.J. (2012). Revisiting the isobole and related quantitative methods for assessing drug synergism. *The Journal of Pharmacology and Experimental Therapeutics* **342**: 2–8.

Tankanow, R., Tamer, H.R., Streetman, D.S. et al. (2003). Interaction study between digoxin and a preparation of hawthorn (*Crataegus oxyacantha*). *Journal Clinical Pharmacology* **43** (6): 637–642.

Tassell, M.C., Kingston, R., Gilroy, D. et al. (2010). Hawthorn (*Crataegus* spp.) in the treatment of cardiovascular disease. *Pharmacognosy Reviews* **4** (7): 32–41.

Valeriote, F. and Lin, H. (1975). Synergistic interaction of anticancer agents: a cellular perspective. *Cancer Chemotherapy Reports* **59**: 95–900.

van Vuuren, S.F. and Viljoen, A.M. (2008). *In vitro* evidence of Phyto-synergy for plant part combinations of *Croton gratissimus* (Euphorbiaceae) used in African traditional healing. *Journal of Ethnopharmacology* **119** (3): 700–704.

Wagner, H. and Ulrich-Merzenich, G. (2009). Synergy research: approaching a new generation of phytopharmaceuticals. *Phytomedicine* **16**: 97–110.

Wang, J., Xiong, X., and Feng, B. (2013). Effect of *Crataegus* usage in cardiovascular disease prevention: an evidence-based approach. *Evidence-Based Complementary and Alternative Medicine* https://doi.org/10.1155/2013/149363. *Epub 2013 Dec 29.*

Webb, J.L. (1963). Effect of more than one inhibitor. In: *Enzymes and Metabolic Inhibitors*, vol. **1** (ed. J.L. Webb), 66–79. New York: Academic Press.

Weinstein, J.N., Bunow, B., Weislow, O.S. et al. (1990). Synergistic drug combinations in AIDS therapy. *Annals of the New York Academy of Sciences* **616**: 367–384.

Wen, L., Guo, X., Liu, R.H. et al. (2015). Phenolic contents and cellular antioxidant activity of Chinese hawthorn '*Crataegus pinnatifida*'. *Food Chemistry* **186**: 54–62.

Williamson, E.M. (2001). Synergy and other interactions in phytomedicines. *Phytomedicine* **8** (5): 401–409.

World Health Organisation (2015). Cardiovascular diseases (CVDs) Fact sheet N°317 [Online]. Available at: https://www.who.int/news-room/fact-sheets/detail/cardiovascular-diseases-(cvds) (accessed 20 November 2019).

Wu, J., Peng, W., Qin, R., and Zhou, H. (2014). *Crataegus pinnatifida*: chemical constituents, pharmacology, and potential applications. *Molecules* **19**: 1685–1712.

Yan, H., Zhang, B., Li, S., and Zhao, Q. (2010). A formal model for analyzing drug combination effects and its application in TNF-α-induced Nfκb pathway. *BMC Systems Biology* **4**: 50–62.

Ye, X.-L., Huang, W.-W., Chen, Z. et al. (2010). Synergetic effect and structure-activity relationship of 3-Hydroxy-3-methylglutaryl coenzyme a reductase inhibitors from *Crataegus pinnatifida* Bge. *Journal of Agricultural and Food Chemistry* **58**: 3132–3138.

Yoo, K.-M., Lee, C.H., Lee, H. et al. (2007). Relative antioxidant and cytoprotective activities of common herbs. *Food Chemistry* **106**: 929–936.

Zhang, Z. (2002a). Hypercholesterolaemic activity of hawthorn fruit is mediated by regulation of cholesterol 7 a hydroxylase and acyl Coa: cholesterol acyltransferase. *Food Research International* **35**: 885–891.

Zhang, Z., Chang, Q., Zhu, M. et al. (2001). Characterization of antioxidants present in hawthorn fruits. *Journal of Nutritional Biochemistry* **12**: 144–152.

Zhang, Z., Ho, W.K.K., Huang, Y. et al. (2002b). Hawthorn fruit is hypolipidemic in rabbits fed a high cholesterol diet. *Journal of Nutrition* **132** (1): 5–10.

Zumdick, S., Deters, A., and Hensel, A. (2012). In vitro intestinal transport of oligomeric procyanidins (DP 2 to 4) cross monolayers of Caco-2 cells. *Fitoterapia* **83**: 1210–1217.

10
Potential Applications of Polyphenols from Herbs and Spices in Dairy Products as Natural Antioxidants

Katerina Tzima[1,2], Nigel P. Brunton[2], Alka Choudhary[1], and Dilip K. Rai[1]

[1]*Department of Food BioSciences, Teagasc Food Research Centre Ashtown, Dublin, D15 KN3K, Ireland*

[2]*School of Agriculture and Food Science, University College Dublin, Dublin, D04 V1W8, Ireland*

10.1 Introduction

In recent years, global demand for milk and dairy products has risen because of the rapid economic growth of developing countries such as China and India (More 2009). However, transport of dairy products to far-off countries has been a challenge due to their short shelf life, associated safety risks, and altered organoleptic characteristics (More 2009; Safer and Al-Nughamish 1999). The main reason is that dairy products have augmented unsaturated fatty acid contents, which are prone to oxidative deterioration. Several external and intrinsic factors drive oxidative deterioration of dairy products, including the existence of O_2 (oxygen), metal ions and enzymes, and also heat and light (Correddu et al. 2015).

Oxidative deterioration of lipids results in the formation of an extensive amount of volatile and non-volatile compounds, with the former being particularly odorous in numerous cases. Hence, an insignificant concentration of secondary fatty acid-derived compounds could be responsible for the development of rancid, metallic, cardboard-like, and fishy off-flavors, as well as discoloration (Siefarth et al. 2014; Frankel 2005). Additionally, lipid oxidation can lead to the modification of vitamins, amino-acids, and proteins and loss of protein functionality as a result of protein denaturation (Frankel 2005). In addition to the nutritional quality deterioration,

Herbs, Spices and Medicinal Plants: Processing, Health Benefits and Safety, First Edition.
Edited by Mohammad B. Hossain, Nigel P. Brunton, and Dilip K. Rai.

another significant issue is safety, as the potentially toxic secondary compounds may result in diabetes, cardiovascular disease, and tumors (Moure et al. 2001; Olmedo et al. 2014).

Despite artificial additives being broadly used in the industry for the prevention of lipid oxidation and microbial growth, the growing concerns of consumers with regard to synthetic chemical residues in food have discouraged the use of synthetic additives (Ayala-Zavala et al. 2011). Commonly used synthetic antioxidants are butylated hydroxyanisole (BHA), butylated hydroxytoluene (BHT), propyl gallate (PG), and *tert*-butyl hydroquinone (TBHQ) (Moure et al. 2001). These synthetic antioxidants are considered to be unstable, as they are volatile and also easily degradable on exposure to high temperatures (Namiki 1990; Martínez-Tomé et al. 2001). Furthermore, regular consumption of foods fortified with synthetic antioxidants could potentially result in health implications such as carcinogenesis and intoxication (Martínez-Tomé et al. 2001).

Therefore, research in the field of natural additives, particularly of plant origin, has increased remarkably (Fernández-López et al. 2005). There are several benefits of their use in food products, including their acceptability for the consumer, safety, organoleptic tolerability, and efficient antioxidant properties (Sacchetti et al. 2005). Phenolic compounds derived from plants have multifunctional roles such as antioxidant and antimicrobial properties (Cicerale et al. 2009), and previous research has demonstrated that polyphenols can reduce oxidation in dairy products (O'Connell and Fox 2001). Among the food plants, herbs and spices have been well documented to possess strong antioxidant properties owing to their rich polyphenol content (Hinneburg et al. 2006; Yanishlieva et al. 2006). However, their application in the production and quality of dairy and milk products has been scarcely reported.

10.2 Implications in the Use of Herbs and Spices as Natural Antioxidants in Milk and Dairy Products

10.2.1 Effect of Phenolic Concentration on Milk and Dairy Products

Incorporation of the essential oils (EOs) of herbs and spices is generally accepted in processed food products (Moro et al. 2015). The normal concentration of herbs and spices in food products ranges between 0.05% and 0.1% (Tajkarimi et al. 2010). However, there are restrictions and limitations on their use in dairy products (Moro et al. 2015; Axten et al. 2008), based on the fact that dairy are relatively complex systems due to high protein (5.55%) and fat (6.82%) contents (Moro et al. 2015).

Milk is a typical example of an oil-in-water emulsion (Alemán et al. 2015), where water is the continuous phase. A significant advantage of water-soluble phenolics is their addition in the emulsion system with a one-step process. However, in parallel, a significant risk of the use of water-soluble antioxidants in oil-in-water emulsions is their exclusive separation into the water phase. Thus, higher concentrations might be required to guarantee adequate availability of antioxidants in the oil–water interface and their antioxidant effectiveness (Liu and Yang 2008).

The high concentrations of polyphenols, however, can lead to interactions with proteins, minerals, and carbohydrates (Karakaya 2004), or pro-oxidative effects in some cases (Shahidi 2015). On the other hand, the lipid-soluble antioxidants need to be initially dissolved in the oil phase, and the oil phase has to be removed subsequently. This multistep processes and its associated costs restrict the industrial usage of lipophilic polyphenols. It is also evident that the antioxidant action of plant extracts is related to the most active phenolic compounds and not their concentration (Abdalla and Roozen 2001), and therefore targeting the most potent phenolic compounds and their use at low concentrations as antioxidants may serve the purpose.

10.2.2 Effect of Phenolics on the Organoleptic Properties of Dairy Products

Polyphenols have a significant role in the organoleptic properties of food products (Rider et al. 1992). Most polyphenols have a distinctive astringency and bitterness (Axten et al. 2008) that result from their interactions, principally of procyanidins, with the glycoproteins of saliva (Rider et al. 1992; Dai and Mumper 2010). As has been reported, astringency stems from water-soluble phenols with molecular weights from 500 to 3000 Da (Bate-Smith and Swain 1962). Apart from their flavor, the aroma of herbs and spices may restrict their use as natural antioxidants (Kiokias et al. 2008; Embuscado 2015). Nonetheless, Ramshaw (1985) has proposed that low concentrations of phenolic compounds could possibly result in anticipated smoky, sweet, or caramel flavors, whereas higher levels impart unpleasant sensory attributes (sharp, sheep yard, medicinal) (Ramshaw 1985).

Although Chilean oregano, summer savory, sage and rosemary possess high antioxidant capacity, their application as food preservatives, even at low concentrations, is restricted due to their characteristic flavor (Madsen et al. 1996; Ibáñez et al. 1999). Similarly, it has been shown by Carrillo and Tena (2006) that the addition of antioxidant extracts of rosemary in food products can lead to unacceptable flavor and aroma due to the presence of residual volatile compounds such as camphor, verbenone, and borneol (Carrillo and Tena 2006).

According to Sawale et al. (2017), the direct addition of herbal bioactive compounds in milk can influence its organoleptic properties, concerning its pH, pigmentation, and flavor. Therefore, their applicability is limited in numerous dairy-based drinks. Their organoleptic properties can further deteriorate throughout storage, resulting in consumer rejection (Sawale et al. 2017). However, the impact of polyphenol addition in dairy has been scarcely investigated. Axten et al. (2008) studied the impact of polyphenolic extracts of apple and grape seed on the properties of a milk-based beverage. Their findings demonstrated a significant impact of apple-seed extract on the bitterness of the product. In parallel, grape-seed extract was preferable to the apple seed and had a little influence on the organoleptic properties of milk. The authors suggested several methods for the creation of an acceptable product, by the addition of flavors along with low amounts of sugars to balance the bitter and astringent flavors, or the addition of cyclodextrin to inhibit the reaction between bitter molecules and taste buds to suppress bitterness. It was also suggested that by adjusting the protein/phenolic content, the astringent flavor could be reduced by the reaction of polyphenols with casein molecules, and complexation of compounds (Axten et al. 2008).

In another study by Bandyopadhyay et al. (2007a), the organoleptic properties of a dairy product (Sandesh) supplemented with aonla, coriander, spinach, turmeric, and curry leaves were examined. The samples with added aonla, coriander, and spinach were preferable compared to the control, whereas the distinctive flavor of curry and turmeric reduced their acceptance (Bandyopadhyay et al. 2007a). In their subsequent study, Bandyopadhyay et al. (2007b) showed that ginger, beet, and their combinations led to better product acceptability compared to mint and its combinations with ginger and beet as natural antioxidants in the same product. The lower acceptance of mint was attributed to the perceived pungency (Bandyopadhyay et al. 2007b).

The sensory evaluation of ice creams flavored with herbal EOs (thyme, basil, and marjoram) resulted in high scores on a scale from 1 (very poor) to 9 (excellent) from all the involved panelists. The examined sensory properties were concerning the appearance, body, and texture, as well as the melting resistance of the samples. The samples with basil oils were less accepted compared to those with thyme and marjoram, and marjoram samples were the most preferred (Ramadan et al. 2013). In an additional study of Karaman and Kayacier (2012), ice cream was supplemented with black tea and herbal tea samples (chamomile, sage, linden). The addition of chamomile resulted in the most accepted product after sensory evaluation. Nonetheless, black tea resulted in dark pigmentation of the products, while sage led to a distinguishable flavor (Karaman and Kayacier 2012).

The addition of sweet potato pulp was examined in terms of sensory acceptance in three types of fermented milk. The fermented milk had the following incorporated matrices: lyophilized extract (1% w/w of 87.5% clove and 12.5% green mate), lyophilized extract and sweet potato pulp, and only sweet potato pulp. The samples were examined in terms of liking (texture, taste, odor, and overall acceptance) using a 9-point hedonic scale (1: extremely disliked, 5: indifferent, and 9: extremely liked). It was revealed that fermented milk supplemented with lyophilized extract (1% w/w) containing 87.5% clove and 12.5% green mate and sweet potato pulp had the best sensory acceptance (Ramos et al. 2017).

Santos et al. (2014) suggested that added aqueous rosemary extract in yogurt, at a concentration of 400 mg/kg, is not considered to have a distinguishable flavor in the product (Santos et al. 2014). In another piece of research, trained panelists evaluated cheddar cheese samples supplemented with green tea aqueous extract at concentrations of 0, 1, and 2 g/kg. With supplementation, cheddar cheese lost its typical flavor and astringency was increased (Giroux et al. 2013).

Hence, based on these research findings, deodorization steps are considered essential for the successful incorporation of natural compounds into dairy products. Deodorized extracts, with no impact on the organoleptic properties of products, are already available in the market. Alternatively, high-purity antioxidant compounds can be generated, which entail usage in low amounts in food products to circumvent the issue of aroma and flavor (Embuscado 2015). Herbal extract encapsulation is considered to be an additional successful method for masking parameters such as astringency, taste, and pigmentation after their addition to dairy drinks (Sawale et al. 2017).

10.2.3 Effect of Phenolics on the Protein Stability of Milk and Dairy Products

Milk proteins are considered the stabilizers of dairy emulsions against flocculation, coalescence, and separation (Zayas 2012). Milk contains two protein fractions, caseins and whey, which constitute 80% and 20% of the whole milk, respectively (Sindayikengera and Xia 2006). Caseins are divided in α-, β-, and κ-caseins, whereas their content is approximately 75%, 22%, and 3%, respectively, of the whole casein fraction (O'Mahony and Fox 2014). Whey proteins consist mainly of α-lactalbumin and β-lactoglobulin and constitute 70–80% of the total whey proteins (Fox 2003). Previous research has demonstrated that molecular interactions can take place into dairy products as phenolic extracts are added, which can consequently stimulate modifications in both extracts and milk components (Hussain et al. 2015).

When natural phenolic extracts are added to milk, there is the probability of the formation of polyphenol–protein complex compounds (Gad and El-Salam 2010; Chaudhuri et al. 2011). Spectroscopic studies have shown that polyphenols interact strongly with casein proteins, and the formed casein–polyphenol complexes result in modifications of both protein and polyphenol structures (Hasni et al. 2011). Phenolic compounds can act as polydentate ligands on the surface area of milk proteins and associate with them through hydrophobic interactions and hydrogen bonding. The interactions are determined by both the category and concentration of milk proteins and phenolics (Gad and El-Salam 2010), and also by the molecular size of polyphenols, as a higher molecular weight compound results in higher polyphenol affinity to protein molecules (De-Fretias and Mateus 2001).

Covalent binding and non-covalent association are the two main mechanisms for protein changes triggered by phenolic compounds (Ozdal et al. 2013). The non-covalent interaction between proteins and polyphenols can occur through hydrogen bonding among electronegative atoms of nitrogen or O_2 (oxygen), mainly amino ($-NH_2$) and hydroxyl (–OH) groups, and a positively charged hydrogen atom from another polyphenol or protein molecule. The interaction can result in the formation of single or multiple bonds and is dependent on the polyphenol structure as well as on the degree of hydroxylation (Haslam 1974).

Additionally, polyphenol autooxidation in the presence of O_2 creates irreversible, covalent bonds with protein molecules and incorporated polyphenols. The autoxidation encompasses one or two steps of electron transfer, where the polyphenolic structure and their capacity for redox cycling contribute as significant parameters in covalent bonding. Subsequently, the formed structures augment antioxidant or pro-oxidant capacities (Brudzynski and Maldonado-Alvarez 2015). In addition, according to Aewsiri et al. (2009), the covalent bonding of phenolic compounds with proteins causes the blocking of hydrophilic groups such as thiol and amino, and there is also an increase of apolar groups and the introduction of polar groups. These processes contribute to the modification of hydrophilic or hydrophobic properties of the protein molecules (Aewsiri et al. 2009).

Protein–polyphenol complexes leading to protein functionality shifting may also result in protein unfolding and precipitation (Hasni et al. 2011; Papadopoulou and Frazier 2004). Additionally, these protein–polyphenol complexes are proposed to reduce the phenolic bioavailability and action, resulting in lower antioxidant capacity (Yuksel et al. 2010) in comparison to the sum of the antioxidant capacities of the individual compounds (Arts et al. 2001).

10.2.4 Effect of Indigenous Antioxidant Compounds (Chlorophyll) on the Color of Milk and Dairy Products

Color poses an additional barrier to the systematic use of herbs and spices as natural additives (Kiokias et al. 2008). Pigments, such as chlorophyll, have a significant effect on the marketability of products, as colors are the initial aspect that consumers observe (Schoefs 2004). Abdalla and Roozen (2001) examined the effect of the addition of plant extracts in salad dressings. Particularly after homogenization of the extracts with olive oil, and subsequent exposure of dressings to light, oxidative deterioration was observed. This was attributed to the content of chlorophylls in plant extracts, as well as in olive oil, and their potential action as photosensitizers (Abdalla and Roozen 2001).

Carocho et al. (2016) examined the effect of basil addition as a functional and preservative agent in "Serra da Estrela" cheese. Dehydrated basil resulted in green pigmentation of the cheese, whereas the samples supplemented with basil decoction had a slightly brighter yellow pigmentation, barely perceptible, compared to the control samples (Carocho et al. 2016). The findings from additional research by Giroux et al. (2013) showed that Cheddar cheese enriched with green tea aqueous extracts was significantly affected in terms of color, where a decreased lightness along with increased redness and yellowness was observed in the product (Giroux et al. 2013).

10.3 Milk and Dairy Products as Carriers of Natural Antioxidants

The action of herbs and spices as antioxidants has also been investigated in dairy beverages and skim milk. O'Connell and Fox (1999) suggested that polyphenol-rich extracts led to increased stability of casein micelles in milk (O'Connell and Fox 1999). As reported by Boroski et al. (2012) oregano extract (*Origanum vulgare*) and EOs of oregano (*Origanum minutiflorum*) decreased photo-oxidation, heat-induced oxidation of omega-3 fatty acids, and color development of dairy beverages. The samples were examined throughout 10-day storage and were supplemented with 2% (w/w) linseed oil. An additional significant aspect was the maintenance of the dairy beverage's physical stability. The samples exposed to heat and light were examined in terms of color, hexanal, propanal, dissolved O_2 (oxygen), and conjugated diene hydroperoxides after the addition of different concentrations of oregano extract and EO of oregano. Oregano extract was found to be more effective in all the evaluated parameters (Boroski et al. 2012).

Gad and El-Salam (2010) examined the antioxidant action of rosemary and green tea water extracts (2%, 4%, 6%, 8%, and 10%) after their individual addition to skim milk. The impact of different processes including pasteurization, homogenization, addition of sodium chloride (NaCl), calcium chloride ($CaCl_2$), and rennet coagulation time were assessed in the reconstituted skim milk. The results indicated that both the phenolic content and antioxidant capacity of milk were significantly increased with the addition of both rosemary and tea extracts. Antioxidant activity was further improved by the addition $CaCl_2$ and pasteurization, whereas rennet coagulation time was also increased by elevating the extract concentration in skim milk. Nonetheless, NaCl reduced the antioxidant action and homogenization was ineffective. Ramos et al. (2017) incorporated phenolic-rich herbal extracts of green mate, clove, and lemongrass in fermented and non-fermented milk, with or without sweet potato pulp. Addition of a lyophilized extract (1% w/w) containing 87.5% clove and 12.5% green mate and sweet potato pulp increased the total phenolic content (TPC) and the antioxidant capacity of fermented milk. The TPC and total reducing capacity had a slight change during 21 days of storage. The data showed that the herbal extracts and sweet potato pulp may be used to develop new dairy foods with potential functional properties (Ramos et al. 2017).

The addition of herb compounds from vidarikand to cow milk at a concentration equal to 0.4% resulted in modified physicochemical properties, but it may be appropriate for low-temperature treated functional dairy products. The milk modifications were evaluated through viscosity measurement, ethanol stability and trolox equivalent antioxidant capacity (TEAC) tests, hydroxy methyl furfural (HMF) content, and color features. It was concluded that the vidarikand-milk model declined in ethanol stability, HMF value, and lightness. However, its redness and yellowness, as well as its antioxidant capacity, were increased in comparison to the control sample (Sawale et al. 2015; 2017).

10.3.1 Butter and Dairy Spreads as Carriers of Natural Antioxidants

The effects of methanolic extracts of Greek sage, rosemary, and oregano on butter stability have been studied by Ayar et al. (2001). After the storage at 5 °C or 25 °C, butter samples incorporated with individual or mixed herb extracts at concentrations of 0.02% or 0.05% were compared with BHA (0.02%) and control samples. As revealed by their peroxide (POVs) and thiobarbituric acid (TBA) values, all the extracts and their mixtures had a better antioxidant capacity than synthetic BHA. Sage extracts displayed the best antioxidant capacity in the butter samples stored at 5 °C in comparison to other extracts (Ayar et al. 2001).

The EOs of *Satureja cilicica* were also used in butter as a natural antioxidant at various concentrations (0.5%, 1.0%, and 2.0% w/w) (Ozkan et al. 2007). The EO incorporated butter samples were stored for 60 days at 4 and 20 °C, and antioxidant analysis was done at day 20, 40, and 60 of the study. A strong antioxidant capacity was observed and was found to be concentration-dependent, as the highest concentration (2%) exhibited the greatest activity. Diterpenes and phenolics, particularly thymol and carvacrol, were reported to be the major antioxidant compounds (Ozkan et al. 2007).

The capacity of the phenolic compounds gallic acid, caffeic acid, and catechin to impede oxidation in butter was examined by Soulti and Roussis (2007). The estimation was carried out through POVs and TBA values throughout storage of butter at 50 and 110 °C. Butter incorporated with 80 mg/l of individual phenolics was compared to butter samples with BHA (200 mg/l). Gallic acid, even at a storage temperature of 110 °C, was found to be more effective than BHA (Soulti and Roussis 2007).

Santos et al. (2014) screened alcoholic extracts of different *Lamiaceae* herbs (rosemary, oregano, sage, thyme, and marjoram) in butter for oxidative stability. The samples at concentration 400 mg/kg of rosemary extract were assessed at two different temperatures (60 and 110 °C). Rosemary was effective in inhibiting lipid deterioration as determined by the low amount of formed and degraded peroxides (Santos et al. 2014).

10.3.2 Cheese as a Carrier of Natural Antioxidants

Han et al. (2011) developed a functional cheese product with the addition of polyphenols. The prepared cheese was supplemented with the phenolics catechin, epigallocatechin gallate, homovanillic acid, hesperetin, tannic acid, and flavones, as well as with crude compounds from grape extract, green tea extract, and dehydrated cranberry powder. It was found that a concentration of 0.5 mg/ml of polyphenols in the cheese curd exhibited an efficacious free radical scavenging capacity (Han et al. 2011). Similarly, Giroux et al. (2013) reported that the incorporation of green tea aqueous extracts at a concentration of 1 or 2 g/kg of milk increased the antioxidant activity of Cheddar cheese (Giroux et al. 2013).

Carocho et al. (2015) suggested basil as a good matrix to be added in food products, due to its high antioxidant capacity, presenting it as a potential functional ingredient or preservative (Carocho et al. 2015). In their subsequent research, Carocho et al. (2016) examined the effects of the addition of basil in "Serra da Estrela" cheese. Basil was added in two different forms in cheese samples (dried leaves and decoctions), at a concentration equal to 1.37 g of dried plant in each sample. The antioxidant capacity of the different cheese samples was determined after approximately one month of maturation. It was demonstrated through antioxidant assays, namely reducing power, β-carotene bleaching inhibition, and thiobarbituric acid reactive substances (TBARS), that the samples supplemented with basil had increased antioxidant capacities. Regarding lipid peroxidation inhibition, basil decoction was more effective; while in reducing power assay, dried basil leaves exhibited considerably higher efficiency compared to the control cheese (Carocho et al. 2016).

Olmedo et al. (2013) reported that the addition of oregano and rosemary EOs 0.2% (w/w) reduced the oxidation and fermented flavors in flavored cream cheese after 35 days, indicating that their addition extended its shelf life (Olmedo et al. 2013). The EOs obtained from oregano hydro-distilled leaves and flowers of different varieties, as well as thymol, were used by Asensio et al. (2015) for the preservation of organic cottage cheese. After the addition of EOs in cottage cheese at a concentration of 0.05% (w/w), and throughout thermal storage for 30 days, lipid oxidation in addition to organic and fatty acid amounts were measured. The addition of oregano EOs in organic cottage cheese effectively retarded lipid-oxidation and consequently quality deterioration during storage (Asensio et al. 2015).

Tooryan and Azizkhani (2016) determined the effect of EOs from clary sage (*Salvia sclarea*) and basil on the storage quality parameters of Iranian white cheese. The samples were supplemented with EOs at three concentration levels (0.5%, 0.75%, 1% w/w) and compared to samples with BHT at a concentration of 0.05% (w/w) after 90 days at 4 °C and 39 days at 26 °C. The high phenolic content of the samples with added EOs was suggested as being responsible for their increased antioxidant capacity as demonstrated through their elevated DPPH (2, 2-diphenyl-1-picryl-hydrazyl-hydrate) free radical activities and reduced TBARS. The samples incorporated with 0.75 and 1% of basil EO exhibited the highest antioxidant action (Tooryan and Azizkhani 2016).

Asensio et al. (2015) examined the effect of Argentinean oregano EOs (Compacto, Cordobes, Criollo, and Mendocino) and thymol on the production of flavored organic cottage cheese. The lipid oxidation products and the modifications in fatty and organic acid profiles were evaluated throughout a 30-day accelerated oxidation test. It was observed that the addition of oregano EO in organic cottage cheese led to reduced chemical degradation throughout storage. Samples supplemented with Cordobes and Compacto EOs significantly reduced the production of organic acids and maintained the stability of polyunsaturated fatty acids and oxidative stability (Asensio et al. 2015).

According to Caleja et al. (2015), the antioxidant capacity of chamomile extracts acquired through decoction is attributed to the presence of phenolic compounds, mainly dicaffeoyl-2,7-anhydro-3-deoxy-2-octulopyranosonic acid and luteolin-*O*-glucuronide. Cottage cheese samples supplemented with chamomile extracts including these compounds were compared with samples with added chamomile powder as well as plain cottage cheese, and different parameters were evaluated (nutritional composition, antioxidant activity, color). It was found that chamomile decoctions did not have a significant effect on the nutritional and fatty acid profiles of the samples, but they increased antioxidant action (Caleja et al. 2015).

10.3.3 Ghee as a Carrier of Natural Antioxidants

The addition of herbs and spices to retain the oxidative stability of Indian clarified butterfat, known as ghee, has been reported by several researchers since the 1990s (Amr 1990; El-Shourbagy and El-Zahar 2014; Gandhi et al. 2013; Merai et al. 2003; Nazz and Prakash 2000; Pankaj et al. 2013; Patel et al. 2013; Pawar et al. 2014; Shende et al. 2014). Oxidative deterioration of ghee occurs throughout storage and deep-frying, with apparent consequences on its main quality factors (color, flavor, aroma, nutritional value) (Pawar et al. 2012).

Recently, Shende et al. (2014) proved that clove extracts, and particularly steam-distilled clove extracts, were effective in inhibiting oxidative deterioration of ghee during accelerated storage conditions and deep-frying. Nonetheless, the synthetic antioxidant BHA exhibited a higher antioxidant capacity under accelerated storage conditions. This was attributed to the phenolic content of the extracts based on the positive correlation between total phenolics and the determined antioxidant activities (Shende et al. 2014).

Pawar et al. (2014) studied the effect of added aqueous and ethanolic herb extracts of vidarikand, shatavari, and ashwagandha on the oxidative stability of ghee through accelerated oxidation. The extracts were assessed in comparison to BHA, with a concentration of 0.5% and 0.02% (w/w), respectively. The antioxidant activities of the samples (β-carotene linoleic acid model assay, DPPH assay) showed that both aqueous and ethanolic extracts had the capacity to inhibit oxidative deterioration in ghee, though not as efficiently as BHA (Pawar et al. 2014).

El-Shourbagy and El-Zahar (2014) used ethanolic extracts of peanut skins, pomegranate peels, and olive pomace to inhibit lipid oxidation in ghee. The natural antioxidants of the plant-waste materials were incorporated at the concentrations of 200, 400, and 600 ppm and compared to samples with incorporated BHA (200 ppm) after accelerated storage conditions. The findings suggested that a concentration of 200 ppm of plant antioxidants is effective in retarding lipid oxidation. Patel et al. (2013) assessed the antioxidant capacity of coriander steam-distilled extract and oleoresin in ghee. After 21 days of storage, both matrices maintained the oxidative stability of ghee in comparison to the control sample. However, relative to BHA, they had lower antioxidant action after storage, and higher action after deep-frying (Patel et al. 2013).

It was suggested by Pankaj et al. (2013) that ethanolic extract (7% w/w) of arjuna bark increased the shelf life of mainly cow, but also buffalo, ghee compared to the control sample throughout storage at accelerated oxidation conditions (80 ± 1 °C). Apart from natural antioxidants, these ethanolic extracts were also suggested to be enhancers of the phytosterol contents of ghee (Pankaj et al. 2013). Gandhi et al. (2013) assessed the antioxidant action of ethanolic and aqueous extracts of vidarikand in ghee and suggested that they were capable of hindering oxidation, but substantially not as efficiently as other natural (rosemary and green tea) and synthetic (BHA and TBHQ) antioxidants. Additionally, it was determined that the ethanolic vidarikand extracts had better antioxidative action relative to aqueous extract in most of the examined parameters (Gandhi et al. 2013).

Merai et al. (2003) also determined the oxidative stability of ghee after the incorporation of antioxidant compounds recovered from two varieties of holy basil (*Ocimum sanctum* and *Ocimum tenuiflorum*) leaf powder. *O. tenuiflorum* exhibited a slightly higher antioxidant activity than *O. sanctum,* and at a concentration of 0.6% (w/v) possessed almost equal antioxidant activity as BHA at a concentration of 0.02% (Merai et al. 2003).

Nazz and Prakash (2000) indicated that ghee prepared with cardamom, clove, fenugreek, pepper, or turmeric in a concentration equal to 1% (w/w) maintained its quality characteristics in comparison to the control samples, where turmeric showed the highest efficiency among all the used spices (Nazz and Prakash 2000). Amr (1990) examined the addition of rosemary, sage, rue, and fennel to inhibit oxidative deterioration of sheep ghee. The ghee samples were prepared with milk, in which 7.5% (w/w) or 250 ppm of (1 : 1) BHA : BHT mixture or no additive, were incorporated. As indicated from the POVs of the samples under accelerated storage conditions, rosemary exhibited an antioxidant activity equivalent to the BHA : BHT mixture, while other herbs were less effective (Amr 1990).

10.3.4 Sandesh as a Carrier of Natural Antioxidants

Sandesh is a widely enjoyed Indian traditional dairy dessert. It is a product of coagulated milk proteins after the appliance of heat dehydration that is similar to cottage cheese (Bandyopadhyay et al. 2007b). Its high content of fat, fat-soluble vitamins, and sucrose (Aneja et al. 2002) make it susceptible to oxidative deterioration. As a result, several researchers examined the effects of the addition of antioxidants from natural sources (herbs and vegetables) in sandesh as means to enhance its oxidative stability (Aneja et al. 2002).

Bandyopadhyay et al. (2007a) attempted the addition of the herbs, turmeric, coriander, curry leaf, spinach, and aonla in the form of a paste at a concentration of 10% (w/w) into sandesh. Subsequently, they were compared to the synthetic antioxidants TBHQ and BHA : BHT (1 : 1) at concentrations of 100 and 200 ppm It was revealed that a 10% (w/w) concentration of the herbal paste enhanced the oxidative stability of sandesh in the order: turmeric > curry leaf > aonla > spinach > coriander leaf. Turmeric, curry leaf, or aonla exhibited analogous activity to that of BHA : BHT mixture, but TBHQ was the most effective antioxidant of all (Bandyopadhyay et al. 2007a).

Bandyopadhyay et al. (2007b) further reported the antioxidant capacities of mint, ginger, and beet as antioxidant sources in sandesh. The herbs were evaluated in four forms (paste, freeze-dried powder, tray-dried powder, ethanolic extract), separately and combined, and after their addition to the initial or final stage of the sample preparation. Subsequently, they were compared to BHA, BHT, and TBHQ. The results showed that the herbal ethanolic extracts exhibited the highest antioxidant action when added at the final preparation stage of sandesh, where ginger and its combination with mint showed exceptional results, demonstrating their ability to substitute TBHQ at an industrial scale. At the same time, all the extracts and their combinations (mint, ginger, and beet) showed the ability to substitute BHA and BHT (Bandyopadhyay et al. 2007b).

In their subsequent research, Bandyopadhyay et al. (2008) examined the same natural antioxidant sources (mint, ginger, and beet) after their addition to sandesh with the use of an accelerated oxidation test. The antioxidant activities of all the used antioxidants (natural/synthetic) were determined based on their capacity to inhibit oxidation of the emulsion β-carotene–linoleic acid system. Their findings indicated that all the natural antioxidants had effectiveness equivalent to that of synthetic antioxidants (TBHQ/combination of BHA and BHT), and ginger demonstrated the highest antioxidant action among all the natural antioxidants. After eight days of oven storage, TBHQ was the most effective antioxidant, and mint showed higher efficiency than ginger and was analogous to that of TBHQ (Bandyopadhyay et al. 2008).

10.3.5 Yogurt as a Carrier of Natural Antioxidants

In a study, Muniandy et al. (2016) examined the antioxidant effect of green, white, or black tea water extracts on yogurt oxidative stability throughout 21 days of storage at 4 °C. The order of the determined phenolic content, as well as the antioxidant action of yogurts incorporated with tea, from the highest to the lowest, was as follows: green tea yogurt > white tea yogurt > black tea yogurt. All the tea yogurts had higher antioxidant action compared to the control sample. An additional significant finding was that in spite of the presence of several phenolic compounds in the tea water extracts, none of the compounds were detected in yogurt samples (Muniandy et al. 2016).

Caleja et al. (2016) determined the effect of chamomile and fennel decoctions as natural antioxidants in yogurts against samples supplemented with the synthetic additive potassium sorbate. In each sample, 0.04% (w/w) natural or synthetic aqueous extract was incorporated. The analysis after three storage periods (0, 7, and 14 days) showed that the natural aqueous extracts improved oxidative stability of yogurts, and their antioxidant action was higher than potassium sorbate (Caleja et al. 2016).

10.3.6 Ice Cream as a Carrier of Natural Antioxidants

Use of thyme, marjoram, and basil EOs containing linalool, thymol, carvacrol, and eugenol in ice cream preparations indicated their effective antioxidant action. The addition of the EOs (10 ppm thyme, 3 ppm basil, and 3 ppm marjoram) in flavored ice cream formulations displayed a superior radical scavenging capacity from 52% to 98% compared to 15% in the control sample (Ramadan et al. 2013).

In a study by Karaman and Kayacier (2012), the addition of black and herbal teas (chamomile, linden, sage) brewed at different temperatures (40 °C, 80 °C) to ice cream revealed that the antioxidant capacity was reliant on both tea variety and temperature. Ice cream samples supplemented with linden or black tea and brewed at 80 °C exhibited the highest antioxidant action in comparison to other samples (Karaman and Kayacier 2012).

Abbreviations

BHA	Butylated hydroxyanisole
BHT	Butylated hydroxytoluene
$CaCl_2$	Calcium chloride
DPPH	2, 2-diphenyl-1-picryl-hydrazyl-hydrate
EO/EOs	Essential Oil/s
HMF	Hydroxy methyl furfural
NaCl	Sodium chloride
NH_2	Amino group
OH	Hydroxyl group
O_2	Oxygen
PG	Propyl gallate
POV	Peroxide values
TBA	Thiobarbituric acid values
TBARS	Thiobarbituric acid reactive substances
TEAC	Trolox equivalent antioxidant capacity
TPC	Total phenolic content
TBHQ	Tert-butyl hydroquinone

References

Abdalla, A.E. and Roozen, J.P. (2001). The effects of stabilised extracts of sage and oregano on the oxidation of salad dressings. *European Food Research and Technology* **212**: 55–560.

Aewsiri, T., Benjakul, S., Visessanguan, W. et al. (2009). Antioxidative activity and emulsifying properties of cuttlefish skin gelatin modified by oxidised phenolic compounds. *Food Chemistry* **117**: 160–168.

Alemán, M., Bou, R., Guardiola, F. et al. (2015). Antioxidative effect of lipophilized caffeic acid in fish oil enriched mayonnaise and milk. *Food Chemistry* **167**: 236–244.

Amr, A.S. (1990). Role of some aromatic herbs in extending the stability of sheep ghee during accelerated storage. *Egyptian Journal of Dairy Science* **18**: 335–344.

Aneja, R.P., Mathur, B.N., Chandan, R.C., and Banerjee, A.K. (eds.) (2002). *Technology of Indian Milk Products: Handbook on Process Technology Modernization for Professionals, Entrepreneurs and Scientists*. Gujarat, India: National Dairy Development Board (NDDB).

Arts, M.J., Haenen, G.R., Voss, H.P., and Bast, A. (2001). Masking of antioxidant capacity by the interaction of flavonoids with protein. *Food and Chemical Toxicology* **39**: 787–791.

Asensio, C.M., Grosso, N.R., and Juliani, H.R. (2015). Quality preservation of organic cottage cheese using oregano essential oils. *LWT-Food Science and Technology* **60**: 664–671.

Axten, L.G., Wohlers, M.W., and Wegrzyn, T. (2008). Using phytochemicals to enhance health benefits of milk: impact of polyphenols on flavor profile. *Journal of Food Science* **73**: H122–H126.

Ayala-Zavala, J.F., Vega-Vega, V., Rosas-Domínguez, C. et al. (2011). Agro-industrial potential of exotic fruit by-products as a source of food additives. *Food Research International* **44**: 1866–1874.

Ayar, A., Özcan, M., Akgül, A., and Akin, N. (2001). Butter stability as affected by extracts of sage, rosemary, and oregano. *Journal of Food Lipids* **8**: 15–25.

Bandyopadhyay, M., Chakraborty, R., and Raychaudhuri, U. (2007a). Incorporation of herbs into sandesh, an Indian sweet dairy product, as a source of natural antioxidants. *International Journal of Dairy Technology* **60**: 228–233.

Bandyopadhyay, M., Chakraborty, R., and Raychaudhuri, U. (2007b). A process for preparing a natural antioxidant enriched dairy product (Sandesh). *LWT-Food Science and Technology* **40**: 842–851.

Bandyopadhyay, M., Chakraborty, R., and Raychaudhuri, U. (2008). Antioxidant activity of natural plant sources in dairy dessert (Sandesh) under thermal treatment. *LWT-Food Science and Technology* **41**: 816–825.

Bate-Smith, E.C. and Swain, T. (1962). Flavonoid compounds. In: *Comparative Biochemistry: A Comprehensive Treatise*, 1e, vol. **4** (eds. H.S. Mason and A.M. Florkin), 755–809. New York: Academic Press.

Boroski, M., Giroux, H.J., Sabik, H. et al. (2012). Use of oregano extract and oregano essential oil as antioxidants in functional dairy beverage formulations. *LWT-Food Science and Technology* **47**: 167–174.

Brudzynski, K. and Maldonado-Alvarez, L. (2015). Polyphenol-protein complexes and their consequences for the redox activity, structure and function of honey. A current view and new hypothesis – a review. *Polish Journal of Food and Nutrition Sciences* **65**: 71–80.

Caleja, C., Barros, L., Antonio, A.L. et al. (2015). Development of a functional dairy food: exploring bioactive and preservation effects of chamomile (*Matricaria recutita* L.). *Journal of Functional Foods* **16**: 114–124.

Caleja, C., Barros, L., Antonio, A.L. et al. (2016). Fortification of yogurts with different antioxidant preservatives: a comparative study between natural and synthetic additives. *Food Chemistry* **210**: 262–268.

Carocho, M. Barros, L. Calhelha, R.C. et al. (2015). Potential of basil (Ocimum basilicum L.) as bioactive ingredient and natural preserver. 5th MoniQA International Conference, Porto, Portugal, 2015.

Carocho, M., Barros, L., Barreira, J.C. et al. (2016). Basil as functional and preserving ingredient in "Serra da Estrela" cheese. *Food Chemistry* **207**: 51–59.

Carrillo, J.D. and Tena, M.T. (2006). Determination of volatile compounds in antioxidant rosemary extracts by multiple headspace solid-phase microextraction and gas chromatography. *Flavour and Fragrance Journal* **21**: 626–633.

Chaudhuri, S., Chakraborty, S., and Sengupta, P.K. (2011). Probing the interactions of hemoglobin with antioxidant flavonoids via fluorescence spectroscopy and molecular modeling studies. *Biophysical Chemistry* **154**: 26–34.

Cicerale, S., Conlan, X.A., Sinclair, A.J., and Keast, R.S.J. (2009). Chemistry and health of olive oil phenolics. *Critical Reviews in Food Science and Nutrition* **49**: 218–236.

Correddu, F., Nudda, A., Manca, M.G. et al. (2015). Light-induced lipid oxidation in sheep milk: effects of dietary grape seed and linseed, alone or in combination, on milk oxidative stability. *Journal of Agricultural and Food Chemistry* **63**: 3980–3986.

Dai, J. and Mumper, R.J. (2010). Plant phenolics: extraction, analysis and their antioxidant and anticancer properties. *Molecules* **15**: 7313–7352.

De-Fretias, N. and Mateus, S. (2001). Structural features of procyanidin interactions with salivary proteins. *Journal of Agricultural and Food Chemistry* **49**: 940–945.

El-Shourbagy, G.A. and El-Zahar, K.M. (2014). Oxidative stability of ghee as affected by natural antioxidants extracted from food processing wastes. *Annals of Agricultural Science* **59**: 213–220.

Embuscado, M.E. (2015). Herbs and spices as antioxidants for food preservation. In: *Handbook of Antioxidants for Food Preservation*, 1e (ed. F. Shahidi), 251–283. Cambridge: Woodhead Publishing.

Fernández-López, J., Zhi, N., Aleson-Carbonell, L. et al. (2005). Antioxidant and antibacterial activities of natural extracts: application in beef meatballs. *Meat Science* **69**: 371–380.

Fox, P.F. (2003). Indigenous enzymes in milk. In: *Advanced Dairy Chemistry*, Proteins, 3e, vol. **1** (eds. P.F. Fox and P.L.H. McSweeney), 447–467. New York: Kluwer Academic/Plenum Publishers.

Frankel, E.N. (ed.) (2005). *Lipid Oxidation*. United Kingdom: Oily Press.

Gad, A.S. and El-Salam, M.H.A. (2010). The antioxidant properties of skim milk supplemented with rosemary and green tea extracts in response to pasteurisation, homogenisation and the addition of salts. *International Journal of Dairy Technology* **63**: 349–355.

Gandhi, K., Arora, S., Nilkanth, P., and Kumar, A. (2013). Effect of Vidarikand (extracts) on oxidative stability of ghee: a comparative study. *Research and Reviews: Journal of Dairy Science and Technology* **2**: 1–11.

Giroux, H.J., De Grandpré, G., Fustier, P. et al. (2013). Production and characterization of Cheddar-type cheese enriched with green tea extract. *Dairy Science & Technology* **93**: 241–254.

Han, J., Britten, M., St-Gelais, D. et al. (2011). Polyphenolic compounds as functional ingredients in cheese. *Food Chemistry* **124**: 1589–1594.

Haslam, E. (1974). Polyphenol-protein interactions. *Biochemical Journal* **139**: 285–288.

Hasni, I., Bourassa, P., Hamdani, S. et al. (2011). Interaction of milk a- and b-caseins with tea polyphenols. *Food Chemistry* **126**: 630–639.

Hinneburg, I., Damien Dorman, H.J., and Hiltunen, R. (2006). Antioxidant activities of extracts from selected culinary herbs and spices. *Food Chemistry* **97**: 122–129.

Hussain, S.A., Panjagari, N.R., Singh, R.R.B., and Patil, G.R. (2015). Potential herbs and herbal Nutraceuticals: food applications and their interactions with food components. *Critical Reviews in Food Science and Nutrition* **55**: 94–122.

Ibáñez, E., Oca, A., De Murga, G. et al. (1999). Supercritical fluid extraction and fractionation of different preprocessed rosemary plants. *Journal of Agricultural and Food Chemistry* **47**: 1400–1404.

Karakaya, S. (2004). Bioavailability of phenolic compounds. *Critical Reviews in Food Science and Nutrition* **44**: 453–464.

Karaman, S. and Kayacier, A. (2012). Rheology of ice cream mix flavoured with black tea or herbal teas and effect of flavouring on the sensory properties of ice cream. *Food and Bioprocess Technology* **5**: 3159–3169.

Kiokias, S., Varzakas, T., and Oreopoulou, V. (2008). In vitro activity of vitamins, flavonoids, and natural phenolic antioxidants against the oxidative deterioration of oil-based systems. *Critical Reviews in Food Science and Nutrition* **48**: 78–93.

Liu, T.T. and Yang, T.S. (2008). Effects of water-soluble natural antioxidants on photosensitized oxidation of conjugated linoleic acid in an oil-in-water emulsion system. *Journal of Food Science* **73**: C256–C261.

Madsen, H.L., Andersen, L., Christiansen, L. et al. (1996). Antioxidative activity of summer savory (*Satureja hortensis* L.) and rosemary (*Rosmarinus officinalis* L.) in minced, cooked pork meat. *Zeitschrift für Lebensmittel-Untersuchung und -Forschung* **203**: 333–338.

Martínez-Tomé, M., Jiménez, A.M., Ruggieri, S. et al. (2001). Antioxidant properties of mediterranean spices compared with common food additives. *Journal of Food Protection* **64**: 1412–1419.

Merai, M., Boghra, V.R., and Sharma, R.S. (2003). Extraction of antioxygenic principles from *Tulsi* leaves and their effects on oxidative stability of ghee. *Journal of Food Science and Technology* **40**: 52–57.

More, S. (2009). Global trends in milk quality: implications for the Irish dairy industry. *Irish Veterinary Journal* **62**: 1–10.

Moro, A., Librán, C.M., Berruga, M.I. et al. (2015). Dairy matrix effect on the transference of rosemary (*Rosmarinus officinalis*) essential oil compounds during cheese making. *Journal of the Science of Food and Agriculture* **95**: 1507–1513.

Moure, A., Cruz, J.M., Franco, D. et al. (2001). Natural antioxidants from residual sources. *Food Chemistry* **72**: 145–171.

Muniandy, P., Shori, A.B., and Baba, A.S. (2016). Influence of green, white and black tea addition on the antioxidant activity of probiotic yogurt during refrigerated storage. *Food Packaging and Shelf Life* **8**: 1–8.

Namiki, M. (1990). Antioxidants/antimutagens in food. *Critical Reviews in Food Science and Nutrition* **29**: 273–300.

Nazz, T. and Prakash, J. (2000). Storage stability of ghee with added spices. *Indian Journal of Nutrition and Dietetics* **37**: 20–27.

O'Connell, J.E. and Fox, P.F. (1999). Effect of extracts of oak (*Quercus petraea*) bark, oak leaves, aloe vera (*Curacao aloe*), coconut shell and wine on the colloidal stability of milk and concentrated milk. *Food Chemistry* **66**: 93–96.

O'Connell, J.E. and Fox, P.F. (2001). Significance and applications of phenolic compounds in the production and quality of milk and dairy products: a review. *International Dairy Journal* **11**: 103–120.

Olmedo, R.H., Nepote, V., and Grosso, N.R. (2013). Preservation of sensory and chemical properties in flavoured cheese prepared with cream cheese base using oregano and rosemary essential oils. *LWT-Food Science and Technology* **53**: 409–417.

Olmedo, R., Nepote, V., and Grosso, N.R. (2014). Antioxidant activity of fractions from oregano essential oils obtained by molecular distillation. *Food Chemistry* **156**: 212–219.

O'Mahony, J.A. and Fox, P.F. (2014). Milk: an overview. In: *Milk Proteins: From Expression to Food*, 2e (eds. M. Boland, H. Singh and A. Thompson), 19–75. New York: Academic Press/Elsevier Science.

Ozdal, T., Capanoglu, E., and Altay, F. (2013). A review on protein–phenolic interactions and associated changes. *Food Research International* **51**: 954–970.

Ozkan, G., Simsek, B., and Kuleasan, H. (2007). Antioxidant activities of Satureja cilicica essential oil in butter and in vitro. *Journal of Food Engineering* **79**: 1391–1396.

Pankaj, P., Khamrui, K., Devaraja, H., and Singh, R. (2013). The effects of alcoholic extract of Arjuna (*Terminalia arjuna* Wight Arn.) bark on stability of clarified butterfat. *Journal of Medicinal Plant Research* **4**: 2545–2550.

Papadopoulou, A. and Frazier, R.A. (2004). Characterization of protein–polyphenol interactions. *Trends in Food Science & Technology* **15**: 186–190.

Patel, S., Shende, S., Arora, S., and Singh, A.K. (2013). An assessment of the antioxidant potential of coriander extracts in ghee when stored at high temperature and during deep fat frying. *International Journal of Dairy Technology* **66**: 207–213.

Pawar, N., Arora, S., Bijoy, R.R., and Wadhwa, B.K. (2012). The effects of *Asparagus racemosus* (shatavari) extract on oxidative stability of ghee, in relation to added natural and synthetic antioxidants. *International Journal of Dairy Technology* **65**: 293–299.

Pawar, N., Gandhi, K., Purohit, A. et al. (2014). Effect of added herb extracts on oxidative stability of ghee (butter oil) during accelerated oxidation condition. *Journal of Food Science and Technology* **51**: 2727–2733.

Ramadan, K.M., Ashoush, I., and El-Batawy, O. (2013). Comparative evaluation of three essential oils as functional antioxidants and natural flavoring agents in ice cream. *World Applied Sciences Journal* **23**: 159–166.

Ramos, L.R., Santos, J.S., Daguer, H. et al. (2017). Analytical optimization of a phenolic-rich herbal extract and supplementation in fermented milk containing sweet potato pulp. *Food Chemistry* **221**: 950–958.

Ramshaw, E.H. (1985). Aspects of the flavor of phenol, methylphenol and ethylphenol. *CSIRO Food Research Quarterly* **45**: 20–22.

Rider, E.D., Ikegami, M., and Jobe, A.H. (1992). Localization of alveolar surfactant clearance in rabbit lung cells. *American Journal of Physiology-Lung Cellular and Molecular Physiology* **263**: 201–209.

Sacchetti, G., Maietti, S., Muzzoli, M. et al. (2005). Comparative evaluation of 11 essential oils of different origin as functional antioxidants, antiradicals and antimicrobials in foods. *Food Chemistry* **91**: 621–632.

Safer, A.M. and Al-Nughamish, A.J. (1999). Hepatotoxicity induced by the anti-oxidant food additive, butylated hydroxytoluene BHT, in rats. An electron microscopical study. *Histology and Histopathology* **14**: 391–406.

Santos, R.D., Shetty, K., and Da Silva Miglioranza, L.H. (2014). Oxidative stability of butter with added phenolics from *Lamiaceae* herbs and in vitro evaluation of potential cytotoxicity of rosemary (*Rosmarinus officinalis* L.) extract. *International Journal of Food Science & Technology* **49**: 768–777.

Sawale, P.D., Singh, R.R.B., and Arora, S. (2013). Stability and quality of herb (*Pueraria Tuberosa*)-milk model system. *Journal of Food Science and Technology* **52**: 1089–1095.

Sawale, P.D., Singh, R.R.B. & Arora, S. (2015). Stability and quality of herb (*Pueraria Tuberosa*)-milk model system. *Journal of Food Science and Technology* **52**: 1089–1095.

Sawale, P.D., Patil, G.R., Hussain, S.A., Singh, A.K. & Singh, R.R.B. (2017). Effect of incorporation of encapsulated and free *Arjuna herb* on storage stability of chocolate vanilla dairy drink. *Food Bioscience* **19**: 142–148.

Schoefs, B.T. (2004). Determination of pigments in vegetables. *Journal of Chromatography A* **1054**: 217–226.

Shahidi, F. (ed.) (2015). *Handbook of Antioxidants for Food Preservation*. United Kingdom: Woodhead Publishing.

Shende, S., Patel, S., Arora, S., and Sharma, V. (2014). Oxidative stability of ghee incorporated with clove extracts and BHA at elevated temperatures. *International Journal of Food Properties* **17**: 1599–1611.

Siefarth, C., Serfert, Y., Drusch, S., and Buettner, A. (2014). Comparative evaluation of diagnostic tools for oxidative deterioration of polyunsaturated fatty acid-enriched infant formulas during storage. *Foods* **3**: 30–65.

Sindayikengera, S. and Xia, W.S. (2006). Nutritional evaluation of caseins and whey proteins and their hydrolysates from Protamex. *Journal of Zhejiang University Science B* **7**: 90–98.

Soulti, K. and Roussis, I.G. (2007). Inhibition of butter oxidation by some phenolics. *European Journal of Lipid Science and Technology* **109**: 706–709.

Tajkarimi, M.M., Ibrahim, S.A., and Cliver, D.O. (2010). Antimicrobial herb and spice compounds in food. *Food Control* **21**: 1199–1218.

Tooryan, F. and Azizkhani, M. (2016). Antioxidant effect of basil and clary sage essential oils on Iranian white cheese. *Iranian Food Science and Technology Research Journal* **13**: 346–362.

Yanishlieva, N.V., Marinova, E., and Pokorný, J. (2006). Natural antioxidants from herbs and spices. *European Journal of Lipid Science and Technology* **108**: 776–793.

Yuksel, Z., Avci, E., and Erdem, Y.K. (2010). Characterization of binding interactions between green tea flavanoids and milk proteins. *Food Chemistry* **121**: 450–456.

Zayas, J.F. (ed.) (2012). *Functionality of Proteins in Food*. Heidelberg: Springer, Science & Business Media.

11
Biotic and Abiotic Safety Concerns for Herbs and Spices

Manja Zec and Maria Glibetic
Center of Research Excellence in Nutrition and Metabolism, Institute for Medical Research, University of Belgrade, Belgrade 11000, Serbia

We are all familiar with the details of Romeo and Juliet's tragedy, where the lovers poisoned themselves and died. The poison in the drama was most certainly a natural, herbal product, indicating the historical timeflow of unsafe uses of natural products. In the modern world, according to the data provided by World Health Organization (WHO), more than 80% of the population consume dietary supplements from herbal plants, in addition to the herbal medicals used as natural products with healing properties. This fact requires interest in the potential safety issues regarding the use and application of herbal products and medicals.

This chapter deals with bi-directional safety concerns regarding herbs and spices. The biotic and abiotic factors influencing the production, processing, and distribution of herbs and spices are covered. The proper handling of herbal products is of crucial importance in order to avoid contamination and further possible intoxication of end-users. In addition, the chapter deals with adverse reactions to herbal product consumption by end-users. Herbals may be applied directly as medical treatments in a complementary/alternative medical approach, or for nutritive purposes, either as dietary supplements or in addition to ready-to-eat foods. Hence, diverse herbal adverse effects, including interactions with concomitant pharmaceutical products, are reviewed in the chapter, with the purpose of drawing attention to the potential deleterious effects of herbal products commonly considered safe and used worldwide. Furthermore, it is of essential importance to establish a regulatory network that can strengthen the quality, safety, and efficacy of herbals used, and empower the overcoming of potential deleterious effects, including herbal toxicity. The regulatory framework in countries and regions worldwide is the final field of discussion in this chapter.

An interesting survey showed that a group of UK herbal users would and would not consider medical advice in the case of an adverse reaction caused by medical treatment

---

Herbs, Spices and Medicinal Plants: Processing, Health Benefits and Safety, First Edition.
Edited by Mohammad B. Hossain, Nigel P. Brunton, and Dilip K. Rai.

and self-care herbal intervention, respectively (Barnes et al. 1997). In contrast with professional healthcare, self-care medicine is based on the use of non-prescription drugs at home, also known as non-legend drugs or OTC (over-the-counter) products (Holt and Chandra 2002), which, among others, include herbal medicines. This fact once again underlines the essential importance of sublimating safety concerns regarding the use of herbs, including spices, as well as their production and processing.

Ernst has defined herbal products as "Herbal preparations produced by subjecting herbal materials to extraction, fractionation, purification, concentration, or other physical or biological process. They may be produced for immediate consumption or as the basis for herbal products. Herbal products may contain excipients, or inner ingredients, in addition to the active ingredients. They are generally produced in larger quantities for the purpose of retail sale" (Ernst 1998). According to the International Standards Organization (ISO), herbs and spices are defined as natural plants, vegetable products, or mixtures thereof, used in whole or in ground form, mainly for imparting flavor, aroma, and pungency to food, for seasoning of food and beverages, and also acting as natural preservatives (Shan et al. 2009; Kanatt et al. 2008). Usually, herbal products are marketed as dietary supplements, and thus conventionally regulated under laws overseeing regulation of dietary supplements release and public use (Alissa 2014).

Herbal interventions refer to the use of medicinal plants, either directly or through dietary supplementation. Currently, there are approximately 70 000 characterized plant species used as medical herbs. The most interesting aspect of herb exploitation relies on their medicinal properties, which can be tracked back to 3000 BCE in ancient Chinese and Indian communities (Alissa 2014). In European countries, Pedanious Dioscorides wrote the oldest known document on the use of medicinal herbs (*De Materia Medica,* first century, AD), which has had an influence on modern taxonomy of medicinal herbs (Holt and Chandra 2002). Herbal medicine may be referred to as complementary medicinal approach if applied concurrently with standard medical therapies, and for purposes of suppression of the disease. Nevertheless, some populations from underdeveloped countries practice the use of herbal intervention for alternative medicine purposes, which is a counterpart to conventional evidence-based medicine and is often disapproved of by the scientific community. Considering medical benefits, herbal medicines are used for their antimicrobial (onion, garlic, ginger, pepper, and mustard, [Chen et al. 1985]), lipid-lowering (ginger, curcumin [Alwi et al. 2008; Alizadeh-Navaei et al. 2008]), antirheumatic (ginger ([Sharma et al. 1994]), antioxidative (clove, cinnamon, oregano, black pepper, turmeric, and ginger ([Shan et al. 2005; Adhikari et al. 2007]), but also anti-inflammatory, antidiabetic, antithrombotic, hepatoprotective, gastroprotective, and antiulcer activities (different spices), antimutagenic and anticancer activities [curcumin (Cai et al. 2009; Ji et al. 2008)], and nephroprotective as well as neuroprotective properties.

Spices are defined as the dry part of the plant, including leaf, roots, etc., used in nutritionally insignificant quantities and contributing to the flavor of food and beverages (Hirasa and Takemasa 1998). Although commonly used for its flavoring properties, including strengthening of food aroma and piquancy, spices exert strong redox-modulating characteristics, due to their enhanced polyphenol content. Spices such as turmeric/curcumin, clove/eugenol, red pepper/capsaicin, black pepper/piperine, ginger/gingerol, garlic, onion, and fenugreek, are predominantly valorized for their natural antioxidative properties. Since spices are cultivated mainly in tropical countries, differences in the production process, pre- and post-harvest period may lead to contamination. Due to this fact, spices are recognized as primary alimentary contaminants, followed by food-borne toxicities and infections (Buckenhiiskes & Rendlen 2004).

11.1 Natural Products in Science – "Generally Recognized as Safe?"

Aspirin is a good example of how natural products serve the population through scientific manipulation (Holt and Chandra 2002), and is one of the oldest examples of the pharmacognosy. Salicin transformed into salicylic acid is the bioactive component of the aspirin. It is used for purposes of pain relief, but also causes mouth, intestine, and blood vessel irritation and thinning. In order to suppress the adverse events of the drug, the Bayer pharmaceutical company launched Aspirin at the end of nineteenth century in the form of acetylsalicylic acid. Aspirin was named after the Spirea plant known for the discovery of salicylic acid (Holt and Chandra 2002). This way, the chemical modification of a natural product led to the development of a strong pharmaceutical based on a herbal plant compound, with medicinal and industrial impact on future population health and pharmacognosy. Aside from salicylic acid, there is a variety of natural compounds used for pharmaceutical purposes. Bioactive compounds from herbs are often a model for the industrial synthesis of bioactive structural analogs (Holt and Chandra 2002), and medical chemistry technologies have facilitated industrial synthesis of compounds, in comparison to the difficulties of isolation and purification from plants. Modern technologies have also paved the way for substances that are naturally toxic, but health-promoting when applied in controlled quantities, such as compounds from Digitalis leaves (Schulz et al. 1998). Some natural bioactive compounds include: cocaine, caffeine, morphine, derived from coca leaves, coffee, and opium poppy, and they are used for anesthetic, stimulative, and analgesic purposes (Holt and Chandra 2002). Well known penicillin is used for antibiotic cases, while atropine and kawain from belladonna and kava are used for the alleviation of neurological disturbances. Colchicine from autumn crocus is used for gout healing, while theophyiline and ephedrine from tea and ephedra shrubs are used as bronchial and blood pressure modulators (Holt and Chandra 2002).

Natural products, including herbal preparations, are considered safe and adverse-event free, but there is a number of alarming examples of incidents suspected to be due to the misuse of herbal products or their careless consumption. Among more than 16 000 suspected herbal adverse events included in the WHO database, the most prominent are blood pressure disturbances, including hypertension, edemas, and thrombocytopenia, viral infections such as hepatitis or dermatitis, as well as fatal outcomes (Uppsala Monitoring Centre 2009). The Committee for Proprietary Medicinal Products (CPMP), in front of the EU Commission, has released a 33-item list of potentially hazardous herbal medicinal plants, including *Aconitum* and *Aristolochia* (all species), *Convovulus scamonia* L., *Ocimum basilicum* L., *Strychnus nux-vomica* L., *Vinca minor* L., etc. (European Medicines Agency 2015).

11.2 Herbs and Spices – Reported Adverse Effects and Adverse Drug Reactions

Herbal adverse events have been confirmed on different levels, spanning molecular implications, clinical manifestations, and drug interactions, and will be reviewed in this order. Pharmacovigilance of herbs and spices has been reviewed in Asiri et al. (2008), and the potential harmful and deleterious health effects of herbal medicines used directly or concomitantly with the drug therapy listed. The authors emphasize the WHO regulative set-up of guidelines on the assessment of the safety, efficacy, and quality of herbal medicines (Asiri et al. 2008).

The toxicity of herbal medicines and spices has been studied at the cellular level and also in experimental models. Although curcumin has been proven for its genotoxic characteristics toward hepatoma G2 and prostate PC12 cells, it also exerts toxicity on normal erythrocytes (Cao et al. 2006; Mendonça et al. 2009; Bentzen et al. 2007). Genotoxicity followed by cytotoxicity, glutathione depletion, and liver cell damage, as well as erythrocyte suicide, has been demonstrated upon elevated concentrations of thymoquinone from *Nigella sativa* (Khader et al. 2009; Qadri et al. 2009). Curcumin (Balaji and Chempakam 2009) and turmeric acid (Kandarkar et al. 1998) are reported for hepatotoxicity in mice experimental models. Adverse weight modulations have been reported upon chronic treatment with high turmeric doses (Deshpande et al. 1998) and *Foeniculum vulgare* ethanolic extracts of fruit (Shah et al. 1991). *Cinnamon zeylanicum, Piper longum,* and *Ruta chalepensis*-treated animals (Shah et al. 1991; Shah et al. 1998) have reported changes in the liver and spleen as well as increase in sperm count and motility.

Clinical case reports indicate a major problem in herbal plant use owing to improper identification of the biological material used for medical purposes. Well known *Aristolochia* species are rich in aristolochic acids, which may induce severe nephrotoxicity and urothelial carcinoma of the upper urinary tract upon long-term consumption (Poon et al. 2013; Hoang et al. 2013). Thus, inadvertently replacing herbal ingredient Stephaniae Tetrandrae Radix (Fangji), derived from *Stephania tetrandra* with Aristolochiae Fangchi Radix (Guangfangji), derived from *Aristolochia fangchi,* has induced progressive renal failure in women taking the pills primarily aimed at weight loss due to the first compound's beneficial properties (Debelle et al. 2008). The occasional misuse of the aristolochic acid-containing herb Aristolochiae Mollissimae Herba (Xungufeng) derived from *Aristolochia mollissima,* instead of non-harmful anticancer herb Solani Lyrati Herba (Baiying), derived from *Solanum lyratum,* has led to nephropathy in three patients ingesting it for a considerable time period (Lo et al. 2005; Li et al. 2011). Since 2004, there has been prohibition of the three medical herbals containing aristolochic acids (AAs): Radix Aristolochiae Fangchi (Guangfangji), Caulis Aristolochiae Manshuriensis (Guanmutong), and Radix Aristolochiae (Qingmuxiang) in China (Sahoo et al. 2010), due to confirmed renal toxicity upon consumption. Those herbal plants that could be confused with *Aristolochiae* spp. are prohibited as well.

Toxicity has also been studied in clinical settings. Although herbal medicals are known for gastro-protective properties, such as treatment of ulceritis and gastric pain (Xia 2004; Chernomorets et al. 1992), a variety of studies report a gastro-toxic effect of spices, such as red and black pepper (Myers et al. 1987), through the modulation of hydrophobic properties of gastric surfaces or the excretion of gastric acids. Additionally, there is a widespread use of commercially available feverfew (*Tanacetum parthenium*), for the purposes of alleviation of menstrual disorders, arthritic conditions, migraines, fevers, etc. Parthenolide is a feverfew's bioactive component, and its daily intake varies, depending on different factors, among other things the type of the feverfew product used (Nelson et al. 2002). However, parthenolide may interfere with the cyclooxygenase and phospholipase A2 enzyme functions, thus interfering the synthesis of biomolecules including lipids and fatty acids, metabolized by the enzymes, and impacting global cellular and physiological homeostasis.

The herbal practice is most prominent in the Chinese and Far East population. Although clinical data and meta-analyses on the herbal medicals' use implications are lacking, there is a retrospective study on a pregnancy cohort from Taipei, indicating potential congenital malformations due to herbal medications (Chuang et al. 2006). The cohort of 14 551 children and mothers' lifestyle during the first trimester was analyzed, and an association was found between increased risk of congenital malformations of the nervous system and use of huanglian (pain reliever).

There is an obvious lack of clinical and toxicological studies and meta-analyses dealing with adverse drug reactions due to the concomitant use of certain herbal interventions, and additional attention in the field is required. Adverse drug reactions upon herbal consumption may appear owing to the disturbed metabolism or drug resistance, due to the pharmacokinetic effect of drug activity decreasing upon herbal treatment. A recent thorough review by Alissa (2014) extensively summarizes the topic. The author covers a wide range of different herbal medicines and spices used for curative purposes (Alissa 2014). The proposed mechanism includes either herbal pharmacokinetic interaction with drug metabolizing enzyme or drug transporter, or pharmacodynamic impact through the additive or antagonistic interaction with drug targets (Alissa 2014). The array of the proposed herbal interactions with drug activity exists and is further speculated. Commercially available feverfew (*T. parthenium*) is used for the purposes of alleviation of menstrual disorders, arthritic conditions, migraines, fevers, etc. Feverfew's products may interfere with the use of warfarin and aspirin (Alissa 2014). Concomitant use of warfarin with *Ginkgo biloba* or ginseng is presumed to increase bleeding as well (Saw et al. 2006). However, contraindications of ginseng have not been proven through clinical trials (Beckert et al. 2007), nor have the scientifically based purposes for which the ginseng is marketed, such as erectile dysfunction, cancer prevention, enhanced physical function, disturbed cognitive functions, etc. (Tyler 1993). Furthermore, results describing *G. biloba* health effects and interactions with platelet drugs are contradictory. There are data indicating no effect of *G. biloba* extracts toward platelet activity *in vivo* and blood coagulation in humans (Bone 2008), but it has also been proven to interact with anticoagulant drugs (Vaes and Chyka 2000), as well as non-steroidal anti-inflammatory drugs (NSAID) and aspirin (Abebe 2002), causing severe intracranial bleeding. Due to this fact, safety precautions must be taken, since Ginkgo is commonly used for cognitive-improving purposes and for the treatment of neurodegenerative conditions, such as Alzheimer's disease (Sastre et al. 1998). The most used herbal dietary supplement is St. John's Wort (Alissa 2014) and this should be taken with caution. It is administered for the treatment of low and mild-stage depression conditions, and its mechanism of action is speculated to interfere with selective-serotonin-uptake-inhibition (Henney 2000), thus potentially interacting with a variety of commonly used antidepressives following the same pattern of action. Additionally, St. John's Wort may interact with anticoagulant warfarin

(Vaes and Chyka 2000), cyclosporines (Ruschitzka et al. 2000), as well as some photosensitizing drugs, such as tetracyclines (Kuhn and Winston 2000). St. John's wort activates the CYP3A family of metabolizing enzymes included in the pharmacodynamics of 50% of modern medication, thus indicating strong herbal interaction with drugs (Wargovich et al. 2001).

Commonly used spices for culinary purposes are garlic and ginger. Aside from its flavoring properties, garlic is used for cholesterol-lowering and atherosclerosis-prevention purposes (Ernst et al. 2008), while ginger is recommended for nausea and vomiting prevention (Ernst et al. 2008), although both spices lack clinical data proving their health promoting efficiency (Tyler 1993). Both herbs have been demonstrated to increase bleeding time and should be taken with precautions for patients waiting for a surgery or in a postoperative period. Both spices interfere with warfarin (Backon 1986), and garlic additionally should be avoided in patients on antiretroviral therapy (Gallicano et al. 2003). Chili pepper, used for analgesic properties, has been shown to interfere with ACE (Angiotensin-converting enzyme) inhibitors and Theophylline, subsequently influencing its activity (Hu et al. 2005; Deahl 1989).

Aside from adverse reactions to herbal medications used concomitantly with drugs, there may also be adverse interactions with other herbal treatments. Thus, fenugreek (*Trigonella foenum-graecum* L., Fabaceae) and *Momordica charantia* L. (Cucurbitaceae) both may modulate blood sugar levels, and must be used with caution in order to obtain a favorable clinical outcome (Raghuram et al. 1994).

On the other hand, there are speculated beneficial directions of herbal–drug interactions. Although potentially causing ulceration and prolonged bleeding, the use of NSAID has been extensively studied for its chemopreventative effects for gastric and colon cancer (Dannhardt and Kiefer 2001). Nevertheless, prolonged use of NSAIDs may lead to toxicity issues, which suggests using structurally similar herbal products with anti-inflammatory activity. Hence, herbal products with NSAID-like anti-inflammatory effects, such as blueberry (*Vaccinium myrtillus*), Devil's claw (*Harpagophytum procumbens*), ginkgo (*G. biloba*), ginger (*Zingiber officinale*), Green tea (*Camellia sinensis*), Red grapes (*Vitus vinifera*), Turmeric (*Curcuma longa*) could have a potentially concomitant beneficial effect in chemoprevention (Wargovich et al. 2001). Additionally, animal studies have demonstrated beneficial effects on skin cancer and its pathophysiological manifestations for green tea catechins (Gensler et al. 1996), resveratrol (Lahiri-Chatterjee et al. 1999), as well as curcumin (Huang et al. 1988) upon topical application in mice.

11.3 (A)Biotic Factors Incorporated in the Foodchain and Influencing the Safety of Herbal Consumption

There is a variety of both biotic and abiotic factors influencing the proper application of plants (Vickers 2007). Abiotic components include non-living factors in the ecosystem, such as light, temperature, energy produced, air current, soil, etc.; while biotic factors include different living organisms taking part in the nutrient and energy chain in nature. This complex network of abiotic and biotic components of an ecosystem influences the quality and safety of food, including herbal products and spices. Thus, the abiotic component represented by the amount of heavy metals in herbal plants is of importance due to the potential gastro-toxicity of non-biodegradable heavy metals. On the other hand, the amount of heavy metals is influenced by abiotic components such as air, water, or soil (Abu-Darwish et al. 2009), but also by direct or indirect biotic components, such as pollution (Abu-Darwish et al. 2009; Angelova et al. 2006), industrial processing, packaging, storage, and transportation (Blagojević et al. 2013). What's more, heavy metals are incorporated into the foodchain through environmental and industrial pollution, including air, soil, and water pollution. There are over 50 published reports on heavy metal toxicity from all over the world, including Australasia, the Indian subcontinent, the Middle East, Western Europe, and North America (Dargan et al. 2008). Permissible levels for heavy metal content in herbal plants are slightly different for the following regulatory agencies: WHO, US Food and Drug Administration (FDA), Department of Ayurveda, Unani, Sidhha, and Homeopathy (AYUSH) India and Health Science Authority (HSA), Singapore (Sahoo et al. 2010), but there is a consensus on the imperative absence of heavy metal at levels that are health threatening.

A survey has analyzed the content of heavy metals including Pb, Hg, As, and Cd in 19 products from a wholesale market in Malaysia (Nordin and Selamat 2013). These metals are known to be neurotoxic and teratogenic (Hg), toxic (As), as well as mutagenic and carcinogenic (Pb and Cd), with a highest daily tolerated dose in human population for Cd while the lowest is for Hg. The analyses of variance on 114 Malaysian products delivering 19 different herbal species has revealed that all of the heavy metals were at detectable levels, with Pb having the greatest variability, from the highest in Vietnamese coriander, to the lowest in garlic. The Cd content was the highest in lemongrass, and the lowest in Philippine wax flower, in contrast to As with the highest concentration in wax flower. The highest value of Hg was found in Kaffir leaf (Nordin and Selamat 2013). Except for Cd, the calculated risk index of these metals for Malaysians was below the PTWI (proposed tolerated weekly intake) established by the FAO/WHO, which is good indicator of Malaysian herbal safety regarding trace metals content. A similar report was provided for the amount of heavy metals, moisture, and ash (total minerals) from the branded spices found at a Serbian market in Belgrade. The research on heavy metal content in different brands of oregano, sweet basil, parsley, and celery found none over limits according to the national laws for Pb and As (Anonymous 2015), and according to the FAO/WHO provisions for Hg (FAO/WHO 2002), indicating the safety of such spices used in the Serbian capital city. On the other hand, there is a range of particularly developing countries, such as Nigeria, where the quality of herbal products available at the market is not legally regulated (Obi et al. 2006). A study on 25 collected and randomly analyzed herbal samples from a Nigerian market revealed alarming results. In 100% of samples, analyzed the nickel, cadmium, lead, selenium, and copper amounts were above maximum permissible levels for nickel (Das and Dasgupta 2002) and copper (National Research Council 1980) and FAO/WHO established PTWI for cadmium (WHO 1989) and lead (FAO/WHO 1993). The findings (Obi et al. 2006), in addition to the lack of Nigerian legislative ground on herbal product use, suggest a great public health hazard in a Nigerian population freely using available herbal products from the market.

There is a commonly reported contamination of herbal medicines by pesticides during agricultural processing. Thus, in a study of 300 samples of traditional Chinese medicine, the presence of hexachlorocyclohexanes residues was demonstrated in every sample (Xue et al. 2008a). At least one of the following organochlorine pesticides – PCNB, aldrin, BHC, or DDT – was found in 75.8% of 280 studied samples of 30 different traditional Chinese medicines (Xue et al. 2008b). The WHO regulates both maximum residue limit (MRL) for pesticides in cultivated or wild medicinal plants, and adequate detection systems in the samples (World Health Organization 2007).

Foodborne pathogens are a public health issue. Food-related contaminations not only break-out quickly, but are also followed by extensive research and detection of the particular source of microbiological contamination. The most prominent vehicles for microbiological contamination of food are herbal products and spices, added for flavoring purposes. The great challenge lies in the discovery of the exact contaminated herbal product, as well as the exact step of the production-to-consumption (Chan 2003; McKee 1995) process where the contamination occurred. In addition, the occurrence of multiresistant bacteria forms in herbal breeds is a great problem, due to the overuse of antimicrobial additives in the herbal agriculture (Hassan and Altalhi 2013).

The microbiological status of herbs and spices used is the dominant biotic factor influencing the safety of herbal products for end-users. Precautionary measures and proper hygiene, as well as strict quality control, processing technology applied, and chemical identification for OTC products cannot be overemphasized. The public health risk lies in the presence of common microorganisms in a foodstuff; particularly pathogen bacteria, mold, and yeast (Sospedra et al. 2010), and herbs and spices are strongly susceptible to microbial contamination. The evidence of salmonella outbreaks was preceded by the contamination of black and white pepper (Anonymous 1994; Gustavsen and Breen 1984), chili and turmeric (Little et al. 2003), and paprika (Lehmacher et al. 1995) used for food flavoring. Aside from *Salmonella* spp., found in the range of 0.6–14% in herbal products, *Bacillus* spp. and spore-forming bacteria including *Bacillus cereus* and *Clostridium perfringens* are found in high and low doses in herbs and spices (Sagoo et al. 2009). The microbiological standards for estimated doses allowed in particular foods, as well as food processing and quality control laws, are declared in the Commission Regulation (EC) No 2073/2005 (European Commission 2005). The criteria should be followed by food business operators at each stage of food production, processing, and distribution. Although there are no microbiological standards for herbal product quality, the Codex Code of Hygienic Practice specifies that pathogenic microorganisms may be present in dried spices and herbs beyond levels that are health threatening (Codex Alimentarius Commission 1995). The Codex also requires the absence of salmonella in treated ready-to-eat spices (Codex Alimentarius Commission 1995). In addition, the absence of salmonella in 25 g of spice (European Spice Association (ESA) 2011), presence of *Escherichia coli* less than 102 ucf/g, and other bacteria requirements agreed between buyer and seller (Muggeridge and Clay 2001), are specified by The European Spice Association (ESA).

Due to its inherent ability to survive extreme desiccation stress, *Salmonella* spp. is commonly found in different forms of spices (Zweifel and Stephan 2012). Historically, *Salmonella* spp. outbreaks occurred at geographically distant locations, and were always followed by the challenge of discovering the exact food source of contamination. The following outbreaks were caused by spice-driven *Salmonella* spp. contamination of food: black, red (CDC 2010), and white (Kennelly 2010) pepper caused outbreaks in the USA, fresh basil in Denmark (Pakalniskiene et al. 2009) and the United Kingdom (Pezzoli et al. 2008), and paprika in Germany (Lehmacher et al. 1995). A review (Zweifel and Stephan 2012) summarizes the different reports on the presence of *Salmonella* spp. in a variety of herbal products in various countries, once again underlining its wide presence, and the necessity for the overall strict regulations toward quality control driven by food business operators. On the other hand, Saudi Arabian research on the selective isolation of bacterial species from 59 dry herbal and spice products from retailers (Hassan and Altalhi 2013) has revealed the presence of *Bacillus* spp., *Acinetobacter* spp., *Pseudomonas aeruginosa*, *Enterobacter* spp., *Erwina* spp., *Klebsiella* spp., *Hafni alvei*, *Shigella* spp., etc., but *Salmonella* spp. was absent (Hassan and Altalhi 2013). The authors found no bacterial contamination within aniseed, cinnamon, thyme, and turmeric (Hassan and Altalhi 2013), which could be attributed to the inherent antimicrobial properties of the particular herbal plants.

Fungal contaminations were studied in 91 herbal samples in the USA, and the results have shown the presence above the allowed limit (2×102 CFU/g of the product; the maximum fungal contamination limit as per US Pharmacopeia) of either genus *Aspergillus* or *Penicillium* in overall 54.9% of samples (Sahoo et al. 2010).

An interesting report on the presence of Hepatitis E virus in various food products in France, including herbs and spices, finds the amount comparable to Hepatitis A virus in pepper (Loisy 2012).

There is a variety of herbs and spices considered for their antimicrobial purposes, and thus found free from microbial contamination in quality control and research studies. Thus, basil (Lachowicz et al. 1998), thyme, and oregano (Sağdıç 2003) have demonstrated antimicrobial activity, while cinnamon has been shown to be a bactericide for *E. coli*, *Listeria monocytogenes*, and *Salmonella* spp. (Friedman et al. 2002) and free of contaminants in the survey of the Spanish market (Sospedra et al. 2010). The same survey (Sospedra et al. 2010) has found the most excessive prevalence of *Shigella* spp. (11% in Spanish herbs and spices) as well as *Acinetobacter calcoaceticus*, considered non-harmful in healthy individuals, and *Enterobacter* spp., especially in paprika and cayenne (Sospedra et al. 2010). The *Enterobacter* spp. are commonly found and studied in infant food, milk powder, cereal products, spices, sugar, and food production (Shaker et al. 2007).

11.4 Herbal Product Safety Concerns – Advances in Identification and Regulatory Framework

The exact methodological techniques used for the purposes of systematic, taxonomic, morphological, chemical, molecular, and genomic identification of herbal products are beyond the scope of this chapter. However, the safe use of herbal products is based on their proper authentication, and advances in molecular identification of herbs deliver progress in the assessment of quality and safety of herbals as well as spices. The state-of-the-art in herbal identification technologies is DNA barcoding of herbal medical ingredients. In addition to the conventional microscopic, morphologic, and chemical assessments of herbal active ingredients, DNA barcoding enables an accurate and precise distinction of even taxonomically close and structurally Analogue molecules, through the identification of species-specific short-term nucleotide sequences/repeats in the DNA molecule (Hebert et al. 2003). DNA barcoding is performed through the input of DNA nucleotide sequence-specific data into the search box through the publicly available database for DNA barcoding for different organisms and taxonomic categories. An array of databases is available for different taxonomic categories and groups of organisms, and in 2010 a specific database for medicinal material was implemented (Lou et al. 2010), including medicinal plant material (Lou et al. 2010). Soon afterwards, identification of herbal material based on DNA barcoding system through the database was established (Chen 2012; Chen et al. 2010; Chen et al. 2013; Xiang et al. 2013; Xin et al. 2013). The distinction between species is based on the intragenetic variation of barcodes inside ITS2 and psbA–trnH nucleotide and plastid DNA sequences, respectively (Chen et al. 2014). In addition, an online database for the identification of certain herbal species is available (www.tcmbarcode.cn), and uses selected ITS2 and psbA–trnH barcode sequences as core and complementary sequence codes (Chen et al. 2014). The database is compliant with Chinese, Japanese, Korean, USA, European, and Indian pharmacopeias, and is comprised of data on medicinal herbs, their adulterants, substitutes, and close relatives as well, in order to provide as accurate a distinction as possible (Chen et al. 2014). This publicly available database enables the prevention of inadvertent or even purposeful use of potentially toxic and harmful medical herbs.

Food safety refers to protection from any unintentional contamination that is likely to appear in food products (i.e. *E. coli, Listeria,* or any physico-chemical contaminants) that may impair human health upon consumption (http://www.usda.gov/wps/portal/usda/usdahome). In contrast, food defense refers to the protection from any intentional biological, physical, chemical, radiological, or any other contamination that is not likely to appear in certain food products (http://www.usda.gov/wps/portal/usda/usdahome). Above all, food security refers to the availability of necessary and sufficient quantitative and qualitative nutrients in the population (http://www.usda.gov/wps/portal/usda/usdahome). Through governmental agencies as well as private stakeholders, countries continually strive to develop and implement regulations and laws with the purpose of improving the food safety and the food industry. Food safety regulations are country specific, and the food allowed in one country may be forbidden in another due to stricter safety requirements. There is variety of the examples of food distribution with fatal health implications (Matthews 2014), but the public also decry certain food additives due to the lack of knowledge, such as ammonium hydroxide – generally recognized as safe by US food safety authorities (Matthews 2014). The above statements regarding food safety, security, and local regulative and guidelines may refer to herbal species as well, although herbals may be used as food, food additives, dietary supplements, or medical plants. Overall, food, herbs, spices, and finally drugs represent four etymologically and semantically different terms, but may be interchangeable for certain natural and commercial products and derivatives. In addition, there may be interchangeable use of certain terminology for a herb and a spice, which is the case with ginger, used as a spice and medical herb at the same time. This poses a great challenge in posting distinctive, precise, and strict regulations on herbal use, and above all harmonization through the worldwide pharmacopeias.

Various definitions of herbal products and particularly herbal medicals exist, implicating diverse legislatives on herbal production, processing, and distribution. The WHO defines herbal medicines as herbs, herbal materials, preparations, and final products and finished herbal products, that's bioactivity is attributed to the plant or its parts (Sahoo et al. 2010). Similarly in the EU, the European Medicines Agency – EMEA defines herbal drugs as the whole, fragmented, or cut plants, parts of plants, algae, fungi, lichen in an unprocessed state, which if treated chemically become herbal drug preparations (Sahoo et al. 2010). The US regulative implies that herbal products fall within the scope of dietary supplements, and thus are regulated as foods, or the Botanical Drug Product (Section 201(g)(1)(B), Federal Food, Drug, and Cosmetic Act), if prepared from one or more plants, algae, or fungi (Sahoo et al. 2010). However, unlike the pharmaceutical developing process, which is amenable to high regulation and quality control, the development of herbal products is not that easy for uniform control – due to the widespread growth of certain botanical species, as well as diversity in its agricultural and geo-climatic developing conditions (Khan and Smillie 2012). The existence of the "quality by design" concept (QbD), introduced by Joseph M. Juran in 1992, paved the way for step-wise strict control from the very beginning of the manufacturing process (Juran 1992). According to QbD, the production of goods and services (including those for therapeutic purpose) should be compliant with high manufacturing standards, which should be fulfilled through adequate checkpoints on every manufacturing step from the outset (Juran 1992; Khan and Smillie 2012). Any potentially occurring safety risk is followed by immediate countermeasures, before the product becomes available for end-users. Although the QbD concept is widely accepted for pharmaceutical products in the USA, its implementation in the field of botanical products is still ongoing (Khan and Smillie 2012).

There is a general belief that all herbal interventions are safe to use, due to the fact that they are natural products. This is not always true, especially when it comes to the potential interaction of medicinal plant interventions with concurrent medical therapy (Alissa 2014). The lack of a concise and unique regulatory network for herbal medicals as well as herbal product use leads to discrepancies in the pharmacovigilance of herbal products (Alissa 2014). A herbal medical should be strictly regulated in terms of the exact ingredients scheme, manufacturer details, contraindications, adulterants – such as presence of heavy metals which may exert a substantial toxic effects – as well as dosage prescription (Barnes 2003).

Aside from the national and international pharmacopeias and monographs, there has been a worldwide effort from the regulatory bodies to critically evaluate novel scientific findings on herbal medicals, toward empowering safety, quality, and efficacy issues. These bodies, among others, include the European Scientific Cooperative on Phytotherapy – ESCOP, EMEA, British Herbal Medicine Association – BHMA, German Commission E, as well as country- and region-specific authorities. Depending on the country, herbal products and herbal medicals are diversely defined and regulated. As mentioned, in the USA, herbs can be considered as drugs, food, or dietary supplements (Samojlik et al. 2013), herbal medicines are regulated under the Dietary Supplement Health and Education Act of 1994 (Sahoo et al. 2010) announced by the FDA, although the FDA itself does not regulate herbals as drugs (Alissa 2014). In the UK, herbal products are referred to as either completely licensed medicines, cosmetics, or food (Mason 2007). The majority of the member states of the European Union classifies herbal plant medicals used for both therapeutic and prophylactic purposes, followed by general regulations applied for pharmaceutical medicals; as well as herbal dietary supplements, which are considered non-medical products (European Commission 2015). EU Directive 2001/83/EC on traditional herbal medicinal products, together with its amendment 2004/24/EC, are aimed at improving public health protection and promoting the safe consumption of traditional medicinal products. In addition, European directives aim to simplify the registration process for traditional herbal medicinal products, thus facilitating the authentication process for food business companies. The Australian legal basis for herbal introduction to the market involves one of the following regulatory bodies, depending on the type of the (herbal) medical used: Office of Complementary Medicines (OCM) for Complementary medicines, Drug Safety and Evaluation Branch (DSEB) for the prescription and other specified medicines, and OTC Medicines in the Therapeutic Goods Administration (TGA) for OTC Medicines. Brazil, the South American leader in herbal products, legally requires phytopharmaceutical drug registration in accordance with Directive 6, issued in 1995 by the Brazilian Drug Division (DIMED) (Sahoo et al. 2010). The Serbian Law on Production and Trade of Medicines, assumes herbal medicals as traditional or homeopathic drugs (Ministry of Health, Republic of Serbia 2010).

The WHO data indicate that nearly 80% of the African and Asian population depends on the herbal tradition medicals for primary healthcare purposes (World Health Organization 2008). In addition, regulation of herbal product use is a critical issue in developing countries, such as Nigeria in Africa, where high contamination of herbal plants by heavy metals has recently been reported (Obi et al. 2006). The National Agency of Food and Drug Administration and Control (NAFDAC) in Nigeria has recently increased efforts in the regulation of herbal use, due to the widespread availability of herbal medicals in the country, especially for the purposes of healing malaria.

Quality and safety control of herbal material, including its proper identification, processing, and consumption is of crucial importance for end-users, and indirectly the food industry. The WHO has developed a range of environmental and agricultural practices involved in the assessment of quality and safety of herbal medicines, including: "Quality Control Methods for Medicinal Plant Materials" (World Health Organization 1998), "Guidelines on good agricultural and collection practices (GACP) for medicinal plants" (published in 2003) and "WHO guidelines for assessing quality of herbal medicines with reference to contaminants and residues" (published in 2007) (World Health Organization 2003). Similar national and regional practices with the purpose of herbal safety and quality assessment have been developed through the EU, China, and Japan (World Health Organization 2007).

Developed countries, such as the USA, import almost 100% of tropical products, including spices, as well as cocoa or tropical fruit, which increases the risk of incorporated/inherited biotic/abiotic components, such as potentially pathogen microorganisms (Matthews 2014). There is a constant problem with safety issues regarding diverse food products, such as spices, due to the uninterrupted mixing of different ethnicities and the complex network of food industry markets. In addition to the diverse regulatory networks listed, and diversity in local quality standards and safety issues, international harmonization of legislatives, quality assurance, and safety assessments are imperative regarding herbal products and herbal medicals. The Medicinal Plant of the Pan American Network of Drug Regulatory Harmonization (PANDRH) is a working group aiming to deliver uniformity in understanding of diverse types, definitions, and terminologies of herbal products, identification of operating procedures and processing, and the minimum requirements for registration of herbal products (Pan American Health Organization 2000). The harmonization efforts are ongoing, and are of invaluable significance all over the world. If taking into account the increasing intake of herbal products – reported to be 1, 0.5, and 4 g/person/day of spices/herbs in Europe, New Zealand, and the United States, respectively (Pan American Health Organization 2000) – there is a crucial need for a uniform regulatory basis underpinning their safe use in the human population.

References

Abebe, W. (2002). Herbal medication: potential for adverse interactions with analgesic drugs. *Journal of Clinical Pharmacy and Therapeutics* **27** (6): 391–401.

Abu-Darwish, M.S., Abu-Dieyeh, Z.H., Mufeed, B. et al. (2009). Trace element contents and essential oil yields from wild thyme plant (*Thymus serpyllum* L.) grown at different natural variable environments, Jordan. *Journal of Food, Agriculture and Environment* **7**: 920–924.

Adhikari, S., Priyadarsini, K.I., and Mukherjee, T. (2007). Physico-chemical studies on the evaluation of the antioxidant activity of herbal extracts and active principles of some Indian medicinal plants. *Journal of Clinical Biochemistry and Nutrition* **40** (3): 174.

Alissa, E.M. (2014). Medicinal herbs and therapeutic drugs interactions. *Therapeutic Drug Monitoring* **36** (4): 413–422.

Alizadeh-Navaei, R., Roozbeh, F., Saravi, M. et al. (2008). Investigation of the effect of ginger on the lipid levels. A double blind controlled clinical trial. *Saudi Medical Journal* **29** (9): 1280–1284.

Alwi, I., Santoso, T., Suyono, S. et al. (2008). The effect of curcumin on lipid level in patients with acute coronary syndrome. *Acta Medica Indonesiana* **40** (4): 201–210.

Angelova, V., Ivanov, K., and Ivanova, R. (2006). Heavy metal content in plants from family Lamiaceae cultivated in an industrially polluted region. *Journal of Herbs, Spices & Medicinal Plants* **11** (4): 37–46.

Anonymous (1994). Salmonella javiana in Europe, European Surveillance: 'Salm-Net'. CDS Weekly Report 4: 61.

Anonymous (2015). Pravilnik o količinama pesticida, metala i metaloida i drugih otrovnih supstancija, hemioterapeutika, anabolika i drugih supstancija koje se mogu nalaziti u namirnicama, Službeni list SRJ br. 5/92, 11/92 - ispr. i 32/2002. Available at: http://fungojug.com/sr/rule_book/pravilnik%20o%20kolicinama%20pesticida,%20metala%20i%20metaloida%20i%20drugih%20otrovnih%20supstancija,%20hemioterapeutika.pdf (accessed 30 June 2015).

Asiri, Y., Al-Dhawailie, A., Alqasoumi, S. et al. (2008). Pharmacovigilance in herbal medicine: a paradigm to drug toxicity monitoring in conventional health care. *Hungarian Medical Journal* **2** (3): 351–363.

Backon, J. (1986). Ginger: inhibition of thromboxane synthetase and stimulation of prostacyclin: relevance for medicine and psychiatry. *Medical Hypotheses* **20** (3): 271–278.

Balaji, S. and Chempakam, B. (2009). Pharmacokinetics prediction and drugability assessment of diphenylheptanoids from turmeric (*Curcuma longa* L.). *Medicinal Chemistry* **5** (2): 130–138.

Barnes, J. (2003). Quality, efficacy and safety of complementary medicines: fashions, facts and the future. Part I. Regulation and quality. *British Journal of Clinical Pharmacology* **55** (3): 226–233.

Barnes, J., Mills, S.Y., Abbot, N.C. et al. (1997). Different standards for reporting ADRs to herbal remedies and conventional OTC medicines: interviews with 515 users of herbal remedies. *Focus on Alternative and Complementary Therapies* **2** (4): 185–185.

Beckert, B.W., Concannon, M.J., Henry, S.L. et al. (2007). The effect of herbal medicines on platelet function: an in vivo experiment and review of the literature. *Plastic and Reconstructive Surgery* **120** (7): 2044–2050.

Bentzen, P.J., Lang, E., and Lang, F. (2007). Curcumin induced suicidal erythrocyte death. *Cellular Physiology and Biochemistry* **19** (1–4): 153–164.

Blagojević, S.M., Blagojević, S.N., Pejić, N.D. et al. (2013). Quality and safety of some commercial spices brands. *Acta Periodica Technologica* **44**: 1–9.

Bone, K.M. (2008). Potential interaction of Ginkgo biloba leaf with antiplatelet or anticoagulant drugs: what is the evidence? *Molecular Nutrition & Food Research* **52** (7): 764–771.

Buckenhiiskes, H.J. and Rendlen, M. (2004). Hygienic problems of phytogenic raw materials for food production m'th special emphasis to herbs and spices. *Food Science and Biotechnology* **13** (2): 262–268.

Cai, X.Z., Wang, J., Xiao-Dong, L. et al. (2009). Curcumin suppresses proliferation and invasion in human gastric cancer cells by down-regulation of PAK1 activity and cyclin D1 expression. *Cancer Biology & Therapy* **8** (14): 1360–1368.

Cao, J., Jia, L., Zhou, H.M. et al. (2006). Mitochondrial and nuclear DNA damage induced by curcumin in human hepatoma G2 cells. *Toxicological Sciences* **91** (2): 476–483.

CDC, Centers for Disease Control and Prevention (2010). Investigation update: Multistate outbreak of human Salmonella Montevideo infections. Available at: http://http://www.cdc.gov/salmonella/montevideo/index.htm.

Chan, K. (2003). Some aspects of toxic contaminants in herbal medicines. *Chemosphere* **52**: 1361–1371.

Chen, S.L. (2012). *DNA Barcoding of Chinese Medicinal Materials*. Beijing: People's Medical Publishing House.

Chen, H.C., Chang, M.D., and Chang, T.J. (1985). [Antibacterial properties of some spice plants before and after heat treatment]. Zhonghua Minguo wei sheng wu ji mian yi xue za zhi=. *Chinese Journal of Microbiology and Immunology* **18** (3): 190–195.

Chen, S., Yao, H., Han, J. et al. (2010). Validation of the ITS2 region as a novel DNA barcode for identifying medicinal plant species. *PLoS One* **5** (1): e8613.

Chen, X., Liao, B., Song, J. et al. (2013). A fast SNP identification and analysis of intraspecific variation in the medicinal Panax species based on DNA barcoding. *Gene* **530** (1): 39–43.

Chen, S., Pang, X., Song, J. et al. (2014). A renaissance in herbal medicine identification: from morphology to DNA. *Biotechnology Advances* **32** (7): 1237–1244.

Chernomorets, N.N., Seleznev, A.V., Revutskiĭ, B.I. et al. (1992). The differentiated phytotherapy of patients with duodenal peptic ulcer. *Likars' ka sprava/Ministerstvo okhorony zdorov'ia Ukrainy* **2**: 112–115.

Chuang, C.H., Doyle, P., Wang, J.D. et al. (2006). Herbal medicines used during the first trimester and major congenital malformations. *Drug Safety* **29** (6): 537–548.

Codex Alimentarius Commission (1995). Code of hygienic practice for spices and dried aromatic plants. CAC/RCP 42–1995 Available at: file:///C:/Users/user/Downloads/CXP_042e_2014.pdf (accessed 30 June 2015).

Dannhardt, G. and Kiefer, W. (2001). Cyclooxygenase inhibitors–current status and future prospects. *European Journal of Medicinal Chemistry* **36** (2): 109–126.

Dargan, P.I., Gawarammana, I.B., Archer, J.R. et al. (2008). Heavy metal poisoning from Ayurvedic traditional medicines: an emerging problem? *International Journal of Environment and Health* **2** (3–4): 463–474.

Das, K.K. and Dasgupta, S. (2002). Effect of nickel sulfate on testicular steroidogenesis in rats during protein restriction. *Environmental Health Perspectives* **110** (9): 923.

Deahl, M. (1989). Betel nut-induced extrapyramidal syndrome: an unusual drug interaction. *Movement Disorders* **4** (4): 330–332.

Debelle, F.D., Vanherweghem, J.L., and Nortier, J.L. (2008). Aristolochic acid nephropathy: a worldwide problem. *Kidney International* **74** (2): 158–169.

Deshpande, S.S., Lalitha, V.S., Ingle, A.D. et al. (1998). Subchronic oral toxicity of turmeric and ethanolic turmeric extract in female mice and rats. *Toxicology Letters* **95** (3): 183–193.

Ernst, E. (1998). Harmless herbs? A review of the recent literature. *The American Journal of Medicine* **104** (2): 170–178.
Ernst, E., Pittler, M.H., Wider, B., and Boddy, K. (2008). *Oxford Handbook of Complementary Medicine*. Oxford, England: Oxford University Press.
European Commission (2005). Official Journal of the European Union. Available at: https://www.fsai.ie/uploadedFiles/Reg2073_2005(1).pdf (accessed 30 June 2015).
European Commission (2015). Herbal medicinal products in the European Union. Available at: http://ec.europa.eu/health/human-use/herbal-medicines/index_en.htm (accessed 25 June 2015).
European Medicines Agency (2015). Committee for Proprietary Medicinal Products. Herbal drugs with serious risks. Doc. Ref. EMEA/HMPC/246736/2005. Available at: (http://www.ema.europa.eu/docs/en_GB/document_library/Scientific_guideline/2010/04/WC500089951.pdf.) (accessed 15 June 2015).
European Spice Association (ESA) (2011). Quality Minima Document Rev. 4. Adopted at the meeting of the Technical Commission on 1st December 2011. Available at: file:///C:/Users/user/Downloads/esaqmdrev1-2nov07.pdf (accessed 30 June 2015).
FAO/WHO (1993). Evaluation of certain food additives and contaminants. WHO Technical Report Series No. 837 1993.
FAO/WHO (2002). Joint FAO/WHO Expert committee on food additives (2002). Available at: www.fao.org. http://www.fao.org/3/a-at881e.pdf.
Friedman, M., Henika, P.R., and Mandrell, R.E. (2002). Bactericidal activities of plant essential oils and some of their isolated constituents against *Campylobacter jejuni*, *Escherichia coli*, *Listeria monocytogenes*, and *Salmonella enterica*. *Journal of Food Protection* **65** (10): 1545–1560.
Gallicano, K., Foster, B., and Choudhri, S. (2003). Effect of short-term administration of garlic supplements on single-dose ritonavir pharmacokinetics in healthy volunteers. *British Journal of Clinical Pharmacology* **55** (2): 199–202.
Gensler, H.L., Timmermann, B.N., Valcic, S. et al. (1996). Prevention of photocarcinogenesis by topical administration of pure epigallocatechin gallate isolated from green tea. *Nutrition and Cancer* **26**: 325–335.
Gustavsen, S. and Breen, O. (1984). Investigation of an outbreak of Salmonella oranienburg infections in Norway, caused by contaminated black pepper. *American Journal of Epidemiology* **119** (5): 806–812.
Hassan, S.A. and Altalhi, A.D. (2013). Safety assessment of spices and herbs consumed in Saudi Arabia: microbiological quality and toxin production. *Life Science Journal* **10**: 2819–2827.
Hebert, P.D., Cywinska, A., and Ball, S.L. (2003). Biological identifications through DNA barcodes. *Proceedings of the Royal Society of London B: Biological Sciences* **270** (1512): 313–321.
Henney, J.E. (2000). Risk of drug interactions with St John's wort. *JAMA* **283** (13): 1679–1679.
Hirasa, K. and Takemasa, M. (1998). *Spice Science and Technology*. CRC Press.
Hoang, M.L., Chen, C.H., Sidorenko, V.S. et al. (2013). Mutational signature of aristolochic acid exposure as revealed by whole-exome sequencing. *Science Translational Medicine* **5** (197): 197ra102.
Holt, G.A. and Chandra, A. (2002). Herbs in the modern healthcare environment-an overview of uses, legalities, and the role of the healthcare professional. *Clinical Research and Regulatory Affairs* **19** (1): 83–107.
Hu, Z., Yang, X., Ho, P.C.L. et al. (2005). Herb-drug interactions. *Drugs* **65** (9): 1239–1282.

Huang, M.T., Smart, R.C., Wong, C.Q., and Conney, A.H. (1988). Inhibitory effect of curcumin, chlorogenic acid, caffeic acid, and ferulic acid on tumor promotion in mouse skin by 12-O-tetradecanoylphorbol-13-acetate. *Cancer Research* **48** (21): 5941–5946.

Ji, C., Cao, C., Lu, S. et al. (2008). Curcumin attenuates EGF-induced AQP3 up-regulation and cell migration in human ovarian cancer cells. *Cancer Chemotherapy and Pharmacology* **62** (5): 857–865.

Juran, J.M. (1992). *Juran on Quality by Design: The New Steps for Planning Quality into Goods and Services*. New York: The Free Press.

Kanatt, S.R., Chander, R., and Sharma, A. (2008). Chitosan and mint mixture: a new preservative for meat and meat products. *Food Chemistry* **107** (2): 845–852.

Kandarkar, S.V., Sawant, S.S., Ingle, A.D. et al. (1998). Subchronic oral hepatotoxicity of turmeric in mice – histopathological and ultrastructural studies. *Indian Journal of Experimental Biology* **36** (7): 675–679.

Kennelly, P. (2010).Salmonella Rissen outbreak associated with white pepper consumption. Available at: http://www.wafdo.org.

Khader, M., Bresgen, N., and Eckl, P.M. (2009). In vitro toxicological properties of thymoquinone. *Food and Chemical Toxicology* **47** (1): 129–133.

Khan, I.A. and Smillie, T. (2012). Implementing a "quality by design" approach to assure the safety and integrity of botanical dietary supplements. *Journal of Natural Products* **75** (9): 1665–1673.

Kuhn, M. and Winston, D. (2000). *Herbal Therapy and Supplements: A Scientific and Traditional Approach*. Philadelphia, PA: JB Lippincott Williams & Wilkins.

Lachowicz, K.J., Jones, G.P., Briggs, D.R. et al. (1998). The synergistic preservative effects of the essential oils of sweet basil (*Ocimum basilicum* L.) against acid-tolerant food microflora. *Letters in Applied Microbiology* **26** (3): 209–214.

Lahiri-Chatterjee, M., Katiyar, S.K., Mohan, R.R., and Agarwal, R. (1999). A flavonoid antioxidant, silymarin, affords exceptionally high protection against tumor promotion in the SENCAR mouse skin tumorigenesis model. *Cancer Research* **59** (3): 622–632.

Lehmacher, A., Bockemühl, J., and Aleksic, S. (1995). Nationwide outbreak of human salmonellosis in Germany due to contaminated paprika and paprika-powdered potato chips. *Epidemiology and Infection* **115** (03): 501–511.

Li, M., Cao, H., BUT, P.P.H., and SHAW, P.C. (2011). Identification of herbal medicinal materials using DNA barcodes. *Journal of Systematics and Evolution* **49** (3): 271–283.

Little, C.L., Omotoye, R., and Mitchell, R.T. (2003). The microbiological quality of ready-to-eat foods with added spices. *International Journal of Environmental Health Research* **13** (1): 31–42.

Lo, S.H., Wong, K.S., Arlt, V.M. et al. (2005). Detection of Herba Aristolochia Mollissemae in a patient with unexplained nephropathy. *American Journal of Kidney Diseases* **45** (2): 407–410.

Loisy, F. (2012). Hepatitis E virus: a new food safety issue? IAFP 2012 Annual Meeting, July 2012.

Lou, S.K., Wong, K.L., Li, M. et al. (2010). An integrated web medicinal materials DNA database: MMDBD (medicinal materials DNA barcode database). *BMC Genomics* **11**: 402.

Mason, P. (ed.) (2007). *Dietary Supplements*, 3e. London: Pharmaceutical Press. ISBN 978 0 85369 653 7.

Matthews, K.R. (2014). Food safety: a global perspective. In: *Practical Food Safety* (eds. R. Bhat and V.M. Gomez-Lopez), 1–9. Hoboken: Wiley.

McKee, L.H. (1995). Microbial contamination of spices and herbs: a review. *LWT- Food Science and Technology* **28** (1): 1–11.

Mendonça, L.M., dos Santos, G.C., Antonucci, G.A. et al. (2009). Evaluation of the cytotoxicity and genotoxicity of curcumin in PC12 cells. *Mutation Research, Genetic Toxicology and Environmental Mutagenesis* **675** (1): 29–34.

Ministry of Health, Republic of Serbia (2010). Zakon o lekovima i medicinskim sredstvima.Službeniglasnik RS, 2010, br. 30 [in Serbian]. Available at: www.zdravlje.gov.rs/downloads/Zakoni/Zakoni/ZakonOLekovimaIMedSredstvima.pdf (accessed 29 June 2015).

Muggeridge, M. and Clay, M. (2001). Quality specifications for herbs and spices. In: *Handbook of Herbs and Spices* (ed. V.K. Peter), 13–22. Cambridge: Woodhead Publishing Ltd.

Myers, B.M., Smith, J.L., and Graham, D.Y. (1987). Effect of red pepper and black pepper on the stomach. *The American Journal of Gastroenterology* **82** (3): 211–214.

National Research Council (1980). *Recommended Dietary Allowances*, 9e. Washington, DC: National Academy of Sciences.

Nelson, M.H., Cobb, S.E., and Shelton, J. (2002). Variations in parthenolide content and daily dose of feverfew products. *American Journal of Health-System Pharmacy* **59** (16): 1527–1531.

Nordin, N. and Selamat, J. (2013). Heavy metals in spices and herbs from wholesale markets in Malaysia. *Food Additives and Contaminants: Part B* **6** (1): 36–41.

Obi, E., Akunyili, D.N., Ekpo, B., and Orisakwe, O.E. (2006). Heavy metal hazards of Nigerian herbal remedies. *Science of the Total Environment* **369** (1): 35–41.

Pakalniskiene, J., Falkenhorst, G., Lisby, M. et al. (2009). A foodborne outbreak of enterotoxigenic *E. coli* and *Salmonella Anatum* infection after a high-school dinner in Denmark, November 2006. *Epidemiology and Infection* **137**: 396–401.

Pan American Health Organization (2000). Regional meeting on regulatory aspects of herbal products, Final report, November 2000, Division of Health Systems and Services Development, Pan American Health Organization, World Health Organization.

Pezzoli, L., Elson, R., Little, C.L. et al. (2008). Packed with salmonella—investigation of an international outbreak of salmonella Senftenberg infection linked to contamination of prepacked basil in 2007. *Foodborne Pathogens and Disease* **5**: 661–668.

Poon, S.L., Pang, S.T., McPherson, J.R. et al. (2013). Genome-wide mutational signatures of aristolochic acid and its application as a screening tool. *Science Translational Medicine* **5** (197): 197ra101.

Qadri, S.M., Mahmud, H., Föller, M., and Lang, F. (2009). Thymoquinone-induced suicidal erythrocyte death. *Food and Chemical Toxicology* **47** (7): 1545–1549.

Raghuram, T.C., Sharma, R.D., Sivakumar, B., and Sahay, B.K. (1994). Effect of fenugreek seeds on intravenous glucose disposition in non-insulin dependent diabetic patients. *Phytotherapy Research* **8** (2): 83–86.

Ruschitzka, F., Meier, P.J., Turina, M. et al. (2000). Acute heart transplant rejection due to Saint John's wort. *The Lancet* **355** (9203): 548–549.

Sağdıç, O. (2003). Sensitivity of four pathogenic bacteria to Turkish thyme and oregano hydrosols. *LWT- Food Science and Technology* **36** (5): 467–473.

Sagoo, S.K., Little, C.L., Greenwood, M. et al. (2009). Assessment of the microbiological safety of dried spices and herbs from production and retail premises in the United Kingdom. *Food Microbiology* **26** (1): 39–43.

Sahoo, N., Manchikanti, P., and Dey, S. (2010). Herbal drugs: standards and regulation. *Fitoterapia* **81** (6): 462–471.

Samojlik, I., Mijatović, V., Gavarić, N. et al. (2013). Consumers' attitude towards the use and safety of herbal medicines and herbal dietary supplements in Serbia. *International Journal of Clinical Pharmacy* **35** (5): 835–840.

Sastre, J., Millan, A., de la Asuncion, J.G. et al. (1998). A Ginkgo biloba extract (EGb 761) prevents mitochondrial aging by protecting against oxidative stress. *Free Radical Biology and Medicine* **24** (2): 298–304.

Saw, J.T., Bahari, M.B., Ang, H.H., and Lim, Y.H. (2006). Potential drug–herb interaction with antiplatelet/anticoagulant drugs. *Complementary Therapies in Clinical Practice* **12** (4): 236–241.

Schulz, V., Hänsel, R., and Tyler, V.E. (1998). *Rational Phytotherapy: A Physician's Guide to Herbal Medicine*, 3e. Springer-Verlag.

Shah, A.H., Qureshi, S., and Ageel, A.M. (1991). Toxicity studies in mice of ethanol extracts of *Foeniculum vulgare* fruit and *Ruta chalepensis* aerial parts. *Journal of Ethnopharmacology* **34** (2): 167–172.

Shah, A.H., Al-Shareef, A.H., Ageel, A.M., and Qureshi, S. (1998). Toxicity studies in mice of common spices, *Cinnamomum zeylanicum* bark and *Piper longum* fruits. *Plant Foods for Human Nutrition* **52** (3): 231–239.

Shaker, R., Osaili, T., Al-Omary, W. et al. (2007). Isolation of Enterobacter sakazakii and other Enterobacter sp. from food and food production environments. *Food Control* **18**: 1241–1245.

Shan, B., Cai, Y.Z., Sun, M., and Corke, H. (2005). Antioxidant capacity of 26 spice extracts and characterization of their phenolic constituents. *Journal of Agricultural and Food Chemistry* **53** (20): 7749–7759.

Shan, B., Cai, Y.Z., Brooks, J.D., and Corke, H. (2009). Antibacterial and antioxidant effects of five spice and herb extracts as natural preservatives of raw pork. *Journal of the Science of Food and Agriculture* **89** (11): 1879–1885.

Sharma, J.N., Srivastava, K.C., and Gan, E.K. (1994). Suppressive effects of eugenol and ginger oil on arthritic rats. *Pharmacology* **49** (5): 314–318.

Sospedra, I., Soriano, J.M., and Mañes, J. (2010). Assessment of the microbiological safety of dried spices and herbs commercialized in Spain. *Plant Foods for Human Nutrition* **65** (4): 364–368.

Tyler, V.E. (1993). *The Honest Herbal*, 3e. New York, NY: Pharmaceutical Products Press.

Uppsala Monitoring Centre (2009). Herbal drug side reactions: 2009 WHO Programme for International Drug Monitoring: https://www.who-umc.org/.

Vaes, L.P. and Chyka, P.A. (2000). Interactions of warfarin with garlic, ginger, ginkgo, or ginseng: nature of the evidence. *Annals of Pharmacotherapy* **34** (12): 1478–1482.

Vickers, A.J. (2007). Which botanicals or other unconventional anticancer agents should we take to clinical trial? *Journal of the Society for Integrative Oncology* **5** (3): 125.

Wargovich, M.J., Woods, C., Hollis, D.M., and Zander, M.E. (2001). Herbals, cancer prevention and health. *The Journal of Nutrition* **131** (11): 3034S–3036S.

WHO. (1989). Evaluation of certain food additives and contaminants (Thirty-third report of the Joint FAO/WHO expert committee on food additives) WHO technical report series No 776. Geneva: World Health Organization.

World Health Organization. (1998). Quality control methods for medicinal plant materials. http://whqlibdoc.who.int/publications/1998/9241545100.pdf (accessed 27 June 2015).

World Health Organization. (2003). Guidelines on good agricultural and collection practices (GACP) for medicinal plants. http://whqlibdoc.who.int/publications/2003/9241546271.pdf (accessed 27 June 2015).

World Health Organization. (2007). WHO guidelines for assessing quality of herbal medicines with reference to contaminants and residues; http://apps.who.int/medicinedocs/index/assoc/s14878e/s14878e.pdf (accessed 28 June 2015).

World Health Organization. (2008). Traditional medicine. http://www.who.int/medicines/areas/traditional/en (accessed 30 June 2015).

Xia, J. (2004). Medicinal herbs used in pairs for treatment of 98 cases of chronic gastritis. *Journal of Traditional Chinese Medicine*= Chung i tsa chih ying wen pan/sponsored by All-China Association of Traditional Chinese Medicine, Academy of Traditional Chinese Medicine **24** (3): 208–209.

Xiang, L., Song, J., Xin, T. et al. (2013). DNA barcoding the commercial Chinese caterpillar fungus. *FEMS Microbiology Letters* **347** (2): 156–162.

Xin, T., Yao, H., Gao, H. et al. (2013). Super food Lycium barbarum (Solanaceae) traceability via an internal transcribed spacer 2 barcode. *Food Research International* **54** (2): 1699–1704.

Xue, J., Liu, D., Chen, S. et al. (2008a). Overview on external contamination sources in traditional Chinese medicines. *World Science and Technology* **10** (1): 91–96.

Xue, J., Hao, L., and Peng, F. (2008b). Residues of 18 organochlorine pesticides in 30 traditional Chinese medicines. *Chemosphere* **71** (6): 1051–1055.

Zweifel, C. and Stephan, R. (2012). Spices and herbs as source of salmonella-related foodborne diseases. *Food Research International* **45** (2): 765–769.

12 Adverse Human Health Effects and Regulation of Metal Contaminants in Terrestrial Plant-Derived Food and Phytopharmaceuticals

Ciara-Ruth Kenny[1,2,3], Brigid Lucey[2], and Ambrose Furey[1,3]

[1] *CREATE BioExplore (Centre for Research in Advanced Therapeutic Engineering), Cork Institute of Technology, Rossa Avenue, Bishopstown, T12 P928, Ireland*

[2] *Department of Biological Sciences, Cork Institute of Technology, Rossa Avenue, Bishopstown, T12 P928, Ireland*

[3] *Deptartment Physical Sciences, Cork Institute of Technology, Rossa Avenue, Bishopstown, T12 P928, Ireland*

12.1 Introduction

Plants can be described as sessile transitional reservoirs through which trace elements (metals, metalloids) from soil, water, and air transfer to humans via nutritional or medicinal avenues. Metals are ubiquitous in nature and can therefore occur as unsolicited residues in plants due to both natural (non-anthropogenic) and human-directed (anthropogenic) processes, with energy conversion and mineral consumption as chief sources of accelerated metal pollution within the biosphere. Metal contaminants can also enter our food during processing, packaging, storage, or preparation (Chan 2003; EFSA 2017b). Metals are non-biodegradable by nature and cause toxicity to eukaryotic organisms even at very low concentrations (Memon and Schröder 2009), thus ingestion of contaminated plant material poses a threat to consumers. Contamination

Herbs, Spices and Medicinal Plants: Processing, Health Benefits and Safety, First Edition.
Edited by Mohammad B. Hossain, Nigel P. Brunton, and Dilip K. Rai.

can compromise the purity of plant material, thus affecting overall quality, safety, and perhaps even their nutritional or medicinal efficacy (Jordan et al. 2010).

Metals can enter plant tissue via (aboveground) atmospheric deposition or uptake through the soil (belowground). Metal concentration in plant-derived foodstuffs (e.g. food crops, vegetables, herbs, spices, teas) is affected by the metal species involved, the plant species itself (e.g. non- or hyper-accumulator), its cultivation environment (e.g. soil profile, irrigation conditions), agrochemical usage, and surrounding anthropogenic contamination levels. Increased metal-uptake by plants grown either for direct human consumption or as feed-plants for animals contributes to the bioaccumulation and persistence of hazardous metals throughout the foodchain. The geographical location of terrestrial produce cultivation directly affects their metal content, further suggesting the need for monitoring. This is important owing to the globalization of plant-based food and medicinal products.

Bioaccumulation and eukaryotic toxicity are the major health threats associated with environmentally persistent metal pollution (Beek 1999; Kabata-Pendias 2010). It is widely accepted that metals above safe threshold concentrations can cause acute toxicity and a range of adverse effects in humans (Tchounwou et al. 2012). Diet is therefore a major factor concerning (oral) human exposure to potentially hazardous metals, whether as a single acute dose or through accumulation. The Agency for Toxic Substances and Disease Registry (ATSDR) lists Aluminum (Al), Arsenic (As), Cadmium (Cd), Chromium (Cr), Lead (Pb), and Mercury (Hg) as top priority metals of human concern; which are further classified as human carcinogens by the International Agency for Research on Cancer (IARC).

Acute toxicity from heavy metal exposure via food (dietary consumption) is an unlikely fate in Europe, presently, based on current exposure assessment data released by the European Food Safety Authority (EFSA). The likelihood of sub-acute or chronic toxicity from continual exposure to low levels of metals and their associated compounds, however, is uncertain (Hartwig and Jahnke 2017) and therefore cannot be ruled out; particularly in vulnerable subgroups. While efforts have been made to establish maximum levels in some foods, recent data suggest that the possibility of adverse effects arising from contaminated foods cannot be excluded. The quality of phytopharmaceuticals is a critical determinant of product safety (Verma 2016). The World Health Organization (WHO) states that metal exposure from the administration or consumption of phytopharmaceuticals or Herbal Medicinal Products (HMP's) is largely insignificant in terms of acute exposure; however, as reflected by the EFSA, chronic exposure contributing to the total bioburden or accumulation of these metals over time cannot be excluded based on current evidence (Hartwig and Jahnke 2017). Minimizing exposure to these metals where possible is therefore a necessary approach to protect public health.

In addition to food, plants are utilized for medicine. There are variable definitions of permissible levels of heavy metals in plants and plant-derived products (medicinal or foodstuff) across geographical locations, because of the non-uniformity of legislation and regulatory standards currently. Although the European Union and several other countries have developed region-specific guidelines, their regulation in developing countries is rarely enforced (Tripathy et al. 2015). To achieve regulatory approval in the EU, all drugs/medicines must be authorized before reaching the market to protect public health and ensure the availability of safe, high-quality, and effective medicines. Phytopharmaceuticals can be marketed upon successful authorization from one of the following application routes: full-, well-established use-, or traditional-use-application, the latter relating to the "Herbal Directive" scheme. General quality requirements are universal regardless of the application route except in the case of metal or elemental impurities and (pre)-clinical efficacy data requirements. The International Conference on Harmonisation (ICH) Q3D guidelines have been implemented verbatim as a replacement for metal impurity specifications in individual monographs in the latest revision of the European Pharmacopoeia (9th Edition). These guidelines, however, are not legally applicable to certain product categories, including herbal or plant-derived products. Several key issues challenging the quality control of phytopharmaceuticals include the lack of product classification or categorization criteria and metal impurity limits. They also include non-enforceable Good Agricultural and Collection Practices (GACP) guidelines and the unregulated practice of wildcrafting (wild plant collection) in non-European countries.

This chapter discusses the many avenues through which we as humans are exposed to non-essential, potentially toxic metal impurities and contaminants in plant-derived food and phytopharmaceuticals. We discuss how metals enter plant tissues, the biological consequences of exposure to the selected metals – Aluminum (Al), Arsenic (As), Cadmium (Cd), Chromium (Cr), Mercury (Hg), and Lead (Pb) – and the regulations that are currently in place to safeguard the general (non-occupationally exposed) European population.

12.2 Sources of Environmental Metal Impurities Contributing to Plant Material Contamination

Plant biomass has the capacity to sequester metals from the environment (environment > plants > humans). Heavy metals, even at trace levels, pose substantial ecological and public health risks due to their toxic and non-biodegradable nature (Singh et al. 2011b). Metal bioavailability to plants (phytoavailability), albeit a non-quantitative concept, refers to an element which is in a chemically acceptable form for plant uptake or absorption (Roberts et al. 2005), and which is influenced by numerous factors including metal species and climatic conditions. In addition to natural (non-anthropogenic) processes, exposure to trace metals has increased with the advent of global anthropogenic activity via agricultural, rural, and industrial pollution. The widespread environmental persistence of heavy metals is widely reported in the literature (Alexander et al. 2009; Singh et al. 2016). The following is a list of common sources of anthropogenic-derived metal contamination and the metals commonly associated with each (Gautam et al. 2014):

- Agrochemicals: As, Cd, Cr, Mo, Pb, U, V, Zn (Nicholson et al. 2003; Otero et al. 2005).
- Waste manures/sewage effluent/sludge: Zn, Cu, Ni, Pb, Cd, Cr, As, Hg (Schmiermund 2004; Walter et al. 2006).
- Landfill leachate: Zn, Cu, Cd, Pb, Ni, Cr, Hg (Kjeldsen et al. 2002; Fernández et al. 2005).
- Metalliferous dust: Cd, Cu, Ni, Cr, Co, Zn, As (Harris et al. 2011).
- Batteries: Pb, Sb, Zn, Cd, Ni, Hg (Naiya et al. 2009).

- Electroplating: Cr, Ni, Zn, Cu (Álvarez-Ayuso et al. 2003; Castelblanque and Salimbeni 2004).
- Electronics: Pb, Cd, Hg, Pt, Au, Cr, As, Ni, Mn (Vegliò et al. 2003).
- Paints and pigments: Pb, Cr, As, Ti, Ba, Zn (Monken 2010).
- Paper and pulp: Zn, Cu, Cd, Pb, Ni, Fe, Mn (Hakeem and Bhatnagar 2010).
- Specialist alloys and steels: Pb, Mo, Ni, Cu, Cd, As, Te, U, Zn (Cheng 2003; Rule et al. 2006).

Consequent contamination of high-value plant material (i.e. crops, vegetables, herbs) arises during plant cultivation, processing, preparation, and/or storage. The following section gives an overview of the origins of environmental metal impurities contributing to plant material contamination: soil, water, and air (see Figure 12.1).

12.2.1 Soil and Surrounding Rhizosphere

Soils contain trace elements of lithogenic (calculi formation) and pedogenic (soil forming) origin. The complexity of soil results largely from its inherent microbiome and trace element diversity (Geldner and Salt 2014). Soil acts as a natural buffer which contributes to elemental transport to the atmosphere, biota, and hydrosphere. Trace elemental concentrations in plants are highly correlated with the chemical makeup of their growth media (i.e. soil and surficial sediments) (Kabata-Pendias 2011); the trace element content of which largely depends on the parent material from which it was derived (Mason and Moore 1982). Subsequent leaching and nutrient cycling (soil–plants–animals) creates horizons exhibiting both depletion and enrichment. The behavior and phytoavailability of each element differs as to their origin – however anthropogenic-derived elements are more mobile and thus more phytoavailable than lithogenic and pedogenic elements (Kuo et al. 1983).

Heavy metals introduced to soil via non-anthropogenic routes are usually related to parent rock weathering and pedogenesis (soil formation) (Ghiyasi et al. 2010). Agrochemical application (fertilizers and pesticides) and sewage-derived products are examples of long-range aerial sources of trace elements which have a capacity to contribute to soil pollution (Bhandari 2014). Elemental mobilization via seepage waters and deposition of organic or inorganic airborne particulates of natural, industrial, or rural origin are predominant sources of surface soil contamination (Pacyna 1995; Eshel and Beeckman 2013).

Within soil solutions, metals can occur as free ions, or be complexed to organic and/or inorganic ligands creating metal–ligand complexes (Roberts et al. 2005). Plant roots can only access total bioavailable metals in soluble metal fractions. Trace metal solubility is often expressed as a function of pH, affected by the type and quantity of organic matter present (Kabata-Pendias 2011). Soil factors which govern the metal proportion in soil solutions, and consequently affect their phytoavailability, include pH, redox conditions, organic matter, clay, moisture, cation exchangeable capacity, and microbiome composition (Micó et al. 2008). Fundamental soil processes which determine the fate of metals in soil include microbial absorption, dissolution, diffusion, (organic and inorganic) complexation, migration, occlusion, precipitation, and volatilization – among others (Kabata-Pendias 2011).

The rhizosphere (endorhizosphere, rhizoplane, and ectorhizosphere) encompasses the area (1–2 mm) of soil around plant roots inhabited by a heterogeneous microbial

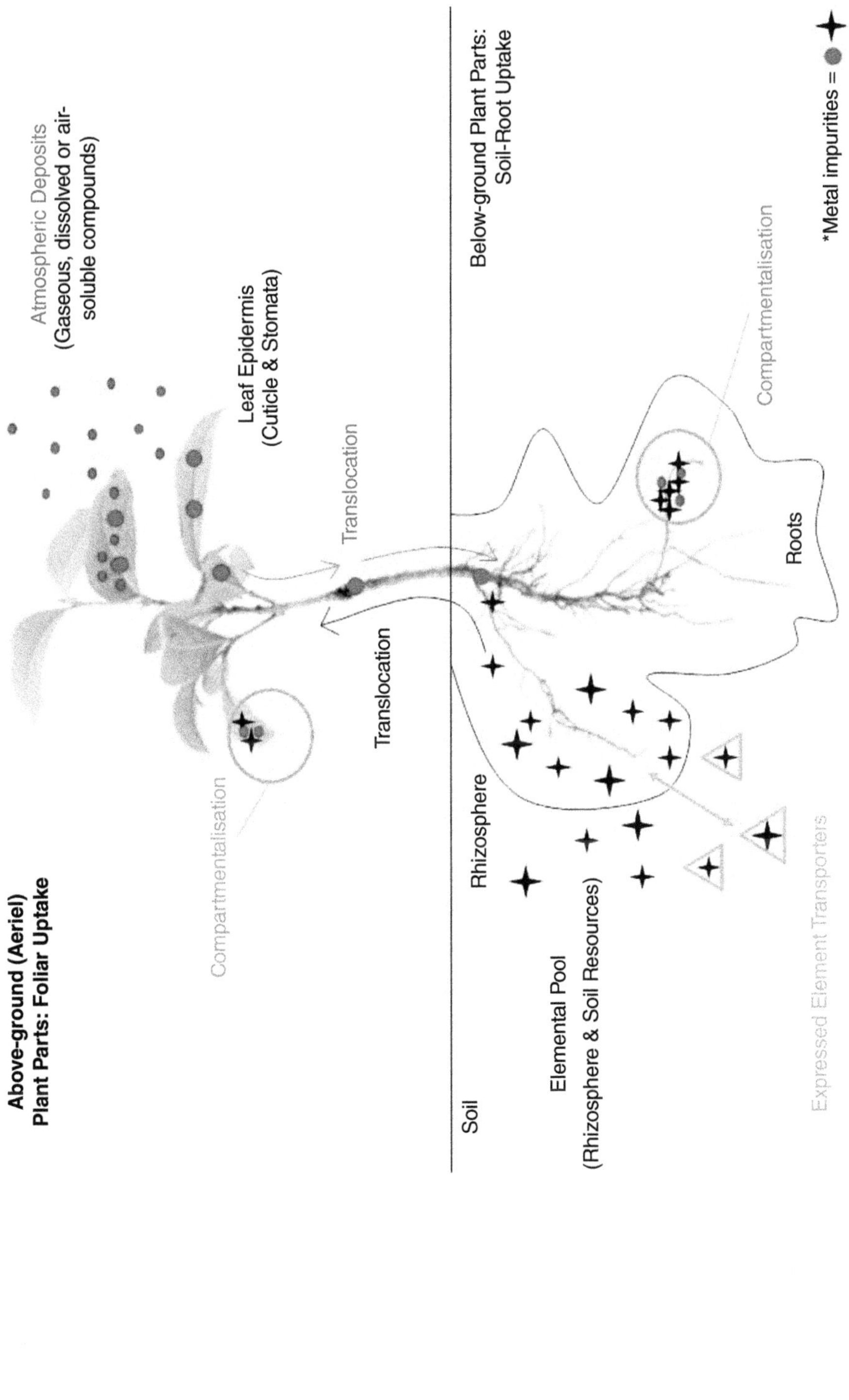

Figure 12.1 Simplified mechanisms of metal uptake in terrestrial plant systems.

population which is influenced by the root exudates (i.e. ions, free oxygen and water molecules, enzymes, and metabolites) (McNear Jr. 2013). Beneficial rhizobacteria can increase root surface area or root hair production thus directly affecting elemental absorption capacity (Dutta and Podile 2010) – a phenomenon triggered by the production of plant growth regulators and ethylene-degrading enzymes to inhibit growth (Lugtenberg and Kamilova 2009), or the acidification of the rhizosphere by rhizobacteria thus producing chelating agents that can enhance metal solubility (Rajkumar et al. 2012; Eshel and Beeckman 2013).

Phytoavailability is influenced by both soil and rhizosphere composition and is strongly correlated to metal speciation, metal solubility, metal mobility (transport, translocation, distribution), surrounding edaphic (soil) factors and microbial associations, plant morphological traits (e.g. root architecture), and biochemical secretion (e.g. root exudates). Soil properties are inversely proportional to the metal bioavailability to plant (roots) (Dghaim et al. 2015). Natural organic matter in the solid phase (e.g. humic substances) strongly retains metals, thus lowering their bioavailability for root uptake (Ross 1994). General phytoavailability of root-acquired trace elements depends on their behavioral properties in soil, where trace element availability to plant roots is strongly correlated with cationic concentration of the liquid soil portion (Kabata-Pendias 2011).

12.2.2 Air

The atmospheric deposition of metal particulates contributes to global biosphere contamination, affecting water, soil, and, consequently, plant systems.

- *Atmospheric particulates* are defined as complex mixtures of air-suspended solid and liquid particles of organic and inorganic substances (WHO 2007a).
- *Particulate matter* (PM) are solid or liquid particles in the air classified in relation to particle size or aerodynamic diameter, for example PM_{10} refers to particles with an aerodynamic diameter of $\leq 10\,\mu m$.

The ubiquitous existence of trace elements suspended within the atmosphere originate from both anthropogenic activities (e.g. metallurgical dust, automobile emissions, combustion emissions, and industrial processes) and natural sources (e.g. mineral aerosol, bio-aerosol, lithic dusts, and volcanic debris) (Pacyna 1995).

- *Primary aerosols:* refer to those that are directly emitted in particulate form, such as automobile emissions.
- *Secondary aerosols:* refer to particles formed from vapor condensation or chemical reactions (Pacyna 1995).

Organic and inorganic aerosol particles (e.g. dust, fume, smoke, fog, smog) range in diameter from 0.001–100 μm in size (Pacyna 1995). Trace elements are absorbed by organic and inorganic particles – the diameter of which affects the overall atmospheric persistence of the pollutant. Larger particles tend to precipitate rapidly near their discharge source, and low-density particles tend to persist and translocate within the atmosphere for varying periods of time (Kabata-Pendias 2011).

Plant foliage acquires metals from atmospheric sources via aerial deposition of gaseous, dissolved, or air-soluble particulate matter, referred to as foliar uptake

(Kannan 1980; Schreck et al. 2012). Absorption of foliar deposited particulates occurs predominantly through stomatal and cuticular openings, ectodesmata/ectocythodes (channels) positioned in the outer epidermal wall, and lenticels in woody stems (Franke 2012). Particulates therefore tend to enter plant tissue as a result of cuticular or stomatal deposition on leaf surfaces followed by upper adaxial sequestration or underground (shoot-to-root) translocation via xylem or phloem vasculature (Shahid et al. 2017). Metabolic routes of entry permit the accumulation of metals against a concentration gradient within plant tissues or organs, referred to as metabolic association. Non-metabolic cuticular penetration (passive diffusion) routes permit the entry of metals through direct superficial contact to exposed aerial foliage (Kabata-Pendias 2011).

12.2.3 Water (Ground-, Surface- and Waste-Water)

Water plays a fundamental role in aerial deposition of trace metals to plants (via rain or irrigation > foliage) and facilitating root acquisition of metals (via groundwater > soil). Both natural processes, including geochemical weathering of rocks and soil leaching, and anthropogenic processes resulting in wastewater effluents (e.g. mining, atomic and municipal waste) steadily contribute to the increased elemental concentration in the hydrosphere (Gautam et al. 2014). Most trace elements, chiefly trace metals, exist predominantly as suspended colloids or are fixed by organic/mineral substances in water. Volatile elements, however, can vaporize under favorable climatic conditions. Furthermore, microbial alkylation of certain metals/metalloids, including As, Hg, Se, Sn, and Te, chiefly occur in water as sediments or suspensions (Bentley and Chasteen 2002). Biogeochemical mechanisms involving microorganisms play a vital role in the transformation between the soluble and insoluble phases of metals/metalloids (White et al. 1997).

12.2.4 Processing, Packaging, Storage, and Preparation

Plant material (starting material, intermediate product, or finished product) is vulnerable to post-harvest contamination throughout industrial processing and packaging (Morgan 1999). Sources of contamination include the transfer from manufacturing infrastructure and equipment used (i.e. metal grinders, reactors, conveyors, rubber septum, or glassware), storage vessels (e.g. lead-lined containers), and decontamination procedures utilized onsite (WHO 2007b). Cross-contamination from the uncontrolled exposure to residues or the release of metallic particulates, gases, or vapors in-process is a constant risk (WHO 2007b).

As an example, most plant material undergoes mechanical grinding processes to produce cut (e.g. tea leaves) or powdered material (e.g. for enhanced extraction efficiency of medicinal plants: (Azwanida 2015)). Li and Qian (2017) reported the migration of heavy metals, including Al, As, and Pb, from pharmaceutical-grade rubber-stoppers during drug manufacture and preparation. Manufacturers are therefore required to comply with specific instructions detailing the process, apparatus specifications and allowable limits for residues. Manufacturing and storage facilities must also undergo periodic environmental monitoring to ascertain the absence of any elemental particulate matter (WHO 2007a,b).

Furthermore, certification of anti-migration packaging and food-contact material is becoming increasingly important. Bruna et al. (2015) reported the Cu, Cr, and Ni transfer from various packaging materials of carbonated soft drinks, exemplifying the influence of packaging material composition and the potential risk of contaminant transfer. In Europe, general requirements and Good Manufacturing Practices (GMPs) for Food Contact Materials (FCMs) are laid out in the European Commission (EC) Regulation No. 1935/2004 and Regulation (EC) No. 2023/2006 (Muncke 2014) respectively. Such legislation prevents the transfer of contaminants from food packaging, utensils, and conveyor belts that may endanger the health of consumers. In-process metal contamination of plants, however, at the time of writing, is certainly not widely reported in the scientific literature.

12.3 Overview of Metal Uptake Systems in Plants

Plants adopt variable and selective absorption patterns. Access is correlated to both the metal bioavailability and the source of uptake (e.g. air- or soil-borne) (Alford et al. 2010). The elemental uptake (absorption) efficiency of plants has been shown to differ between plant species (Schönherr and Luber 2001). Hyperaccumulators, for example, function to maintain characteristic high metal concentrations, and sustained metal accumulation in plant aerial tissue thus are becoming increasingly lucrative for their eco-toxicological uses, such as phytoremediation, phytomining, biomonitoring, and rhizofiltration (Krämer 2010; Rascio and Navari-Izzo 2011). Modifications in elemental concentrations in plants can change depending on several other variable factors, including variations (Baxter 2009) in:

- site of metal acquisition (i.e. root or aerial);
- soil-chemical profile and surrounding environmental conditions;
- plant morphological and physiological states;
- plant vegetative or reproductive stage of growth;
- plant uptake capacity (i.e. relating to transporter channels or cell wall composition);
- chelator accumulation in plant tissues and organs;
- intracellular element compartmentalization and subsequent concentration (e.g. vacuolar or mitochondrial sequestration).

Many factors influence the fate of absorbed metals within plant tissue, as summarized in Table 12.1.

12.4 Human Exposure to Metals in Plant-Derived Food and Associated Regulation

Long-term, low-dose exposure is a more likely route of metal exposure through dietary means, resulting in systemic accumulation over time (Goyer et al. 2004). Evaluating plant-derived food as sources of human exposure to non-essential metals, their associated compounds, and the formation of reactive metabolites contributes to a more unified understanding of the effects of aggregated exposure (Thomas

Table 12.1 Factors affecting the various metal fates in plants both pre- and post-entry

Metal uptake systems		Key points	References
Metal availability (Phyto-availability)	Soil composition	• Parent material composition • Soil pH • Organo-metallic complex formation • Oxidation-reduction states • Metal sorption reactions	Ross (1994), Rieuwerts et al. (1998), Michalke (2003), Roberts et al. (2005), Dghaim et al. (2015)
	Rhizosphere composition	• Rhizobacterial and mycorrhizal enhanced root architecture • Metal (de-)mobilizing root exudates (e.g. oxalic and malic acids, glomalin secretion)	Leyval et al. (1997), Hall (2002), Carter (2008), Lugtenberg and Kamilova (2009), Dutta and Podile (2010), Rajkumar et al. (2012), Eshel and Beeckman (2013), McNear Jr. (2013), Kushwaha et al. (2016)
Metal absorption	Air–foliage	• Environmental temperature and humidity • Leaf morphology • Cuticular and stomatal permeability • Ectodesmata (ectocythodes) • Phyllosphere microbiota interactions	Kannan (1980), Schreiber and Schönherr (1990), Prasad (2004), Eichert and Goldbach (2008), Birbaum et al. (2010), Eichert and Fernández (2012)
	Soil–root	• Root branching • Selective foraging • Root hair formation • Root morphological modulation • Root exudate and membrane transporter expression	Alford et al. (2010), Tangahu et al. (2011), Atkinson et al. (2014), Giehl and von Wirén (2014), Zelazny and Vert (2014), Montiel-Rozas et al. (2016)

(continued)

Table 12.1 *(continued)*

Metal uptake systems		Key points	References
Translocation/mobility/ distribution	Xylem (Apoplastic)	• Cation complexation with organic acids facilitates root-to-shoot translocation	Marschner (1995), Prasad (2004), Riesen and Feller (2005), Colangelo and Guerinot (2006), Liang et al. (2009), Rascio and Navari-Izzo (2011), Page and Feller (2015), Singh et al. (2016)
	Phloem (symplastic)	• Metal-binding compounds (e.g. nicotianamine) facilitates aerial-to-source organ (e.g. senescing leaves) or -sink organ translocation (e.g. maturing fruit)	
	Metal transporter proteins (MTP)	• Govern metal uptake, efflux, translocation/ distribution	
Biomolecular interactions	Complexation Chelation Immobilization Sequestration Compartmentalization	• Low-molecular mass (e.g. organic acids, amino acids) and high-molecular mass ligands (e.g. proteins, polysaccharides) • Categorized as oxygen-, sulfur-, or nitrogen-donor-based ligands	Baker et al. (2000), Haydon and Cobbett (2007), Husted et al. (2011), Timerbaev (2012), Leitenmaier and Kupper (2013), Mehes-Smith et al. (2013), Alvarez-Fernández et al. (2014)
Adaptive responses to metal stress	Hyperaccumulation	• Ability to retain high metal concentrations without exhibiting phytotoxicity • Enhanced metal uptake, translocation, and compartmentalization • Upregulation of metal transport genes	White et al. (2002), Alford et al. (2010), Krämer (2010), Rascio and Navari-Izzo (2011), Eshel and Beeckman (2013), Leitenmaier and Kupper (2013), Giehl and von Wirén (2014), Viehweger et al. (2014), Kushwaha et al. (2016), Singh et al. (2016)

Homeostatic maintenance	• Selective resource acquisition via root absorption stimulation or suppression • Rhizospheric, physiochemical, and microbial adaptions • Metal sequestration, precipitation, and exclusion	Clemens (2001), Puig and Peñarrubia (2009), Haydon et al. (2011), Assunção et al. (2013), Eshel and Beeckman (2013), Leitenmaier and Kupper (2013)
Detoxification strategies	• *Uptake restrictions (pre-entry):* avoidance phenomena, translocation restriction, exudate immobilization, rhizospheric pH alteration, mycorrhizal association, membrane alterations • *Defense strategies (post-entry):* complex formation, sequestration, efflux pump activation, cell wall modification, apoplastic exclusion, aerial leaching, phytovolatilization, redox mechanisms, hormone-mediated tolerance	Hall (2002), Haydon and Cobbett (2007), González-Mendoza and Zapata-Pérez (2008), Kabata-Pendias (2011), Mehes-Smith et al. (2013), Emamverdian et al. (2015)

and Bradham 2016) to multiple contaminants. The severity of the toxicity varies depending on the metal species involved, chronicity and exposure, gender, genetics, and lifestyle (Tchounwou et al. 2012). Nutritional status plays an irrefutable role in metal toxicity. Nutrient deficiency predisposes people to increased risk of toxicity from non-essential metals (Peraza et al. 1998). Adequate nutrient levels can decrease the bioavailability of certain metals from food in humans thus reducing the risk of toxicity (e.g. cadmium in iron deficiency), and vice versa. The species (chemical form/oxidation state/valency) of metals needs consideration, as some metal species are more potently toxic than others (e.g. hexavalent chromium (Cr (VI)) is more toxic than its trivalent (Cr (III)) form). Molecular or ionic mimicry describes situations where a metal complexes with an endogenous intracellular ligand and the end-product of this complex mimics the behavior of the normal substrate but alters its typical function (Goyer et al. 2004; Bridges and Zalups 2005). Such interactions are crucial to the understanding of metal uptake, kinetics, and ultimately metal toxicity in humans (Goyer et al. 2004).

When interpreting metal toxicity data from food, it is vital to include the rate of metal absorption and intake frequency as it may not be the food commodities with the highest metal level(s), but the foods which are more regularly consumed in larger quantities, which pose the greatest risk to consumers over time. Dietary exposure is assessed based on the metal concentration present in foods and associated food consumption estimates which includes both the consumption patterns of the food/ingredient and the probability of the consumer ingesting the food (Kroes et al. 2002). Various exposure assessment methodologies used to estimate potential health impacts of residues and contaminants in food have been reviewed elsewhere (Kroes et al. 2002; EFSA, 2011). Examples of calculation used to identify the transfer risk of plant-derived metals to humans include the Daily Dietary Index (DDI), Daily Intake of Metals (DIM), Hazard Index (HI), Hazard Quotient (HQ) and Hazard Risk Index (HRI) (Gall, Boyd and Rajakaruna, 2015). Such techniques are necessary to quantify the extent of exposure to consumers in relation to health-based guidance values (EFSA, 2011).

Furthermore, where genetic predisposition to micronutrient-associated disease is considered, the concentration of certain heavy metals in food and medicine can adversely affect certain subpopulations – an important parameter not to be overlooked. The clinical testing of human samples does not include the assessment of the concentration of heavy metals except in exceptional circumstances. Therefore, the contribution of these elements to individual human pathologies is almost always unknown. Nevertheless, the limits allowable through regulation, combined with what has been reported in the scientific literature of the pathological effects of these individual elements, have provided us with considerable information, which is reviewed below. The authors suggest that clinical metal toxicity should be diagnosed through laboratory testing, particularly among patients lacking a diagnosis while suffering from chronic symptoms.

Table 12.2 summarizes the target systems for As, Cd, Hg, and Pb toxicity and the current carcinogenic classification of these metals. It is necessary to control the levels of metal contaminants or impurities in our food and medicinal products to safeguard the public from exposure to potentially harmful metals.

Table 12.2 Symptoms of acute and chronic exposure to selected metals and their associated limits (Tolerable Weekly Intake (TWI); Benchmark Dose Lower Level (BMDL); Tolerable Daily Intake (TDI)) in food

Hazardous metal	Symptoms of exposure		Dietary limits (EU)	References
	Acute	Chronic		
Aluminum (Al)	*Not documented*	• Aluminosis • Neurotoxicity (Dementia syndrome, encephalopathy) • Breast cancer	TWI: 1 mg/kg body weight (bw)	Klotz et al. (2017)
Arsenic (As)[a]	• Gastrointestinal • Hematological • Neuropathy • Encephalopathy	• Carcinogenicity • Hyper-keratosis • Hyper-pigmentation	$BMDL_{01}$: 0.3–8 μg/kg bw	ATSDR (2007a)
Cadmium (Cd)[a]	• Pneumonitis • Renal damage • Steroidogenesis alteration	• Lung cancer • Osteomalacia • Ita-Itai disease • Proteinuria	TWI: 2.5 μg/kg bw	Godt et al. (2006), ATSDR (2012a)
Chromium (Cr)	• Gastrointestinal hemorrhage • Hemolysis • Reproductive toxicity • Dermal effects	• Pulmonary fibrosis • Carcinogenicity • Mutagenicity • Genotoxicity	TDI: 0.3 mg/kg/bw/day (CrIII)	ATSDR (2012b)

(continued)

Table 12.2 *(continued)*

Hazardous metal	Symptoms of exposure		Dietary limits (EU)	References
	Acute	Chronic		
Mercury (Hg)[c,d]	• Renal necrosis • Caustic gastroenteritis • Paraesthesia	• Neurological and psychological disturbances • Reproductive toxicity • Hypersensitivity/acrodynia (Pink Disease) • Minamata disease • Gingivo-stomatitis • Nephrotic syndrome • Visual and auditory damage	TWI: 1.6–4 μg/kg bw	Takeuchi et al. (1962), Järup et al. (1998), ATSDR (1999), Lash et al. (2007), Dufault et al. (2009), CDC (2016)
Lead (Pb)[b]	• Gastrointestinal effects • Encephalopathy • Renal and hepatic damage • Acute psychosis	• Hematological effects (anaemia) • Nephropathy • Reproductive toxicity • Deposition in bones and teeth • Arterial hypertension	$BMDL_{01}$: 1.5 μg/kg bw	Jarup (2003), ATSDR (2007b), Poręba et al. (2011), Jan et al. (2015)

IARC (International Agency for Research on Cancer) classifies As (IARC 2012) and Cd (IARC 2012) as Group 1 carcinogens [a] (*carcinogenic to humans*); Pb as Group 2A carcinogen [b] (*probably carcinogenic to humans*) (IARC 2006); Me-Hg as Group 2B carcinogen [c] (*possibly carcinogenic to humans*); and Inorganic Me-Hg as Group 3 carcinogens [d] (*unclassifiable as to its carcinogenicity to humans*) (IARC 1993).

12.4.1 Aluminum (Al)

12.4.1.1 Human Health Effects Al (3+ oxidation state) occurs naturally in our environment and is the most abundant metal component of the Earth's crust (ATSDR 2008; Jaishankar et al. 2014). It is frequently combined with fluorine (aluminum fluoride), oxygen (aluminum oxide), and silicon for industrial uses. Despite being an experimentally demonstrated neurotoxin (Tomljenovic and Shaw 2011), it is commonly used in medical and personal care products such as antacids, astringents, antiperspirants, buffered aspirin, food additives (ATSDR 2008), vaccine adjuvants (e.g. al-hydroxyphosphate and boehmite) (Lindblad 2004), and food-contact materials (Klotz et al. 2017). The nervous system is a well-known target for Al toxicity, in addition to the musculoskeletal and respiratory systems (ATSDR 2008). While Al could be a potentially toxic co-factor in neurodegenerative conditions, one must acknowledge that these diseases are likely the result of multiple etiologies (Tomljenovic and Shaw 2011), and further research is required. Al is non-carcinogenic *in vitro;* however, human trials have not yet been conducted. Al is unlikely to accumulate in most plants or animals (ATSDR 2008).

12.4.1.2 Dietary Exposure

12.4.1.2.1 Occurrence, Prevalence, and Regulatory Limits in Plant-Based Food While most unprocessed products contain ≤5 mg/kg of Al (FSAI 2016), EFSA have reported that tea leaves, herbs and spices, soy, and cocoa products contain high concentrations of Al (EFSA 2008). Bakery foodstuffs (e.g. cereals, cakes, pastries, breads) containing Al food-additives, such as sodium aluminum phosphate, similarly contain higher Al concentrations. Recent restrictions on the use of Al-containing food additives were introduced by the European Commission (Commission Regulation (EU) No 380/2012) to reduce consumer exposure (FSAI 2016). Considering a mean dietary exposure of ≤2.3 mg/kg, EFSA established a Tolerable Weekly Intake (TWI) of 1 mg/kg bw/week for Al in unprocessed food, with higher permissible concentrations in baked goods (EFSA 2008). This is lower than the provisional TWI of 2 mg/kg established by the Joint Food and Agriculture Organization/World Health Organization Expert Committee on Food Additives (JECFA) (JECFA 2011). The US Food and Drug Administration (FDA) regards Al as safe for use as food additives (e.g. in cereals and cheese products), food-contact materials, or medicinal excipients e.g. buffered analgesics and antacids (ATSDR 2008). A TDS conducted by the FDA estimated average Al intake ranges from 0.7 mg/day in infants, 11.5 mg/day in male teens, 8–9 mg/day in male adults, and 7 mg/day in female adults (Pennington and Schoen 1995). The US Environmental Protection Agency (EPA) recommends a Secondary Maximum Contaminant Level (SMCL) of 0.05–0.2 mg/l for Al in potable water, while EU limits are 200 μg/l for Al (ATSDR 2008). Dietary Al exposure is within the TWI range; however, while average exposure is below the TWI, it is still close to the TWI for Al. While orally ingested Al is poorly absorbed, once within the body, it has a whole-body half-life of approximately 50 years (FSAI 2016). Taking this into account, an attempt should be made to reduce Al exposure, particularly for infants, toddlers, and children (Hartwig and Jahnke 2017).

12.4.2 Arsenic (As)

12.4.2.1 Human Health Effects As is a naturally occurring metalloid present in groundwater, soil, and air. It exists in organic and inorganic structural forms and various oxidation states (−3, 0, +3, +5) (Hughes 2002). Natural sources include volcanic emissions, weathering of rocks, and natural springs (Zhao et al. 2010). Historically As has been used as a therapeutic agent in products such as Fowler's solution (*potassium arsenite:* $AsKO_2$) and Salvarsan, and in modern medicine as an approved chemotherapeutic agent (*arsenic trioxide:* As_2O_3) in acute promyelocytic leukemia (Murgo 2001; Tchounwou et al. 2012). Evidence of the environmental persistence of arsenate residues as a result of previously accepted agricultural practices are reported in the literature (Hood 2006), following the application of arsenic-based agrochemicals such as Paris-green insecticides (*copper acetoarsenite:* $Cu(C_2H_3O_2)_2 \cdot 3Cu(AsO_2)_2$) and pesticides (*lead hydrogen arsenate:* $PbHAsO_4$; *monosodium methanearsonate:* CH_4AsNaO_3; *cacodylic acid:* $Cu_3(AsO_4)_2$). Other environmental sources of As include copper smelting industries, wood preservation (*chromated copper arsenate*: $Cu_3(AsO_4)_2$), glass, and semi-conductor production (Hughes 2002; Hughes et al. 2011a). Three further classes of arsenical compounds of toxicologic concern, predominantly present in seafood, are the complex organic arsenicals (Borak and Hosgood 2007; Thomas and Bradham 2016): arseno-lipids, -sugars, and trimethylarsonium. These compounds are characterized by the occurrence of a di- or tri-methylated As-containing moiety in an aliphatic or aromatic molecule, and contribute to the aggregate exposure to As in the human population (Thomas and Bradham 2016). Primary dietary sources include fish, fish oil supplements, and macroalgae (i.e. seaweed).

The toxic potencies of As compounds depend on its chemical form, oxidation state, and effects of mammalian metabolism, including reduction to a trivalent state and oxidative methylation to a pentavalent state (Thomas et al. 2001; Hughes 2002). In essence, As metabolism involves a cascade of events from pentavalency to trivalency (reduction) catalyzed by As^{13}-methyltransferase, and back to pentavalency (oxidative methylation) (Hughes et al. 2011a). Toxicologically relevant forms of inorganic As (see Figure 12.2) are pentavalent arsenate ($AsO_4{}^{3-}$) and trivalent arsenite ($AsO_3{}^{3-}$) (Tchounwou et al. 2012). Monomethylarsonic acid (MMA), dimethylarsinic acid (DMA), and trimetylarsine oxide are stable methylated mammalian metabolites of inorganic As (Hughes 2002), often referred to as the organic forms of As.

Genetic polymorphisms associated with increased susceptibility to inorganic As-induced disease have been reported (McCarty et al. 2007; Steinmaus et al. 2007; De Chaudhuri et al. 2008; Wang et al. 2009; Porter et al. 2010). Genotypic variation in the *As3MT* (As^{3+} Methyltransferase) genotype can alter methylation profiles for inorganic As, referred to as the As methylation phenotype (Hughes et al. 2011a). Studies show that persistently high urinary MMA concentrations associated with the *M287T* (Methionine 287 Threonine) genotype, which affects the As methylation phenotype, is potentially linked with increased risk of As-induced adverse health effects (Chung et al. 2009; Fujihara et al. 2009; Valenzuela et al. 2009; Rodrigues et al. 2012).

Exposure to As compounds is explicably linked to cancer; As compounds are classified as Group 1 carcinogens (carcinogenic in humans) by the IARC and EPA (IARC 2012). Consumption of As-contaminated foodstuffs is a potential contributor to the global cancer epidemic (Oberoi et al. 2014; Thomas and Bradham 2016).

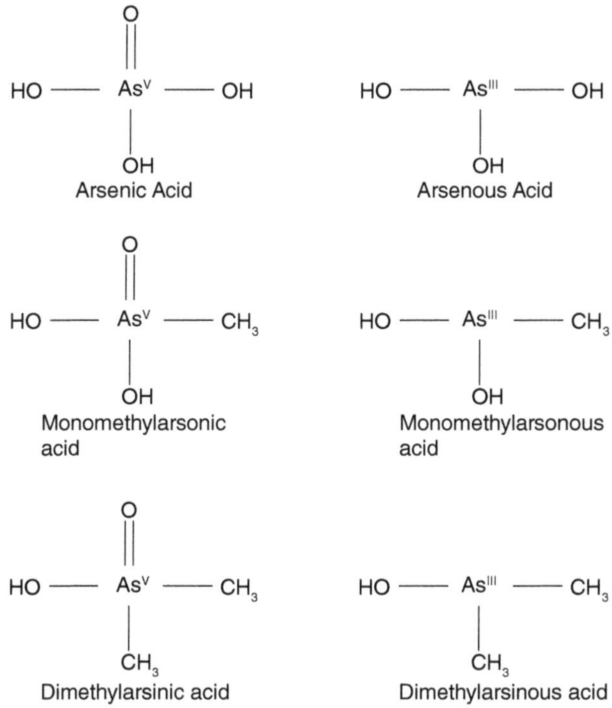

Figure 12.2 Toxicologically relevant forms of As (Hughes 2002).

Associated adverse effects are well established. Acute toxicity arising from trivalent As exposure is greater than that arising from pentavalent ion (Hughes 2002), due to its reactivity with sulfur and cellular generation of Reactive Oxygen Species (ROS) (Hughes et al. 2011a). Methylated trivalent intermediates of As are more acutely (geno)toxic than arsenite (Mass et al. 2001). Symptoms of acute As toxicity are centered around gastrointestinal (GIT) disorders, whereas symptoms of chronic As toxicity affect multiple systems including the integumentary, cardiovascular, nervous, excretory (renal), and endocrine systems (Hughes 2002). Adverse effects associated with long-term consumption of inorganic As in humans are abnormal glucose metabolism, diabetes, cancer, cardiovascular disease, developmental toxicity, neurotoxicity, and skin lesions (EFSA-CONTAM 2009). The development of skin lesions characterized by hyper-keratosis and hypo- and hyper-pigmentation are a distinctive characteristic of chronic oral exposure to As (Hughes 2002; Paul et al. 2015). Based on frequency, toxicity, and likelihood of human exposure, As ranks first on the priority list of hazardous substances published by the ATSDR, ahead of Pb and Hg (ATSDR 2017).

The toxicological profiles of As compounds are discussed in detail by the ATSDR (ATSDR 2007a). The mechanism(s) of action (MoA) responsible for these effects, however, are complex and still poorly understood (Shen et al. 2013). Potential MoA for As compounds has been extensively reviewed in the literature (Kitchin 2001; Hughes 2002; Tapio and Grosche 2006; Platanias 2009; Kitchin and Conolly 2010; Singh et al. 2011a). The toxicity of As-contaminated potable water is acknowledged worldwide (NRC 1999; Zhao et al. 2010; Thomas and Bradham 2016), and further elucidation of this is outside the scope of this chapter. Dietary exposure to As through food is, however, just as prevalent (Kurzius-Spencer et al. 2014; Wilson 2015; Thomas and Bradham 2016).

12.4.2.1.1 Interactions with Endogenous Oxyanions Inorganic arsenate ($HAsO_4^{2-}$) is a molecular analogue of phosphate (HPO_4^{2-}). Structural similarities and comparable dissociation constants thereby permit inorganic arsenate to compete for phosphate anion transporters (Shen et al. 2013) and replace phosphate in biochemical reactions such as the *in vitro* uncoupling of ATP; coined "arsenolysis." Arsenolysis weakens the *in vitro* formation of ATP at both substrate (glycolysis) and mitochondrial levels (oxidative-phosphorylation) by substituting phosphate with arsenate in enzymatic reactions creating unstable arsenate anhydrides (Crane and Lipmann 1953; Gresser 1981; Dixon 1996). Ultimately, the binding of pentavalent arsenicals in phosphate-utilizing enzymes that typically alkylate, acylate, or phosphorylate the phosphate (Dixon 1996), confers biological alterations (Shen et al. 2013). The similarities between these two oxyanions may explain its prevalence in marine organisms. Evidence suggests that marine algae cannot distinguish between them and unintentionally uptake arsenate instead of the essential nutrient phosphate which subsequently leads to the production of toxic methylated organo-arsenic compounds which bioaccumulate throughout the foodchain. Studies have also demonstrated arsenite as a functional mimic of estrogen (estradiol) which could suggest its potential role in the etiology of breast cancer or hormone-related disease (Bridges and Zalups 2005).

12.4.2.1.2 Altered Glucose Metabolism The cellular binding location of As species is an important determinant of toxicity. The integration of trivalent arsenicals to specific functional groups within (co)-enzymes or receptors would likely result in adverse metabolic function, whereas binding to non-essential protein sites may be a necessary cellular detoxification mechanism (Aposhian 1997). MMA^{III} inhibits pyruvate dehydrogenase (PDH) activity by binding to the lipoic acid moiety which contains vicinal dithiols (Petrick et al. 2001), thereby interfering with pyruvate oxidation to acetyl-coA in the citric-acid cycle (Hughes 2002). This enzymatic interference may cause decreased ATP production and altered glucose metabolism. Recent studies suggest that exposure to inorganic As can worsen diabetogenic effects in type-2 patients (Liu et al. 2014a). The results of one study showed that inorganic As altered lipid metabolism and pancreatic β-cell dysfunction, increased gluconeogenesis and oxidative hepatic damage in mice, and additionally worsened glucose tolerance in diabetic mice (Liu et al. 2014a).

12.4.2.1.3 Oxidative Stress and ROS Generation Cellular ROS generation is a prominent inducer of toxicity and disease in humans (Jomova et al. 2011). Arsenic species associated with ROS generation include: As-centered and As-peroxyl radicals, hydrogen peroxide, hydroxyl radical, superoxide anion, and reactive nitrogen species (Kitchin 2001). Chronic, low-dose As exposure alters oxidative stress and inflammation-associated genes and the proteins and transcriptional regulators of the resulting altered genes are redox-sensitive (ATSDR 2007a). As-induced oxidative stress has been confirmed both *in vitro* and *in vivo,* and is often implicated in the inhibition of numerous enzymes (Shen et al. 2013). Arsenite constrains PDH activity upon both the direct binding to inherent vicinal sulfhydryl groups within the enzyme, and/or by generating ROS which ultimately inactivates the enzyme (Samikkannu et al. 2003). As-induced ROS play a role in a number of hypothesized MoA, such as altered signal transduction, altered DNA repair, cell proliferation, and genotoxicity (Hughes et al. 2011b); however, the mechanisms by which As form ROS are poorly understood. Proposed metabolic events leading to ROS generation include the metabolic oxidation of arsenite to arsenate (Del Razo et al. 2001), the production of arsenic metabolites (Yamanaka and Okada 1994), NADH or NADPH oxidase activation (Chou et al. 2004), thiol chelation/complexation in dithiol-containing enzymes (Shen et al. 2013), and ferritin iron release in the presence of ascorbic acid (Ahmad et al. 2000). Oxidative stress may be involved in As-induced cytotoxicity (Yedjou et al. 2006; Jomova et al. 2011), while ROS-mediated genomic mutation is a likely initiation step of As-induced carcinogenicity (Li and Chen 2016; Wei et al. 2005).

12.4.2.1.4 Carcinogenicity As is classified as a Group 1 carcinogen (IARC 2012) based on several epidemiological studies. Current evidence suggests that As may be a co-carcinogen, a promoter, or a progressor of carcinogenesis (Tchounwou et al. 2012). Proposed mechanisms of carcinogenesis include altered cell proliferation and DNA methylation, co-mutagenesis (Hughes et al. 2011b), genotoxicity, oxidative stress, and tumor protection (Hughes 2002; Martinez et al. 2011). As-induced epigenetic effects, such as DNA methylation, post-translational histone modification, and miRNA interference, play a role in As toxicity (Li and Chen 2016; Bjørklund et al. 2017a; Paul et al. 2017). Key pathways involved in As-induced carcinogenesis have reportedly been modulated as a result of such epigenetic alterations. Research has shown that As alters genomic methylation profiles within human cells, leading to anomalous gene expression resulting in various pathophysiological outcomes including genomic instability and oncogenesis (Paul et al. 2017). There is emerging evidence to support the hypotheses that the interactions of As compounds with chemical compounds (Pershagen et al. 1984) or UV radiation (Rossman et al. 2001) causes a co-carcinogenic effect (Hughes 2002). As can interfere with cell signaling pathways implicated in tumor progression, e.g. suppression of p53 (Tchounwou et al. 2012), intracellular kinases, and transcription factor signaling pathways (Huang et al. 2004). The ability of As species to modulate gene expression contributes to the carcinogenic potential of these compounds (Tchounwou et al. 2012). Given the carcinogenic potential of As and As compounds, it is vital to minimize human exposure where possible – starting with food.

12.4.2.2 Dietary Exposure

12.4.2.2.1 Occurrence, Prevalence, and Regulatory Limits in Plant-Based Foods Predominant As compounds routinely present in food are MMA, DMA^{V}, arsenobetaine, arsenocholine, arsenosugars, and arsenolipids, which are of course dependent on the food type (Hughes et al. 2011b). Organic As species, such as arsenobetaine and arsenosugars, are most frequently present in seafood, while inorganic As forms predominate in plant-derived foods, including As (V), As (III), methylarsonate, methylarsenite, and DMA (EFSA 2014). Contaminated water used in agricultural irrigation of dietary crops accelerates the introduction of As into the foodchain via plant uptake. Plant-derived food products generally contain low levels of total and inorganic As (≤ 0.25 mg/kg). Foods such as rice, seafood, algae, and animal offal are the main dietary contributors (EFSA-CONTAM 2009). Dietary intake of inorganic

As from plants is generally low except for populations who consume rice as a dietary staple (Schoof et al. 1999).

EFSA lists processed grain-based products, such as rice grains and derivatives, wheat bread, dairy, and potable water as the chief sources of As exposure for the general European population (European Commission 2017a). Other specific food groups, including fish, vegetables, algae, coffee, and special dietary food, are also significant contributors to the daily dietary exposure of the general European population to inorganic As (European Commission 2017a). Estimates of dietary inorganic As intake levels vary worldwide (Hughes et al. 2011b). Recently, EFSA estimated that dietary intake of As for average consumers in European populations ranged from 0.2–1.37 μg/kg bw/day among infants and young children, with the 95th percentile estimates ranging from 0.36–2.09 μg/kg bw/day (EFSA 2014). Average dietary exposure among the adult population was much lower, ranging from 0.09–0.38 μg/kg bw/day, with the 95th percentile estimates ranging from 0.14–0.64 μg/kg bw/day (EFSA 2014).

Currently, no maximum concentration levels (MCLs) or tolerable intake values have been defined for As compounds in dietary foodstuffs (Sun et al. 2008), except for rice and rice-based products (see Table 12.3). In 2009, the European Commission revoked the PTWI (Provisional Tolerable Weekly Intake) for inorganic As of 15 μg/kg bw, established by the JECFA, based on reported data confirming the respiratory-, skin-, and urinary-carcinogenic potential of inorganic As at exposures lower than the current PWTI (European Commission 2015). The CONTAM panel recommends a Benchmark Dose (Lower Limit) $BMDL_{01}$ values of 0.3–8 μg/kg bw/day to be used in place of a singular reference point in risk characterization for inorganic As. In 2011, JECFA established $BMDL_{0.5}$ values of 3 μg/kg bw/day (lung cancer), 5.2 μg/kg bw/day (bladder cancer), and 5.4 μg/kg bw/day (skin lesions) (FSAI 2016). The EFSA scientific opinion concluded that the estimated dietary exposure to inorganic As for European consumers, while within the range, is close to the $BMDL_{01}$ values. Thus, there is little or no safe margin of exposure and the possibility of risk to some consumers cannot be excluded (European Commission 2015). For As compounds, benchmark calculations suggest that increased risk of cancer related to the dietary intake of inorganic As cannot be ruled out, taking the current exposure levels into account (EFSA-CONTAM 2009; CONTAM 2014; Hartwig and Jahnke 2017).

Children ($\leq$3 years) are the most exposed subpopulation to inorganic As (European Commission 2017a), with estimated two- to three-fold higher exposure rates than adults (EFSA-CONTAM 2009; European Commission 2015). Based on available evidence, vegetarians are not at an increased risk of dietary exposure to As compared to

Table 12.3 Maximum limits of inorganic As in rice and rice products reported in Regulation (EC) No. 2015/1006 (amending 1881/2006) (European Commission 2015)

Food commodities	Permissible limit(s) of As (mg kg[a])
Milled rice (non-parboiled, polished/white)	0.20
Parboiled and husked rice	0.25
Rice cakes/crackers/waffles/wafers	0.30
Rice intended for infant/children food products	0.10

[a] Wet weight.

the general population, unless large amounts of algae-derived products are consumed (European Commission 2017a). Alternating patterns of food usage has been suggested as a strategy to decrease exposure to vulnerable subpopulations (Gundert-Remy et al. 2015). Alternatively, As limits for specific, frequently consumed food commodities should exist where possible.

As accumulation in marine organisms, including fish, algae, and seaweed, is widely reported in the literature (Thomas and Bradham 2016). With increasing interest in algae as a source of bioactive natural products for use in pharmaceuticals, nutraceuticals, dietary supplements, novel, and functional foods (Fan et al. 2014; Cardoso et al. 2015; Abdul et al. 2016), levels in the starting materials of these marine-derived products should be monitored to ensure consumer safety. In a bid to reduce As accumulation in plants, the use of phosphorous fertilizers has been employed as a semi-successful treatment. Phosphate competes with arsenate for root uptake and adsorption on Fe oxides and/or hydroxides (Zhao et al. 2010), thereby limiting the success of these fertilizers. Alternative solutions are to increase the cellular concentration of phosphorous as a detoxification mechanism, the use of silicon fertilizers, sulfur supplementation or Fe-reducing microbes (Zhao et al. 2010).

12.4.2.2.2 Rice and Rice-Based Products It is becoming increasingly acknowledged worldwide that inorganic As accumulation in plant-based dietary staples, such as rice (*Oryza sativa* L.), poses a tangible risk to populations with high levels of daily rice consumption (Zhao et al. 2010), particularly in susceptible subpopulations such as infants and young children (Signes-Pastor et al. 2017). Rice is a staple foodstuff for more than half the world's population (Muthayya et al. 2014). Kitchen preparation techniques have been explored as a means of reducing As load in foods such as rice (Carey et al. 2015). Undissociated arsenite and methylated As species enter plant tissues through nodulin 26-like (NIP) aquaporin channels, whereas arsenate enters via phosphate transporters. Silic acid and arsenous acid share similarities which permit the entry of the latter via the silicon transport pathway. Arsenite enters plant tissue via the silicon transport pathway, which then leads to arsenite mobilization. Arsenate can be reduced to arsenite, which complexes with thiol-rich peptides such as phytochelatins and/or vacuolar sequestration as a means of cellular detoxification *in planta*. Complexation with sulfur may restrict As mobility from the root as a detoxification mechanism (Zhao et al. 2010)

A recent study showed that 73% of rice-based products targeted at infants and young children exceeded the stipulated EU limit of 0.1 mg/kg for inorganic As (Signes-Pastor et al. 2017). As for all contaminants, actual risk is based on mg/kg/day intake (Sun et al. 2008); therefore, based on infants' size alone, they are more sensitive to exposure to elevated levels of inorganic As in comparison with children or adults. This means that they are relatively exposed to higher levels of inorganic As from the same food item on a bodyweight basis. This study illustrates non-compliance of rice-based products on the current EU market, thus justifying current advice against the consumption of rice-based products (e.g. non-dairy infant formula, milk, puddings, crackers/cakes) in infants and young children (Signes-Pastor et al. 2017).

In situ distribution and localization of As within the actual rice grain should not be overlooked (Zhao et al. 2010) as it is a factor contributing to the bioavailability of As in the foodchain (Lombi et al. 2009). Elemental mapping of rice grains shows prominent As accumulation alongside the margin of the rice grain, which corresponds to the ovular vascular trace containing vascular tissue responsible for nutrient transport (Meharg et al. 2008; Lombi et al. 2009; Zhao et al. 2010). Studies have shown that rice bran is more enriched with As than the polished endosperm (Rahman et al. 2007; Sun et al. 2008), with some studies reporting As concentrations 10-fold higher in whole-grain bran (brown rice) at 1.9 mg/kg As compared to the processed endosperm (white rice) at 0.21 mg/kg As (Sun et al. 2008). Considering a recommended serving of 20 g/day, this equates to 0.012–0.038 mg dietary intake of inorganic As from one food source. Furthermore, these findings are a concern where such products, rice hull (husk) or soluble rice bran (milled hull), are marketed as "superfoods" in developed counties, as a source of soluble fiber (Sun et al. 2008). Even more concerning is the use of stabilized rice bran as a staple dietary supplement for malnourished children through humanitarian food-aid programs (Meharg et al. 2008; Sun et al. 2008; FedEx 2009; Kinyuru et al. 2015).

12.4.3 Cadmium

12.4.3.1 Human Health Effects The ATSDR ranks Cd as the seventh leading contaminant on its priority list of hazardous substances, ahead of benzo(α)pyrene and polycyclic aromatic compounds (ATSDR 2017). Chief industrial and manufacturing sources that contribute to the anthropogenic Cd burden in our environment include: non-ferrous metal mining (Cu, Pb, Zn), phosphate agri-fertilizers, alkaline (Ni-Cd-hydroxide) rechargeable batteries (electrode component), Cd-based pigments (Jaishankar et al. 2014), and anti-corrosion applications (Jarup 2003). Indirect food-associated sources of Cd include Cd-coated utensils, pottery, ceramics, and as a plastic stabilizer in FCMs (Galal-Gorchev 2009). Volcanic activity and weathering of rocks account for the natural emission of inorganic Cd into the environment (EFSA 2012a). Cd binds to organic matter within soil matrices which enhances Cd uptake in plant roots (ATSDR 2012a). Soil contamination thus leads to increased Cd-uptake by food crops and vegetables grown either for direct human consumption (Jarup 2003), or as feed-plants for animals, thereby contributing to bioaccumulation of this metal within the foodchain. Cd-uptake (via plant roots) is further enhanced at acidic soil pH (Järup et al. 1998).

Cd is classified by the IARC as a Group 1 carcinogen based on increased human risk of bladder, breast, endometrium, and lung cancer (IARC 2012). Proposed mechanisms of Cd carcinogenesis include induced oxidative stress, inactivation of DNA-repair proteins, enzymes, altered cell proliferation and signal transduction, tumor-suppressor protein inactivation (e.g. p53), upregulation of ROS tolerance genes, and epigenetic alterations (Stohs et al. 2001; Potts et al. 2003; Waisberg et al. 2003; Joseph 2009; Wang et al. 2012; Rani et al. 2014; Venza et al. 2015; Vilahur et al. 2015). The generation of ROS and oxidative damage is associated with the inhibition of antioxidant enzymes (Stohs et al. 2001; Valko et al. 2006; IARC 2012).

Dietary (oral) exposure through food is the most likely route of exposure for the general population (ATSDR 2012a). Major food sources are fruits and vegetables due to its soil-to-root transfer (Satarug et al. 2010). Risk of Cd exposure through the food supply is secondary for smokers, and primary for non-smokers (ATSDR 2012a). Direct consumption of Cd-containing food and water accounts for 1–10% of the total exposure to Cd (ATSDR 2012a). Cd levels vary depending on the food group in question, and are influenced by soil and irrigation conditions, agrochemical usage, and atmospheric deposition rates in the surrounding environment. Potatoes and grains, soybeans, leafy vegetables, soybeans, and oilseeds (e.g. sunflower) generally contain high levels of Cd (ATSDR 2012a). Cd has a low intestinal absorption rate in humans (approx. 6.5%) (Horiguchi et al. 2004), or ≤ 10% from food (Flanagan et al. 1978).

The kidneys and bones are the primary sites of oral toxicity resulting from chronic, low-levels of exposure to Cd (ATSDR 2012a), with a long half-life (10–30 years) in renal organs (kidneys) and skeletal tissue (bones) (Mamtani et al. 2011). Renal sensitivity to Cd is related to the *de novo* synthesis of metallothionein in the kidneys (ATSDR 2012a). Acute oral toxicity causes severe GIT disturbances (Liu et al. 2014b) and even death, depending on the dosage (ATSDR 2012a). Other adverse effects include hematological, hepatic, reproductive, and immunological effects, and nephropathy (ATSDR 2012a). Chronic, low-level exposure to Cd in food combined with inhalation from cigarettes can cause asymptomatic accumulation in target organs leading to the onset of non-reversible adverse effects, such as renal dysfunction or osteoporosis, over time (Järup et al. 1998; Goyer et al. 2004). Low-level exposure causes nephrotoxicity for certain subgroups, particularly infants and children (Hartwig and Jahnke 2017) and subgroups at risk of co-exposure with tobacco smoking (ATSDR 2012a).

The ATSDR state that the toxicological properties of Cd salts and oxides are similar to those of (elemental) Cd. Not all forms of Cd are equally absorbed in humans, and this variation in absorption and distribution consequently leads to differences in biological effects (ATSDR 2012a). Ionic Cd is more readily absorbed from the GIT compared to Cd-bound complexes in food (ATSDR 2012a). Soluble Cd exists as the Cd^{+2} ion, irrespective of the original salt. Cd exists in the free-ionic form in water, while in food matrices the Cd ion complexes with a number of organic ligands, such as metallothionein (Stillmanso et al. 1987). Similar absorption patterns are observed for the Cd ion and inorganic Cd-complexes in food (e.g. proteins) (McKenzie-Parnell et al. 1988).

The nutritional status of an individual is an important parameter not to be overlooked when interpreting toxicity data from food. Individuals deficient in calcium (Ca) or iron (Fe) are more susceptible to Cd toxicity (Hartwig and Jahnke 2017). The relationship between Cd absorption and Fe deficiency has been experimentally confirmed (Alexander et al. 2009). Fe deficiency upregulates the expression of Divalent Metal Transporter 1 (DMT1), which also has a high affinity for Cd (Kim et al. 2007; Kayaaltı et al. 2015), which may explain the enhanced intestinal absorption of Cd in Fe-deprived states. As exemplified by Reeves and Vanderpool (1997), high habitual intakes of sunflower kernels not only increased Cd intake, but also Cu and phytate – the presence of which reduces the bioavailability (and thus toxicity) of the ingested Cd. Thus, adequate nutrient levels, such as Fe, can decrease the bioavailability of Cd from food in humans (ATSDR 2012a). Conversely, micronutrient-associated disease can also affect the bioavailability and thus resulting toxicity from ingested Cd.

12.4.3.1.1 Renal Nephropathy Toxicity is dependent on renal Cd concentrations within the kidney(s) (ATSDR 2012a). The development of kidney stones, related to increased urinary excretion of Ca, has been demonstrated in numerous studies (Hossny et al. 2001). Studies have established an association between Cd exposure and (chronic) End-Stage Renal Disease (ESRD) (Hellström et al. 2001). Events of acute oral toxicity are rare; however, renal nephropathy can occur in conditions of chronic low-level exposure to Cd and Cd compounds (Hartwig and Jahnke 2017), because accumulation can lead to eventual renal failure.

Cd binds to metallothionein (via the blood), undergoes glomerular filtration and reabsorption in the proximal tubule, within which the Cd–metallothionein complex is degraded, resulting in the release of unbound Cd which stimulates metallothionein synthesis in the tubular cells (Dorian et al. 1992). Unbound Cd levels above 50–300 μ/g (wet weight) initiate tubular damage (ATSDR 2012a). The cellular uptake of Cd may be related to ionic mimicry of Zn (Goyer et al. 2004). Both Zn and Cd induce metallothionein-synthesizing genes through MTF-1 regulation (Alexander et al. 2009). There are seven Zn atoms shared between two clusters of the metallothionein monomer, and Cd can replace Zn in either of these clusters (Nordberg et al. 1971a; Foulkes 1978; Alexander et al. 2009), which consequently prevents free-radical scavenging activity (Ruttkay-Nedecky et al. 2013) of metallothionein, among other effects. Further proposed MoAs include the inactivation of metalloenzymes, activation of calmodulin, and ROS-induced cellular damage (ATSDR 2012a).

The secretion of low molecular weight proteins (e.g. β2-microglobulin, α1-microglobulin [pHC], and retinol-binding protein) are known proteinaceous biomarkers indicative of Cd-induced kidney damage in humans (Jarup 2003). Other indicative signs include the increased urinary concentration of the intercellular tubular enzyme N-acetyl-β-glycosaminidase (NAG), amino-acids, albumin, cysteine-rich (sulfur) metallothioneins, and increased excretion of Ca, sodium, and potassium (Nordberg et al. 1971b; Alexander et al. 2009; ATSDR 2012a). Cd–sulfhydryl complexes interfere with MAP kinases and Na^+-K^+-ATPase activity (Chunhabundit 2016). There is some evidence to suggest that diabetic (Type II) subgroups may be more sensitive to renal nephropathy associated with Cd toxicity (Buchet et al. 1990; Åkesson et al. 2005; Haswell-Elkins et al. 2008; Edwards and Prozialeck 2009), and may benefit from Zn supplementation (Anetor et al. 2016). Studies have also shown that Cd-induced hepatoxicity can occur in the general population at urinary Cd levels of 2–3 μg Cd/g creatinine (Buchet et al. 1990; Jarup et al. 2000; Jarup 2003).

12.4.3.1.2 Skeletal Abnormalities Cd-induced renal dysfunction is directly linked to adverse skeletal damage. Altered renal metabolism of Vitamin D, and the reduced assimilation of Ca and phosphate compounds, accelerates the onset of bone disease (Hossny et al. 2001; Jarup 2003; ATSDR 2012a). Itai-Itai disease is a Cd-induced illness prevalent in nutrient-deprived populations with a high consumption of Cd-contaminated rice and water (ATSDR 2012a). Factors such as multiple pregnancies and nutrient deficiencies (i.e. Ca, Vitamin D, Fe, Zn) as a result of inadequate diet, contribute to the etiology of this disease (ATSDR 2012a). The first reports of Itai-Itai disease were recorded in Japan from Cd-contaminated water intake. Recent studies have indicated that chronic Cd exposure causes skeletal abnormalities, as evidenced by bone demineralization and fractures (Staessen et al. 1999; Alfvén et al. 2000; Nordberg et al. 2002). Cd-induced hypercalciuria from renal tubular dysfunction indirectly decreases bone density (Chunhabundit 2016). Other bone-related effects include osteomalacia, osteoporosis, increased risk of fractures, and decreased bone densities (ATSDR 2012a). Proposed MoAs include signal transduction pathways (e.g. inositol polyphosphate formation), elevated cystolic Ca levels, and Ca channel disruption (Tchounwou et al. 2012).

12.4.3.2 Dietary Exposure

12.4.3.2.1 Occurrence, Prevalence, and Regulatory Limits in Plant-Based Foods Low levels of Cd are present in meat and marine organisms with the exception of certain shellfish and organ meats (e.g. kidney, liver) which accumulate Cd (IARC 2012). High levels of Cd have been observed in crustaceans, edible offal, fungi, oilseeds (e.g. sunflower), seaweed, water mollusks, algae-derived, and cocoa-based products (including bitter chocolate) and identified (EFSA 2012a). It is important to note that it may not be the food commodities with the highest Cd levels, but the foods which are more regularly consumed (intake frequency) in large quantities, which pose the greatest risk of Cd exposure over time (EFSA 2012a). By analyzing consumption data, the major food groups which contribute to dietary exposure were determined. A recent scientific report by the EFSA (2012a) listed the following food commodities as the principal dietary sources of Cd in adults: cereals/grains and associated products, potatoes and tubers, and vegetables. Major dietary sources for children and adolescents were similar, with the addition of confectionary as a primary source of dietary exposure. For children and infants, major food sources were the same as the adult population with the addition of dairy products and infant formulae (milk and soya). The EFSA concluded that dietary contribution to oral Cd exposure is spread out over a variety of different food groups (EFSA 2012a; European Commission 2014), which appears contrary to the recommendations of Gundert-Remy et al. (2015) for alternating patterns of food consumption as a strategy to reduce the risk of accumulative dietary exposure.

In a scientific opinion on Cd in food, mean dietary exposures to Cd for the general European population are between 2.5 and 4.8 μg/kg bw (adults), which are close to or slightly above the TWI of 2.5 μg/kg bw established by the EFSA (Alexander et al. 2009). In the report, mean dietary exposure to Cd for children and adults (smokers) currently exceeds the TWI. The CONTAM panel suggested a reduction in the exposure to Cd at the population level (Alexander et al. 2009).

Maximum levels of Cd for individual food groups were therefore established by the European Commission in Regulation (EC) No. 488/2014 ("Maximum levels of Cadmium in foodstuffs") (European Commission 2014), as modified in Table 12.4, as a step toward reducing exposure. The risk of adverse effects for the general population through dietary exposure is unlikely because the TWI is based on early biomarkers of toxicity; however, a reduction in Cd exposure at the population level is encouraged by the CONTAM panel (EFSA 2017b). A limit of 0.3 mg/L for Cd is permitted to transfer from ceramic FCMs or 0.1 mg/L from cooking utensils, packaging, or storage vessels ($\geq$ 3 l capacity), as outlined in the Directive 84/500/EEC (FSAI 2016). In contrast, JECFA established a Provisional Tolerable Monthly Intake (PTMI) of 25 μg/kg/bw/month (JECFA 2013), which is considerably higher than EFSA's acceptable limit.

Immobilized Cd uptake from contaminated soil and water can accumulate in plants and organisms, consequently entering the food supply (ATSDR 2012a). Cd concentration in soils is not the sole determinant of Cd uptake in plant roots, as Cd concentration in plant-derived foodstuffs is affected by the Cd species involved, the plant species itself (e.g. non- or hyper-accumulator), its Cd species involved, plant species-specific characteristics (e.g. non- or hyper-accumulator), cultivation environment, agrochemical usage (e.g. phosphate fertilizer application), and surrounding anthropogenic contamination levels (e.g. soil and water (IARC 2012)).

It has been suggested that because Cd accumulates predominantly in the liver and kidneys and is poorly absorbed in the intestines and muscles of vertebrates, that the risk of biomagnification may therefore be an insignificant risk to human health. Nevertheless, the ATSDR state that there is strong evidence to prove Cd

Table 12.4 Limits of Cd in a range of terrestrial plant-derived food commodities reported in Regulation (EC) No. 488/2014 (as amended) (European Commission 2014)

Food commodities	Permissible limit(s) of Cd (mg/kg[a])
Specific vegetables	
• Leafy vegetables (e.g. leafy *Brassica*)	0.20
• Celery (*Apium gaveolens*) and Celeriac (*A. gaveolens* var. *rapaceum*)	
• Parsnip *(Pastinaca sativa)*	
• Salsify (*Tragopogon porrifolius*)	
• Horseradish (*Armoracia rusticana*)	
• Fresh culinary herbs	
Root and tuber vegetables (excluding the above)	0.10
Vegetables and fruit (excluding all the above, stem vegetables and seaweed)	0.05
Cereal grains (excluding rice, wheat)	0.10
Wheat, rice, rice-bran, soy beans	0.20

[a] Wet weight.

bioaccumulation throughout the foodchain, which has important implications for human exposure (ATSDR 2012a).

12.4.4 Chromium (Cr)

12.4.4.1 Human Health Effects Cr is an abundant element of the Earth's crust which exists in multiple oxidation or valence states, with trivalent [Cr(III)] and hexavalent Cr [Cr(VI)] being the most biologically relevant in terms of human dietary exposure (Tchounwou et al. 2012). Industrial sources of Cr include metallurgy, electroplating (Jaishankar et al. 2014), wood preservation (Cu-dichromate), leather tanning (Cr-sulfate), textiles, and stainless steel production (ATSDR 2012b). Cr (III) is naturally present in many fresh foods, while Cr (VI) is considered a toxic environmental pollutant present in terrestrial-derived foods only as a consequence of anthropogenic contamination (CONTAM 2014).

The ATSDR ranks Cr (VI) as the seventeenth contaminant on its priority list of hazardous substances (ATSDR 2017). The IARC classifies Cr (VI) as a Group 1 carcinogen based on its ability to form respiratory-targeted cancers (IARC 1993; CONTAM 2014). Unlike Cr (III), a TDI for Cr (VI) could not be established based on its associated carcinogenicity. Cr (III) is postulated as an essential nutrient required for macromolecular metabolism and insulin efficiency (e.g. chromodulin) (Pechova and Pavlata 2007), although its essentiality as a dietary nutrient has been questioned based on a lack of appropriate evidence of any physiological function or symptoms of dietary deficiency (Stearns 2000; Di Bona et al. 2011; Vincent and Love 2012). Regardless, EFSA established a TDI of 0.3 mg/kg bw for Cr (III) to ensure consumer safety. Dietary exposure to Cr (III) in the general European population is well below the established TDI for all age groups, thus Cr (III) is of negligible concern for public health, according to EFSA experts (CONTAM 2014).

12.4.4.1.1 Cr Absorption and Metabolism Cr (VI) can enter cells via non-specific anion channels, whereas Cr (III) cannot (Witt et al. 2013; Sun et al. 2015). Cr (III) generally presents lower dietary toxicity compared to Cr (VI) (Jennette 1981; Goyer et al. 2004). In general, Cr has a low intestinal absorption rate – less than 10% of the ingested dose, which is largely dependent on its oxidation state and the presence of ligands (e.g. phytate, oxalate, amino acids) (CONTAM 2014). The onset of adverse effects depends on whether the ingested Cr (VI) is intra- or extra-cellularly reduced, the efficacy of which essentially determines the outcome of oral Cr-toxicity. The extracellular reduction of Cr (VI) to Cr (III) in saliva or gastric fluid in the stomach (Guertin 2004; Sun et al. 2015) reduces its bioavailability, and consequently its potential to confer toxicity, since the reduced Cr (III) cannot gain entry to the cell. Remaining water-insoluble chromate by-products are phagocytosed, while water-soluble chromates are taken up by sulfate channels based on their iso-structural similarity to phosphate and sulfate (Costa 1997). Both the entry of Cr (VI) into the cell and the location of cellular reduction is crucial when considering the likelihood of Cr toxicity via food. Recent evidence, however, suggests that while the biological effects of Cr (VI) oral exposure are alleviated upon extracellular gastrointestinal reduction, a percentage of the ingested Cr (VI) evades this detoxification and reaches target organs (Witt et al. 2013) of the hematological, hepatic, renal, and gastrointestinal systems. If ingested Cr (VI) enters the cell, it is intracellularly reduced by ascorbate, reduced glutathione GSH, and cysteine (Zhitkovich 2005, 2011; Sun et al. 2015) creating reactive intermediates which alter cellular function (O'Brien et al. 2003; De Mattia et al. 2004; Tchounwou et al. 2012). Studies have shown that intracellular Cr (III) may contribute to the genotoxicity of Cr (VI) (Zhitkovich 2005; Nickens et al. 2010; Sun et al. 2015). Uncertainty prevails regarding the rate, extent, and location of Cr (VI) metabolism, as the possibility cannot be excluded that a small percentage of ingested Cr (VI), even at low dosages, may penetrate cellular membranes and confer adverse biological effects (CONTAM 2014).

Intracellular Cr (III) binds to the Fe circulating protein apo-transferrin (Vincent and Love 2012). There is evidence, albeit contradictory, to suggest that Cr (III) may interfere with Fe absorption (Stearns 2000) caused by antagonistic competitive binding to apo-transferrin (Ani and Moshtaghie 1992; Bjørklund et al. 2017b). While the hematological effects of ingested Cr remains to be determined, caution should be exercised in patients presenting with hypoferremia and Fe-deficiency anemia on the possibility that trace-metal interactions could potentially affect Fe status (Bjørklund et al. 2017b).

12.4.4.2 Dietary Exposure

12.4.4.2.1 Occurrence, Prevalence, and Regulatory Limits in Plant-Based Foods The leading source of Cr exposure in the general population is from food and Cr-containing dietary supplements, followed by drinking water. Typical levels of Cr in food ranges from < 10–1300 μg/kg (ATSDR, 2012b). In a 2014 study published by the CONTAM panel, the food groups exhibiting the highest levels of detectable Cr were vegetables and fungi, vegetable/animal fats and oils, herbs, spices, condiments, and confectionary foods (CONTAM 2014). All analytical results in the above food samples were considered as Cr (III) and the panel concluded that the presence of Cr (VI) in foods is uncommon (CONTAM 2014). Estimated chronic dietary exposure levels ranged from 0.6–5.9 μg/kgbw/day. Toddlers displayed the highest chronic exposure levels out of all the age groups, averaging 2.3–5.9 μg/kg bw/day. The main contributors to elevated Cr (III) exposure were infant and follow-on formulae, milk and dairy products, and grain products. Food preparation may also contribute to the total Cr content in foods (CONTAM 2014). The transfer of Cr (III) from stainless steel via harvesting, processing, or cooking utensils to (acidic) foods has been documented in the literature (Offenbacher and Pi-Sunyer 1983; Anderson 1997; Kamerud et al. 2013).

Cr (VI) exists under oxidizing conditions as CrO_4^{2-} and $HCrO_4$, both of which are mobile within soil matrices (James et al. 1997). Cr (III), however, is the predominant species found in soils but has limited mobility, which explains the inefficient root-to-shoot translocation of Cr in plants. The bioaccumulation of Cr in the aerial plant parts, and subsequent biomagnification of Cr along the foodchain, is therefore unlikely (Langård 1982; Petruzzelli et al. 1987).

Maximum Levels (MLs) for Cr in foodstuffs have not been established (CONTAM 2014). The EFSA current opinion on Cr (VI) in food is that the hexavalent ion is of negligible concern to the general population – however, more speciation data is required on the Cr (III) and Cr (VI) content in food and drinking water across Member States and greater insight into the gastrointestinal detoxification of Cr (VI) at doses relevant for human exposure (CONTAM 2014).

12.4.5 Lead (Pb) and Mercury (Hg)

Lead (Pb) and mercury (Hg) are both significant environmental contaminants and are ranked second and third, respectively, on the ATSDR's priority list of hazardous substances. The exclusion of a discussion of Pb and Hg in this chapter, however, is based on their unlikeliness to exceed safe (oral) limits.

A recent Scientific Opinion published by EFSA (European Commission 2011) concluded that cereals/grains, leafy vegetables, and (peeled) potatoes were the main plant-derived contributors to dietary Pb exposure to the general European population. Maximum levels for Pb permitted in various terrestrial-derived foods range from 0.05–0.30 mg/kg wet weight, as per Commission Regulation (EU) 2015/1005 (Amending Regulation (EC) No 1881/2006) (European Commission 2015). The original PTWI of 25 μg/kg bw established by the JECFA was withdrawn based on evidence of developmental neurotoxicity (children), cardio, renal, and nephron toxicity (adults) associated with Pb exposure (EFSA CONTAM 2010). EFSA established a $BMLD_{01}$ and $BMDL_{10}$ of 1.5 and 0.6 μg/kg bw/day, respectively. The Margins of Exposure (MoE) calculated by the CONTAM panel suggested that the possibility of adverse effects from Pb cannot be excluded, particularly in young children (EFSA CONTAM 2010). As a result, a $BMDL_{01}$ of 50 μg/kg bw/day was developed to ensure the safety of young children. By implementing a lower $BMDL_{01}$, EFSA are safeguarding children against the risk of neurodevelopmental effects, which is a sequential protective measure for all other adverse effects in all other populations (EFSA CONTAM 2010). Nonetheless, EFSA also established a $BMLD_{01}$ (cardiovascular) and $BMDL_{10}$ (nephrotoxicity) of 1.50 and 0.63 μg/kg bw/day, respectively, for the adult population (EFSA CONTAM 2010). In Europe, mean dietary intake is within the range of the calculated benchmark dose and acute toxicity to Pb has been reported as being improbable (Hartwig and Jahnke 2017) – however, neurotoxicity (in fetuses, infants, and children) cannot be ruled out even at current exposures. Pb levels should be limited at all stages of life, but most importantly during pregnancy and early childhood (EFSA 2017b).

For Hg compounds, no maximum permissible concentrations have been set in terrestrial-derived foods since they typically contain low concentrations (ATSDR 1999; Francesconi 2007), supported by recent data indicating that the average dietary exposure is within the TWI of 1.6–4 μg/kg bw for Hg (and Hg compounds) across all age groups (EFSA 2012b). The current opinion adopted by EFSA concludes that the occurrence of Hg in foods, except for marine-soured organisms, are of negligible concern to the European population.

12.5 Metals in Phytopharmaceuticals and Associated Regulation

12.5.1 Phytopharmaceuticals

Phytopharmaceuticals is a collective term for botanical drugs, herbal drugs, or herbal medicines intended for human use. Official definitions of phytopharmaceutical products include (EMA 2010):

- Herbal substance: all whole, fragmented, or cut starting material in an unprocessed (fresh or dried) form (e.g. leaf, root, berry). Defined by the binomial system (genus, species, variety and author) and plant part used.
- Herbal preparation: obtained by subjecting herbal substances to treatments such as solvent extraction, purification, expression, concentration, distillation, or fermentation (e.g. comminuted/powdered material, extracts, essential oils).
- Herbal Medicinal Product (HMP) (finished herbal drug): any medicinal product, exclusively containing as active agents, one or more herbal substance(s), or herbal preparation(s) individually or in combination.

12.5.2 Current European Regulatory Guidelines: The Herbal Directive Scheme

To achieve regulatory approval in the EU, all drugs must be authorized before reaching the market to protect public health and ensure the availability of safe, high-quality, and effective medicines (EMA 2016b). The EU regulatory system for human medicines is collaboratively governed by the European Commission (EC), European member states, and the European Medicines Agency (EMA) who control and monitor both the initial market authorization and post-authorization of human medicines, including phytopharmaceuticals, for sale in European member states. Harmonization is achieved by implementing and enforcing the same set of rules and regulations.

In the European system, phytopharmaceuticals can be marketed upon successful authorization from one of the following application routes: full-, well-established-use, or traditional-use-application (Poveda 2015). General quality requirements are universal regardless of the application route with the exception of metal or elemental impurities (EMA 2016a,b) and (pre)-clinical efficacy data requirements, which differ in the dossier depending on the application route. The pre-clinical, or non-clinical, stages refer to laboratory-based *in vitro* and *in vivo* studies, including compound screening, pharmacological (pharmacodynamic and pharmacokinetic), and toxicity data. The clinical development stages refer to human studies or trials intended to prove the safety of the drug in humans (Hughes et al. 2011b).

Products outside of the well-established or traditional-use categories must comply with all relevant quality, safety, and efficacy criteria that are required for any drug product. For traditional products, a simplified registration process has been adopted by the European Committee since 2004, known as the Herbal Directive (Directive 2004/24/EC) (European Commission 2017b). This scheme was established to overcome issues encountered in the application of pharmaceutical legislation to THMPD, by providing a simplified regulatory approval process for the authorization of THMPD to the EU market (European Commission 2017b). Prior to this, no formal authorization process existed in the EU and consequently products were regulated at a national level which introduced disharmony in the market.

The Committee for Herbal Medicinal Products (HMPCs) was established by the EMA in accordance with the Herbal Directive and Regulation (EC) 726/2004 to support harmonization within the European market, thereby replacing the former Committee for Proprietary Medicinal Products' (CPMP) working party on HMPs. By evaluating available scientific data, the HMPC is responsible for preparing the EMA's scientific opinions on herbal substances, preparations, and combinations thereof, with the intention of establishing official (EU) herbal (formerly community) monographs and a comprehensive (EU) list of herbal substances with a long tradition of recommended and safe usage (EMA 2017b).

The Herbal Directive is aimed at HMP that have either a long tradition of use or have a well-established record of use. In simple terms, the entry of HMP deficient of published scientific evidence, tests for safety and efficacy, and pre-clinical and clinical trial data is permitted based on sufficient (ethno)pharmacological evidence of medicinal use throughout a period of ≥ 30 years, including ≥ 15 years in the European Community, i.e. a product which is generally considered safe under normal conditions of use and without medical supervision (European Commission 2017b). As per Article 16(a), there are several conditions which must be met for a product to be granted authorization. The medicinal indication of use must not require medical intervention (i.e. non-prescription only); only oral, dermal, and/or inhalation route of administration are permitted; the posology and strength must be specified and derived from traditional documents (e.g. monographs); and the safety/efficacy must be justified based on long-term use in Europe.

This scheme therefore justifies less stringent regulation of THMPD (Mosihuzzaman and Choudhary 2008), in comparison to conventional pharmaceuticals, by permitting an exemption of pharmacological, toxicological, and clinical data (Qu et al. 2014), following careful assessment of the quality and credibility of the ethnopharmacological or bibliographic evidence provided. Monographs established by The European Scientific Cooperative on Phytotherapy (ESCOP), WHO, and the German Commission E are used as a source of bibliographic evidence on various medicinal plants (Verma 2016). For HMP that fall outside the category of THMPD, like any other pharmaceutical drug, must acquire market authorisation or registration from a Competent Authority as a pre-requisite for entry to the EU market.

12.5.2.1 Non-European Traditional Products (e.g. Chinese, Ayurvedic) The Herbal Directive has been a vital initiative to protect public health against unauthorized phytopharmaceuticals by clarifying the status of THMPD. By harmonizing registration rules and regulations, the directive has consequently eased the importation and exportation of such products within member states (European Commission 2017b). While the scheme has demonstrated success, challenges regarding the registration of non-European THMPD, e.g. Chinese or Ayurvedic traditions, has received some criticism particularly among the alternative and complementary therapy communities (Qu et al. 2014). A strict requirement of the directive is to provide evidence of safe medicinal use over a minimum 15-year period in the EU as per Article 16a (1d and 1e). The absence of this ultimately impedes the successful registration of a non-European THMPD. Current export data for the sale of traditional Chinese HMPs to the EU suggest that unauthorized non-European THMPD remain on the EU market without appropriate legal compliance, which is a potential concern for the public who have access to these unauthorized products (Qu et al. 2014). Caution is expressed concerning the procurement of unlicensed or unregulated products online. Consumers are encouraged to familiarize themselves with the official list of approved online vendors monitored by the EMA (EMA 2017a).

The (EC) Rapid Alert System for Food and Feed (RASFF) database collates relevant information for every notification of non-conformance throughout Europe (Leuschner et al. 2013). As an example, Table 12.5 lists all 17 documented notifications of heavy metal contaminants present in herbs and spices between 1994 and 2019, which includes cases of As, Cd, Pb, Hg, and Pb-oxide contamination. The following criteria were searched on the RASFF Database on 03/05/2019 (Product category = herbs and spices; Hazard Category = Heavy Metals).

12.5.3 Current Quality Criteria for Metal Impurities

Included in the quality criteria for pharmaceuticals is the control of inorganic elemental impurities in both the starting materials and the finished product. All manufactured pharmaceuticals can become contaminated with metals throughout the process in numerous ways. Potential origins of contamination include the raw materials, air-borne particulates, metal reagents, or metal catalysts used during synthesis, excipients, or from vessels, equipment, or probes (Wang et al. 2000). Monitoring of both the finished product and process intermediates is therefore necessary to ensure the manufacture of quality medicinal products (Wang et al. 2000; EMA 2011; Balaram 2016). Compendial texts, such as the European Pharmacopoeia (Ph. Eur.), detail legally binding quality standards which include specifications, general texts, and general methods.

In the latest edition (Ph. Eur., 9th Edition), individual monographs no longer specify heavy metal tests; instead, implementation of International Conference of Harmonisation (ICH) principles is now enforced. Advantages and challenges of these newly addressed changes are reviewed elsewhere (Balaram 2016; Pohl et al. 2017). General methods for quality and control of impurities that have been recently revised in the European Pharmacopoeia (Ph. Eur., 9th Edition) include chapter 2.4.20: Detection of metal impurities (formerly "Detection of metal catalysts or metal reagent residues"), and chapter 5.20: Elemental impurities (formerly "Metal catalysts or metal reagent residues") which replaces the EMA Guideline on

Table 12.5 Record of cross-border "herbs and spices" product refusals in Europe identified as potentially hazardous to consumers (1994–2019)

Plant material	Heavy metal(s) identified and Concentration (mg/kg)	Country of origin	Notifying country	Date of case
Burdock root	Pb (11)	Bulgaria	France	15/09/2017
Organic turmeric	Pb (58)	India	U.K.	02/05/2017
Garcinia powder	Pb (2.4)	Sri Lanka	Finland	05/07/2016
Dried nettle	Pb (9.9)	Germany	Finland	31/01/2014
Raw ground nutmeg	Hg (0.21)	Indonesia via Italy	Greece	24/03/2011
Szechuan flower pepper	As (10.2); Cd (0.35); Pb (76.8)	Singapore	U.K.	21/01/2011
Arthemisia absinthium	Cd (0.113); Pb (0.6)	Serbia	Italy	02/10/2007
Ginseng root	Pb (0.208 and 0.334)	China	Italy	19/09/2007
Peppers	Pb (1.3)	Turkey	U.K.	04/06/2007
Table salt	Pb (0.42; 0.59)	Netherlands	Belgium	30/06/2006
Spirulina platensis	Cd (24)	China	Germany	14/06/2005
Garlic powder	Pb (2.926)	China via the U.K.	Belgium	18/03/2005
Meat and vegetable masala mix	Pb (62; 38)	Bangladesh	U.K.	11/05/2004
Salt	Cu (0.3)	Malta	Italy	18/10/2002
Herbal products	Unspecified	Unspecified	Italy	24/09/1998
(unspecified)	Unspecified	Unspecified	Italy	11/05/1998
Paprika	Pb-oxide (Unspecified concentration)	Unspecified	Germany	03/10/1994

specification limits for residues of metal catalyst and metal reagents (EMA 2008) with the principles of the harmonized guideline: ICH Q3D for elemental impurities (ICH 2014; EMA 2016a). The current guideline adopted by the EMA ICH Q3D: elemental impurities is legally enforceable from December 2017 onwards for both new marketing authorization applicants and authorized medicinal products. This document details the assessment and control of elemental impurities in drugs using the ICH principles of risk management (ICH Q9). The document, however, does not apply to herbal products. The ICH commented that herbal products are commonly subject to region-specific regulations rather than harmonized guidance. The ICH state that the application of the Q3D to herbal products will likely be addressed by regional regulatory authorities in the future (ICH 2016).

12.5.3.1 Starting Materials (Herbal Substances) Considering the ability of many plant species to (hyper)accumulate metals within their tissue, either directly from the soil or rhizosphere, air, or water, it seems logical to enforce environmental monitoring specifications for plant cultivators. The metal content of plant material is therefore directly influenced by the environment in which they are cultivated. Geographical location, soil profile, cultivation methods, and harvesting and post-harvesting conditions not only affect the metabolite profile (active constituent(s)) between batches but also the purity of the resulting intermediate or final product (Wah et al. 2012). The first step in reducing public risk and eliminating the possibilities of human exposure to medicinal plants (and products thereof) containing harmful metal impurities is the quality control of the starting material. This is not a straightforward task and requires agricultural and environmental monitoring (WHO 2007b).

Consequently, the WHO originally established the following technical documents: GACP guidelines for medicinal plants (WHO 2003), Assessing the quality of plant materials with reference to contaminants and residues (WHO 2007b), and Quality control methods for medicinal plant materials (WHO 1998), among others. The WHO states that the GACP should be implemented only as guidelines in national and/or regional quality control of herbal medicines (WHO 2007b). Unfortunately, GACP is therefore not currently enforceable by law, it is simply an optional checklist (Verma 2016). Both GACP and GMP compliance is critical for the manufacture of high-quality medicinal plant products, from cultivation to the final product (WHO 2007b; Heinrich 2015).

There are no universal limits for metal impurities in medicinal plants or products thereof. Acceptance criteria differ based on both the matrix (e.g. soil, water, starting materials, finished products) in question and the regulations implemented at a regional and/or national level (see Table 12.6). Countries including Canada, China, Australia and New Zealand, India, Malaysia, Singapore, and Thailand, all implement their own national limits to ensure safety and quality of medicinal plants (WHO 2007c; Sahoo et al. 2010; Tripathy et al. 2015). The legal diversity between national laws jeopardizes the harmonization of the quality of medicinal plants and products thereof (Govindaraghavan and Sucher 2015) and could ultimately threaten the international trade of high-value plants. Unifying regulatory requirements will result in the production of globally acceptable, safe products for human consumption (Sharma 2015). This, however, is a complex task and it should be noted that uniformity may never be achieved.

Table 12.6 Various national permissible limits for As, Cd, Pd and Hg in medicinal plants (Tripathy et al. 2015)

Location	As (mg/kg)	Cd (mg/kg)	Pb (mg/kg)	Hg (mg/kg)
WHO	10.0	0.30	10.0	1.00
FDA	10.0	0.30	10.0	1.00
Ph. Eur.	—	1.00	5.00	0.10
Singapore (HAS*)	5.00	0.05	20.0	0.50
Ph. China	2.00	0.30	5.00	0.50
India (AYUSH†)	10.0	0.30	1.00	1.00
Canada	5.00	0.30	10.0	0.20
Malaysia (FoSIM)‡	5.00	—	10.0	0.50
Thailand	4.00	0.30	10.0	—

**Health Sciences Authority (HAS)*; †Ministry of Ayurveda, Yoga and Naturopathy, Unani, Siddha and Homeopathy (AYUSH); ‡Food Safety Information System of Malaysia (FoSIM).

12.5.3.2 Extracts (Herbal Preparations) and HMPs (Finished Products) Current European guidelines for metal impurities in herbal products are outlined in Heavy metals in herbal drugs and fatty oils (8th Edition; chapter 2.4.27), which describes recommended tests. Included are general maximum limits in herbal products for Cd, Hg, and Pb at 1.0, 0.1, and 5 ppm, respectively (Bouin and Wierer 2014). Limited exceptions include willow bark, tormentil, fumitory, kelp, and linseed oil. Recommended maximum or permissible limits are clearly deficient from compendial texts. Further to this, legislation differs between countries outside of the EU. An extended suite of limits for a greater number of toxicologically significant elements in herbal products is therefore desirable. Additionally, as per EMA guidelines, the testing of HMPs for metal impurities is not required if metal impurity levels of the herbal substance(s) and/or preparation(s) used to prepare HMP are satisfactory (EMA 2011). This consequently excludes the possibility that extracts or HMPs may become contaminated with metal residues throughout the various stages of processing and/or packaging.

12.5.4 Key Issues

12.5.4.1 Product Classification or Categorization The classification of a health product ultimately determines the route of entry for that product to the European market, and thus the quality requirements. Health products that are plant-derived can essentially be marketed as either herbal medicines, food supplements, functional foods, or novel ingredients in different regions (Chan et al. 2009), as exemplified by *Ginkgo biloba* L. Ginkgo is registered as a food supplement or traditional medicine in the UK, as a dietary supplement in the US, as a medicine in Germany, and as a listed medicine in Australia (Heinrich 2015). The herbal medication market is more stringently monitored than food supplements, which may encourage enterprises to seek food supplementation status for plant-derived products over herbal registration (Wah et al. 2012). Both the EFSA and EMA clearly state that it is not their role to determine the classification of a botanical as either a medicine or food supplement (EFSA 2017a). Without clear requirements for product classification, however, difficulty in distinguishing between a dietary supplement versus a medicinal product of plant origin exists (Wah et al. 2012; Ekor 2014). Product categorization is primarily dependent on the product's claims, whether health-related or otherwise. Products devoid of any claim to prevent disease or ailment can be regulated as a food (including spices) or dietary supplement (Wah et al. 2012).

12.5.4.2 Non-universal Metal Impurity Limits Food and pharmaceutical safety standards within the EU are stringently controlled, thanks to the suite of EU legislation implemented. Quality, however, remains a key concern with respect to plant material outside the EU (Mukherjee et al. 2015). Our analysis of data collected from the RASFF database, concluded that the China, India, and the US were the top three countries from which repeated cases of metal contamination of plant products originated between 1994 and European Commission, 2019. This highlights the issue of quality-related problems inherent throughout the supply chain, resulting in plant material and plant-derived products which do not meet the quality standards of similar commodities produced under EU legislation (Mukherjee et al. 2015). Over time this non-uniformity may result in trading constraints between countries.

Recommendations for the implementation of an international monitoring body for the surveillance of contamination (e.g. biological, chemical, or metal) have been previously proposed (Tripathy et al. 2015); however, the cost-effectiveness of such a program is questionable. Furthermore, some authors have expressed concern that legally imposing more stringent regulations in developing countries may not be feasible due to insufficient resources or expertise in the area (Wah et al. 2012).

As stated in the WHO Guidelines for Assessing Quality of Herbal Medicines (with reference to contaminants and residues), it would be "desirable to harmonize limits for toxic metals and standards, as this would have many benefits including the facilitation of global trade." To initiate change, the establishment of universal acceptance criteria and universal analytical detection methods for elemental impurities in phytopharmaceuticals needs to be agreed upon and legally enforced. The expansion of international trade further emphasizes the necessity of global standards for human medicines (Rose 2016).

12.5.4.3 Non-enforceable GACP Guidelines Manufacturing facilities are legally obliged to conform to GMP for the authorized manufacture of medicinal plant products. GACP guidelines, however, are non-enforceable by law for cultivators/farmers supplying manufacturers (Wah et al. 2012). At a minimum, mandatory plant cultivation criterion, such as selection of non-hazardous soil profiles and use of irrigation water free from or within the acceptable limits of toxic heavy metals, needs to be enforced along with GACP guidelines.

12.5.4.4 Non-regulated Wildcrafting Practices The gathering of botanicals from the wild (i.e. wildcrafting), without either the implementation of GACP guidelines or onsite expertise in botanical taxonomy, immediately compromises plant quality in terms of correct species authentication and traceability (Govindaraghavan and Sucher 2015). Evidence suggests that wild-collected plant material is more likely to contain higher levels of contaminants than their selectively cultivated counterparts (Harris et al. 2011). For example, organic powdered turmeric (root) sourced from India reached the UK where it was found to contain 58 mg/kg Pb (European Commission 2019), which is five times the recommended limit as per WHO guidelines (see Table 12.5).

In India alone, 90% of plant materials and their derivatives are collected from the wild (Mukherjee et al. 2015), i.e. non-regulated environments. Additionally, wildcrafting in India by untrained personnel has consequently endangered 20–25% of existing plant species due to over-collection of economically and medicinally valuable plant material biomass (Laloo et al. 2006; Mosihuzzaman and Choudhary 2008). Ethical sourcing of plants and maintenance of biodiversity is regulated by the Convention on International Trade in Endangered Species of Wild Fauna (CITES) (Mosihuzzaman and Choudhary 2008). CITES also provides details on prohibited or restricted botanicals and information concerning necessary export/import permits (Mosihuzzaman and Choudhary 2008). Enforcing responsible farming will have a positive outcome on the quality of raw starting materials before reaching the manufacturing and processing stages of production, while also safeguarding plant biodiversity.

12.6 Metal Contaminants in Supplements: An Overview

As with any healthcare product, the degree of regulatory control imposed depends on how the product is originally classified, which is based on any direct product health claims (Wah et al. 2012). In the US, herbal products are generally marketed as food supplements, and specific health claims must be authorized by the FDA (Verma 2016). In Europe, the quality requirements for food supplements are based on food legislation, which is less stringent than medicinal or pharmaceutical legislation in terms of composition and quality requirements (Heinrich 2015). Marketing claims on botanical ingredients in food supplements are not yet harmonized under EU law. Consequently, the regulation of therapeutic claims is monitored at a national level which, similarly to the lack of uniform acceptable metal levels in products, leads to under- and over-regulation between countries. BELFRIT, a draft decree, has been developed through joint efforts from Belgium, France, and Italy to provide a harmonized list of ($\geq$1000) established botanicals approved for use in food supplements. The use of health-maintaining (i.e. non-therapeutic) claims on food supplement labels or packaging requires authorization by the European Commission through EFSA, provided satisfactory data is presented to substantiate said claim(s) (Miroddi et al. 2013). The EC and EFSA have not yet established maximum limits of elemental impurities in dietary supplements, fortified foods, novel foods, or food ingredients – which highlights a gap in legislation.

Additionally, the EC has not yet established a universal authorization process for the use of botanicals or derived preparations (i.e. plants, algae, fungi or lichens) in dietary (food) supplements, such as St. John's Wort, ginseng, ginkgo, garlic, or echinacea (EFSA 2017a). EFSA provides science-based safety criteria to organizations involved in the safety assessment of botanical ingredients to establish the safe usage of botanicals or derived preparations used in dietary (food) supplements. EFSA published a "toolkit" for risk assessors and food manufacturers which provides guidance documents, reports, and a "Compendium of botanicals" database. Nevertheless, dietary food supplements containing botanical ingredients must comply with European food supplement legislation (Directive 2002/46/EC) and general European Food Law (Regulation (EC) No 178/2002). The use, safety, and permitted health claims of botanical ingredients in dietary supplements is currently under review by EFSA (EFSA 2017a).

12.7 Conclusion

Metals can enter plant tissue from the environment. Plants are consecutively consumed as dietary foodstuffs and/or phytopharmaceuticals containing plants as active ingredients. Because the levels of metals within these foods or medicinal products are not routinely analyzed, it is difficult to know if we are subjecting ourselves to any form of acute or chronic metal exposure – symptomatic or asymptomatic. Diet has been shown to be a risk factor for human exposure to heavy metals, whether as a single dose or through accumulation. Above safe threshold concentrations, metals can cause a range of deleterious adverse effects in humans. Stringent regulatory controls are currently in place in European member states to safeguard the general population against exposure to hazardous heavy metals in food. While regulatory measures are enforced, there are apparent pitfalls, since current dietary exposure data published by scientific expert groups at the EFSA acknowledge that the risks of adverse health effects from certain metals in food cannot be excluded. The authors suggest that maximum limits for frequently consumed foodstuffs should be established where possible to safeguard public health. Furthermore, advocating alternate patterns of food consumption by introducing variety and implementing safe kitchen preparation techniques are recommended to reduce metal load in food. Regarding phytopharmaceuticals, the adapted ICH Q3D guidelines published by the EMA define limits for a total of 24 elements; however, these limits are not currently applicable to phytopharmaceuticals. In contrast, compendial (Ph. Eur.) limits for herbal products exist for only Cd, Hg, and Pb. Two possible solutions to consider include extending the application of ICH Q3D guidelines to phytopharmaceuticals or, alternatively, establishing a defined set of general permissible elemental limits for a greater suite of toxicologically significant metals applicable to herbal products. Harmonization of quality requirements for these products is a necessity, particularly in the context of international trade and to reduce human exposure to potentially dangerous impurities.

Declaration of Interest

The authors declare that there is no conflict of interest in this work.

Funding and Acknowledgments

CRK is in receipt of a RISAM postgraduate scholarship (2015) from the Cork Institute of Technology. The author also acknowledges the funding of a High-Resolution Sector-Field Inductively Coupled Plasma Mass Spectrometer (HR-ICP-SFMS) under the Science Foundation Ireland (SFI) Research Infrastructure Call 2012 [Proposal #12/RI/2335 (2)].

References

Abdul, Q.A., Choi, R.J., Jung, H.A., and Choi, J.S. (2016). Health benefit of fucosterol from marine algae: a review. *Journal of the Science of Food and Agriculture* https://doi.org/10.1002/jsfa.7489.

Agency for Toxic Substances and Disease Registry (ATSDR) (2008). *Toxicological Profile for Aluminum*. Atlanta, GA: U.S. Department of Health and Human Services, Public Health Service Retrieved July 11, 2017, from https://www.atsdr.cdc.gov/toxfaqs/tf.asp?id=190&tid=34.

Ahmad, S., Kitchin, K.T., and Cullen, W.R. (2000). Arsenic species that cause release of iron from ferritin and generation of activated oxygen. *Archives of Biochemistry and Biophysics* **382** (2): 195–202. https://doi.org/10.1006/abbi.2000.2023.

Åkesson, A., Lundh, T., Vahter, M. et al. (2005). Tubular and glomerular kidney effects in Swedish women with low environmental cadmium exposure. *Environmental Health Perspectives* **113** (11): 1627–1631. https://doi.org/10.1289/ehp.8033.

Alexander, J., Benford, D., Cockburn, A. et al. (2009). Cadmium in food: scientific opinion of the panel on contaminants in the food chain. *EFSA Journal* **980**: 1–139.

Alford, É.R., Pilon-Smits, E.A.H., and Paschke, M.W. (2010). Metallophytes-a view from the rhizosphere. *Plant and Soil* **337** (1): 33–50. https://doi.org/10.1007/s11104-010-0482-3.

Alfvén, T., Elinder, C.G., Carlsson, M.D. et al. (2000). Low-level cadmium exposure and osteoporosis. *Journal of Bone and Mineral Research* **15** (8): 1579–1586. https://doi.org/10.1359/jbmr.2000.15.8.1579.

Álvarez-Ayuso, E., García-Sánchez, A., and Querol, X. (2003). Purification of metal electroplating waste waters using zeolites. *Water Research* **37** (20): 4855–4862. https://doi.org/10.1016/j.watres.2003.08.009.

Alvarez-Fernández, A., Díaz-Benito, P., Abadía, A. et al. (2014). Metal species involved in long distance metal transport in plants. *Frontiers in Plant Science* **5** (105) https://doi.org/10.3389/fpls.2014.00105.

Anderson, R.A. (1997). Chromium as an essential nutrient for humans. *Regulatory Toxicology and Pharmacology* **26** (1): S35–S41. https://doi.org/10.1006/rtph.1997.1136.

Anetor, J.I., Uche, C.Z., Ayita, E.B. et al. (2016). Cadmium level, glycemic control, and indices of renal function in treated type II diabetics: implications for polluted environments. *Frontiers in Public Health* **4** (114) https://doi.org/10.3389/fpubh.2016.00114.

Ani, M. and Moshtaghie, A. (1992). The effect of chromium on parameters related to iron metabolism. *Biological Trace Element Research* **32**: 57–64.

Aposhian, H.V. (1997). Enzymatic methylation of arsenic species and other new approaches to arsenic toxicity. *Annual Review of Pharmacology and Toxicology* **37**: 397–419. https://doi.org/10.1146/annurev.pharmtox.37.1.397.

Assunção, A.G.L., Persson, D.P., Husted, S. et al. (2013). Model of how plants sense zinc deficiency. *Metallomics: Integrated Biometal Science* **5** (9): 1110–1116. https://doi.org/10.1039/c3mt00070b.

Atkinson, J.A., Rasmussen, A., Traini, R. et al. (2014). Branching out in roots: uncovering form, function, and regulation. *Plant Physiology* **166** (2): 538–550. https://doi.org/10.1104/pp.114.245423.

ATSDR. (1999). Toxicological profile: mercury. Available at: https://www.atsdr.cdc.gov/toxprofiles/tp.asp?id=115&tid=24 (accessed 27 January 2017).

ATSDR. (2007a). Toxicological profile: arsenic. Available at: https://www.atsdr.cdc.gov/toxprofiles/tp.asp?id=22&tid=3 (accessed 27 January 2017).

ATSDR. (2007b). Toxicological profile: lead. Available at: https://www.atsdr.cdc.gov/toxprofiles/tp.asp?id=96&tid=22 (accessed 27 January 2017).

ATSDR. (2012a). Toxicological profile: cadmium. Available at: https://www.atsdr.cdc.gov/toxprofiles/tp.asp?id=48&tid=15 (accessed 27 January 2017).

ATSDR. (2012b). Toxicological profile: chromium. Available at: https://www.atsdr.cdc.gov/toxprofiles/tp.asp?id=62&tid=17 (accessed 27 January 2017).

ATSDR. (2017). Priority list of hazardous substances: ATSDR. Available at: https://www.atsdr.cdc.gov/spl/index.html (accessed 20 July 2017).

Azwanida, N.N. (2015). A review on the extraction methods use in medicinal plants, principle, strength and limitation. *Medicinal & Aromatic Plants* **4** (196) https://doi.org/10.4172/2167-0412.1000196.

Baker, A., McGrath, S., Reeves, R., and Smith, J. (2000). Metal hyperaccumulator plants: a review of the ecology and physiology of a biological resource for phytoremediation of metal-polluted soils. In: *Phytoremediation of Contaminated Soil and Waters* (eds. N. Terry and G.S. Banuelos), 85–107. Danvers, MA: CRC https://doi.org/10.1.1.467.809.

Balaram, V. (2016). Recent advances in the determination of elemental impurities in pharmaceuticals – status, challenges and moving frontiers. *TrAC Trends in Analytical Chemistry* **80**: 83–95. https://doi.org/10.1016/J.TRAC.2016.02.001.

Baxter, I. (2009). Ionomics: studying the social network of mineral nutrients. *Current Opinion in Plant Biology* **12** (3): 381–386. https://doi.org/10.1016/j.pbi.2009.05.002.

Beek, B. (1999). Bioaccumulation New Aspects and Developments. In: . Berlin, Hiedelberg: Springer.

Bentley, R. and Chasteen, T.G. (2002). Microbial methylation of metalloids: arsenic, antimony, and bismuth. *Microbiology and Molecular Biology Reviews* **66** (2): 250–271. https://doi.org/10.1128/mmbr.66.2.250-271.2002.

Bhandari, G. (2014). An overview of agrochemicals and their effects on environment in Nepal. *Applied Ecology and Environmental Sciences* **2** (2): 66–73. https://doi.org/10.12691/aees-2-2-5.

Birbaum, K., Brogioli, R., Schellenberg, M. et al. (2010). No evidence for cerium dioxide nanoparticle translocation in maize plants. *Environmental Science and Technology* **44** (22): 8718–8723. https://doi.org/10.1021/es101685f.

Bjørklund, G., Aaseth, J., Chirumbolo, S. et al. (2017a). Effects of arsenic toxicity beyond epigenetic modifications. *Environmental Geochemistry and Health* https://doi.org/10.1007/s10653-017-9967-9.

Bjørklund, G., Aaseth, J., Skalny, A.V. et al. (2017b). Interactions of iron with manganese, zinc, chromium, and selenium as related to prophylaxis and treatment of iron deficiency. *Journal of Trace Elements in Medicine and Biology* **41**: 41–53. https://doi.org/10.1016/j.jtemb.2017.02.005.

Borak, J. and Hosgood, H.D. (2007). Seafood arsenic: implications for human risk assessment. *Regulatory Toxicology and Pharmacology* **47** (2): 204–212. https://doi.org/10.1016/j.yrtph.2006.09.005.

Bouin, A.-S. and Wierer, M. (2014). Quality standards of the European Pharmacopoeia. *Journal of Ethnopharmacology* **158**: 454–457. https://doi.org/10.1016/J.JEP.2014.07.020.

Bridges, C. and Zalups, R. (2005). Molecular and ionic mimicry and the transport of toxic metals. *Toxicology and Applied Pharmacology* **204** (3): 274–308.

Bruna, B., Francisco, A., Brum, D.M., and Cassella, R.J. (2015). Determination of metals in soft drinks packed in different materials by ETAAS. *Food Chemistry* **185**: 488–494. https://doi.org/10.1016/j.foodchem.2015.04.020.

Buchet, J.P., Lauwerys, R., Roels, H. et al. (1990). Renal effects of cadmium body burden of the general population. *Lancet* **336** (8717): 699–702. https://doi.org/10.1016/0140-6736(90)92201-R.

Cardoso, S.M., Pereira, O.R., Seca, A.M.L. et al. (2015). Seaweeds as preventive agents for cardiovascular diseases: from nutrients to functional foods. *Marine Drugs* **13** (11): 6838–6865. https://doi.org/10.3390/md13116838.

Carey, M., Jiujin, X., Gomes Farias, J., and Meharg, A.A. (2015). Rethinking rice preparation for highly efficient removal of inorganic arsenic using percolating cooking water. *PLoS One* **10** (7): e0131608. https://doi.org/10.1371/journal.pone.0131608.

Carter, M.R. (2008). Soil sampling and methods of analysis. *Experimental Agriculture* **44** (03): 823. https://doi.org/10.1017/S0014479708006546.

Castelblanque, J. and Salimbeni, F. (2004). NF and RO membranes for the recovery and reuse of water and concentrated metallic salts from waste water produced in the electroplating process. *Desalination* **167** (1–3): 65–73. https://doi.org/10.1016/j.desal.2004.06.114.

CDC. (2016). NBP Factsheet: mercury. Available at: https://www.cdc.gov/biomonitoring/Mercury_FactSheet.html (accessed 27 January 2017).

Chan, K. (2003). Some aspects of toxic contaminants in herbal medicines. *Chemosphere* **52** (9): 1361–1371. https://doi.org/10.1016/S0045-6535(03)00471-5.

Chan, K., Leung, K.S.-Y., and Zhao, S.S. (2009). Harmonization of monographic standards is needed to ensure the quality of Chinese medicinal materials. *Chinese Medicine* **4**: 18. https://doi.org/10.1186/1749-8546-4-18.

Cheng, S. (2003). Heavy metal pollution in China: origin, pattern and control. *Environmental Science and Pollution Research International* **10** (3): 192–198. https://doi.org/10.1065/espr2002.11.141.1.

Chou, W.-C., Jie, C., Kenedy, A.A. et al. (2004). Role of NADPH oxidase in arsenic-induced reactive oxygen species formation and cytotoxicity in myeloid leukemia cells. *Proceedings of the National Academy of Sciences of the United States of America* **101** (13): 4578–4583. https://doi.org/10.1073/pnas.0306687101.

Chung, C.J., Hsueh, Y.M., Bai, C.H. et al. (2009). Polymorphisms in arsenic metabolism genes, urinary arsenic methylation profile and cancer. *Cancer Causes and Control* **20** (9): 1653–1661. https://doi.org/10.1007/s10552-009-9413-0.

Chunhabundit, R. (2016). Cadmium exposure and potential health risk from foods in contaminated area, Thailand. *Toxicology Research* **32** (1): 65–72. https://doi.org/10.5487/TR.2016.32.1.065.

Clemens, S. (2001). Molecular mechanisms of plant metal tolerance and homeostasis. *Planta* **212** (4): 475–486. https://doi.org/10.1007/s004250000458.

Colangelo, E.P. and Guerinot, M.L. (2006). Put the metal to the petal: metal uptake and transport throughout plants. *Current Opinion in Plant Biology* **9** (3): 322–330. https://doi.org/10.1016/j.pbi.2006.03.015.

CONTAM (2014). Scientific opinion on the risks to public health related to the presence of chromium in food and drinking water. *EFSA Journal* **12** (3): 3595. https://doi.org/10.2903/j.efsa.2014.3595.

Costa, M. (1997). Toxicity and carcinogenicity of Cr(VI) in animal models and humans toxicity and carcinogenicity of Cr(VI) in animal models and humans. *Critical Reviews in Toxicology* **27** (275): 431–442. https://doi.org/10.3109/10408449709078442.

Crane, R.K. and Lipmann, F. (1953). The effect of arsenate on aerobic phosphorylation. *The Journal of Biological Chemistry* **201** (1): 235–243.

De Chaudhuri, S., Ghosh, P., Sarma, N. et al. (2008). Genetic variants associated with arsenic susceptibility: study of purine nucleoside phosphorylase, arsenic (+3) methyltransferase, and glutathione S-transferase omega genes. *Environmental Health Perspectives* **116** (4): 501–505. https://doi.org/10.1289/ehp.10581.

De Mattia, G., Bravi, M.C., Laurenti, O. et al. (2004). Impairment of cell and plasma redox state in subjects professionally exposed to chromium. *American Journal of Industrial Medicine* **46** (2): 120–125. https://doi.org/10.1002/ajim.20044.

Del Razo, L.M., Quintanilla-Vega, B., Brambila-Colombres, E. et al. (2001). Stress proteins induced by arsenic. *Toxicology and Applied Pharmacology* **177** (2): 132–148. https://doi.org/10.1006/taap.2001.9291.

Dghaim, R., Al Khatib, S., Rasool, H., and Khan, M.A. (2015). Determination of heavy metals concentration in traditional herbs commonly consumed in the United Arab Emirates. *Journal of Environmental and Public Health* **2015**: 1–6. https://doi.org/10.1155/2015/973878.

Di Bona, K.R., Love, S., Rhodes, N.R. et al. (2011). Chromium is not an essential trace element for mammals: effects of a "low-chromium" diet. *JBIC Journal of Biological Inorganic Chemistry* **16** (3): 381–390. https://doi.org/10.1007/s00775-010-0734-y.

Dixon, H.B.F. (1996). The biochemical action of arsonic acids especially as phosphate analogues. *Advances in Inorganic Chemistry* **44** (C): 191–227. https://doi.org/10.1016/S0898-8838(08)60131-2.

Dorian, C., Gattone, V.H., and Klaassen, C.D. (1992). Accumulation and degradation of the protein moiety of cadmium-metallothionein (CdMT) in the mouse kidney.

Toxicology and Applied Pharmacology **117** (2): 242–248. https://doi.org/10.1016/0041-008X(92)90243-L.
Dufault, R., Schnoll, R., Lukiw, W.J. et al. (2009). Mercury exposure, nutritional deficiencies and metabolic disruptions may affect learning in children. *Behavioral and Brain Functions* **5** (1): 44. https://doi.org/10.1186/1744-9081-5-44.
Dutta, S. and Podile, A.R. (2010). Plant growth promoting rhizobacteria (PGPR): the bugs to debug the root zone. *Critical Reviews in Microbiology* **36** (3): 232–244. https://doi.org/10.3109/10408411003766806.
Edwards, J.R. and Prozialeck, W.C. (2009). Cadmium, diabetes and chronic kidney disease. *Toxicology and Applied Pharmacology* **238** (3): 289–293. https://doi.org/10.1016/j.taap.2009.03.007.
EFSA (2008). Safety of aluminium from dietary intake – scientific opinion of the panel on food additives, flavourings, processing aids and food contact materials (AFC). *EFSA Journal* **6** (7): 754. https://doi.org/10.2903/j.efsa.2008.754.
EFSA (2011). Overview of the procedures currently used at EFSA for the assessment of dietary exposure to different chemical substances. *EFSA Journal* **9** (12): 2490. https://doi.org/10.2903/j.efsa.2011.2490.
EFSA (2012a). Cadmium dietary exposure in the European population. *EFSA Journal* **10** (1): 1–37. https://doi.org/10.2903/j.efsa.2012.2551.
EFSA (2012b). Compendium of botanicals reported to contain naturally occuring substances of possible concern for human health when used in food and food supplements. *EFSA Journal* **10** (5): 2663–2723. https://doi.org/10.2903/j.efsa.2012.2663.
EFSA (2014). Dietary exposure to inorganic arsenic in the European population. *EFSA Journal* **12** (3) https://doi.org/10.2903/j.efsa.2014.3597.
EFSA. (2017a). Botanicals: European Food Safety Authority. Available at: https://www.efsa.europa.eu/en/topics/topic/botanicals (accessed 6 May 2017).
EFSA. (2017b). Metals as contaminants in food: European Food Safety Authority. Available at: https://www.efsa.europa.eu/en/topics/topic/metals-contaminants-food (accessed 6 May 2017).
EFSA CONTAM (2010). Scientific opinion on lead in food. *EFSA Journal* **8** (4): 1570. https://doi.org/10.2903/j.efsa.2010.1570.
EFSA Panel on Contaminants in the Food Chain (CONTAM) (2009). Scientific opinion on arsenic in food. *EFSA Journal* **7** (10): 1351. https://doi.org/10.2903/j.efsa.2009.1351.
Eichert, T. and Fernández, V. (2012). *Marschner's Mineral Nutrition of Higher Plants*. Elsevier https://doi.org/10.1016/B978-0-12-384905-2.00004-2.
Eichert, T. and Goldbach, H.E. (2008). Equivalent pore radii of hydrophilic foliar uptake routes in stomatous and astomatous leaf surfaces – further evidence for a stomatal pathway. *Physiologia Plantarum* **132** (4): 491–502. https://doi.org/10.1111/j.1399-3054.2007.01023.x.
Ekor, M. (2014). The growing use of herbal medicines: issues relating to adverse reactions and challenges in monitoring safety. *Frontiers in Pharmacology* **4** (177) https://doi.org/10.3389/fphar.2013.00177.
EMA. (2008). Committee for Medicinal Products for Human Use (CHMP): Guideline of the specification limits for residues of metal catalysts or metal reagents (Vol. 21). London. Available at: http://www.emea.europa.eu (accessed 16 November 2017).
EMA. (2010). Guideline on declaration of herbal substances and herbal preparations in herbal medicinal products. London, U.K. Available at: http://www.ema.europa.eu/docs/en_GB/document_library/Scientific_guideline/2009/09/WC500003272.pdf (accessed 9 November 2017).
EMA. (2011). Guideline on specifications: test procedures and acceptance criteria for herbal substances, herbal preparations and herbal medicinal products/traditional

herbal medicinal products. London. Available at: http://www.ema.europa.eu/docs/en_GB/document_library/Scientific_guideline/2011/09/WC500113210.pdf (accessed 16 November 2017).

EMA. (2016a). ICH guideline Q3D on elemental impurities (Step 5). London. Available at: http://www.ema.europa.eu/docs/en_GB/document_library/Scientific_guideline/2015/01/WC500180284.pdf (accessed 16 November 2017).

EMA. (2016b). The European regulatory system for medicines: A consistent approach to medicines regulation across the European Union. London, UK. Available at: http://www.ema.europa.eu/docs/en_GB/document_library/Leaflet/2014/08/WC500171674.pdf (accessed 9 November 2017).

EMA. (2017a). Buying medicines online. Available at: http://www.ema.europa.eu/ema/index.jsp?curl=/pages/regulation/general/general_content_000630.jsp (accessed 16 November 2017).

EMA. (2017b). European Medicines Agency - Committees - Committee on Herbal Medicinal Products (HMPC). Available at: http://www.ema.europa.eu/ema/index.jsp?curl=pages/about_us/general/general_content_000264.jsp (accessed 31 May 2017).

Emamverdian, A., Ding, Y., Mokhberdoran, F., and Xie, Y. (2015). Heavy metal stress and some mechanisms of plant defense response. *The Scientific World Journal* **2015**: 7–9. https://doi.org/10.1155/2015/756120.

Eshel, A. and Beeckman, T. (2013). *Plant Roots: The Hidden Half*. CRC Press LLC.

European Commission (2011). EFSA Panel on Contaminants in the Food Chain (CONTAM); scientific opinion on tolerable weekly intake for cadmium. *EFSA Journal* **9** (2) https://doi.org/10.2903/j.efsa.2011.1975.

European Commission. (2014). Commission Regulation (EU) No 488/2014: Maximum levels of cadmium in foodstuffs. Available at: https://www.fsai.ie/uploadedFiles/Reg488_2014.pdf (accessed 10 August 2017).

European Commission. (2015). Commission Regulation (EU) 2015/1006: amending Regulation (EC) No 1881/2006 as regards maximum levels of inorganic arsenic in foodstuffs. Available at: http://eur-lex.europa.eu/legal-content/EN/TXT/?uri=CELEX:32015R1006 (accessed 18 July 2017).

European Commission. (2017a). Arsenic - European Commission. Available at: https://ec.europa.eu/food/safety/chemical_safety/contaminants/catalogue/arsenic_en (accessed 18 July 2017).

European Commission. (2017b). Herbal medicinal products - European Commission. Available at: https://ec.europa.eu/health/human-use/herbal-medicines_en (accessed 31 May 2017).

European Commission. (2019). RASFF Portal. Available at: https://webgate.ec.europa.eu/rasff-window/portal (accessed 16 November 2019).

Fan, X., Bai, L., Zhu, L. et al. (2014). Marine algae-derived bioactive peptides for human nutrition and health. *Journal of Agricultural and Food Chemistry* **62** (38): 9211–9222. https://doi.org/10.1021/jf502420h.

FedEx. (2009). NutraCea, FedEx and Feed The Children Team Up to Provide Food Aid to Families in Need in Brazil. Available at: http://about.van.fedex.com/newsroom/latin-america-english/nutracea-fedex-and-feed-the-children-team-up-to-provide-food-aid-to-families-in-need-in-brazil (accessed 18 July 2017).

Fernández, Y., Marañón, E., Castrillón, L., and Vázquez, I. (2005). Removal of cd and Zn from inorganic industrial waste leachate by ion exchange. *Journal of Hazardous Materials* **126** (1): 169–175. https://doi.org/10.1016/j.jhazmat.2005.06.016.

Flanagan, P.R., McLellan, J.S., Haist, J. et al. (1978). Increased dietary cadmium absorption in mice and human subjects with iron deficiency. *Gastroenterology* **74** (5 Pt 1): 841–846. https://doi.org/10.4319/lo.2013.58.2.0489.

Foulkes, E.C. (1978). Renal tubular transport of cadmium-metallothionein. *Toxicology and Applied Pharmacology* **45** (2): 505–512. https://doi.org/10.1016/0041-008X(78)90112-6.

Francesconi, K. (2007). Toxic metal species and food regulations–making a healthy choice. *The Analyst* **132** (1): 17–20. https://doi.org/10.1039/b610544k.

Franke, W. (2012). The entry of residues into plants via ectodesmata (ectocythodes). *Residue Reviews/Rückstands-Berichte* **38**: 81–115.

FSAI. (2016). Report of the Scientific Committee of the Food Safety Authority of Ireland: Metals of Toxicological Importance in the Irish Diet. Dublin.

Fujihara, J., Fujii, Y., Agusa, T. et al. (2009). Ethnic differences in five intronic polymorphisms associated with arsenic metabolism within human arsenic (+ 3 oxidation state) methyltransferase (AS3MT) gene. *Toxicology and Applied Pharmacology* **234** (1): 41–46. https://doi.org/10.1016/j.taap.2008.09.026.

Galal-Gorchev, H. (2009). Dietary intake, levels in food and estimated intake of lead, cadmium, and mercury. *Food Additives and Contaminants* **10** (1): 115–128. https://doi.org/10.1080/02652039309374135.

Gall, J.E., Boyd, R.S., and Rajakaruna, N. (2015). Transfer of heavy metals through terrestrial food webs: a review. *Environmental Monitoring and Assessment* **187** (201) https://doi.org/10.1007/s10661-015-4436-3.

Gautam, R.K., Mudhoo, A., Lofrano, G., and Chattopadhyaya, M.C. (2014). Biomass-derived biosorbents for metal ions sequestration: adsorbent modification and activation methods and adsorbent regeneration. *Journal of Environmental Chemical Engineering* **2** (1): 239–259. https://doi.org/10.1016/j.jece.2013.12.019.

Geldner, N. and Salt, D.E. (2014). Focus on roots. *Plant Physiology* **166** (2): 453–454. https://doi.org/10.1104/pp.114.900494.

Ghiyasi, S., Karbassi, A., Moattar, F. et al. (2010). Origin and concentrations of heavy metals in agricultural land around aluminium industrial complex. *Journal of Food. Agriculture and Environment* **8** (3–4 Part 2): 1237–1240.

Giehl, R.F.H. and von Wirén, N. (2014). Root nutrient foraging. *Plant Physiology* **166** (2): 509–517. https://doi.org/10.1104/pp.114.245225.

Godt, J., Scheidig, F., Grosse-Siestrup, C. et al. (2006). The toxicity of cadmium and resulting hazards for human health. *Journal of Occupational Medicine and Toxicology (London, England)* **1**: 22. https://doi.org/10.1186/1745-6673-1-22.

González-Mendoza, D. and Zapata-Pérez, O. (2008). Mecanismos de tolerancia a elementos potencialmente tóxicos en plantas. *Boletín de la Sociedad Botánica de México* **82**: 53–61.

Govindaraghavan, S. and Sucher, N.J. (2015). Quality assessment of medicinal herbs and their extracts: criteria and prerequisites for consistent safety and efficacy of herbal medicines. *Epilepsy and Behavior* **52**: 363–371. https://doi.org/10.1016/j.yebeh.2015.03.004.

Goyer, R., Golub, M., Choudhury, H. et al. (2004). Issue paper on the human health effects of metals. US Environmental Protection Agency Risk Assessment Forum. Available at: https://www.epa.gov/sites/production/files/2014-11/documents/human_health_effects.pdf (accessed 10 July 2017).

Gresser, M.J. (1981). ADP-arsenate. Formation by submitochondrial particles under phosphorylating conditions. *Journal of Biological Chemistry* **256** (12): 5981–5983. https://doi.org/10.1017/CBO9781107415324.004.

Guertin, J. (2004). Toxicity and health effects of chromium (all oxidation states). In: *Chromium(VI) Handbook*, 1e (eds. J. Guertin, C.P. Avakian and J.A. Jacobs), 215–234. CRC Press https://doi.org/https://doi.org/10.1201/9780203487969.ch6.

Gundert-Remy, U., Damm, G., Foth, H. et al. (2015). High exposure to inorganic arsenic by food: the need for risk reduction. *Archives of Toxicology* **89** (12): 2219–2227. https://doi.org/10.1007/s00204-015-1627-1.

Hakeem, A.S. and Bhatnagar, S. (2010). Heavy metal reduction of pulp and paper mill effluent by indigenous microbes. *Asian Journal of Experimental Biological Sciences* **1** (1): 201–203.

Hall, J.L. (2002). Cellular mechanisms for heavy metal detoxification and tolerance. *Journal of Experimental Botany* **53** (366): 1–11. https://doi.org/10.1093/jexbot/53.366.1.

Harris, E.S.J., Cao, S., Littlefield, B. et al. (2011). Heavy metal and pesticide content in commonly prescribed individual raw Chinese Herbal Medicines. *Science of the Total Environment* **409** (20): 4297–4305. https://doi.org/10.1016/j.scitotenv.2011.07.032.

Hartwig, A. and Jahnke, G. (2017). Metalle und ihre Verbindungen als Kontaminanten in Lebensmitteln. *Bundesgesundheitsblatt - Gesundheitsforschung - Gesundheitsschutz* **60** (7): 715–721. https://doi.org/10.1007/s00103-017-2567-0.

Haswell-Elkins, M., Satarug, S., O'Rourke, P. et al. (2008). Striking association between urinary cadmium level and albuminuria among Torres Strait Islander people with diabetes. *Environmental Research* **106** (3): 379–383. https://doi.org/10.1016/j.envres.2007.10.004.

Haydon, M.J. and Cobbett, C.S. (2007). Transporters of ligands for essential metal ions in plants. *The New Phytologist* **174** (3): 499–506. https://doi.org/10.1111/j.1469-8137.2007.02051.x.

Haydon, M.J., Bell, L.J., and Webb, A.A.R. (2011). Interactions between plant circadian clocks and solute transport. *Journal of Experimental Botany* **62** (7): 2333–2348. https://doi.org/10.1093/jxb/err040.

Heinrich, M. (2015). Quality and safety of herbal medical products: regulation and the need for quality assurance along the value chains. *British Journal of Clinical Pharmacology* **80** (1): 62–66. https://doi.org/10.1111/bcp.12586.

Hellström, L., Elinder, C.G., Dahlberg, B. et al. (2001). Cadmium exposure and end-stage renal disease. *American Journal of Kidney Diseases: The Official Journal of the National Kidney Foundation* **38** (5): 1001–1008. https://doi.org/10.1053/ajkd.2001.28589.

Hood, E. (2006). The apple bites back: claiming old orchards for residential development. *Environmental Health Perspectives* **114** (8): A470–A476.

Horiguchi, H., Oguma, E., Sasaki, S. et al. (2004). Dietary exposure to cadmium at close to the current provisional tolerable weekly intake does not affect renal function among female Japanese farmers. *Environmental Research* **95** (1): 20–31. https://doi.org/10.1016/S0013-9351(03)00142-7.

Hossny, E., Mokhtar, G., El-Awady, M. et al. (2001). Environmental exposure of the pediatric age groups in Cairo City and its suburbs to cadmium pollution. *Science of the Total Environment* **273** (1–3): 135–146. https://doi.org/10.1016/S0048-9697(00)00848-2.

Huang, C., Ke, Q., Costa, M., and Shi, X. (2004). Molecular mechanisms of arsenic carcinogenesis. *Molecular and Cellular Biochemistry* **255** (1/2): 57–66. https://doi.org/10.1023/B:MCBI.0000007261.04684.78.

Hughes, M.F. (2002). Arsenic toxicity and potential mechanisms of action. *Toxicology Letters* **133**: 1–16.

Hughes, M.F., Beck, B.D., Chen, Y. et al. (2011a). Arsenic exposure and toxicology: a historical perspective. *Toxicological Sciences* **123** (2): 305–332. https://doi.org/10.1093/toxsci/kfr184.

Hughes, J.P., Rees, S.S., Kalindjian, S.B., and Philpott, K.L. (2011b). Principles of early drug discovery. *British Journal of Pharmacology* **162** (6): 1239–1249. https://doi.org/10.1111/j.1476-5381.2010.01127.x.

Husted, S., Persson, D.P., Laursen, K.H. et al. (2011). Review: the role of atomic spectrometry in plant science. *Journal of Analytical Atomic Spectrometry* **26** (1): 52–79. https://doi.org/10.1039/C0JA00058B.

IARC (1993). *IARC Monographs on the Evaluation of Carcinogenic Risks to Humans: Beryllium, Cadmium , Mercury, and Exposures in the Glass Manufacturing Industry*, 58. Lyon, France: IARC/WHO Press.

IARC (2006). *IARC Monographs on the Evaluation of Carcinogenic Risks to Humans: Inorganic and Organic Lead Compounds*, vol. **87**. Lyon, France: IARC/WHO Press Available at: http://monographs.iarc.fr/ENG/Monographs/vol87/mono87.pdf (accessed 26 July 2017).

IARC (2012). *Arsenic, Metals, Fibres, and Dusts: A Review of Human Carcinogens*, vol. **100**. Lyon, France: IARC/WHO Press.

ICH. (2014). ICH Harmonised Guide: Guideline for Elemental Impurities Q3D (Step 4). Available at: https://www.ich.org/fileadmin/Public_Web_Site/ICH_Products/Guidelines/Quality/Q3D/Q3D_Step_4.pdf (accessed 27 July 2017).

ICH. (2016). ICH Q3D Elemental Impurities: Frequently Asked Questions. Available at: http://www.ich.org/products/guidelines/quality/article/quality-guidelines.html (accessed 16 November 2017).

Jaishankar, M., Tseten, T., Anbalagan, N. et al. (2014). Toxicity, mechanism and health effects of some heavy metals. *Interdisciplinary Toxicology* **7** (2): 60–72. https://doi.org/10.2478/intox-2014-0009.

James, B.R., Petura, J.C., Vitale, R.J., and Mussoline, G.R. (1997). Oxidation-reduction chemistry of chromium: relevance to the regulation and remediation of chromate-contaminated soils. *Soil and Sediment Contamination* **6** (6): 569–580. https://doi.org/10.1080/15320389709383590.

Jan, A.T., Azam, M., Siddiqui, K. et al. (2015). Heavy metals and human health: mechanistic insight into toxicity and counter defense system of antioxidants. *International Journal of Molecular Sciences* **16**: 29592–29630. https://doi.org/10.3390/ijms161226183.

Jarup, L. (2003). Hazards of heavy metal contamination. *British Medical Bulletin* **68** (1): 167–182. https://doi.org/10.1093/bmb/ldg032.

Järup, L., Berglund, M., Elinder, C.G. et al. (1998). Health effects of cadmium exposure–a review of the literature and a risk estimate. *Scandinavian Journal of Work, Environment & Health* **24** (Suppl 1): 1–51.

Jarup, L., Hellstrom, L., Alfven, T. et al. (2000). Low level exposure to cadmium and early kidney damage: the OSCAR study. *Occupational and Environmental Medicine* **57** (10): 668–672. https://doi.org/10.1136/oem.57.10.668.

JECFA. (2011). Aluminium. Available at: http://apps.who.int/food-additives-contaminants-jecfa-database/chemical.aspx?chemID=298 (accessed 10 August 2017).

JECFA. (2013). Cadmium. Available at: http://apps.who.int/food-additives-contaminants-jecfa-database/chemical.aspx?chemID=1376 (accessed 10 August 2017).

Jennette, K.W. (1981). The role of metals in carcinogenesis: biochemistry and metabolism. *Environmental Health Perspectives* **40**: 233–252. Retrieved from http://www.ncbi.nlm.nih.gov/pubmed/7023933.

Jomova, K., Jenisova, Z., Feszterova, M. et al. (2011). Arsenic: toxicity, oxidative stress and human disease. *Journal of Applied Toxicology* **31** (2): 95–107. https://doi.org/10.1002/jat.1649.

Jordan, S.A., Cunningham, D.G., and Marles, R.J. (2010). Assessment of herbal medicinal products: challenges, and opportunities to increase the knowledge base for safety assessment. *Toxicology and Applied Pharmacology* **243** (2): 198–216. https://doi.org/10.1016/j.taap.2009.12.005.

Joseph, P. (2009). Mechanisms of cadmium carcinogenesis. *Toxicology and Applied Pharmacology* **238** (3): 272–279. https://doi.org/10.1016/j.taap.2009.01.011.

Kabata-Pendias, A. (2010). *Trace Elements in Soils and Plants*, 4e. CRC Press.

Kabata-Pendias, A. (2011). *Trace Elements in Soils and Plants*, vol. **5**. CRC Press.

Kamerud, K.L., Hobbie, K.A., and Anderson, K.A. (2013). Stainless steel leaches nickel and chromium into foods during cooking. *Journal of Agricultural and Food Chemistry* **61** (39): 9495–9501. https://doi.org/10.1021/jf402400v.

Kannan, S. (1980). Mechanisms of foliar uptake of plant nutrients: accomplishments and prospects. *Journal of Plant Nutrition* **2** (6): 717–735. https://doi.org/10.1080/01904168009362810.

Kayaaltı, Z., Akyüzlü, D.K., and Söylemezoğlu, T. (2015). Evaluation of the effect of divalent metal transporter 1 gene polymorphism on blood iron, lead and cadmium levels. *Environmental Research* **137**: 8–13. https://doi.org/10.1016/j.envres.2014.11.008.

Kim, D.-W., Kim, K.-Y., Choi, B.-S. et al. (2007). Regulation of metal transporters by dietary iron, and the relationship between body iron levels and cadmium uptake. *Archives of Toxicology* **81** (5): 327–334. https://doi.org/10.1007/s00204-006-0160-7.

Kinyuru, J.N., Borresen, E.C., and Ryan, E.P. (2015). Nutritional and safety evaluation of heat-stabilized rice bran for supplementary feeding of malnourished children in nutritional and safety evaluation of heat-stabilized rice bran for supplementary feeding of malnourished children in Kenya. *International Journal of Food Sciences and Nutrition* **04** (6): 226–232. https://doi.org/10.19070/2326.

Kitchin, K.T. (2001). Recent advances in arsenic carcinogenesis: modes of action, animal model systems, and methylated arsenic metabolites. *Toxicology and Applied Pharmacology* **172** (3): 249–261. https://doi.org/10.1006/taap.2001.9157.

Kitchin, K.T. and Conolly, R. (2010). Arsenic-induced carcinogenesis–oxidative stress as a possible mode of action and future research needs for more biologically based risk assessment. *Chemical Research in Toxicology* **23** (2): 327–335. https://doi.org/10.1021/tx900343d.

Kjeldsen, P., Barlaz, M.A., Rooker, A.P. et al. (2002). Present and long-term composition of MSW landfill leachate: a review. *Critical Reviews in Environmental Science and Technology* **32** (4): 297–336. https://doi.org/10.1080/10643380290813462.

Klotz, K., Weistenhöfer, W., Neff, F. et al. (2017). The health effects of aluminum exposure. *Deutsches Arzteblatt International* **114**: 653–659. https://doi.org/10.3238/arztebl.2017.0653.

Krämer, U. (2010). Metal hyperaccumulation in plants. *Annual Review of Plant Biology* **61**: 517–534. https://doi.org/10.1146/annurev-arplant-042809-112156.

Kroes, R., Müller, D., Lambe, J. et al. (2002). Assessment of intake from the diet. *Food and Chemical Toxicology* **40**: 327–385. https://doi.org/10.1016/S0278-6915(01)00113-2.

Kuo, S., Heilman, P.E., and Baker, A.S. (1983). Distribution and forms of copper, zinc, cadmium, iron, and manganese in soils near a copper smelter. *Soil Science* https://doi.org/10.1097/00010694-198302000-00004.

Kurzius-Spencer, M., Burgess, J.L., Harris, R.B. et al. (2014). Contribution of diet to aggregate arsenic exposures-an analysis across populations. *Journal of Exposure Science & Environmental Epidemiology* **24** (2): 156–162. https://doi.org/10.1038/jes.2013.37.

Kushwaha, A., Rani, R., Kumar, S. et al. (2016). Heavy metal detoxification and tolerance mechanisms in plants: implications for phytoremediation. *Environmental Reviews* **24** (1): 39–51. https://doi.org/10.1139/er-2015-0010.

Laloo, R.C., Kharlukhi, L., Jeeva, S. et al. (2006). Status of medicinal plants in the disturbed and the undisturbed sacred forests of Meghalaya, northeast India: population structure and regeneration efficacy of some important species. *Current Science* **90** (2): 225–232.

Langård, S. (1982). *Biological and Environmental Aspects of Chromium*. Elsevier Biomedical Press.
Lash, L.H., Putt, D.A., Hueni, S.E. et al. (2007). Interactive toxicity of inorganic mercury and trichloroethylene in rat and human proximal tubules: effects on apoptosis, necrosis, and glutathione status. *Toxicology and Applied Pharmacology* **221** (3): 349–362. https://doi.org/10.1016/j.taap.2007.03.023.
Leitenmaier, B. and Kupper, H. (2013). Compartmentation and complexation of metals in hyperaccumulator plants. *Frontiers in Plant Science* **4** (374) https://doi.org/10.3389/fpls.2013.00374.
Leuschner, R.G.K., Hristova, A., Robinson, T., and Hugas, M. (2013). The Rapid Alert System for Food and Feed (RASFF) database in support of risk analysis of biogenic amines in food. *Journal of Food Composition and Analysis* **29** (1): 37–42. https://doi.org/10.1016/j.jfca.2012.09.004.
Leyval, C., Turnau, K., and Haselwandter, K. (1997). Effect of heavy metal pollution on mycorrhizal colonization and function: physiological, ecological and applied aspects. *Mycorrhiza* **7** (3): 139–153. https://doi.org/10.1007/s005720050174.
Li, L. and Chen, F. (2016). Oxidative stress, epigenetics, and cancer stem cells in arsenic carcinogenesis and prevention. *Current Pharmacology Reports* **2** (2): 57–63. https://doi.org/10.1007/s40495-016-0049-y.
Li, X. and Qian, P. (2017). Identification of an exposure risk to heavy metals from pharmaceutical-grade rubber stoppers. *Journal of Food and Drug Analysis* **25** (3): 723–730. https://doi.org/10.1016/j.jfda.2016.07.008.
Liang, H.M., Lin, T.H., Chiou, J.M., and Yeh, K.C. (2009). Model evaluation of the phytoextraction potential of heavy metal hyperaccumulators and non-hyperaccumulators. *Environmental Pollution* **157** (6): 1945–1952. https://doi.org/10.1016/j.envpol.2008.11.052.
Lindblad, E.B. (2004). Aluminium compounds for use in vaccines. *Immunology and Cell Biology* **82** (5): 497–505. https://doi.org/10.1111/j.0818-9641.2004.01286.x.
Liu, S., Guo, X., Wu, B. et al. (2014a). Arsenic induces diabetic effects through beta-cell dysfunction and increased gluconeogenesis in mice. *Scientific Reports* **4**: 6894. https://doi.org/10.1038/srep06894.
Liu, Y., Li, Y., Liu, K. et al. (2014b). Exposing to cadmium stress cause profound toxic effect on microbiota of the mice intestinal tract. *PLoS One* **9** (2): e85323. https://doi.org/10.1371/journal.pone.0085323.
Lombi, E., Scheckel, K.G., Pallon, J. et al. (2009). Speciation and distribution of arsenic and localization of nutrients in rice grains. *New Phytologist* **184** (1): 193–201. https://doi.org/10.1111/j.1469-8137.2009.02912.x.
Lugtenberg, B. and Kamilova, F. (2009). Plant-growth-promoting rhizobacteria. *Annual Review of Microbiology* **63**: 541–556. https://doi.org/10.1146/annurev.micro.62.081307.162918.
Mamtani, R., Stern, P., Dawood, I., and Cheema, S. (2011). Metals and disease: a global primary health care perspective. *Journal of Toxicology* **2011** 319136. https://doi.org/10.1155/2011/319136.
Marschner, H. (1995). *Mineral Nutrition of Higher Plants*, vol. **1**, 889. San Diego: Academic Press.
Martinez, V.D., Vucic, E.A., Becker-Santos, D.D. et al. (2011). Arsenic exposure and the induction of human cancers. *Journal of Toxicology* **2011** 431287. https://doi.org/10.1155/2011/431287.
Mason, B. and Moore, C.B. (1982). *Principles of Geochemistry*. New York: Wiley.
Mass, M.J., Tennant, A., Roop, B. et al. (2001). Methylated trivalent arsenic species are genotoxic. *Chemical Research in Toxicology* **14** (4): 355–361. https://doi.org/10.1021/TX000251L.

McCarty, K.M., Chen, Y.C., Quamruzzaman, Q. et al. (2007). Arsenic methylation, GSTT1, GSTM1, GSTP1 polymorphisms, and skin lesions. *Environmental Health Perspectives* **115** (3): 341–345. https://doi.org/10.1289/ehp.9152.

McKenzie-Parnell, J.M., Kjellstrom, T.E., Sharma, R.P., and Robinson, M.F. (1988). Unusually high intake and fecal output of cadmium, and fecal output of other trace elements in New Zealand adults consuming dredge oysters. *Environmental Research* **46** (1): 1–14. https://doi.org/10.1016/S0013-9351(88)80054-9.

McNear, D.H. Jr. (2013). The rhizosphere – roots, soil and everything in between. *Nature Education Knowledge* **4** (3): 1.

Meharg, A.A., Lombi, E., Williams, P.N. et al. (2008). Speciation and localization of arsenic in white and brown rice grains. *Environmental Science & Technology* **42** (4): 1051–1057. https://doi.org/10.1021/es702212p.

Mehes-Smith, M., Nkongolo, K., and Cholew, E. (2013). Coping mechanisms of plants to metal contaminated soil. *Environmental Change and Sustainability*: 53–90. https://doi.org/10.5772/55124.

Memon, A.R. and Schröder, P. (2009). Implications of metal accumulation mechanisms to phytoremediation. *Environmental Science and Pollution Research* **16** (2): 162–175. https://doi.org/10.1007/s11356-008-0079-z.

Michalke, B. (2003). Element speciation definitions, analytical methodology, and some examples. *Ecotoxicology and Environmental Safety* **56** (1): 122–139. https://doi.org/10.1016/S0147-6513(03)00056-3.

Micó, C., Li, H.F., Zhao, F.J., and McGrath, S.P. (2008). Use of co speciation and soil properties to explain variation in co toxicity to root growth of barley (*Hordeum vulgare* L.) in different soils. *Environmental Pollution* **156** (3): 883–890. https://doi.org/10.1016/j.envpol.2008.05.017.

Miroddi, M., Mannucci, C., Mancari, F. et al. (2013). Research and development for botanical products in medicinals and food supplements market. *Evidence-Based Complementary and Alternative Medicine: ECAM* **2013** 649720. https://doi.org/10.1155/2013/649720.

Monken, A. (2010). Water pollution control for paint booths. *Metal Finishing* **108** (11–12): 323–329. https://doi.org/10.1016/S0026-0576(10)80245-4.

Montiel-Rozas, M.M., Madejón, E., and Madejón, P. (2016). Effect of heavy metals and organic matter on root exudates (low molecular weight organic acids) of herbaceous species: an assessment in sand and soil conditions under different levels of contamination. *Environmental Pollution* **216**: 273–281. https://doi.org/10.1016/j.envpol.2016.05.080.

Morgan, J.N. (1999). Effects of processing of heavy metal content of foods. In: *Advances in Experimental Medicine and Biology* (eds. L.S. Jackson, M.G. Knizem and J.N. Morgan), 196–211. Boston: Springer.

Mosihuzzaman, M. and Choudhary, M.I. (2008). Protocols on safety, efficacy, standardization, and documentation of herbal medicine. *Pure and Applied Chemistry* **80** (10): 2195–2230. https://doi.org/10.1351/pac200880102195.

Mukherjee, P.K., Bahadur, S., Chaudhary, S.K. et al. (2015). Quality related safety issue-evidence-based validation of herbal medicine farm to pharma. In: *Evidence-Based Validation of Herbal Medicine* (ed. P.K. Mukherjee), 1–28. https://doi.org/10.1016/B978-0-12-800874-4.00001-5.

Muncke, J. (2014). Hazards of food contact material: food packaging contaminants. In: *Encyclopedia of Food Safety*, vol. **2** (ed. Y. Motarjemi), 430–437. Elsevier https://doi.org/10.1016/B978-0-12-378612-8.00218-3.

Murgo, A.J. (2001). Clinical trials of arsenic trioxide in hematologic and solid tumors: overview of the National Cancer Institute Cooperative Research and Development

Studies. *The Oncologist* **6** (90002): 22–28. https://doi.org/10.1634/theoncologist.6-suppl_2-22.

Muthayya, S., Sugimoto, J.D., Montgomery, S., and Maberly, G.F. (2014). An overview of global rice production, supply, trade, and consumption. *Annals of the New York Academy of Sciences* **1324** (1): 7–14. https://doi.org/10.1111/nyas.12540.

Naiya, T.K., Chowdhury, P., Bhattacharya, A.K., and Das, S.K. (2009). Saw dust and neem bark as low-cost natural biosorbent for adsorptive removal of Zn(II) and Cd(II) ions from aqueous solutions. *Chemical Engineering Journal* **148** (1): 68–79. https://doi.org/10.1016/j.cej.2008.08.002.

Nicholson, F.A., Smith, S.R., Alloway, B.J. et al. (2003). An inventory of heavy metals inputs to agricultural soils in England and Wales. *Science of the Total Environment* **311** (1–3): 205–219. https://doi.org/10.1016/S0048-9697(03)00139-6.

Nickens, K.P., Patierno, S.R., and Ceryak, S. (2010). Chromium genotoxicity: a double-edged sword. *Chemico-Biological Interactions* **188** (2): 276–288. https://doi.org/10.1016/j.cbi.2010.04.018.

Nordberg, G.F., Piscator, M., and Lind, B. (1971a). Distribution of cadmium among protein fractions of mouse liver. *Acta Pharmacologica et Toxicologica* **29** (5): 456–470. http://www.ncbi.nlm.nih.gov/pubmed/5171119.

Nordberg, G.F., Piscator, M., and Nordberg, M. (1971b). On the distribution of cadmium in blood. *Acta Pharmacologica et Toxicologica* **30** (3–4): 289–295. https://doi.org/10.1111/j.1600-0773.1971.tb00660.x.

Nordberg, G., Jin, T., Bernard, A. et al. (2002). Low bone density and renal dysfunction following environmental cadmium exposure in China. *Ambio* **31** (6): 478–481. https://doi.org/10.1579/0044-7447-31.6.478.

NRC (1999). *Arsenic in Drinking Water*. Washington, D.C.: National Academies Press https://doi.org/10.17226/6444.

Oberoi, S., Barchowsky, A., and Wu, F. (2014). The global burden of disease for skin, lung, and bladder cancer caused by arsenic in food. *Cancer Epidemiology Biomarkers and Prevention* **23** (7): 1187–1194. https://doi.org/10.1158/1055-9965.EPI-13-1317.

O'Brien, T.J., Ceryak, S., and Patierno, S.R. (2003). Complexities of chromium carcinogenesis: role of cellular response, repair and recovery mechanisms. *Mutation Research - Fundamental and Molecular Mechanisms of Mutagenesis* **533**: 3–36. https://doi.org/10.1016/j.mrfmmm.2003.09.006.

Offenbacher, E.G. and Pi-Sunyer, F.X. (1983). Temperature and pH effects on the release of chromium from stainless steel into water and fruit juices. *Journal of Agricultural and Food Chemistry* **31** (1): 89–92. https://doi.org/10.1021/jf00115a024.

Otero, N., Vitòria, L., Soler, A., and Canals, A. (2005). Fertiliser characterisation: major, trace and rare earth elements. *Applied Geochemistry* **20** (8): 1473–1488. https://doi.org/10.1016/j.apgeochem.2005.04.002.

Pacyna, J.M. (1995). Sources, particle size distribution and transport of aerosols. In: *Airborne Particulate Matter*, vol. **4/4D** (eds. T. Kouimtzis and C. Samara), 69–97. Berlin, Heidelberg: Springer https://doi.org/10.1007/978-3-540-49145-3.

Page, V. and Feller, U. (2015). Heavy metals in crop plants: transport and redistribution processes on the whole plant level. *Agronomy* **5** (3): 447–463. https://doi.org/10.3390/agronomy5030447.

Paul, S., Majumdar, S., Giri, A.K. et al. (2015). Genetic susceptibility to arsenic-induced skin lesions and health effects: a review. *Genes and Environment* **37** (1): 23. https://doi.org/10.1186/s41021-015-0023-7.

Paul, S., Bhattacharjee, P., Giri, A.K., and Bhattacharjee, P. (2017). Arsenic toxicity and epimutagenecity: the new LINEage. *Biometals* **30** (4): 505–515. https://doi.org/10.1007/s10534-017-0021-2.

Pechova, A. and Pavlata, L. (2007). Chromium as an essential nutrient: a review. *Veterinární Medicína* **52** (1): 1–18. Retrieved from http://vri.cz/docs/vetmed/52-1-1.pdf.

Pennington, J.A.T. and Schoen, S.A. (1995). Estimates of dietary exposure to aluminium. *Food Additives and Contaminants* **12** (1): 119–128. https://doi.org/10.1080/02652039509374286.

Peraza, M.A., Ayala-Fierro, F., Barber, D.S. et al. (1998). Effects of micronutrients on metal toxicity. *Environmental Health Perspectives* **106**: 203–216. Retrieved from http://ehpnetl.niehs.nih.gov/docs/1998/Suppl-1/203-216peraza/abstract.html.

Pershagen, G., Nordberg, G., and Björklund, N.E. (1984). Carcinomas of the respiratory tract in hamsters given arsenic trioxide and/or benzo[a]pyrene by the pulmonary route. *Environmental Research* **34** (2): 227–241. Retrieved from http://www.ncbi.nlm.nih.gov/pubmed/6086305.

Petrick, J.S., Jagadish, B., Mash, E.A., and Aposhian, H.V. (2001). Monomethylarsonous acid (MMA III) and Arsenite: LD 50 in hamsters and in vitro inhibition of pyruvate dehydrogenase. *Chemical Research in Toxicology* **14** (6): 651–656. https://doi.org/10.1021/tx000264z.

Petruzzelli, G., Lubrano, L., and Cervelli, S. (1987). Heavy metal uptake by wheat seedlings grown in fly ash-amended soils. *Water, Air, and Soil Pollution* **32** (3–4): 389–395. https://doi.org/10.1007/BF00225123.

Platanias, L.C. (2009). Biological responses to arsenic compounds. *The Journal of Biological Chemistry* **284** (28): 18583–18587. https://doi.org/10.1074/jbc.R900003200.

Pohl, P., Bielawska-Pohl, A., Dzimitrowicza, A. et al. (2017). Impact and practicability of recently introduced requirements on elemental impurities. *TrAC Trends in Analytical Chemistry* **88**: 119–133. https://doi.org/10.1016/J.TRAC.2017.09.011.

Poręba, R., Gać, P., Poręba, M., and Andrzejak, R. (2011). Environmental and occupational exposure to lead as a potential risk factor for cardiovascular disease. *Environmental Toxicology and Pharmacology* **31** (2): 267–277. https://doi.org/10.1016/j.etap.2010.12.002.

Porter, K.E., Basu, A., Hubbard, A.E. et al. (2010). Association of genetic variation in cystathionine-beta-synthase and arsenic metabolism. *Environmental Research* **110** (6): 580–587. https://doi.org/10.1016/j.envres.2010.05.001.

Potts, R.J., Watkin, R.D., and Hart, B.A. (2003). Cadmium exposure down-regulates 8-oxoguanine DNA glycosylase expression in rat lung and alveolar epithelial cells. *Toxicology* **184** (2–3): 189–202. https://doi.org/10.1016/S0300-483X(02)00579-6.

Poveda, R. (2015). Regulation of herbal (traditional) medicinal products in the European Union. *Pharmaceutical Regulatory Affairs: Open Access* **04** (02) https://doi.org/10.4172/2167-7689.1000142.

Prasad, M.N.V. (2004). *Heavy Metal Stress in Plants: From Biomolecules to Ecosystems*. Berlin, Heidelberg: Springer.

Puig, S. and Peñarrubia, L. (2009). Placing metal micronutrients in context: transport and distribution in plants. *Current Opinion in Plant Biology* **12** (3): 299–306. https://doi.org/10.1016/j.pbi.2009.04.008.

Qu, L., Zou, W., Zhou, Z. et al. (2014). Non-European traditional herbal medicines in Europe: a community herbal monograph perspective. *Journal of Ethnopharmacology* **156**: 107–114. https://doi.org/10.1016/j.jep.2014.08.021.

Rahman, M.A., Hasegawa, H., Rahman, M.M. et al. (2007). Accumulation of arsenic in tissues of rice plant (*Oryza sativa* L.) and its distribution in fractions of rice grain. *Chemosphere* **69** (6): 942–948. https://doi.org/10.1016/j.chemosphere.2007.05.044.

Rajkumar, M., Sandhya, S., Prasad, M.N.V., and Freitas, H. (2012). Perspectives of plant-associated microbes in heavy metal phytoremediation. *Biotechnology Advances* **30** (6): 1562–1574. https://doi.org/10.1016/j.biotechadv.2012.04.011.

Rani, A., Kumar, A., Lal, A., and Pant, M. (2014). Cellular mechanisms of cadmium-induced toxicity: a review. *International Journal of Environmental Health Research* **24** (4): 378–399. https://doi.org/10.1080/09603123.2013.835032.

Rascio, N. and Navari-Izzo, F. (2011). Heavy metal hyperaccumulating plants: how and why do they do it? And what makes them so interesting? *Plant Science* **180** (2): 169–181. https://doi.org/10.1016/j.plantsci.2010.08.016.

Reeves, P.G. and Vanderpool, R.A. (1997). Cadmium burden of men and women who report regular consumption of confectionery sunflower kernels containing a natural abundance of cadmium. *Environmental Health Perspectives* **105** (10): 1098–1104. Retrieved from http://www.ncbi.nlm.nih.gov/pubmed/9349833.

Riesen, O. and Feller, U. (2005). Redistribution of nickel, cobalt, manganese, zinc, and cadmium via the phloem in young and maturing wheat. *Journal of Plant Nutrition* **28** (3): 421–430. https://doi.org/10.1081/PLN-200049153.

Rieuwerts, J.S., Thornton, I., Farago, M.E., and Ashmore, M.R. (1998). Factors influencing metal bioavailability in soils: preliminary investigations for the development of a critical loads approach for metals. *Chemical Speciation & Bioavailability* **10** (2): 61–75. https://doi.org/10.3184/095422998782775835.

Roberts, D., Nachtegaal, M., and Sparks, D.L. (2005). *Chemical Processes in Soils*. SSSA Books.

Rodrigues, E.G., Kile, M., Hoffman, E. et al. (2012). GSTO and AS3MT genetic polymorphisms and differences in urinary arsenic concentrations among residents in Bangladesh. *Biomarkers* **17** (3): 240–247. https://doi.org/10.3109/1354750X.2012.658863.

Rose, U. (2016). Participation of industry experts in the elaboration of monographs and chapters of the European Pharmacopoeia. *European Journal of Pharmaceutical Sciences* **93**: 504–506. https://doi.org/10.1016/j.ejps.2016.01.030.

Ross, S. (1994). *Toxic Metals in Soil Plant Systems*. Wiley.

Rossman, T.G., Uddin, A.N., Burns, F.J., and Bosland, M.C. (2001). Arsenite is a cocarcinogen with solar ultraviolet radiation for mouse skin: an animal model for arsenic carcinogenesis. *Toxicology and Applied Pharmacology* **176** (1): 64–71. https://doi.org/10.1006/taap.2001.9277.

Rule, K.L., Comber, S.D.W., Ross, D. et al. (2006). Diffuse sources of heavy metals entering an urban wastewater catchment. *Chemosphere* **63** (1): 64–72. https://doi.org/10.1016/j.chemosphere.2005.07.052.

Ruttkay-Nedecky, B., Nejdl, L., Gumulec, J. et al. (2013). The role of metallothionein in oxidative stress. *International Journal of Molecular Sciences* **14** (3): 6044–6066. https://doi.org/10.3390/ijms14036044.

Sahoo, N., Manchikanti, P., and Dey, S. (2010). Herbal drugs: standards and regulation. *Fitoterapia* **81** (6): 462–471. https://doi.org/10.1016/j.fitote.2010.02.001.

Samikkannu, T., Chen, C.-H., Yih, L.-H. et al. (2003). Reactive oxygen species are involved in arsenic trioxide inhibition of pyruvate dehydrogenase activity. *Chemical Research in Toxicology* **16** (3): 409–414. https://doi.org/10.1021/tx025615j.

Satarug, S., Garrett, S.H., Sens, M.A., and Sens, D.A. (2010). Cadmium, environmental exposure, and health outcomes. *Environmental Health Perspectives* **118** (2) https://doi.org/10.1289/ehp.0901234.

Schmiermund, R.L. (2004). Mineral resources management and the environment. *Eos, Transactions American Geophysical Union* **85** (46): 485. https://doi.org/10.1029/2004EO460007.

Schönherr, J. and Luber, M. (2001). Cuticular penetration of potassium salts: effects of humidity, anions, and temperature. *Plant and Soil* **236** (1): 117–122. https://doi.org/10.1023/A:1011976727078.

Schoof, R., Yost, L., Eickhoff, J. et al. (1999). A market basket survey of inorganic arsenic in food. *Food and Chemical Toxicology* **37** (8): 839–846. https://doi.org/10.1016/S0278-6915(99)00073-3.

Schreck, E., Foucault, Y., Sarret, G. et al. (2012). Metal and metalloid foliar uptake by various plant species exposed to atmospheric industrial fallout: mechanisms involved for lead. *Science of the Total Environment* **427–428**: 253–262. https://doi.org/10.1016/j.scitotenv.2012.03.051.

Schreiber, L. and Schönherr, J. (1990). Phase transitions and thermal expansion coefficients of plant cuticles: the effects of temperature on structure and function. *Planta* **182** (2): 186–193. https://doi.org/10.1007/BF00197109.

Shahid, M., Dumat, C., Khalid, S. et al. (2017). Foliar heavy metal uptake, toxicity and detoxification in plants: a comparison of foliar and root metal uptake. *Journal of Hazardous Materials* **325**: 36–58. https://doi.org/10.1016/j.jhazmat.2016.11.063.

Sharma, S. (2015). Current status of herbal product: regulatory overview. *Journal of Pharmacy & Bioallied Sciences* **7** (4): 293–296. https://doi.org/10.4103/0975-7406.168030.

Shen, S., Li, X.-F., Cullen, W.R. et al. (2013). Arsenic binding to proteins. *Chemical Reviews* **113** (10): 7769–7792. https://doi.org/10.1021/cr300015c.

Signes-Pastor, A.J., Woodside, J.V., McMullan, P. et al. (2017). Levels of infants' urinary arsenic metabolites related to formula feeding and weaning with rice products exceeding the EU inorganic arsenic standard. *PLoS One* **12** (5): e0176923. https://doi.org/10.1371/journal.pone.0176923.

Singh, A.P., Goel, R.K., and Kaur, T. (2011a). Mechanisms pertaining to arsenic toxicity. *Toxicology International* **18** (2): 87–93. https://doi.org/10.4103/0971-6580.84258.

Singh, R., Gautam, N., Mishra, A., and Gupta, R. (2011b). Heavy metals and living systems: an overview. *Indian Journal of Pharmacology* **43** (3) https://doi.org/10.4103/0253-7613.81505.

Singh, N.K., Raghubanshi, A.S., Upadhyay, A.K., and Rai, U.N. (2016). Arsenic and other heavy metal accumulation in plants and algae growing naturally in contaminated area of West Bengal, India. *Ecotoxicology and Environmental Safety* **130**: 224–233. https://doi.org/10.1016/j.ecoenv.2016.04.024.

Staessen, J., Roels, H., Emelianov, D. et al. (1999). Environmental exposure to cadmium, forearm bone density, and risk of fractures: prospective population study. *The Lancet* **353** (9159): 1140–1144. https://doi.org/10.1016/S0140-6736(98)09356-8.

Stearns, D.M. (2000). Is chromium a trace essential metal? *BioFactors* **11** (3): 149–162. https://doi.org/10.1002/biof.5520110301.

Steinmaus, C., Moore, L.E., Shipp, M. et al. (2007). Genetic polymorphisms in MTHFR 677 and 1298, GSTM1 and T1, and metabolism of arsenic. *Journal of Toxicology and Environmental Health. Part A* **70** (2): 159–170. https://doi.org/10.1080/15287390600755240.

Stillmanso, M.J., Cais, W., and Zelazowskis, A.J. (1987). Cadmium binding to metallothioneins. *The Journal of Biological Chemistry* **262** (10): 4538–4548. Retrieved from http://www.jbc.org/content/262/10/4538.full.pdf.

Stohs, S.J., Bagchi, D., Hassoun, E., and Bagchi, M. (2001). Oxidative mechanisms in the toxicity of chromium and cadmium ions. *Journal of Environmental Pathology, Toxicology and Oncology: Official Organ of the International Society for Environmental Toxicology and Cancer* **20** (2): 77–88. https://doi.org/10.1615/JEnvironPatholToxicolOncol.v20.i2.10.

Sun, G.-X., Williams, P.N., Carey, A.-M. et al. (2008). Inorganic arsenic in rice bran and its products are an order of magnitude higher than in bulk grain. *Environmental Science & Technology* **42** (19): 7542–7546. https://doi.org/10.1021/es801238p.

Sun, H., Brocato, J., and Costa, M. (2015). Oral chromium exposure and toxicity. *Current Environmental Health Reports* **2** (3): 295–303. https://doi.org/10.1007/s40572-015-0054-z.

Takeuchi, T., Morikawa, N., Matsumoto, H., and Shiraishi, Y. (1962). A pathological study of Minamata disease in Japan. *Acta Neuropathologica* **2** (1): 40–57. https://doi.org/10.1007/BF00685743.

Tangahu, B.V., Sheikh Abdullah, S.R., Basri, H. et al. (2011). A review on heavy metals (As, Pb, and Hg) uptake by plants through phytoremediation. *International Journal of Chemical Engineering* **2011**: 1–31. https://doi.org/10.1155/2011/939161.

Tapio, S. and Grosche, B. (2006). Arsenic in the aetiology of cancer. *Mutation Research - Reviews in Mutation Research* **612** (3): 215–246. https://doi.org/10.1016/j.mrrev.2006.02.001.

Tchounwou, P.B., Yedjou, C.G., Patlolla, A.K., and Sutton, D.J. (2012). Heavy metal toxicity and the environment. *EXS* **101**: 133–164. https://doi.org/10.1007/978-3-7643-8340-4_6.

Thomas, D.J. and Bradham, K. (2016). Role of complex organic arsenicals in food in aggregate exposure to arsenic. *Journal of Environmental Sciences (China)* https://doi.org/10.1016/j.jes.2016.06.005.

Thomas, D.J., Styblo, M., and Lin, S. (2001). The cellular metabolism and systemic toxicity of arsenic. *Toxicology and Applied Pharmacology* **176** (2): 127–144. https://doi.org/10.1006/taap.2001.9258.

Timerbaev, A.R. (2012). Determination of metal species in biological samples: from speciation analysis to metallomics. *Journal of Analytical Chemistry* **67** (2): 179–185. https://doi.org/10.1134/S106193481202013X.

Tomljenovic, L. and Shaw, C.A. (2011). Aluminum vaccine adjuvants: are they safe? *Current Medicinal Chemistry* **18** (17): 2630–2637. Retrieved from http://www.ncbi.nlm.nih.gov/pubmed/21568886.

Tripathy, V., Basak, B.B., Varghese, T.S., and Saha, A. (2015). Residues and contaminants in medicinal herbs – a review. *Phytochemistry Letters* **14**: 67–78. https://doi.org/10.1016/j.phytol.2015.09.003.

Valenzuela, O.L., Drobná, Z., Hernández-Castellanos, E. et al. (2009). Association of AS3MT polymorphisms and the risk of premalignant arsenic skin lesions. *Toxicology and Applied Pharmacology* **239** (2): 200–207. https://doi.org/10.1016/j.taap.2009.06.007.

Valko, M., Rhodes, C.J., Moncol, J. et al. (2006). Free radicals, metals and antioxidants in oxidative stress-induced cancer. *Chemico-Biological Interactions* https://doi.org/10.1016/j.cbi.2005.12.009.

Vegliò, F., Quaresima, R., Fornari, P., and Ubaldini, S. (2003). Recovery of valuable metals from electronic and galvanic industrial wastes by leaching and electrowinning. *Waste Management* **23** (3): 245–252. https://doi.org/10.1016/S0956-053X(02)00157-5.

Venza, M., Visalli, M., Biondo, C. et al. (2015). Epigenetic effects of cadmium in cancer: focus on melanoma. *Current Genomics* **15** (6): 420–435. https://doi.org/10.2174/138920291506150106145932.

Verma, N. (2016). Current regulatory challenges and approaches in the registration of herbal drugs in Europe. *Clinical Research and Regulatory Affairs* **33** (1): 9–24. https://doi.org/10.3109/10601333.2016.1130717.

Viehweger, K., Agrawal, G., Jwa, N. et al. (2014). How plants cope with heavy metals. *Botanical Studies* **55** (1): 35. https://doi.org/10.1186/1999-3110-55-35.

Vilahur, N., Vahter, M., and Broberg, K. (2015). The epigenetic effects of prenatal cadmium exposure. *Current Environmental Health Reports* **2** (2): 195–203. https://doi.org/10.1007/s40572-015-0049-9.

Vincent, J.B. and Love, S.T. (2012). The need for combined inorganic, biochemical, and nutritional studies of chromium(III). *Chemistry and Biodiversity* **9** (9): 1923–1941. https://doi.org/10.1002/cbdv.201100440.

Wah, C. L., Hock, S. C., & Yun, T. K. (2012). Current scientific status and regulatory control of traditional/herbal medicinal products: Globalization challenges. *Scopus*. Available at: http://scholarbank.nus.edu.sg/handle/10635/106638 (accessed 8 June 2017).

Waisberg, M., Joseph, P., Hale, B., and Beyersmann, D. (2003). Molecular and cellular mechanisms of cadmium carcinogenesis. *Toxicology* **192** (2–3): 95–117. https://doi.org/10.1016/S0300-483X(03)00305-6.

Walter, I., Martínez, F., and Cala, V. (2006). Heavy metal speciation and phytotoxic effects of three representative sewage sludges for agricultural uses. *Environmental Pollution* **139** (3): 507–514. https://doi.org/10.1016/j.envpol.2005.05.020.

Wang, T., Wu, J., Hartman, R. et al. (2000). A multi-element ICP-MS survey method as an alternative to the heavy metals limit test for pharmaceutical materials. *Journal of Pharmaceutical and Biomedical Analysis* **23** (5): 867–890.

Wang, Y.-H., Yeh, S.-D., Shen, K.-H. et al. (2009). A significantly joint effect between arsenic and occupational exposures and risk genotypes/diplotypes of CYP2E1, GSTO1 and GSTO2 on risk of urothelial carcinoma. *Toxicology and Applied Pharmacology* **241** (1): 111–118. https://doi.org/10.1016/j.taap.2009.08.008.

Wang, B., Li, Y., Shao, C. et al. (2012). Cadmium and its epigenetic effects. *Current Medicinal Chemistry* **19** (16): 2611–2620. Retrieved from http://www.ncbi.nlm.nih.gov/pubmed/22471978.

Wei, M., Arnold, L., Cano, M., and Cohen, S.M. (2005). Effects of co-administration of antioxidants and arsenicals on the rat urinary bladder epithelium. *Toxicological Sciences* **83** (2): 237–245. https://doi.org/10.1093/toxsci/kfi033.

White, C., Sayer, J.A., and Gadd, G.M. (1997). Microbial solubilization and immobilization of toxic metals: key biogeochemical processes for treatment of contamination. *FEMS Microbiology Reviews* **20** (3–4): 503–516. https://doi.org/10.1016/S0168-6445(97)00029-6.

White, P.J., Whiting, S.N., Baker, A.J.M., and Broadley, M.R. (2002). Does zinc move apoplastically to the xylem in roots of *Thlaspi caerulescens*? *New Phytologist* **153** (2): 201–207. https://doi.org/10.1046/j.0028-646X.2001.00325.x.

WHO (1998). *Quality Control Methods for Medicinal Plant Materials*. Geneva: World Health Organization.

WHO (2003). *WHO Guidelines on Good Agricultural and Collection Practices (GACP) for Medicinal Plants*. Geneva: World Health Organization.

WHO. (2007a). Health risks of heavy metals from long-range transboundary air pollution (2007).

WHO. (2007b). WHO guidelines for assessing quality of herbal medicines with reference to contaminants and residues. Guidelines. I. World Health Organization, 1. Available at: http://apps.who.int/medicinedocs/documents/s14878e/s14878e.pdf (accessed 2 June 2017).

WHO. (2007c). WHO Guidelines for Assessing Quality of Herbal Medicines with Reference to Contaminants and Residues. Available at: http://apps.who.int/medicinedocs/en/m/abstract/Js14878e (accessed 27 January 2017).

Wilson, D. (2015). Arsenic consumption in the United States. *Journal of Environmental Health* **78** (3): 8–14. quiz 44.

Witt, K.L., Stout, M.D., Herbert, R.A. et al. (2013). Mechanistic insights from the NTP studies of chromium. *Toxicologic Pathology* **41** (2): 326–342. https://doi.org/10.1177/0192623312469856.

Yamanaka, K. and Okada, S. (1994). Induction of lung-specific DNA damage by metabolically methylated arsenics via the production of free radicals. *Environmental Health Perspectives* **102**: 37–40. https://doi.org/10.1289/ehp.94102s337.

Yedjou, C.G., Moore, P., and Tchounwou, P.B. (2006). Dose- and time-dependent response of human leukemia (HL-60) cells to arsenic trioxide treatment. *International Journal of Environmental Research and Public Health* **3**: 136–140. https://doi.org/10.3390/ijerph2006030017.

Zelazny, E. and Vert, G. (2014). Plant nutrition: root transporters on the move. *Plant Physiology* **166** (2): 500–508. https://doi.org/10.1104/pp.114.244475.

Zhao, F.-J., McGrath, S.P., and Meharg, A.A. (2010). Arsenic as a food chain contaminant: mechanisms of plant uptake and metabolism and mitigation strategies. *Annual Review of Plant Biology* **61** (1): 535–559. https://doi.org/10.1146/annurev-arplant-042809-112152.

Zhitkovich, A. (2005). Importance of chromium–DNA adducts in mutagenicity and toxicity of chromium(VI). *Chemical Research in Toxicology* **18** (1): 3–11. https://doi.org/10.1021/tx049774.

Zhitkovich, A. (2011). Chromium in drinking water: sources, metabolism, and cancer risks. *Chemical Research in Toxicology* **24** (10): 1617–1629. https://doi.org/10.1021/tx200251t.

Index

Herbs, Spices and Medicinal Plants: Processing, Health Benefits and Safety, First Edition.
Edited by Mohammad B. Hossain, Nigel P. Brunton, and Dilip K. Rai.

www.ingramcontent.com/pod-product-compliance
Ingram Content Group UK Ltd.
Pitfield, Milton Keynes, MK11 3LW, UK
UKHW050943290926
15470UKWH00005B/1606

9 781119 036616